Epidemiology and the People's Health

Epidemiology and the People's Health
Theory and Context

Nancy Krieger

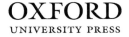

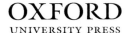

OXFORD
UNIVERSITY PRESS

Oxford University Press, Inc., publishes works that further
Oxford University's objective of excellence
in research, scholarship, and education.

Oxford   New York
Auckland   Cape Town   Dar es Salaam   Hong Kong   Karachi
Kuala Lumpur   Madrid   Melbourne   Mexico City   Nairobi
New Delhi   Shanghai   Taipei   Toronto

With offices in
Argentina   Austria   Brazil   Chile   Czech Republic   France   Greece
Guatemala   Hungary   Italy   Japan   Poland Portugal   Singapore
South   Korea   Switzerland   Thailand   Turkey   Ukraine   Vietnam

Published by Oxford University Press, Inc.
198 Madison Avenue, New York, New York 10016
www.oup.com

Library of Congress Cataloging-in-Publication Data

Krieger, Nancy, author.
Epidemiology and the people's health : theory and context / Nancy Krieger.
p. ; cm.
Includes bibliographical references and index.
ISBN 978-0-19-538387-4
1. Epidemiology. 2. Epidemiology—Methodology. I. Title.
[DNLM: 1. Epidemiology. 2. Epidemiologic Methods. WA 105]
RA651.K75 2011
614.4—dc22

2010049897

9 8 7 6 5 4

Printed in the United States of America
on acid-free paper

Epidemiology at any given time is something more than the total of its established facts. It includes their orderly arrangement into chains of inference, which extend more or less beyond the bounds of direct observation. Such of these chains as are well and truly laid guide investigations to the facts of the future; those that are ill made fetter progress. But it is not easy, when divergent theories are presented, to distinguish between those which are sound and those which are merely plausible.

Wade Hampton Frost
"Introduction" to *Snow on Cholera*
New York: Commonwealth Fund, 1936; ix.

Both thinking and facts are changeable, if only because changes in thinking manifest themselves in changed facts. Conversely, fundamentally new facts can be discovered only through new thinking.

Ludwick Fleck
Genesis and Development of a Scientific Fact
Chicago: University of Chicago Press,
1979 (1935); 50–51.

Once we recognize the state of the art is a social product, we are freer to look critically at the agenda of our science, its conceptual framework, and accepted methodologies, and to make conscious research choices.

Richard Levins and Richard Lewontin
"Conclusion" of *The Dialectical Biologist*
Cambridge, MA: Harvard University Press,
1987; 286.

Preface

Why a Book on Epidemiologic Theory?

Epidemiologic theory. As a phrase, it sounds at once dry and arcane. Yet, in reality, it is vital and engaging. Epidemiologic theory is about explaining the people's health. It is about life and death. It is about biology and society. It is about ecology and the economy. It is about how the myriad activities and meanings of people's lives—involving work, dignity, desire, love, play, conflict, discrimination, and injustice—become literally incorporated into our bodies—that is, embodied—and manifest in our health status, individually and collectively. It is about why rates of disease and death change over time and vary geographically. It is about why different societies—and within societies, why different societal groups—have better or worse health than others. And it is about essential knowledge critical for improving the people's health and minimizing inequitable burdens of disease, disability, and death.

In other words, epidemiologic theory is about the health status of populations—in societal and ecological context. It is not about why specific individuals become ill or stay healthy. Epidemiologic theory instead seeks to explain extant and changing population distributions of health, disease, and death, within and across societies, over time, space, and place. To fulfill this expansive mandate, epidemiologic theory necessarily must engage with a whole host of other theories relevant to explaining society, biology, population dynamics, the mechanisms of disease causation, and the processes that promote health—along with theories pertaining to probability, statistics, and causal inference. And it does so to tackle epidemiologic theory's defining question: Who and what determines population rates and distributions of morbidity, mortality, and health?

Not that there is one answer to this question—or one theory to tackle it, let alone one disciplinary approach. Instead, a wide array of academic fields, in the "social," "natural," public health, and biomedical sciences have engaged in asking questions about aspects of population health. What distinguishes the epidemiologic theories and approaches is their obligate engagement with defining and measuring health outcomes and exposures in populations and empirically testing hypotheses to explain the observed population rates and risks of the outcomes under study.

Accordingly, epidemiologic theory is a particular *type* of theory, concerned with explaining the distribution and causes of population patterns of health, disease, and well-being–that is, the substantive phenomena that comprise the domain of epidemiologic inquiry (Krieger, 1994; Krieger, 2001). Thus, just as evolutionary *theory* encompasses a variety of complementary and competing theories to explain the *fact* of biological evolution (Mayr, 1982; Eldredge, 1999; Gould, 2002), so too does epidemiologic *theory* include myriad complementary and competing theories to explain the *fact* of differential distributions of population health. Although sharing a common focus on the population patterning of health, the specific explanations nevertheless depend on choice of epidemiologic theory. Are the explanations to be found in individuals' choices? In the actions of institutions? In the interactions of nations? In the characteristics of particular pathogens, toxins, or other biophysical exposures? In the nucleotide sequences of the genome? In how work, the economy, and political systems are organized and families and relationships are constituted? In how people interact with the rest of the ecosystem? Or somewhere else?

One might consider the sorts of questions posed by epidemiologic theory to be compelling. As a practicing epidemiologist, I certainly do. As would, I imagine, many others concerned about people's health—whether in terms of disparate burdens of disease, of premature mortality, or of harmful social, physical, chemical, and biological exposures encountered at home, at school, at work, in the neighborhood, or other contexts.

And yet.

Meaning: given the issues at stake, one would think there would be plenty of books—or even just articles—on the topic of epidemiologic theory. But there aren't.

I provide the evidence for this assertion in Chapter 1, along with my thoughts on why this gap in the literature exists. And throughout I make the case that analysis and development of epidemiologic theory is essential for two reasons: one intellectual, one empirical.

—The *intellectual argument* is that epidemiology, like any science, needs theory to explain the phenomena in its specified domain. For epidemiology, this means theory to explain extant and changing population health profiles, so as to inform efforts to prevent disease, improve population health, and reduce health inequities. Understanding the strengths and limitations of diverse epidemiologic theories, and their origins and applications, is essential for improving the intellectual rigor, moorings, and creativity of the field.

—The *empirical argument* is that without explicit and transparent theory—as is currently the case in most epidemiologic textbooks and articles—we are likely to pose poorly-conceived hypotheses, inadequately interpret our findings, and potentially generate dangerously incomplete or wrong answers.

The overall premise is that theoretical clarity about the substantive questions epidemiology poses can improve the odds of generating valid—and potentially useful—knowledge. Theory is essential for formulating, testing, and assessing competing explanations—in other words, for good science. And good science, in turn, is a precondition for science that can make a difference for the good.

The book begins by arguing, in Chapter 1, that epidemiologic theory is a practical necessity for thinking about and explaining disease distribution. Chapter 2, concerned with theories about disease occurrence in various ancient and also contemporary traditional societies, introduces a range of ways that diverse peoples in various contexts, over time, have sought to explain their society's patterns of health and disease, as influenced by both their societal and ecologic context. Chapter 3 applies this analytic perspective to the emergence of epidemiology as a self-designated discipline and considers the range of competing theories of disease distribution employed between 1600 and 1900, with a focus on poison, filth, class, and race. Chapter 4 extends these analyses to encompass the first half of the twentieth century, whose theories focused on germs, genes, and the (social) environment. Chapter 5 then turns critical attention to the biomedical and lifestyle approaches dominating epidemiologic theorizing and research since the mid-twentieth century. Chapter 6 offers a systematic summary of the main alternatives to the dominant framework, as provided by the theories of the two main trends in social epidemiology: its sociopolitical and psychosocial frameworks. Chapter 7 introduces a newer variant of social epidemiologic theory: ecologically informed approaches, in particular the ecosocial theory of disease distribution that I first proposed in 1994 (Krieger, 1994) and its systematic linking of social and biological processes across levels and in relation to diverse spatiotemporal scales, as informed by both political economy and political ecology. As a final argument for why epidemiologic theory matters, Chapter 8 presents four cases examples illustrating how people's health can be harmed—or aided—depending on choice of epidemiologic theory and concludes by arguing that the science of epidemiology can be improved by consciously embracing, developing, and debating epidemiologic theories of disease distribution.

The impetus for me to write this book is the same as that for the course I first created and taught in 1991 to address the issue of epidemiologic theory in societal context and which I have been teaching, with modification, ever since. Recognizing the strengths and gaps in my own training as an epidemiologist (having obtained my master degree in 1985 and my Ph.D in 1989), and drawing on my background in biochemistry and biology, my interest in the history and philosophy of science, and my commitment to research and activism regarding the profound links between social justice and public health, I wanted to create a course that would address what I perceived as a huge lacuna in my education: a profound silence on the topic of epidemiologic theory. I accordingly designed my course to introduce others to ideas and literatures that I found relevant for my conceptual and empirical work as an epidemiologist. This path of inquiry has been, and continues to be, an ongoing intellectual journey, informed by the stark circumstances of people's lives I have encountered via my work and also the colleagues I have met along the way. The goal throughout has been to attain a better understanding of the realities of—and the possibilities for—the people's health.

While engaged in writing this book, I have of course been conscious that its content inevitably reflects my individual interests, experiences, and limitations as a scholar. In particular, I am acutely aware that my fluency only in English, coupled with my passable ability to read scientific texts in Spanish and French, restricts the primary literature I can analyze, such that I must rely on expert translation of works in all other languages. That said, English currently is, for good or for bad, the dominant language of scientific texts on epidemiologic theory and research. My hope is that my linguistic limitations nevertheless do not unduly restrict the ideas presented or their relevance to the majority of the world's people who speak languages other than English. To help ensure the cited texts speak in their own voice, and also to acquaint readers with the variety of expressions and ideas employed, I frequently use textboxes to accompany the analysis I present in my own words. Any errors in fact or interpretation are my responsibility alone.

Finally, I end this preface by acknowledging my debt to the many whose work, lives, and thoughts inform this text and the research on which it is based. Their contributions only just begin to summarized by the book's bibliography. In particular, I offer deep thanks to my mentors: Ruth Hubbard, who taught me it was not only possible but essential to think critically and historically about science and its inextricable links to concerns about social justice, while still doing—and not only critiquing—the science; Noel S. Weiss, who taught me to be an epidemiologist; and S. Leonard Syme, who gave full support to my becoming a social epidemiologist.

With regard to institutional support, I first thank Lisa Berkman, who served as chair of my department from 1995 to 2008, was enthusiastic about this project from the start, and who permitted me to work on it in lieu of teaching my course during the 2009 to 2010 academic year. I likewise thank the many students who, as my successive literature search assistants, have tracked down many an obscure book and article; they include, in chronological order since 2002, when I began more concretely planning for this project: David Rehkopf, David Chae, Malavkia Subramanyam, Shalini Tendulkar, and Marlene Camacho. I also thank the editors I have worked with at Oxford University Press—Jeffrey House, William J. Lamsback, Regan Hofmann, and Maura Roessner—for their interest and encouragement.

The making of a book, however, is not simply an academic enterprise. I thank my friends and colleagues who over the years have engaged with me on and off about the ideas I present in this book and who at various points have given invaluable support as I worked on it: Mary Bassett, George Davey Smith, Sofia Gruskin, Lisa Moore, Anne-Emanuelle Birn, Rosalyn Baxandall, and Jason Beckfield, and also my core team members, Jarvis T. Chen and Pamela D. Waterman, whose wonderful daily work on our many theoretically-grounded empirical epidemiologic investigations has bolstered, extended, and given space for my thinking. To the extent that my own epidemiologic investigations inform the content of this book, I thank, for the studies that enrolled participants, the individuals who agreed to share information about their lives to inform the public understanding of health and disease, and for the studies that relied on vital statistics and other public health surveillance data, I thank the staff of the agencies involved who diligently transform information from people's medical records, birth and death certificates, and other such resources into usable data for understanding population health.

I conclude with a final set of thanks that transcend words. I begin with thanks to my parents, Dorothy T. Krieger (1927–1985) and Howard P. Krieger (1918–1992), who taught me to value learning and apply that knowledge to making the world a better place; to my brother, Jim Krieger, who is simultaneously friend, family, and a public health inspiration, connecting social justice and public health through his tangible work to reduce health inequities and promote the public's health; to Mrs. Montez Davis (1914–1997), who helped raise me; and to my three cats, who have been my constant companions since I first conceived this project: Emma (1981–1996), Samudra (b. 1996), and her brother Bhu (1996–2010). And to Lis Ellison-Loschmann: thank you.

REFERENCES

Eldredge N. *The Pattern of Evolution*. New York: W.H. Freeman & Co., 1999.

Gould SJ. *The Structure of Evolutionary Theory*. Cambridge, MA: The Belknap Press of Harvard University Press, 2002.

Krieger N. Epidemiology and the web of causation: has anyone seen the spider? *Soc Sci Med* 1994; 39:887–903.

Krieger N. Theories for social epidemiology in the 21st century: an ecosocial perspective. *Int J Epidemiol* 2001; 30:668–677.

Mayr E. *The Growth of Biological Thought: Diversity, Evolution, and Inheritance*. Cambridge, MA: The Belknap Press of Harvard University Press, 1982.

Table of Contents

Epidemiology and the People's Health

1

Does Epidemiologic Theory Exist?

On Science, Data, and Explaining Disease Distribution

Theory. Traced to its Greek roots, "theory" means to see inwards; to theorize is to use our mind's eye systematically, following articulated principles, to discern meaningful patterns among observations and ideas (Oxford English Dictionary [OED] 2008). The implication is that without theory, observation is blind and explanation is impossible.

In this chapter, I will make the argument that epidemiologic theory is a practical necessity for thinking about and explaining disease distribution. What could be more obvious?

Yet, apparently refuting what ought to be this simple self-evident claim is the curious fact that epidemiologic textbooks have, for the past several decades—as I discuss below—offered little or no guidance on what an epidemiologic theory is, let alone why such theory is important or how it can be used (Krieger, 1994). Sorting out this conundrum requires considering what scientific theory is—and what place it might have in epidemiologic thinking and research.

Figuring Out the People's Health: Theory and the Stories (About) Data (that People) Tell

First: Why even posit that epidemiologic theory is a practical necessity? Consider the epidemiologic data shown in **Figures 1–1** through **1–7**. Together, they illustrate population distributions of disease—over time, space, and social group—in the United States and globally.

Figure 1–1 presents data from a study titled "The fall and rise of US inequities in premature mortality: 1960–2002" (Krieger et al., 2008). These data show that between 1960 and 2002, as rates of U.S. premature mortality (**Figure 1–1a**, deaths before age 65 years) and infant death (**Figure 1–1b**, deaths before age 1 year) declined in all county income quintiles, socioeconomic and racial/ethnic inequities in premature mortality and infant death (both relative and absolute) *shrank* between 1966 and 1980, especially for U.S. populations of color, but from 1980 onward, the relative health inequities *widened* and the absolute differences barely changed. Why?

3

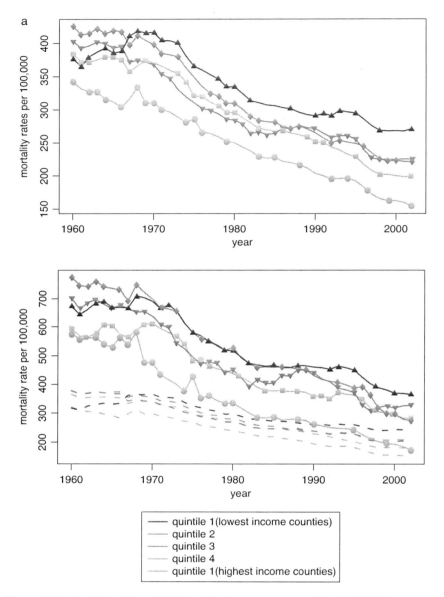

Figure 1–1. The fall and rise of U.S. inequities in premature mortality, 1960–2002, by county median income quintile. (Krieger et al., 2008)

Figure 1–1a. The fall and rise of U.S. inequities in premature mortality: deaths before age 65 years, 1960–2002, by county median income quintile, for: (A) total population by county median income quintile, and (B) the US White population (dashed lines) and populations of color (solid lines).

b

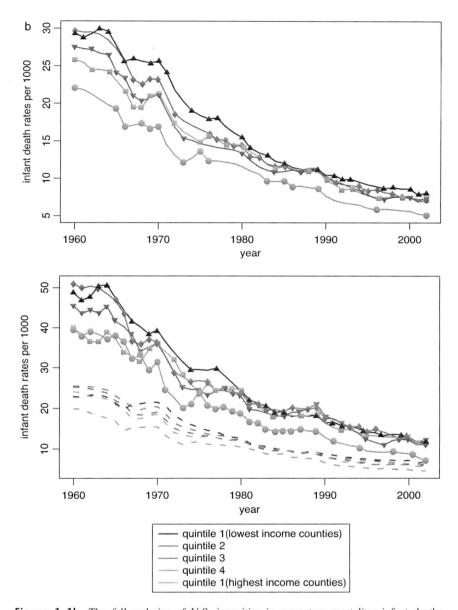

Figure 1–1b. The fall and rise of U.S. inequities in premature mortality: infant deaths, 1960–2002, by county median income quintile, for: (A) total population, and (B) the US White population (dashed lines) and populations of color (solid lines).

Figure 1–1 Technical Considerations

1. U.S. counties are politically defined geographic areas within United States. As explained by the U.S. Census, "states and counties are the major legally defined political and administrative units of the United States" (U.S. Census Geographic Areas Reference Manual 2008, p. 4-1). More specifically, counties are "a type of governmental unit that is the primary legal subdivision of every State except Alaska and Louisiana" (the former uses "borough" and the latter uses "parish" instead of "county") (U.S. Census Geographic Areas Reference Manual 2008, p. G-17).

2. The county income quintiles are based on county median family income, referring to the income level at which half the families in the county are below this level and half are above. The lowest income county quintile (the darkest line) contains the bottom fifth of counties, and the highest income county quintile (the lightest line) contains the top fifth of counties, as ranked by their county median family income.

3. In Figure 1–1 the death rates are age-standardized to permit meaningful comparison of death rates by county income level over time and across counties (Anderson & Rosenberg 1998; Krieger & Williams 2001). In this approach, each and every county in each and every year is treated as if it had the exact same age distribution, such that any county differences in the age-standardized death rates are not simply a result of the population of one county being younger or older than another but, rather, because the county mortality rates differ within specific age groups. For example, a county with many retirees would be expected to have a higher death rate than a county consisting chiefly of young families with young children, simply because older people are more likely to die than younger people. Age-standardization avoids this problem by taking into account whether, at each and every age, from young to old, the deaths rates are similar or different. Stated more technically, the age-standardized death rate is computed by applying each county's age-specific mortality rates (e.g., for persons ages 0–4, 5–9, 10–19,…, 65–69, 70–75, 75–78, and 80+ years) to a specified "standard population," determining the number of persons in each age group who would have died (given the county age-specific mortality rates), summing them up, and dividing by the total size of the "standard population." If the age-standardized rate for the counties differs, then by definition it differs because of something other than the counties' age structure. In the hypothetical example below, two populations have similar crude death rates ([total of deaths divided by total population]*100,000) but the age-standardized death rate of Population 2 is 1.3 times higher than that of Population 1, because in every age strata, Population 2 has higher age-specific death rates than Population 1, which is masked by the crude death rate, given the younger age structure of Population 2 compared to Population 1 combined with lower mortality rates at younger ages.

Age group (years)	Population 1			Population 2			US 2000 standard million population	Population 1	Population 2
	Deaths(N)	Population(N)	Age-specific death rate per 100,000	Deaths (N)	Population(N)	Age-specific death rate, per 100,000		Number of deaths if apply their death rates to the same standard population	
	(A)	(B)	(C) = ((A)/(B)) * 100,000	(D)	(E)	(F) = ((D)/(E)) * 100,000		(C) * standard population	(F) * standard population
<1	99	17,150	577.3	202	15,343	1,316.6	13,818	79.8	181.9
1–4	22	67,265	32.7	27	64,718	41.7	55,317	18.1	23.1
5–14	32	200,511	16.0	51	170,355	29.9	145,565	23.3	43.5
15–24	134	174,405	76.8	200	181,677	110.1	138,646	106.5	152.6
25–34	118	122,567	96.3	296	162,066	182.6	135,573	130.6	247.6
35–44	210	113,616	184.8	421	139,237	302.4	162,613	300.5	491.7
45–54	426	114,265	372.8	895	117,811	759.7	134,834	502.7	1,024.3
55–64	784	91,481	857.0	1,196	80,294	1,489.5	87,247	747.7	1,299.5
65–74	1,374	61,192	2,245.4	1,471	48,426	3,037.6	66,037	1,482.8	2,005.9
75–84	1,766	30,112	5,864.8	1,117	17,303	6,455.5	44,842	2,629.9	2,894.8
85+	1,042	7,436	14,012.9	360	2,770	12,996.4	15,508	2,173.1	2,015.5
Total	6,007	1,000,000		6,236	1,000,000		1,000,000	8,195.0	10308.04

Death rates (per 100,000)

Population	Crude	Age-standardized
Population 1	600.7	819.5
Population 2	623.6	1,038.0

Ratio of death rates: Population 2/Population 1

	Crude	Age-standardized
	1.04	1.27

Figure 1–2 depicts age-specific trends in U.S. breast cancer incidence rates among U.S. White women from 1937 to 2003 (Krieger, 2008). It reveals a marked jump in incidence among women age 55 years and older starting in 1980, with rates then falling after 2002. Why?

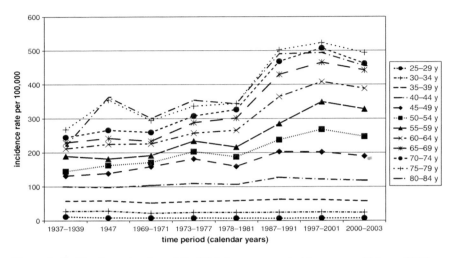

Figure 1–2. The rise and perhaps fall of U.S. breast cancer incidence rates. (Krieger, 2008)

Figure 1–3 is the graph of changing trends in mortality among women and men ages 55 to 64 years in England and Wales from 1850 to 1950 that Jerry Morris (1910–2009) used in his classic 1955 article on "Uses of Epidemiology" (Morris, 1955) and with which he opened his pathbreaking 1957 textbook by the same name (Morris, 1957). During this time period, mortality rates fell in both groups, but not evenly so: whereas the male:female mortality ratio was approximately 1.1 in 1850, it was 1.3 in 1920, and 1.9 in 1950. The growing divergence, Morris noted, resulted chiefly from the "emergence of three diseases from obscurity to become exceedingly common, disease which particularly affect men and are very frequent in middle-age: duodenal ulcer, cancer of the bronchus and coronary thrombosis" (Morris, 1957, pp. 1–2). As Morris also wondered: Why?

Figure 1–4 shows maps from the "Worldmapper" project, in which the size of countries is scaled to the size of the outcome depicted: population size, economic resources, and health status (Worldmapper, 2008). **Figure 1–4a** provides the conventional map of the world, with countries scaled to land size; in **Figure 1–4b,** the countries are scaled to the size of their population. **Figure 1–4c** shows the data for "absolute poverty," defined by the World Bank as living on an income of at most $2 per day; **Figure 1–4d** displays the data for wealth, as measured by the gross domestic product (GDP). In the former, the African continent and Asian subcontinent loom large; in the latter, the United States, Europe, and Japan are bloated, and the Asian subcontinent shrinks and the African continent dwindles to the merest strand. **Figure 1–4e** presents data on infant mortality; **Figure 1–4f** provides data on lung cancer deaths; **Figure 1–4g** shows data on "often preventable deaths," defined

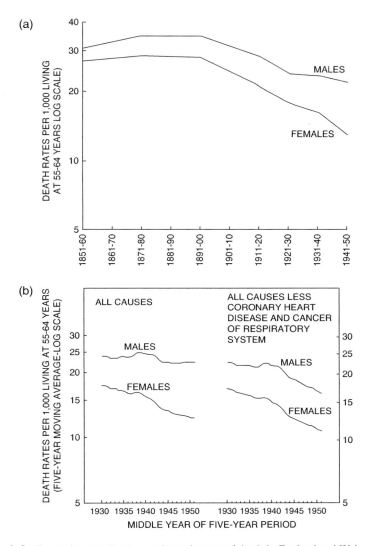

Figure 1–3. Trends in mortality by gender and cause of death in England and Wales, 1850–1950, as presented in Morris's 1955 article on "Uses of Epidemiology" (Morris, 1955) and incorporated into his 1957 pathbreaking textbook *Uses of Epidemiology* (Morris, 1957, pp. 1–2).

in relation to communicable infections and maternal, perinatal, and nutritional conditions and accounting for one-third of the world's deaths in 2002; and **Figure 1–4h** depicts data on sewerage sanitation. In **Figures 1–4e** and **1–4g**, the African continent and Asian subcontinent again loom large, whereas the United States, Europe, and Japan are massively shrunk. In **Figures 1–4f** and **1–4h**, the reverse occurs. Why?

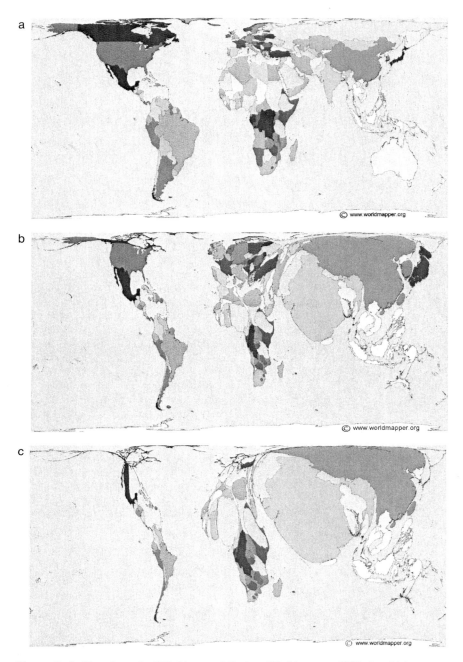

Figure 1–4. Maps from the "Worldmapper" Project (Worldmapper, 2008), in which country size is scaled in relation to the outcome depicted. © Copyright 2006 SASI Group (University of Sheffield) and Mark Newman (University of Michigan).

Figure 1–4a. Countries scaled to land size.

Figure 1–4b. Countries scaled to population size (2002).

Figure 1–4c. Absolute poverty (up to $2 per day) (2002).

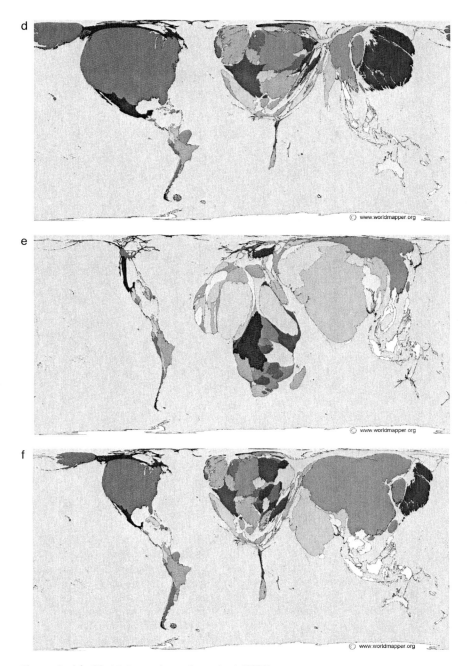

Figure 1–4d. Wealth (gross domestic product) (2002).

Figure 1–4e. Infant mortality (2002).

Figure 1–4f. Lung cancer deaths (2002).

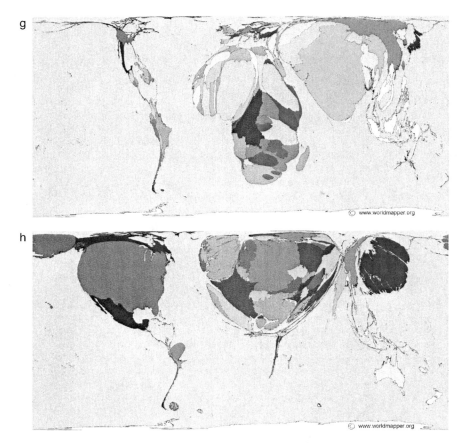

Figure 1–4g. Often preventable deaths (communicable infections, maternal, perinatal, and nutritional conditions) (2002)

Figure 1–4h. Sewerage sanitation (1999).

Finally, **Figures 1–5, 1–6,** and **1–7** display data from the "Gapminder" project regarding associations between child survival (children dying before age 5 years per 1000 live births) and Gross National Income per capita (Gapminder, 2008). **Figure 1–5** depicts these country-level associations for 2006, with the size of each country's data point scaled to population size, and countries within the same global region shaded the same color. Although it shows an overall robust direct association between child survival and income (the lower the income, the poorer the survival), as underscored in **Figure 1–6,** at any given level of per capita income, countries vary considerably in their rates of child survival (e.g., South Africa fares worse than Malaysia, despite similar per capita income), and at any given level of child survival, countries vary considerably in their per capita income (e.g., Malaysia fares as well as the United States, despite its lower per capita income). **Figure 1–7** in turn presents data on within-region distributions of income in 2000, along with data on within-countries inequities in child survival and income in 2003, for India, Bangladesh, Peru, Guatemala, Yemen, South Africa, and Vietnam. Illuminating

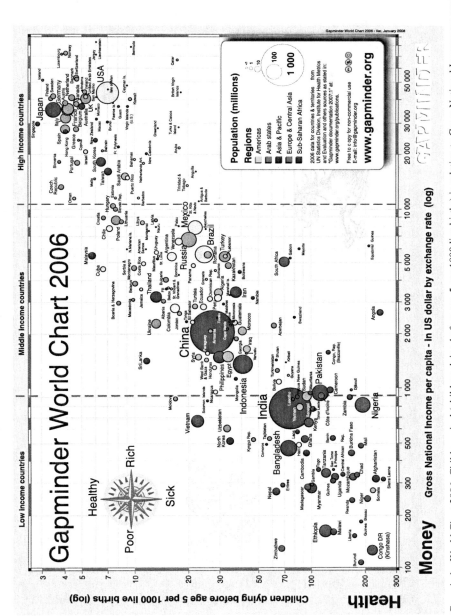

Figure 1–5. Gapminder World Chart 2006: Child survival (children dying before age 5 per 1000 live births) in relation to Gross National Income per capita.

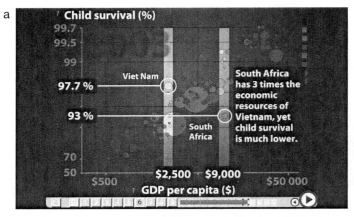

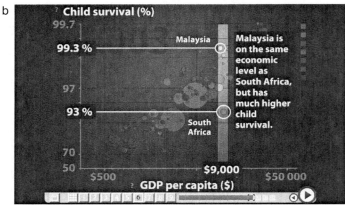

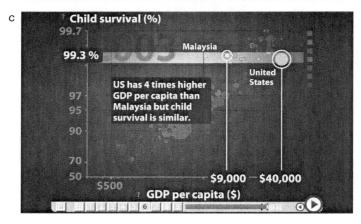

Figure 1–6. Between-country comparisons of child survival and per capita income, by level of child survival and by per capita income, excerpted from the Gapminder Human Development 2005 presentation (Gapminder, 2008).

Figure 1–6a. Income and child survival inequities: South Africa and Vietnam (2003)

Figure 1–6b. Income and child survival inequities: South Africa and Malaysia (2003)

Figure 1–6c. Income and child survival inequities: Malaysia and the United States (2003)

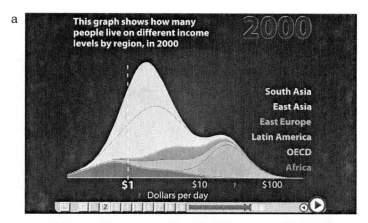

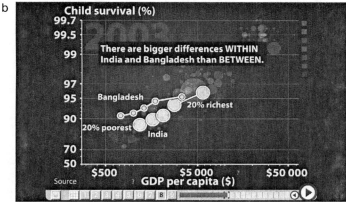

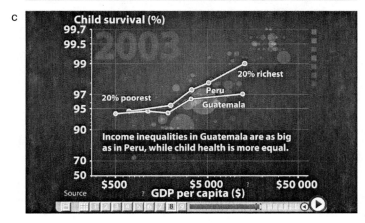

Figure 1–7. Within-country inequities in child survival and per capita income, excerpted from the Gapminder Human Development 2005 presentation (Gapminder, 2008)

Figure 1–7a. Income distribution by global region

Figure 1–7b. Income and child survival inequities: within Bangladesh and India (2003)

Figure 1–7c. Income and child survival inequities: within Peru and Guatemala (2003)

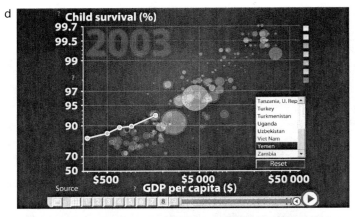

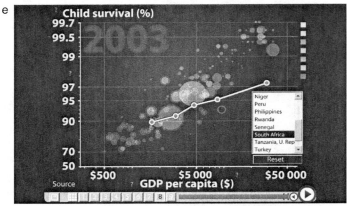

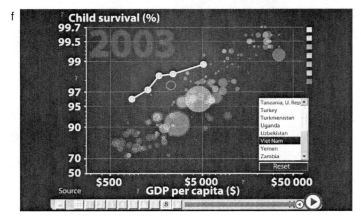

Figure 1–7d. Income and child survival inequities: Yemen (2003)

Figure 1–7e. Income and child survival inequities: South Africa (2003)

Figure 1–7f. Income and child survival inequities: Vietnam (2003)

the variability behind the on-average values, these figures show that within-country differences in income and child survival can dwarf between-country differences. Once again: Why?

Before even considering the role of theory in answering these "whys," it is important to step back and ask: What is the thinking that leads to data allowing these questions even to be posed? And where does theory fit into this process?

One place to begin is to realize that **Figures 1–1** through **1–7** are premised on a host of assumptions. What ideas are built into these figures? To start: population rates of disease—a phrase that requires understanding *population*, *rate*, and *disease*. Other ideas at play include: changing incidence rates over time; geographic variation in disease occurrence; and differences in disease rates by social group. None of these ideas are intuitively obvious. They make sense only if one already has a theoretical orientation that finds it compelling and reasonable to think abstractly about populations, about individuals in numerators and denominators, about averages and distributions, about disease occurrence in space and time, and about disease as a definable entity apart from (as opposed to uniquely residing in) the individual persons in whom it is experienced—and hence diseased persons as countable cases.

Prelude, then, to **Figures 1–1** through **1–7** are the ideas that would compel someone to collect and display their data. Also notable is who and what is omitted, not simply who and what is included—for example, if the data are or are not separately shown by such social categories as social class, gender, race/ethnicity, sexuality, or by subtypes of disease.

In other words, data are not simply "observed": there is active thinking behind the act of data acquisition. Not to mention the active thinking that guides data analysis, display, and interpretation.

And this active thinking is the stuff of theory.

Meaning: contrary to its etymologic origins, data are not a "given" ("datum" is the past participle of the Latin verb "dare," "to give" [OED, 2008; Krieger, 1992]). Nor do data tell stories. People do. An important caveat, however, is that the stories that people who are scientists tell are not simply or simple "stories": they are (or are supposed to be) transparent accounts, informed by theory, and premised on the public testing of ideas and explanations, using explicitly defined concepts and methods.

So What Is a Scientific Theory?

To appreciate what an epidemiologic theory is (or ought to be), it helps first to have a sense of what counts as a scientific theory—and also: what counts as science. The literature on these topics is vast, contentious, and complex (Mendelsohn et al., 1997; Archer et al., 1998; Ziman, 2000; Collins, 2001; Gould, 2002; Grene & Depew, 2004; Daston & Galison, 2007; Sober, 2008). That said, some common contemporary criteria for science and scientific theories do exist (*see* **Textboxes 1–1** and **1–2**).

To begin, most current scholarship would agree that scientific theories, in contemporary terms, are coherent and presumptively testable sets of inter-related ideas that enable scientists to describe, explain, and predict features of a commonly shared biophysical reality in which cause-and-effect exists (Mendelsohn et al., 1997; Ziman, 2000; Krieger, 2001a). Science, in turn, is both a human activity and a body of knowledge premised on the thinking and action of people to describe and to test their explanations and predictions about features of their commonly shared reality. Particular fields of scientific inquiry are, in turn, distinguished by the domains they seek to understand, the substantive and explanatory

Textbox 1–1. Contested Definitions: Science, Theory, and Hypothesis

Term   Definition

science   *Oxford English Dictionary* **(OED, 2008):**
            —etymology: "(a. F. *science* = Pr. *sciensa*, Sp. *ciencia*, Pg. *sciencia*, It. *scienza*, ad. L. *scientia* knowledge, f. *scient-em*, pr. pple. of *sc re* to know.)"
            —definition:
            4a. In a more restricted sense: A branch of study which is concerned either with a connected body of demonstrated truths or with observed facts systematically classified and more or less colligated by being brought under general laws, and which includes trustworthy methods for the discovery of new truth within its own domain.
            5. ...In mod. use chiefly: The sciences (in sense 4) as distinguished from other departments of learning; scientific doctrine or investigation.
            5b. In modern use, often treated as synonymous with "Natural and Physical Science," and thus restricted to those branches of study that relate to the phenomena of the material universe and their laws, sometimes with implied exclusion of pure mathematics. This is now the dominant sense in ordinary use.

            Oxford Dictionary of Science **(2005) (Daintith,** 2005): no definition (!)
            —and worth considering what it means the term is considered to be self-evident...

            Oxford Dictionary of Sociology **(2005) (Scott & Marshall,** 2005): no definition (!)—ditto...

            Keywords **(1983) (Williams,** 1983): (*italics* and **bold** in the original; C = century (e = early, m = mid))
            p. 277: "**Science** came into English in C14, from fw *science*, F., *scientia*, L–knowledge. Its earliest uses were very general... often interchangeably with art, to describe a particular body of knowledge or skill..."
            p. 278: "The key distinction was not a first in **science** but in the crucial C18 distinction between *experience* and *experiment*. This supported a distinction between *practical* and *theoretical* knowledge, which was then expressed as a distinction between *art* and **science** in their C17 and C18 general senses... The distinction hardened in eC19 and mC19... we can find by 1867 the significantly confident, yet also significantly conscious, statement: 'we shall... use the word 'science' in the sense which Englishmen so commonly give to it .. as expressing physical and experimental science, to the exclusion of theological and metaphysical.'"

            New Keywords **(2005) (Shapin,** 2005) (*italics* and **bold** in the original; C = century)
            p. 314: "In the early modern period, the L *scientia* just mean knowledge, usually in the sense of a systematically organized body of knowledge, acquired through a course of study... During the course of the C19 and C20, 'science' came overwhelmingly to pick out those practices proceeding by observation and experiment, thus jettisoning history and philosophy and leaving the social sciences a courtesy title, with limited credibility in the general cultural or among natural scientists 'proper.'"

            p. 315: "Linguistically, this more restrictive sense of 'science' was an artifact of the way English usage developed and changed in recent centuries... by the C19 'science' did not usually need the qualifying

'natural' to summon up the idea of organized methodological research into the things, phenomena, and capacities belonging to nature as opposed to culture. How this shift occurred is still little understood..."
p. 317: "Talk about the 'scientific method' is predicated upon some version of the 'unity' of science... Disunity theorists doubt that there are any methodological procedures held in common by invertebrate zoology, seismology, microbial genetics, and any of the varieties of particle physics, which are *not* to be found in non-scientific forms of culture. How can the human sciences coherently either embrace or reject "the natural science model" when the natural sciences themselves display such conceptual and methodological heterogeneity?"

theory   *Oxford English Dictionary* **(OED, 2008):**
—etymology: "(ad. late L. theōria (Jerome in Ezech. XII. xl. 4), a. Gr. θεωρία a looking at, viewing, contemplation, speculation, theory, also a sight, a spectacle, abstr. n. f. spectator, looker on, f. stem of to look on, view, contemplate. In mod. use prob. from med.L. transl. of Aristotle. Cf. It. *teoria* (Florio 1598 *theoría*), F. *théorie* (15. in Godef. *Compl.*).)"
—definition:
3. A conception or mental scheme of something to be done, or of the method of doing it; a systematic statement of rules or principles to be followed.
4a. A scheme or system of ideas or statements held as an explanation or account of a group of facts or phenomena; a hypothesis that has been confirmed or established by observation or experiment, and is propounded or accepted as accounting for the known facts; a statement of what are held to be the general laws, principles, or causes of something known or observed.
4b. That department of an art or technical subject which consists in the knowledge or statement of the facts on which it depends, or of its principles or methods, as distinguished from the practice of it.

Oxford Dictionary of Science **(2005) (Daintith, 2005):**
p. 464: "A description of nature that encompasses more than one law but has not achieved the uncontrovertible status of a law is sometimes called a **theory.**"

Oxford Dictionary of Sociology **(2005) (Scott & Marshall, 2005):**
p. 662: "A theory is an account of the world which goes beyond what we can see and measure. It embraces a set of interrelated definitions and relationships that organizes our concepts and understanding of the empirical world in a systematic way, Generally speaking, there are three different conceptions of theory in sociology. Some think of theory as generalization about, and classification of, the social world. The scope of generalization varies from theorizing about a particular range of phenomena to more abstract and general theories about society and history as a whole. Others believe that theoretical statements should be translated into empirical, measurable, or observable propositions, and systematically tested... Finally, yet others argue that theory should explain phenomena, identifying causal mechanisms and processes which, although they cannot be observed directly, can be seen in their effects."

Keywords **(1983) (Williams, 1983):** (*italics* and **bold** in the original; C = century [l = late])

p. 316: "**Theory** has an interesting development and range of meanings, and a significant distinction from (later an opposition to) practice.

The earliest English form was *theorique* (C14), followed by *theory* (C16), from fw *theoria*, lL, *theoria*, Gk–contemplation, spectacle, mental conception (from *theoros*, Gk–spectator, rw *thea*, Gk–sight; cf *theatre*)... A distinction between **theory** and *practice* was widely made in C17, as in Bacon (1626)."

p. 317: "But **theory** in this important sense is always in active relation to *practice*: an interaction between things done, things observed and (systematic) explanation of these. This allows a necessary distinction between **theory** and *practice*, but does not require their opposition."

New Keywords **(2005) (Frow, 2005)** (*italics* and **bold** in the original; C = century)

p. 347: "In its modern sense the word **theory** probably entered English from medieval translations of Aristotle. Etymologically it has the same root (*theoros*, spectator, from rw *thea*, sight) as the word *theatre*; Gk *theorie* is a sight of spectacle, and the literal sense of looking has then been metamorphosized to that of contemplating or speculating... . In a more general philosophical and scientific sense, a theory is:

> a scheme or system of ideas or statements held as an explanation or account of a group of facts or phenomena; a hypothesis that has been confirmed or established by observation or experiment, and is propounded or accepted as accounting for the known facts; a statement of what are held to be the general laws, principles, or causes of something known or observed.
>
> Central to this definition is the notion of the systematic relations holding between the components of an explanatory model, and the differentiation of theory from the more tentative conception of a hypothesis."

p. 348: "The account of **scientific theorization** in the C20, dominated by the logical positivism of Rudolf Carnap, Karl Popper, and others, attempts to reduce the speculative dimension of theorization by requiring the use of rigorous correspondence rules between observation statements and theoretical meta-languages. A more positive view of theory particularly in the social sciences, however, has stressed that observation statements in the natural sciences are always theory-laden and are meaningful in relation to a particular theoretical framework . . . In contemporary usage in the humanities and social sciences, 'theory' designates less any particular set of systematic ideas than a politically contested attitude toward the use of abstract explanatory models in humanistic and social inquiry."

hypothesis *Oxford English Dictionary* **(OED, 2008):**
—etymology: (a. Gr. ὑπόθεσις foundation, base; hence, basis of an argument, supposition, also, subject-matter, etc., f. ὑπό under + θέσις placing.)

—definition:
2. A proposition or principle put forth or stated (without any reference to its correspondence with fact) merely as a basis for reasoning or argument, or as a premiss from which to draw a conclusion; a supposition.
3. A supposition or conjecture put forth to account for known facts; *esp.* in the sciences, a provisional supposition from which to draw conclusions that shall be in accordance with known facts, and which serves as a starting-point for further investigation by which it may be proved or disproved and the true theory arrived at.

Oxford Dictionary of Science **(2005) (Daintith, 2005):**
p. 464: "A **hypothesis** is a theory or law that retains the suggestion that it may not be universally true."

Oxford Dictionary of Sociology **(2005) (Scott & Marshall, 2005):**
p. 285: "A hypothesis is an untested statement about the relationship (usually of association or causation) between concepts within a given theory."

Keywords **(1983) (Williams, 1983):** no entry

New Keywords **(2005) (Bennett et al., 2005):** no entry

---

concepts they use, and the metaphors and mechanisms they employ for their causal explanations (*see* **Textbox 1–2**) (Martin & Harré, 1982; Ziman, 2000; Krieger, 2001a). Additionally, those sciences whose domains encompass non-deterministic phenomena (e.g., excluding what are held to be invariant "natural laws," such as the law of thermodynamics) can further be characterized by historical contingency (meaning what occurs depends on context, hence is not universally invariant)—and among these are the subset of reflexive sciences, which are focused on phenomena that can be influenced by human action (e.g., societal characteristics), such that the explanation adduced can be used to transform that which is being explained (Lieberson, 1992; Archer, 1998; Gannett, 1999; Ziman, 2000; Gadenne, 2002; Krieger, 2001a).

Core to the theorizing and conduct of science are a host of assumptions (Lieberson, 1992; Mendelsohn et al., 1997; Archer et al., 1998; Ziman, 2000; Collins, 2001; Gould, 2002; Grene & Depew, 2004; Daston & Galison, 2007; Sober, 2008). One such assumption is that we humans live in a commonly shared biophysical (including social) world—and, more broadly, universe—which provides the referent for what we term *reality*. Another is that this commonly shared biophysical world encompasses diverse processes, structures, and events that are in principal knowable by humans and amenable to scientific investigation. A third is that the existence of this commonly shared knowable biophysical world can be investigated by—and is independent of—any particular human individual. A fourth is that independent humans (in solo and in groups) can independently formulate and test their ideas about "how the world works" and collectively compare ideas, methods, and results. All four of these assumptions are preconditions for the existence and evaluation of scientific theories. More bluntly, no postulated referent reality shared by and accessible to independent humans, no science.

Equally essential is the assumption that causal processes exist. Whether these processes are "deterministic" or "probabilistic" is another question entirely. I note only in passing that debates have raged for millennia over the meaning of causality—and, more recently, within a variety of scientific disciplines, over connections between "chance" and "necessity," and whether "randomness" is "real" or simply a reflection of ignorance of otherwise deterministic causes (Moyal, 1949; Monod, 1972; Stigler, 1986; Desrosières, 1988; Hacking, 1990; Daston, 1994; Gannett, 1999; Weber, 2001; Gadenne, 2002; Russo & Williamson, 2007; Machamer & Wolters, 2007; Groff, 2008). Regardless of the positions argued in these debates, however, the basic point remains that the scientific work of causal inference necessarily presumes that some sort of underlying causal relationship exists, either of the inevitable or contingent variety. Hence, one key corollary to the assumption about a referent reality: no causal processes, no science—and no scientific explanations.

This is all very abstract. It is supposed to be. Science and scientific theories require abstract thinking: to imagine and discern the causal processes behind the observed and postulated specifics, to derive meaning from pattern, and, as the poet William Blake (1757–1827) put it so well, "[t]o see a world in a grain of sand/And a heaven in a wild flower/Hold infinity in the palm of your hand/And eternity in an hour" (Blake, 1977, p. 506). Or, as stated more prosaically by Stanley Lieberson (b. 1933) in a 1991 presidential address to the American Sociological Association: "[T]heory involves generating principles that explain existing information; but it also goes beyond those observations to integrate and account for a variety of other phenomena in ways that would not otherwise be apparent" and would further "'predict' all sorts of observations not yet made" (Lieberson, 1992, p. 4).

Why bother with these abstract assertions? Because to understand and evaluate epidemiologic theories, it is important to know what science and scientific theories presume—and what they do not.

First, scientific theories are, by definition, conceptual. But they are not about just any set of ideas. They are instead sets of inter-related ideas intended to explain phenomena in specified domains of the commonly shared biophysical world. Additionally, both the ideas and what they refer to are capable of being independently evaluated and employed by different individuals. Accordingly, some of the concepts in scientific theories pertain to the phenomena that are being described and explained. Others pertain to the causal processes that are theorized to explain the selected phenomena. And both kinds of concepts— substantive and explanatory—are essential for scientific theory; neither alone suffices. What is being explained and how it is being explained are constituent and complementary—and often contested—aspects of scientific theory. Within any given discipline, different theories can exist, simultaneously or successively, offering different and debated explanatory accounts; across disciplines, theories additionally differ because of their respective focus on different aspects of what nevertheless is presumed to be a shared referent reality— whether physical, chemical, biological, or social. A theory of biological evolution, for example, needs not only the concepts of organism, environment, reproduction, and heredity (all of which presumably can in some way be studied by independent investigators) but also the causal ideas (which may be convergent, competing, or complementary) that tie these concepts together to explain the occurrence of evolution (Mayr, 1982; Eldredge, 1999; Gould, 2002; Grene & Depew, 2004; Sober, 2008).

Moreover, to express the ideas at play, scientific theories inevitably employ a combination of metaphor and mechanisms—metaphor to convey concepts describing both phenomena and causal processes and mechanisms to explain the pathways between cause and effect (Lakoff, 1980; Osherson et al., 1981; Martin & Harré, 1982; MacCormac, 1985; Young, 1985; Holton, 1988; Krieger, 1994; Keller, 1995; Krieger, 2001a; Keller, 2002). As I have noted in prior essays, this use of metaphor in scientific theories—essential for enabling the "unknown" to be comprehended in terms of the "known"—can simultaneously free and constrain thought (Krieger, 1994). A salient example, relevant to epidemiology, concerns the widespread—and now increasingly contested—metaphor of DNA as the "blueprint" or "master program" for the organism (Watson, 1968). This conceit, as pointed out by the biologist Richard Lewontin (b. 1929) (Lewontin, 2000, pp. 10–11), has dominated the genetics research agenda since the mid-twentieth century. Attesting to its widespread acceptance are the statements of prominent scientists, such as Sydney Brenner (b. 1927; Brenner, 2002), who in 1968 asserted, "The goal of molecular biology is to be able to compute an organism from a knowledge of its genes" (Melnechuk, 1968), and Walter Gilbert (b. 1932; Gilbert, 1980), who in 1992 declared that the complete sequencing of the human genome will enable us to know "what makes us human" (Gilbert, 1992, p. 84). Explicit articulation of the "blueprint" metaphor, moreover, was likewise provided in 1992 by James D. Watson (b. 1928), one of the co-discoverers of the double-helical form of DNA, who declared that the human genome constitutes "the complete genetic blueprint of man (*sic*)," arguing, "if you can study life from the level of DNA, you have a real explanation for its processes" (Watson, 1992, p. 164), a statement echoed in one newspaper account of the first full sequencing of the human genome on June 26, 2000: "The blueprint of humanity, the book of life, the software for existence—whatever you call it, decoding the entire three billion letters of human DNA is a monumental achievement." (Carrington, 2000). Although this architectural/computer programming conceit may initially have fruitfully guided genetic research (with the idea of DNA being "in command"), it is increasingly understood to disregard how DNA—and biological development—is dependent on and subject to myriad exogenous influences on gene regulation and expression (Keller, 1992; Keller, 1995; Gilbert, 2000; Lewontin, 2000; Keller, 2002; Van Speybroeck et al., 2002). The key point is that the concepts employed by scientific theories—whether to describe phenomena or causal processes—are not simply self-evident terms. Instead, they are usually rife with connections to other concepts—which is only to be expected, as theories, by definition, must employ interrelated ideas, and the people who use and develop these theories must employ words and symbols that convey these ideas to others interested in understanding them.

Second, the scientific assumption that there is a commonly shared biophysical world is a precondition for science—even as this assumption does *not* presume this referent reality is commonly perceived or understood by all individuals. Depending on people's specific characteristics and worldviews, individuals within and across different societies and time periods may vary in their perceptions and interpretations of any given biophysical phenomenon. At a fairly trivial level, color-blindness in particular individuals does not mean the absence of reflected light at the frequency at which these individuals are color-blind (Gibson, 1979). At a more profound level, different individuals may agree on the existence of the same set of associations—for example, when the sun passes below the horizon, it gets dark—and yet may have completely different interpretations of why these associations exist (e.g., because the sun is passing through the underworld; because the sun revolves around the Earth and has moved to location where it is not observable by the person on Earth; or because the Earth revolves around the sun and has rotated to a point where the sun is no longer observable by a person on that point of the Earth's surface; Hanson, 1958). Or, more epidemiologically, the shared observation of an association between two variables—say, race/ethnicity and disease—does not mean the variables or their association are comprehended in the same way. Whereas some might deem "race" a biological characteristic that explains the observed association (Burchard et al., 2003), others might argue instead that racism, and its associated socially-constructed categories of race/ethnicity, is what has causal relevance (Krieger, 2005). That said, disputes over the causal ideas at issue—and the substantive phenomena under study—nevertheless presume that there is a common reality to which they refer; otherwise, attempting to elucidate the reasons for disagreement—and testing competing hypotheses—would be impossible.

Third, scientific observation is not a passive phenomenon: what we "see" and apprehend depends on the ideas we have about we expect—and do not expect—to "see" and our technical capacity to do so (Fleck, 1935 [1979]; Hanson, 1958; Daston & Gallison, 2007). In one sense, this means meaningful observation is, at some level, theory-laden: what we "see" depends in part on what our ideas are about what we expect to see and what assumptions underlie the methods used to "observe" the data. If our theoretical ideas do not include micro-organisms, we would not devise methods to see them—and if offered a microscope, we would not know what we are seeing, regardless of the magnification employed. Similarly, if we do not have the idea of birth cohort effects, we will not "see" their impact on a population's age-specific disease incidence rates. For example, whereas Johannes Clemmesen (b. 1908) in the late 1940s (Clemmesen, 1948) saw the slight dip in the period's breast cancer incidence rates after age 50 as evidence that the risk of the disease was lower in women just older than 50 compared to those just younger than 50 and those in their late 50s and older (**Figure 1–8a**), Brian MacMahon (1923–2007) in the late 1950s saw this same pattern as evidence of a change in risk among women who reached age 50 before rather than after the mid-twentieth century (**Figures 1–8b** to **1–8d**; MacMahon, 1957)—and others since have explored the impact of age–period–cohort effects on the observed yearly incidence of breast cancer (Krieger et al., 2003; Chia et al., 2005).

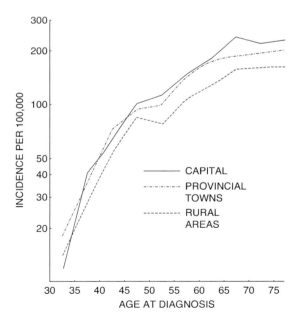

Figure 1–8. Data on breast cancer incidence: differing interpretations by Clemmesen and MacMahon (MacMahon, 1957)

Figure 1–8a. Clemmesen's age-specific breast cancer incidence data for Denmark (1943–1947)

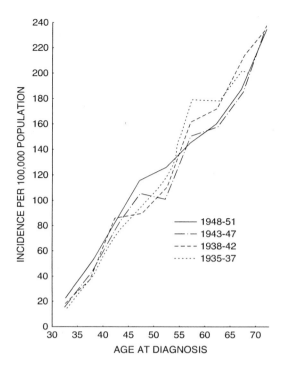

Figure 1–8b. MacMahon's analogous age-specific breast cancer incidence data for Connecticut (1935–1951)

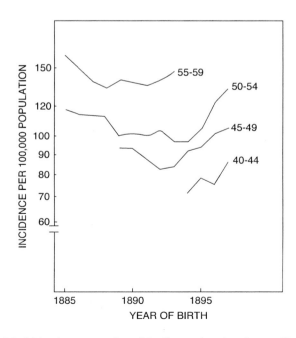

Figure 1–8c. MacMahon's re-expression of the Connecticut data for specific age groups, by birth cohort

25

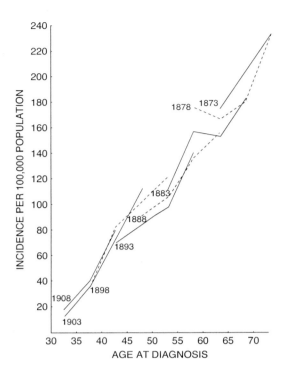

Figure 1–8d. MacMahon's re-expression of the Connecticut age-specific incidence data, by birth cohort

In another sense, meaningful observation is experience-laden: we need familiarity not only with the concepts at issue but also the experience of looking at the data themselves and working with the methods to do so. In other words, trained judgment (Daston & Gallison, 2007). Or, as Ludwig Fleck (1896–1961) wrote in the early twentieth century, even with the expectation that when we look through a microscope we will see cells and micro-organisms, we need to learn to prepare the sample with appropriate methods (e.g., stains) and likewise need to learn to "see," to decipher what is "signal" and what is "noise" (based on theory-laden ideas about what is being observed) (Fleck, 1929; Daston, 2008); the same holds for when we look at epidemiologic data. These statements do not mean that when we do science, we can "see" just anything we please. What counts as scientific evidence is not idiosyncratic; it is instead bound to the assumption of a shared biophysical world and the replicable, contestable, and debatable work of scientists, conducted in the public domain and collectively interpreted and argued.

Fourth, science is by definition fallible—in part because the testing of evidence and ideas, with or without new technologies, can result in the refinement and at times partial (and occasionally wholesale) replacement of explanatory theories, leading to new insights and new predictions as well as new interpretations (or dismissals) of prior observed associations (Fleck, 1935 [1979]; Cohen, 1985; Mendelsohn et al., 1997; Ziman, 2000; Sober, 2008). The recognition that science yields provisional and fallible knowledge, however, does not render all scientific knowledge equally tentative: some theories and their diverse predictions have withstood repeated tests; some hypotheses have been tested only a handful of times. For example, the scientific evidence that biological evolution occurs is rich and robust to the point where scientists concur its existence is a fact—even as lively scientific controversies exist over the causal processes at play (Mayr, 1982; Eldredge, 1999; Gould, 2002; Grene & Depew, 2004; Eldredge, 2005; Sober, 2008).

The testing and evaluation of scientific theories, however, as recognized by an enormous literature, is multifaceted and complex and involves debates over methods as well as substance (Fleck, 1935 [1979]; Lieberson, 1992; Mendelsohn et al., 1997; Ziman, 2000; Gadenne, 2002; Grene & Depew, 2004; Daston & Gallison, 2007; Archer et al., 1998; Sober, 2008). Rarely, if ever, does it simply follow the pristine hypothetico-deductive logic of particular observations refuting entire theories—a stance famously postulated by influential philosopher of science, Sir Karl Popper (1902–1994; Popper, 1959, 1985), and one that has been subjected to serious critique in contemporary philosophy of science (Hacking, 2001; Collins, 2001; Mjøset, 2002; Sober, 2008) (even as it has had its share of adherents in epidemiology [Rothman, 1986; Rothman, 1988; MacClure, 1995]) as well as some epidemiologic critics [Susser, 1986; Pearce & Crawford-Brown, 1989; Krieger, 1994; Greenland, 1998]). The theory of general relativity, for example, does not mean Newtonian mechanics are wrong, but rather that the latter is a subset of the former, applicable only at certain spatiotemporal scales (Hanson, 1958; Holton & Brush, 2001). Moreover, an important asymmetry exists between evaluating results from a particular study to (*1*) decide if they are compatible with a particular theory versus (*2*) determine how much they strengthen or weaken confidence in a theory (Lieberson, 1992). In part, this is because even if the study results are accurate and valid, it is highly implausible a given data set contains enough elements to test all competing hypotheses (especially under alternative sets of conditions). Thus, as noted by Lieberson, in the case of probabilistic theories, "a theory may be correct even if there is negative evidence" (Lieberson, 1992, p. 1)—and understanding why this can occur requires in-depth consideration of the conditions under which certain associations would or would not be expected.

More deeply, however, science is fallible because as historians and other analysts of science have extensively documented (Fleck, 1935 [1979]; Rose & Rose, 1980; Desrosières, 1988; Holton, 1988; Hubbard, 1990; Rosenberg & Golden, 1992; Keller, 1995; Massen et al., 1995; Mendelsohn et al., 1997; Lock & Gordon, 1988; Ziman, 2000; Keller, 2002; Harraway, 2004; Longino, 2006), scientists are part of the societies in which they are raised and work and, consequently, both think with—and sometimes challenge—the ideas and beliefs of their times. The eighteenth to nineteenth century scientific shift from a constrained biblical time-scale to expansive notions of "deep time" not only reflected fundamental changes in theories of geology, cosmology, physics, and biology but also constituted a profound rupture with dominant and deeply held religious views (Mayr, 1982; Gould, 1987; Holton, 1988; Eldredge, 2005). Closer to home for epidemiology are the powerful and painful connected examples of scientific racism and eugenics and their views of innately biologically inferior and superior "races"—which, far from being "crackpot" theories, were widely accepted and promoted by leading scientists in the nineteenth and the first half of the twentieth centuries (Chase, 1977; Harraway, 1989; Harding, 1993; Kevles, 1995; Gould, 1996; Banton, 1998; Harris & Ernst, 1999; Allen, 2001; Proctor, 2003; Lewontin et al., 1984; Jackson & Weidman, 2004; Stern, 2005a). Their lingering influence on how epidemiologists and others analyze racial/ethnic—and also socioeconomic—health inequities remains a topic of considerable concern (Krieger, 1987; Muntaner et al., 1996; Stern, 2005b; Krieger, 2005; Duster, 2006; Braun et al., 2007).

Fifth and finally, science is not the sole arbiter of knowledge, and scientific theories are not the only path to wisdom. It would be hubris to think otherwise (and not just because of myriad changes in what is "scientifically known"). Knowledge and insights generated and obtained from the arts, the humanities, healing practices, and religious and spiritual beliefs can be of profound importance—and, like scientific knowledge, can be profoundly destructive as well. Although these alternative approaches to different kinds of knowledge are not, by definition, premised on the scientific approach of the testing ideas by independent individuals using methods and data that in principle are public, they can—on other grounds—question whether particular scientific studies are immoral, unethical, or in violation of human rights and hence should not be done (Chase, 1977; Kevles, 1995; Proctor, 2003; Gould, 2003; Lavery et al., 2007). Beyond this, they can challenge underlying assumptions that scientific theories posit about "how the world is" or "works"—and, hence, potentially raise critical questions that can be addressed empirically. Challengers engaged in the repeated waves of effort to discredit scientific racism, for example, by and large came from outside the ranks of science, even as some of these critics worked with scientists to make the scientific case (Chase, 1977; Krieger, 1987; Harding, 1993; Kevles, 1995; Allen, 2001; Jackson, & Weidman, 2004). In this example and many others (Longino, 2006), the "non-science" criticisms of scientific theories and purported evidence were brought into the public domain of debate about publicly testable ideas. Recent contentious debates over scientific evidence (e.g., in the case of so-called "creationist science" or "abstinence-only" sex education) additionally underscore there is a world of difference in testing hypotheses about and debating the evidence and its implications—versus ignoring, distorting, or fudging the evidence or contriving invalid "tests" of ideas (Mooney, 2005; Schulman, 2006; Sober, 2008). Unsubstantiated opinion is insufficient to counter the empirical findings produced by science; valid counter-evidence matters.

A useful metaphor, employed by John Ziman (1925–2005; Ziman, 2000), accordingly posits scientific theory is a map: one can never map reality *per se*, but one can construct and test different representations of this reality. Defining aspects of any given scientific discipline thus include: the domain of phenomena it seeks to explain, the theories it uses to explain and predict the phenomena within the specified domain, and the methods employed to test competing and potentially refutable hypotheses suggested by these theories.

What Is Epidemiologic Theory?

Enough about science in general. What about the science of epidemiology? What would considerations about the nature of science and of scientific theories (as listed in **Textbox 1–2**) lead us expect to be key features of epidemiologic theory?

First and foremost: that epidemiologic theory would exist. (This would seem to be an obvious statement—yet, as I discuss below, it is, in fact, a contentious one.)

Second: that the content of epidemiologic theory, like that of any scientific theory, would be premised on the domain it seeks to explain. In the case of epidemiology, this domain concerns "population distributions of disease, disability, death, and health and their determinants and deterrents, across time and space" (Krieger, 2001b; *see* **Textbox 1–2**). A corollary is that if the types, rates, or distributions of diseases and causes of death change over time, it would follow that epidemiologic theories would need account for these changes in their explanations of the population patterning of health.

Third: that epidemiologic theory would necessarily employ domain-specific substantive concepts and explanatory concepts relevant to describing and analyzing extant and changing population distributions of health, disease, and well-being (*see* **Textbox 1–2**).

Textbox 1–2. General Features of Scientific Theories and as Applied to Epidemiologic Theories of Disease Distribution.

Scientific theory: constituent features

—All scientific theories

1. **Domain:** phenomena to be explained

2. **Objectives:** types of causal explanations sought

3. **Substantive concepts:** pertaining to the actual entities considered to be the phenomena of interest and their causes

4. **Explanatory concepts:** pertaining to the types of causal pathways posited to explain the phenomena of interest

5. **Metaphors and mechanisms:** employed to explain how things occur, with metaphor aiding comprehension of the "unknown" via the "known"

—Unique to scientific theories focused on context-dependent phenomena

6. **Historical contingency:** relevant to phenomena for whom the causal pathways (whether probabilistic or deterministic) depend on initial conditions and/or the temporal sequencing of non-deterministic events

—Unique to scientific theories focused on causal pathways that can be affected by human action

7. **Reflexivity:** explanation has the objective of transforming that which is being explained

Specific features of epidemiologic theories of disease distribution

EPIDEMIOLOGIC THEORIES OF DISEASE DISTRIBUTION

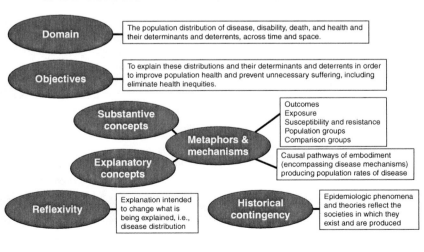

An additional expectation is that both types of concepts—substantive and explanatory—would be informed by metaphors, which in turn would influence the kinds of causal mechanisms proposed.

Fourth: that there would not be "one" epidemiologic theory but, rather, many—even as they all would share the common domain-specific focus of explaining the population occurrence of disease, disability, death and health. Given diverse and changing societal and technological contexts, it would be expected that different epidemiologic theories, employing different substantive and explanatory concepts, would exist, within and across different time periods and societies.

Fifth: that the process of developing, testing, refining, and at times replacing epidemiologic theories would involve data ("observations") that are theory-laden and whose use and interpretation is experience-laden. And it would likewise involve methods that are themselves theory-laden and whose use and interpretation is likewise experience-laden. That said, the conceptual ideas of epidemiologic theory—both substantive and explanatory (i.e., causal)—would be distinguishable from the methods (and their underlying theories) used to test epidemiologic theories and hypotheses.

Sixth: that epidemiologic theories would be influenced by—even as they might contest—the ideas and beliefs of the societies in which they are formulated. The implication is that epidemiologic theory would reflect not only the theorizing conducted within the field of epidemiology but also likely the responses to and engagement with epidemiologic theory by the diverse sectors of the populations and societies whose health is being described and analyzed.

One implication of these statements for the scope and mandate of epidemiologic theory is that they clarify that epidemiologic theories are, in essence, what I have termed *theories of disease distribution*—a shorthand phrase meant to be inclusive of the population occurrence of not only disease but also of disability, death, health, and well-being (Krieger, 2001c). They accordingly cannot be reduced to—even as they must incorporate—explanations of disease mechanisms (Krieger, 1994; Krieger, 2000; Krieger, 2001a; Krieger, 2001b). Consider, for example, the epidemiology of diseases related to tobacco use. It is unlikely that the mechanisms by which cigarette smoking causes lung cancer have notably changed between the early and late twentieth century (plus or minus alterations in cigarette additives) (Brandt, 2007, pp. 360, 393; Rabinoff et al., 2007); by contrast, the social patterning of cigarette smoking in the United States and many Western European countries changed dramatically, from initially being more common among professionals and affluent populations to becoming increasingly concentrated among working class and impoverished populations, a pattern emerging in other regions of the world as well (Barbeau et al., 2004; Graham, 2007; Davis et al., 2007). The implication is that explanations of the changing epidemiology of lung cancer and other smoking-related disease requires considering not only specific disease mechanisms but also factors leading to the changing and differential distribution of the exposure.

Consequently, explaining disease distribution is *not* the same as explaining disease mechanism. By the same token, theories of disease distribution are *not* the same as theories of disease causation. Nevertheless—and this is key—epidemiologic theories of disease distribution require appraising whether postulated disease mechanisms are compatible or not with observed spatiotemporal and social patterns of disease distribution. In other words, can the hypothesized mechanisms account for increases, declines, or stagnation of rates over time, space, and social group? If not, is this because still other mechanisms contribute to the observed disease distribution? Is it because the wrong time-scale was used to evaluate the exposure–outcome association? Or, alternatively, is the posited mechanism simply (or not so simply) wrong? The thinking enabling the triangulation of disease distribution data with hypothesized disease mechanisms is yet another reason why epidemiologic theories of disease distribution are essential (Davey Smith & Egger, 1996; Krieger, 2001a).

The mandate of epidemiology, however, imposes yet one more requirement for epidemiologic theory, one not necessarily shared by sciences unconcerned with human (or other living) populations. As articulated by Morris, writing a half-century ago in his now classic text, *Uses of Epidemiology* (Morris, 1957), the promise—and responsibility—of epidemiology was clear: to generate scientific knowledge about the "presence, nature, and distribution of health and disease among the population" (Morris, 1957, p. 96), ultimately to "*abolish the clinical picture*" (Morris, 1957, p. 98). Stated another way, the objective of epidemiology, as long-argued by many leading epidemiologists (Morris, 1957; Terris, 1979; Lilienfeld & Lilienfeld, 1982; Susser, 1989), and as underscored in the "Ethics Guidelines" issued by the American College of Epidemiology in 2000 (American College of Epidemiology, 2000), is to create knowledge relevant to improving population health and preventing unnecessary suffering, including eliminating health inequities (Krieger, 1994; Krieger, 2001a; Krieger, 2000; Krieger, 2007a; Krieger, 2007b).

Hence, an additional reflexive feature of epidemiologic theory is that it seeks to generate valid knowledge that people can use to change the distribution of disease, the very phenomenon that the theory seeks to understand (an intellectual challenge and tension also evident in many of the social sciences; Lieberson, 1992). Not that all epidemiologists would agree: in 1998, some prominent epidemiologists felt impelled to assert, in the face of rising epidemiologic discussions about investigating societal determinants of health, that although "moral purpose of epidemiology is to alleviate the human burden of disease," epidemiologists should nevertheless be free "to pursue knowledge for its own sake without fear of being badgered about the practical relevance of their work" (Rothman et al., 1998). Granted, the biological fact that we are mortal creatures, who are born and who die, means it is not in the scope of epidemiology—or any science—to eliminate the world of all morbidity and mortality. Yet, to the extent there is spatiotemporal and/or social variation in the age-specific patterns of any particular health outcome, it suggests modifiable causes are at play, whose mechanisms could presumably be altered by informed action.

In summary, key features of any epidemiologic theory, as one type of scientific theory and as summarized in **Textbox 1–2**, necessarily include *interrelated sets of ideas—including both substantive and explanatory concepts—for describing, explaining, and ultimately transforming population distributions of health, disease, and well-being*. It can likewise be expected that the ideas of epidemiologic theories, and the metaphors through which they are expressed and the mechanisms they propose, are influenced by the historical and societal context in which the epidemiologic theories are formulated, debated, and bolstered, modified, or rejected. A robust analysis of epidemiologic theory accordingly requires attention to each key aspect, in context, as the next few chapters will show.

And yet this listing of expected characteristics of epidemiologic theory, derived from analysis of critical aspects of science and scientific theories, rests on one very big "if." It is premised on the logic that *if* epidemiology is a science, then it must have a scientific theory, hence epidemiologic theory must exist. But this holds ONLY *if* epidemiology *is* a science. Conversely, if epidemiology is *not* a science, but is instead something else, then there need not be any epidemiologic theory. The standard hypothetico-deductive approach would accordingly posit that if evidence of epidemiologic theory cannot be found, then epidemiology is not a science. The next section considers whether this is a reasonable approach.

Epidemiologic Theory in Practice: "Lost-and-Found" or Something Else?

A logical place to look for discussion of epidemiologic theory—that is, theories of disease distribution—is in epidemiologic textbooks. This is because textbooks, a key sign of disciplinary institutionalization (Altbach et al., 1991; Apple & Christian-Smith, 1991; Keith & Ender, 2004; Topham, 2000; Morning, 2008), are designed by one generation of scholars to train the next in the fundamental issues of their field: the accumulated body of knowledge, the relevant theories, important controversies, and, in the case of science, the diverse methods used to generate evidence and test hypotheses (Krieger, 1994). Also shaping the content of textbooks is the context of their times, referring not only to the extant state of knowledge but also societal attitudes about what is being taught—especially regarding such controversial topics as the origins and evolution of life, sexuality, and the structure of human societies (Altbach et al., 1991; Apple & Christian-Smith, 1991; Keith & Ender, 2004; Mooney, 2005; Roughgarden, 2004; Morning, 2008). In the case of textbooks for health professionals, for example, recent content analyses have explored ways in which content has been affected by implicit and explicit assumptions about gender, race/ethnicity, sexuality, disability, and aging (Lawrence & Bendixen, 1992; Mendelsohn et al., 1994; Rabow et al., 2000; Byrne, 2001; Tompkins et al., 2006; Macgillivray & Jennings, 2008). A related but different question is how textbooks portray the theories of their fields.

In 1994, I conducted the first systematic evaluation of the coverage of epidemiologic theory in epidemiologic textbooks (Krieger, 1994). My search began with the first generation of books published as epidemiologic textbooks, which appeared in the late 1950s (all in the English language) and extended up to the early 1990s (with my search limited to books published in English, still the dominant scientific language for epidemiology). My strategy was to see how much text, if any, each textbook devoted to epidemiologic concepts pertaining to explaining disease distribution and also the history of ideas in the field. **Table 1–1** shows both the original results (**Table 1–1a**), to which I have now added my findings for additional textbooks, including those published through 2007 (**Table 1–1b**), and I supplement both sets of results by newly adding, in the last column, the definition of epidemiology offered by each text, if any. All textbooks appearing in **Tables 1–1a** and **1–1b** were published in English, with several of them translated into multiple languages and serving as foundational texts for epidemiology courses worldwide.

A curious pattern emerges. It would seem that from the late 1950s up to about 1980, epidemiologic textbooks, although not featuring overt discussion of epidemiologic theory as such, nevertheless typically did include sections on the history of epidemiologic thinking about disease in populations and the kinds of concepts needed to generate epidemiologic hypotheses. Exemplifying this approach was the stance Morris took in his 1957 text, *Uses of Epidemiology*, in which he wrote (Morris, 1957, p. 3):

> In this book I am concerned mainly with epidemiology as a way of learning, of asking questions, and getting answers that raise further questions: that is, as a *method*.

From 1980 until the mid-to-late 1990s, this type of discussion virtually disappeared, with the emphasis instead shifting to a different sort of epidemiologic methods: technical methods, understood in relation to study design, data analysis, and causal inference. Since the latter part of the 1990s, however, several of the newer epidemiologic textbooks have again begun to include text on ideas germane to epidemiologic theories of disease distribution. Nevertheless, considering the last half-century of influential and mainstream epidemiologic textbooks, it is striking to note that none of these texts has a section explicitly focused on epidemiologic theories of disease distribution.

One interpretation of the evidence presented in **Table 1–1** is that the lack of serious attention to epidemiologic theory means epidemiology is actually *not* a science and hence has no need of domain-specific explanatory theories. The most usual form that this argument takes is that epidemiology is about methods, meaning it offers a "toolkit" of methodological approaches for obtaining and analyzing data on disease in populations, with epidemiological concepts equated with concepts referring to epidemiologic methods (Rothman, 1988; Mawson, 2002; Morabia, 2004). In keeping with the Popperian tradition of treating the origins of scientific hypotheses and theories as outside of the bounds of scientific inquiry (Popper, 1959, 1985), this orientation holds that asking whence epidemiologic questions arise is not in epidemiology's domain. The focus is on applying methods, rather than on the source(s) of the questions being asked to which these methods are being applied. Less philosophically, another plausible reason that the origins of epidemiologic questions get little special attention is of the "it's obvious" variety: epidemiologic questions simply build off the extant evidence—including its contradictions, gaps, and need for replication.

An alternative interpretation might start with a "lost-and-found" approach, recognizing the typically less-than-linear development of scientific thought (Mayr, 1982; Ziman, 2000; Krieger, 2000; Keller, 2002; Gould, 2002). That is, when the field of epidemiology was first producing textbooks, those epidemiologists who wrote their groundbreaking texts had inklings of theories of disease distribution—if not in whole, then in part. Subsequent textbooks then somehow either took for granted or lost these theoretical bearings in the 1980s, only to start to find them again in the latter part of the 1990s.

Offering some evidence in support of this latter interpretation are two different bursts of articles in the epidemiologic literature. Thus, around the time that epidemiologic textbooks began shifting in the late 1970s and early 1980s to their more technical methodological orientation, several articles written by leading epidemiologists trained in an earlier generation began to raise alarm at the increasingly technical bent of the field, which they felt was losing sight of the public health import of the questions being asked (Terris, 1979; Stallones, 1980; Najman, 1980; Lilienfeld & Lilienfeld, 1982; Susser, 1985; Susser, 1989). Also during the late 1970s, a brief flurry of articles and letters debated definitions of epidemiology, including its status as a science (Lilienfeld, 1978; Frerichs & Neutra, 1978; Abramson, 1979; Evans, 1979). Subsequently, starting in the mid-1990s, a new round of epidemiologists, many trained by and reacting to their heavily methodological textbooks, began to publish articles calling for the development of explicit epidemiologic theory (Krieger, 1994; McMichael, 1995; Link & Phelan, 1995; Susser, 1996; Pearce, 1996; Davey Smith & Egger, 1996; Victora et al., 1997; Berkman & Kawachi, 2000; Ben-Shlomo & Kuh, 2002; Carpiano & Daley, 2006; Popay, 2006; Dunn, 2006; Vågerö, 2006), with their arguments reflected in the newer textbooks published in the early part of the twenty-first century (*see* **Table 1–1b**).

If correct, however, this alternative "lost-and-found" interpretation raises more questions than it answers. First, how can a science misplace its domain-specific theories? Second, given that epidemiologists were nevertheless busily—and fruitfully—conducting studies to describe population patterns of disease and to generate evidence to test etiologic hypotheses about these patterns throughout this entire period, from whence did their hypotheses come? And on what sorts of ideas and theories were epidemiologists drawing before 1950?

To answer these questions, and those I posed at the outset about the ideas animating and spurred by **Figures 1** to **7**, a more nuanced approach to epidemiologic theory is warranted. In the following chapters, I will accordingly examine the diverse array of ideas that people have elaborated, in different places and different times, to explain the population patterning of health—including during the latter half of the twentieth century, when epidemiology seemingly was "atheoretical." And the three-pronged argument I will make is that:

1. theories of disease distribution are vital to the conduct of epidemiology;
2. these theories all too often inform epidemiologic research implicitly, rather than explicitly; and
3. analysis of epidemiologic theories of disease distribution can improve the intellectual rigor of the field.

In other words, theory is a practical necessity, not an obscure luxury.

Table 1–1. Analysis of English-Language Epidemiologic Textbooks for Content on Epidemiologic Theory: 1922 to 2007

Table 1–1a. Initial Survey of U.S. Epidemiologic Textbooks and Anthologies Published Since 1960: Content on Epidemiologic History and Theory*, and Diagram of "Web of Causation" (Krieger, 1994)

Text	Total Pages	Percent of pages			New addition: definition of epidemiology
		History	Theory	Diagram of web	
MacMahon B, Pugh TF, Ipsen J. *Epidemiologic Methods.* Boston: Little, Brown, & Co. 1960.**	302	0	11.6	+	p. 3: "Epidemiology is the study of the distribution and determinants of disease prevalence in man."
Fox JP, Hall CE, Elveback. *Epidemiology: Man and Disease.* New York: Macmillan, 1970.	339	3.5	44.8	—	p. 1: "Epidemiologic curiosity centers about the causation of disease in human populations."
Susser M. *Causal Thinking in the Health Sciences: Concepts and Strategies of Epidemiology.* New York: Oxford University Press, 1973.	181	12.2	8.3	—	p. 1: "In a current definition, epidemiology is the study of distribution and determinants of states of health in human populations. This definition has room for most present-day activities of epidemiologists. Some prefer to add that these activities are for the purpose of prevention, surveillance, and control of health disorders in populations. This addition emphasizes a determinant of health that weighs heavily in public health and medicine, namely, such conscious intervention in health matters as societies elect to undertake."

Text	Total Pages	Percent of pages			New addition: definition of epidemiology
		History	Theory	Diagram of web	
Mausner JS, Bahn AK. Epidemiology: An Introductory Text. Phelapdelphia: Saunders, 1974.	377	0.0	4.0	+	p. 3: "Epidemiology may be defined **as the study of the distribution and determinant of diseases and injuries in human populations.**" (bold in original)
Friedman G. *Primer of Epidemiology*. New York: McGraw-Hill, 1974.	230	0.0	0.9	+	p. 1: "Epidemiology is the study of disease occurrence in human populations."
White KL, Henderson M (eds). *Epidemiology as a Fundamental Science: Its Uses In Health Services Planning, Administration, and Evaluation*. New York: Oxford University Press, 1976.	235	0.9	0.9	—	p. 19: "However defined, epidemiology implies methods and strategies used to identify and study that which determines the level and distribution of health and disease in the community."
Lilienfeld A, Lilienfeld D. *Foundations of Epidemiology*. New York: Oxford University Press, 1980.	375	6.1	5.1	—	p. 3: "Epidemiology is concerned with the patterns of disease occurrence in human populations and of the factors that influence these patterns."
Kleinbaum DG, Kupper LL, Morgenstern H (eds). *Epidemiologic Research: Principles and Quantitative Methods*. Belmont, CA: Lifetime Learning Publications, 1982.	529	0.0	1.1	—	p. 2: "As exemplified by John Snow's famous work on cholera, epidemiology was initially concerned with providing a methodological basis for the study and control of population epidemics. Currently, however, *epidemiology* (italics in the original) has a much broader scope—namely, the study of health and illness in human populations."
Schlesselman J. *Case–Control Studies: Design, Conduct, Analysis*. New York: Oxford University Press, 1982.	354	0.6	0.0	—	None provided.
Kahn HA. *An Introduction to Epidemiologic Methods*. New York: Oxford University Press, 1983.	166	0.0	0.0	—	None provided.
Miettinen OS. *Theoretical Epidemiology: Principles of Occurrence Research in Medicine*. New York: Wiley, 1985.	359	0.0	1.4	—	p. vii: "This text treats theoretical epidemiology as *the discipline of how to study the occurrence of phenomena of interest in the health field.*" (italics in the original)

Text	Total Pages	Percent of pages			New addition: definition of epidemiology
		History	Theory	Diagram of web	
Feinstein AR. *Clinical Epidemiology: The architecture of Clinical Research*. Philadelphia: W B Saunders Co., 1985.	812	1.1	1.2	—	p. 1: "Clinical epidemology is concerned with studying groups of people to achieve the background evidence needed for clinical decisions in patient care."
Weiss N. *Clinical Epidemiology: The Study of the Outcome of Illnesses*. New York: Oxford University Press, 1986.	144	0.0	0.0	—	pp. 3–4: "Epidemiology per se is the study of variation in the occurrence of disease, and the reasons for that variation . . . Clinical epidemiology is defined here in a parallel way: It is the study of variation in the *outcome* (italics in the original) of illness and of reasons for that variation."
Rothman K. *Modern Epidemiology*. Boston: Little, Brown, 1986.	358	1.7	0.0	—	p. 23: "The clearest of many definitions of epidemiology that has been proposed has been attributed to Gaylord Anderson. His definition is: 'Epidemiology: the study of the occurrence of illness.' Other sciences are also directed toward the study of illness, but in epidemiology the focus is on the *occurrence* (italics in the original) of illness."
Kelsey J, Thompson WD, Evans AS. *Methods in Observational Epidemiology*. New York: Oxford University Press, 1986.	366	0.0	7.4	—	p. 3: "Epidemiology, the study of the occurrence and distribution of disease and other health-related conditions in populations, is used for many purposes."
Hennekens CH, Buring JE. *Epidemiology in Medicine*. Boston: Little, Brown, 1987.	383	2.6	3.9	—	p. 3: " . . . a useful and comprehensive definition of epidemiology : 'the study of the distribution and determinants of disease frequency' in human populations."
Abramson JH. *Making Sense of Data: A Self-Instruction Manual on the Interpretation of Epidemiologic Data*. New York: Oxford University Press, 1988.	326	0.0	0.6	—	None provided.

Text	Total Pages	Percent of pages			New addition: definition of epidemiology
		History	Theory	Diagram of web	
Anthologies					
Winklestein W Jr, French FE, Lane JM (eds.). *Basic Readings in Epidemiology*. New York: MSS Educational Pub. Co., 1970.	193	13.9	27.8	—	"Epidemiology may be defined as the study of disease distributions and the factors that influence them. Epidemiology shares with other disciplines an interest in the natural history of disease and the utilization of the scientific method. Its distinctiveness is more related to the design and execution of studies than to content and conclusions."
Greenland S (ed). *Evolution of Epidemiologic Ideas: Annotated Readings on Concepts and Methods*. Chestnut Hill, MA: Epidemiology Resources, Inc., 1987.	190	7.9	0.0	—	None provided.
Buck C, Llopis A, Najera E, Terris M (eds). *The Challenge of Epidemiology: Issues and Selected Readings*. Washington, DC: Pan American Health Organization, 1988.	989	14.8	24.9	—	p. x: "Besides its importance and usefulness in disease surveillance and prevention, epidemiology has an even more critical function to carry out—the gathering of knowledge for understanding the health-disease process. It can anticipate needs, identify risk conditions, and orient the definition of priorities and the use of available resources for planning and administering health systems. In short, by analyzing and evaluating health problems and health services, and their contexts, epidemiology can go beyond considering just specific health problems: it can help bring us closer to considering society as the source for explaining health problems and their solutions."
Rothman K (ed). *Causal Inference*. Chestnut Hill, MA: Epidemiology Resources, Inc., 1988.	207	0.0	0.0	—	None provided.

Table 1–1b. Additional Selected Introductory and Advanced Textbooks Not Included in the Original Review (1922–2007)

Text	Total Pages	Percent of pages			New addition: definition of epidemiology
		History	Theory	Diagram of web	
Vaughan VC. *Epidemiology and Public Health: A Text and Reference Book for Physicians, Medical Students and Health Workers. Vol. 1: Respiratory Infections.* St Louis, MO: CV Mosby, 1922.	683	34.0	7.8	—	p. 23: "We may be asked for a definition of epidemiology. It is the science of epidemic diseases, and these may appear in any given community at any given time singly or by the hundreds."
Greenwood M. *Epidemics and Crowd-Diseases: An Introduction to the Study of Epidemiology.* New York: Macmillan, 1937.	378	32.5	5.0	—	p. 10: "Epidemiology came to mean the study of disease, any disease, as a mass phenomenon . . . the epidemiologist's unit is not a single human being but an aggregation of human beings, and since it is impossible to hold in mind distinctly a separate mass of the particulars he (*sic*) forms a general picture, on average of what is happening, and what works upon that."
Taylor I, Knowelden J. *Principles of Epidemiology.* Boston: Little Brown & Co., 1957.	292	1.4	7.9	—	p. 1: "One of the most fundamental tasks of the epidemiologist is to describe the pattern of disease in communities, whether national or some smaller groups . . . (in relation to 'which diseases,' 'what *persons* are most affected., '*when* the disease occurs,' and '*where* the disease is found') . . . Armed with answers to these questions, which together describe the pattern of disease in a community, the epidemiologist may postulate theories of the mode of spread of the disease he (*sic*) finds, and these theories may be put to the test by clinical, field, or laboratory studies . . . Finally, having made his (*sic*) epidemiological diagnosis, he (*sic*) may be able to put forward logical ideas for the control of those diseases he (*sic*) describes" (italics in the original).

Text	Total Pages	Percent of pages			New addition: definition of epidemiology
		History	Theory	Diagram of web	
Morris JN. *Uses of Epidemiology.* Edinburgh: Churchill Livingston, 1957.	131	6.9	15.3	—	p. 5: "Epidemiology may be further defined as *the study of health and disease of population and groups in relation to their environment and ways of living*" (italics in the original).
Kark SL. *Epidemiology and Community Medicine.* New York: Appleton-Century Crofts, 1974.	463	2.6	14.3	—	p. 1: "The function of epidemiology is to study health in population groups."
Barker DJP, Rose G. *Epidemiology and Medical Practice.* 2nd ed. Edinburgh: Churchill Livingston, 1979.	148	0.0	4.7	—	p. v: "Epidemiology, the study of the distribution and determinants of disease in human populations, has always been an integral part of medical practice."
Ahlbom A, Norell S. *Introduction to Modern Epidemiology.* Chestnut Hill, MA: Epidemiology Resources, 1990.	100	0.0	2.0	+	p. 1: "Epidemiology is the science of occurrence of diseases in human populations."
Walker AM. *Observation and Inference: An Introduction to the Methods of Epidemiology.* Chestnut Hill, MA: Epidemiology Resources, 1991.	165	0.0	0.0	—	None provided.
Beaglehole R, Bonita R, Kjellstrom T. *Basic Epidemiology.* Geneva: World Health Organization, 1993.	153	1.3	4.6	—	p. 3: "Epidemiology has been defined as 'the study of the distribution of health-related states or event in specified populations, and the application of this study to the control of health problems'" (citing definition from Last J (ed). *A Dictionary of Epidemiology.* 2nd ed. New York: Oxford, 1988).
Friis RH, Sellers TA. *Epidemiology for Public Health Practice.* Gaithersburg, MD: Aspen Publishers, 1996.	406	2.5	4.2	—	p. 4: "Epidemiology is concerned with the distribution and determinants of health and disease, morbidity, injuries, disabilities, and mortality in populations."

Text	Total Pages	Percent of pages			New addition: definition of epidemiology
		History	Theory	Diagram of web	
Young TK. *Population Health: Concepts and Methods*. New York: Oxford University Press, 1998.	306	3.6	4.7	—	p. 7: "*The Dictionary of Epidemiology* defines epidemiology as 'The study of the distribution and determinants of health-related states or events in specified populations, and the application of this study to control health problems.'
Brownson RC, Petitti DB (eds). *Applied Epidemiology: Theory to Practice*. New York: Oxford University Press, 1998.	387	1.0	1.3	—	p. ix: "In our view, applied epidemiology synthesizes and applies the results of etiologic studies to set priorities for interventions; it evaluates public health interventions and policies; it measures the quality and outcome of medical care; and it effectively communicates epidemiologic findings to health professionals and the public."
Berkman LF, Kawachi I (eds). *Social Epidemiology*. New York: Oxford University Press, 2000.	382	6.0	16.2	—	p. 3: "Epidemiology is the study of the distribution and determinants of states of health in populations."
Rothman K. *Epidemiology: An Introduction*. New York: Oxford University Press, 2002.	217	0.9	1.8	—	p. 1: "Often considered the core science of public health, epidemiology involves 'the study of the distribution and determinants of disease frequency,' or, put even more simply, 'the study of the occurrence of illness.'"
Bhopal RS. *Concepts of Epidemiology: An Integrated Introduction to the Ideas, Theories, Principles, and Methods of Epidemiology*. Oxford: Oxford University Press, 2002.	296	1.0	16.6	+	p. xxii: " . . . in short it (epidemiology) is the science and craft that studies the patterns of disease (and health, though usually indirectly) in populations to help understand both their causes and the burden they impose. This information is applied to prevent, control or manage the problems under study."
Aschengrau, A, Seage GR. *Essentials of Epidemiology in Public Health*. Sudbury, MA: Jones and Bartlett, 2003.	447	5.1	3.1	+	p. 6: "*The study of the distribution and determinants of disease frequency in human populations and the application of this study to control health problems.*" (italics in the original)

Text	Total Pages	Percent of pages			New addition: definition of epidemiology
		History	Theory	Diagram of web	
Gordis L. *Epidemiology*, 3rd ed. Philadelphia, PA: WB Saunders, 2004.	323	1.2	1.5	—	p. 3: "Epidemiology is the study of how disease is distributed in populations and the factors that influence or determine this distribution."
Webb P. *Essential Epidemiology: An Introduction for Students and Health Professionals.* New York: Cambridge University Press, 2005.	323	2.5	1.8	—	pp. 1–2: "Epidemiology . . . is about measuring health, identifying the causes of ill-health, and intervening to improve health . . . Perhaps epidemiology's most fundamental role is to provide a logic and structure for the analyses of health problems both great and small."
Fletcher RH, Fletcher SW. *Clinical Epidemiology: The Essentials.* 4th ed. Baltimore, MD: Lippincott Williams & Wilkins, 2005.	243	0.0	1.1	—	p. 3: "**Epidemiology** is the 'study of disease occurrence in human populations.'" (bold in the original)
Oakes JM, Kaufman JS (eds). *Methods in Social Epidemiology.* San Francisco, CA: Jossey-Bass, 2006.	460	5.0	20.4	—	p. 3: "Epidemiology is the study of the distribution and determinants of states of health in populations."
Yarnell J (ed). *Epidemiology and Prevention: A Systems-Based Approach.* Oxford: Oxford University Press, 2007.	275	1.1	2.5	—	p. 5: "At the beginning of the twenty-first century, **epidemiology is a broad-based population science**, drawing on many disciplines from biology and sociology to biostatistics and philosophy of science, which investigates **the causes of human disease** and **methods for their control**." (bold in the original)
Szklo M, Nieto FJ. *Epidemiology: Beyond the Basics.* 2nd ed. Sudbury, MA: Jones and Bartlett, 2007.	482	0.6	0.6	—	p. 3: "*Epidemiology* is traditionally defined as the study of the distribution and determinants of health-related states or events in specified populations and the application of this study to the control of health problems." (italics in the original)

* Epidemiologic theory: defined as explicit discussion of theories of disease causation and/or epidemiologic concepts (e.g., "time, place, person") (NB: This footnote is per the 1994 text; I would now instead refer to "theories of disease distribution" [rather than "theories of disease causation"], and I would further clarify that the text pertaining to epidemiologic theory is that which provides guidance on theories and concepts required to generate epidemiologic hypotheses, to develop substantive explanations for patterns of disease distribution [as distinct from the methods to test the ideas]).

** In the original 1994 table, I cited the 1970 version of MacMahon et al.; I have changed it to the 1960 version in this table.

2

Health in the Balance

Early Theories About Patterns of Disease Occurrence

Curiosity about the causes and occurrence of disease is not unique to epidemiologists. After all, who wouldn't be interested in knowing about how to live a healthy life—or how to predict and ward off sickness, injury, and death? As the myriad histories of medicine and public health attest and the work of innumerable archeologists and anthropologists reveals (Ackerknecht, 1946; Sigerist, 1951; Rosen, 1958 [1993]; Hughes, 1963; Feierman & Janzen, 1992; Bannerman et al., 1983; Porter, 1997; Porter, 1999; Baer et al., 1997; Green, 1999; Bynum, 2008), from the earliest documented eras to the present, people have experienced the joys and tribulations of living in our bodies—alive with senses, thoughts, and emotions, daily engaged with the people and world around us, interacting, eating, working, sleeping, having sex, sometimes procreating, sometimes fighting, vulnerable to physical and mental ailments and injuries, and ultimately confronting mortality.

But as the historical record also makes clear, we do more than simply experience or witness health, disease, injury, and death—we also try to make sense of them: for ourselves, personally, and in relation to the ills we see around us. Two recurrent themes stand out. The first is that whether we hold that existence is senseless or pre-ordained (or something in between), people *do* try to explain disease occurrence: both individual cases and population patterns. The second is that no matter how varied the causal accounts, whether within a particular society or across times and cultures, the etiologic explanations that people offer, and their inclination and ability to put these ideas to the test, are deeply enmeshed—however clearly or muddled—with extant views about the nature of the world, how it works, and our place in it.

Seeing causal ideas in context is not easy to do, especially when steeped in the mix of one's own times. Stepping back to gain perspective—and even perhaps to learn something new—is a useful way to start. Hence: welcome to selected examples of ancient and current theories of disease distribution included in ancient texts and oral traditions.

Health in the Balance: Bodies, Society, and Nature in Ancient Texts and Current Oral Traditions

Humors, Democracy, Slavery, and Health: Theories of Disease Distribution in Ancient Greece

Epidemiology. The word itself hearkens—deliberately—back to ancient Greece. After all, as recounted in any introductory epidemiology course, the etymology of "*epidemic*" is: *epi* ("upon") + *demos* ("the people") (Oxford English Dictionary [OED], 2008). The word "epidemic" was used, as such, in ancient Greece in fifth century BCE (Lloyd, 1983a, pp. 87–138), including in the Hippocratic corpus, the classic texts of Greek medicine and public health (Lloyd 1983a; Nutton, 2004; Jouanna, 1999). It denoted episodes of mass disease and, by extension, disease occurrence among populations. However, the *demos* in ancient Greece were not just any group of people (Beckfield & Krieger, 2009). Instead, the term was inherently political and referred to the "people or commons of an ancient Greek state, esp. of a democratic state, such as Athens" (OED, 2008). Not that Athenian democracy (*demos* ["people"] + *-cracy* ("politically who rules") (OED, 2008) was particularly democratic by contemporary standards, as only free male citizens (less than 10% of the population) could vote; free women, metics, and slaves were not enfranchised (Pomeroy, 1975; Austin & Vidal-Naquet, 1977; Murray, 1978 [1993]; Powell, 1988; Sealey, 1990; King, 1998; Lloyd & Sivin, 2002, pp. 82–95). Tellingly, these latter two groups—accounting for upward of 75% of the population—were described in the Hippocratic treatise *On Diet* as "the mass of people who are obliged to work," "who drink and eat what they happen to get," and so "who cannot, neglecting all, take care of their health" (Sigerist, 1961, p. 240; *see also*: Wilkins, 2005, p. 127). As the Hippocratic texts repeatedly emphasized, the pursuit of health required leisure, property, and freedom (Sigerist, 1961; Lloyd, 1983a; Jouanna, 1999; Nutton, 2004; Wilkins, 2005). In other words: awareness that social position affects health is ancient; whether this association was deemed unjust or amenable to change is another question entirely (Beckfield & Krieger, 2009).

Pivotal to the Hippocratic analyses of health—in individuals and in populations—was the notion of *balance*. This *balance*, as revealed by a person's bodily and mental state of health, itself reflected the interplay of factors in and outside the body. If a person was healthy, all was in balance; if ill, then an imbalance existed. As to the source of the imbalance—here, the population patterning of health provided a critical clue. For example, as argued in the Hippocratic text, "The Nature of Man"(*sic*) (Lloyd, 1983a, pp. 260–271; quote: p. 266):

> Some diseases are produced by the manner of life that is followed; others by the life-giving air we breathe. That there are these two types may be demonstrated in the following way. When a large number of people all catch the same disease at the same time, the cause must be ascribed to something common to all and which they all use; in other words to what they all breathe. In such a disease, it is obvious that the individual bodily habits cannot be responsible because the malady attacks one after another, young and old, men and women alike, those who drink their wine neat and those who drink only water; those who eat barley-cake as well as those who live on bread, those who take a lot of exercise and those who take but little. The regime cannot therefore be responsible where people who live very different lives catch the same disease.
>
> However, when many different diseases appear at the same time, it is plain that the regimen is responsible in individual cases.

As argued by this excerpt, some mass exposure must be the cause of any imbalance leading to mass diseases that strike everyone at the same time, regardless of their bodily types, habits, age, or gender—with the most likely culprit being the air that everyone breathed (water, by contrast, was not necessarily a shared resource, given reliance on individual wells [Austin & Vidal-Naquet, 1977; Murray, 1978 (1993)]). Alternatively, explanations for diverse manifestations of ill health among individuals in a given place at a given point in time resided in differences in individuals' constitutions and how they lived their lives, under the assumption that they were all presumed to be equally exposed to their ostensibly shared environs.

What, then, were the factors inside and outside the body that made for being healthy or in ill health? Reflecting the diverse authorship of the Hippocratic corpus—a collection of about 60 medical treatises influenced by (and some perhaps written by) the famous physician Hippocrates of Cos (born c. 460 BCE) and the naturalistic school of medicine associated with him (Sigerist, 1961; Lloyd, 1983a, pp. 6–90; Nutton, 1992; Jouanna, 1999; Nutton, 2004; King, 2005; van der Eijk, 2005)—there is no single answer. Nevertheless, four sets of factors appear repeatedly in the different treatises [Sigerist, 1961; Lloyd, 1983a; Longrigg, 1993; Edelstein, 1967a; Jouanna, 1999; Nutton, 2004; van de Eijk, 2005]:

1. *innate constitution*, affecting how people respond to factors both within and outside their body;
2. *bodily humors*, variously including blood, phlegm, yellow bile, and black bile, viewed as actual substances that could be seen—for example, when people bled, coughed, sneezed, vomited, urinated, and defecated;
3. *the regimen people follow*—that is, their practices regarding eating, exercising, resting, sleeping, and having sex, all of which were held to affect how people replenished (or "concocted") their humors; and
4. *the physical environs*, especially the air, water, weather, temperature, altitude, soil, and vegetation.

The interactions between this foursome of factors were, in turn, deeply linked to three other sets of four widely discussed and debated in the Greek science and philosophy of the time: the four elements (fire, air, water, earth), the four qualities (hot, moist, cold, dry), and, reflecting their mix, the four seasons (summer, spring, winter, autumn) (Sigerist, 1961; Edelstein, 1967b; Lloyd, 1983a; Lloyd, 1979; Lloyd, 1987; Nutton, 1992; Longrigg, 1993; Nutton, 2004; King, 2005; van de Eijk, 2005). Although there existed competing theories (Jouanna, 1999; Nutton, 2004; van der Eijk, 2005), varying in the number and types of constituent components at play in people's health and disease, all of the naturalistic theories nevertheless relied on notions of balance, with the human body part of and subject to impersonal cosmic forces (as opposed to the vagaries of divine intervention). As shown in **Figure 2–1**, which represents the schematic that has endured, in part because of its embrace by Galen, the influential and prolific Roman physician whose writings dominated medical discourse for millennia (Sigerist, 1961; Edelstein, 1967b; Lloyd, 1983a; Lloyd, 1979; Lloyd, 1987; Nutton, 1992; Longrigg, 1993; Nutton, 2004; King, 2005), the correspondences—and imbalances—between the quartet of the humors, elements, qualities, and seasons set the basis for observed individual and population manifestations of health and disease.

Thus, as argued by "The Nature of Man" (Lloyd, 1983a, pp. 260–271), health is what people experience when the humors "are in the correct proportion to each other, both in strength and quantity, and are well-mixed" (Lloyd, 1983a, p. 262), whereas pain and

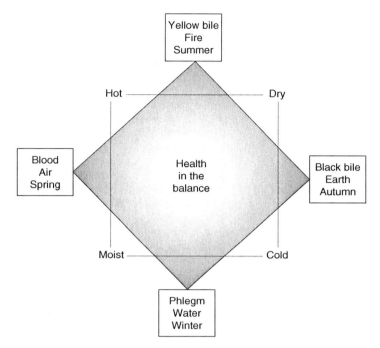

Figure 2–1. Greek humoral theory of disease causation: schematic of dominant view of relationships between the four elements, humors, qualities, and seasons. (Adapted from Sigerist, 1961, p. 323).

disease result "when one of these substances presents either a deficiency or an excess, or is separated in the body and not mixed with the others" (Lloyd, 1983a, p. 262). Taking this logic one step further, the text further averred that the four major types of fever—the "continued, quotidian, tertian, and quartan" (Lloyd, 1983a, p. 270), each distinguished by its duration, periodicity ("critical days"), and intensity—resulted from differing degrees of excess bile. "Airs, Waters, and Places" (Lloyd 1983a, pp. 148–169) likewise attributed the appearance of diverse diseases within a locale to combinations of weather, seasons, humors, constitution, and age (Lloyd, 1983a, p. 158):

> If the summer is rainy with southerly winds and the autumn similar, the winter will necessarily be unhealthy. Those of phlegmatic constitution and those over forty years may suffer from *causus* [a febrile malady], while those who are full of bile suffer from pleurisy and pneumonia ... If the autumn is rainless with northerly winds ... this weather suits best those who are naturally phleg-matic and of a watery constitution and also women. But it is most inimical to those of a bilious disposition because they become dried up too much. This produces dry ophthalmia and sharp fevers which last a long time and also, in some cases, 'black bile' or melancholy. The reason for this is found in the drying up of the more fluid part of the bile while the denser and more bitter part is left behind. The same is true of the blood. But these changes are beneficial to those of phlegmatic habit so that they become dried up and start the winter braced up instead of relaxed.

From this standpoint, disease was not a separate entity that could be understood apart from the body in which it occurred. Instead, it was an embodied expression of imbalance—of the humors, in context.

It is important to situate the science of the Hippocratic corpus. First, it was written at a time when technology was at the human scale: there existed no instruments to see inside the body or to measure minute quantities of substances (Jouanna, 1999; Nutton, 2004). As stated in the Hippocratic text, "Tradition in Medicine" (Lloyd, 1983a, pp. 70–86; quote: p. 75): "One aims at some criterion as to what constitutes a correct diet, but you will find neither number nor weight to determine what this exactly, and no other criterion than bodily feeling." The balance discussed was thus balance inferred, not balance measured: insight into the inner world of bodily processes was metaphorically transported from the observed patterns and phenomena of the outer world and its seasons, cycles, qualities, and elements. Although the treatises made appeals to the evidence to support their etiologic arguments, actual measurement to provide data germane to the theory was limited at best (Lloyd, 1979; Lloyd, 1983a; Lloyd, 1987).

A reliance on abstract reasoning, despite scant empirical evidence, however, was an acceptable practice among the literate Greek citizens (a tiny fraction of the population) who enjoyed debating topics in their academies and who considered manual work (including the work of touching patients) to be beneath them (Edelstein, 1967c; Lloyd, 1983a; Lloyd, 1990; Nutton, 1992; Jouanna, 1999; Lloyd & Sivin, 2002; Nutton, 2004). In the words of GER Lloyd, an eminent historian of ancient Greek science and medicine, "[a]nyone who earned money by practicing a skill was liable to be treated as a social inferior by men whose leisure was guaranteed by inherited, usually landed, wealth" (Lloyd, 1983a, p. 18). Thus, in contrast to the acutely observed case reports appearing in such Hippocratic treatises as "Epidemics, Book I" and "Epidemics, Book II" (Lloyd, 1983a, pp. 87–138), which likely were written by practicing physicians (most of whom had the rank of metic, not free citizen [Jouanna, 1999; Nutton, 2004]), the primarily philosophical and speculative Hippocratic treatises typically were more concerned with the logical validity of their argument than with the truth of its premises (Edelstein, 1967b; Lloyd, 1990; Longrigg, 1993; Lloyd & Sivin, 2002; Nutton, 2004). Not that these texts were prepared to argue just anything, for as noted by Mirko Grmek, in his book *Diseases in the Ancient Greek World* (Grmek, 1983 [1989], pp. 1–2):

> ... The theory of humors is at once the logical consequence of Ionian philosophy and a faithful reflection of the pathological and clinical features of the ills actually suffered by Mediterranean populations. If the Hippocratic doctrine of critical days can reasonably be interpreted as the result of a desire to introduce number into the explanation of nature, it is no less true that such a notion was well supported in a region where the majority of patients suffer from malaria or pneumonia ... A medical practitioner in Scandinavia would never have devised a theory of acute fevers comparable to the Hippocratic one.

In other words, people not surprisingly develop theory to explain the phenomena at hand—as well as those they may predict or imagine.

From this perspective, Greek humoral theory (in its different variants) can be seen as an elegant and ambitious attempt to explain individual episodes of illness and the variations in health status observed in populations in relation to underlying principles and environmental exposures, powerfully linking the events of the microcosm and macrocosm (Sigerist, 1961; Edelstein, 1967b; Lloyd, 1983a, pp. 9–60; Nutton, 1992; Longrigg, 1993; Jouanna, 1999; Nutton, 2004; van den Eijk, 2005). Hewing to naturalistic explanations at a time when the majority of the Greek population routinely supplicated major and minor gods alike to ward off and heal illness (Edelstein, 1967d; Lloyd, 1983a, pp. 9–60; Lloyd, 1979; Nutton, 1992; Jouanna, 1999; Nutton, 2004; King, 2005), it should be no surprise that the Hippocratic corpus—and especially the treatise "Airs, Waters, Places"—is conventionally touted as the foundation of epidemiologic thinking and public health more generally (Greenwood, 1932; Buck et al., 1988; Schneider et al., 2008; Susser & Stein, 2009) (*see* **Textbox 2–1**, however, on the nevertheless circuitous history of Hippocratic thought in Western science, traveling from ancient Greece to imperial Rome to Arabic countries and thence, via Islamic medicine, re-introduced to European thought as part of the European Renaissance) (Gremk, 1998; Porter, 1997; Saliba, 2007; Poormann & Savage-Smith, 2007; Bynum, 2008).

Yet to leave the discussion at the level of nature and philosophy would be to omit still another important influence on Greek humoral theory: Greek politics. During the latter part of the fifth century BCE, when the Hippocratic texts first began to be formulated (Sigerist, 1961; Lloyd, 1983a, pp. 9–60; Jouanna, 1999; Nutton, 2004; van der Eijk, 2005), the intellectual and cultural center of Greece was Athens, a prosperous coastal city-state (Sigerist, 1961; Webster, 1973; Austin & Vidal-Naquet, 1977; Murray, 1978 [1993]; Powell, 1988; Lloyd & Sivin, 2002). Overturning prior traditions of monarchy, and in contrast to the more militarized city-state of Sparta, one distinctive feature of Athenian political life was the participatory nature of the Athenian assembly, in which the male citizens of Athens debated and enacted laws and policies; another was that this democratic form of governance existed side-by-side with extensive reliance on slave labor (Webster, 1973; Pomeroy, 1975; Austin & Vidal-Naquet, 1977; Murray, 1978 [1993]; Powell, 1988; Sealey, 1990; Lloyd & Sivin, 2002). Commenting on this apparent paradox, two historians of ancient Greece, M.M. Austin and P. Vidal-Naquet, have observed "the Greek point of view was different: the freedom of some could not be imagined without the servitude of others, and the two extremes were not thought of as contradictory, but as complementary and interdependent" (Austin & Vidal-Naquet, 1977, p. 19).

The influence of the particular version of democracy espoused in ancient Greece on theories of distribution was twofold: on what was considered—and what was ignored. Not only nature but politics informed the conceptualization of "balance" in Greek humoral theory (Murray, 1978 [1993], p. 279; Lloyd, 1979, pp. 240–248; Lloyd, 1983a, pp. 9–60; Powell, 1988, p. 83; Longrigg, 1993, p. 52; Jouanna, 1999, p. 347; Nutton, 2004, pp. 47–48; King in King, 2005, pp. 151–152); in the fifth century BCE, the influential Greek physician-philosopher Alcmaeon openly stated (Sigerist, 1961, p. 103):

> Health is maintained by the [*isonomia*], the equality of rights, of the qualities wet, dry, cold, hot, bitter, sweet, and the rest; but the [*monarchia*], the single rule among them, causes disease, for the single rule of either pair of opposites causes disease.

A link between forms of political rule, character, and environment was likewise central to the last section of "Airs, Waters, Places" (Lloyd, 1983a, pp. 148–169). Premised on the general rule the "greater the variations in climate, so much will be the differences in character" (Lloyd, 1983a, p. 161), the text contrasted what it asserted to be the "feebleness of the Asiatic race" (Lloyd, 1983a, p. 159), as compared to the "keener" and more "sinewy" Greeks (Lloyd, 1983a, p. 169), and attributed this difference to the combination of climate (Asia's being more "blended" compared to the Greek "extremes of hot and cold") and to the "greater part of Asia" being "under monarchial rule" (Lloyd, 1983a, p. 159).

Textbox 2-1. The Circuitous Route from Hippocratic Thinking in Ancient
Greece to Contemporary Epidemiology—Via Galenic to Islamic
Medicine to the European Renaissance.

Despite conventional epidemiologic accounts that imply there is an unbroken link
between Hippocratic thought in the fifth century BCE and contemporary epidemiology
and medicine (Greenwood, 1932; Buck et al., 1988; Schneider et al., 2008), the historical record makes clear the connections are far more circuitous. As numerous scholars
have documented, the Hippocratic corpus and "school" was one—but not the only—
approach to medical thought and practice in ancient Greece (Sigerist, 1961; Lloyd,
1983a; Jouanna, 1999; Nutton, 2004; King, 2005). One step in its rise to prominence
was the adoption and extension of Hippocratic thought, in the first century CE, by the
prominent and prolific Greek-born Roman physician Galen (129–200 CE), who
worked his way up from treating gladiators to becoming physician to two Roman
emperors, Marcus Aurelius and Septimus Severus, and who wrote many of his volu-
minous treatises while residing in the Roman imperial court (Sigerist, 1961; Temkin,
1973; Porter, 1997; Nutton, 2004; King, 2005).

With the decline of the Roman empire, however, and the rise of the authority of the
Catholic church and contingent emergence of monasteries as centers of knowledge
and learning, both Hellenistic and Roman scholarship became not only less relevant
but also suspect, in part because of their pagan origins. The preservation, interpretation, and extension of Hippocratic and Galenic medicine (and other scientific works)
subsequently and consequently shifted to Arabic countries, where the texts were
translated into Arabic and informed the development of Islamic medicine, which both
built upon and extended the discoveries of its Hellenic predecessors (Hodgson, 1993;
Grmek, 1998; Porter, 1997; Poorman & Savage-Smith, 2007; Saliba, 2007; Bynum,
2008, Masood, 2009)

Starting in the eleventh century CE, Latin translations of Islamic medical texts and
other Greek and Roman scientific writings preserved and amplified by Arabic scholars
were re-introduced to Western Europe. They thereby helped not only to re-establish
the authority of Galenic medicine but also to spark the European Renaissance, which
ironically led to the rise of physicians, scientists, and other scholars, such as Paracelsus
(1493–1541) and Andreas Vesalius (1514–1564), who then challenged the intellectual
underpinnings and evidence of Galenic and, by extension, Hippocratic medicine
(Porter, 1997; Nutton, 2004; Bynum, 2008; Masood, 2009). Thus, no unbroken lineage
in Hippocratic thought extends from ancient Greece to contemporary epidemiology.
Instead, had the ancient Greek texts not been preserved and incorporated into Islamic
medicine, it is likely that the Hippocratic tradition would have endured in Europe only
as a type of uneducated "folk medicine," given Church suppression of pagan writings—
and not deemed a source of scholarly wisdom.

Notably, awareness of the broken chain of thought—between ancient Greece and
modern Europe—was evident to participants in the early days of epidemiology's emergence as science in the early nineteenth century (as discussed in **Chapter 3**). For
example, one of the era's leading investigators, William Farr (1807–1883) (Eyler, 1979),
in an article appearing in *The Lancet* in 1835–1836, urged fellow epidemiologists to
once again familiarize themselves with the Hippocratic texts and their understanding
of links between health, hygiene, and the environment (Farr 1835–1836). By the early
twentieth century, the transformation was complete: epidemiologic writings presented Hippocratic texts as foundational to the field. Exemplifying this approach was
one of the first books to focus on the history of epidemiology, *Epidemiology: Historical
and Experimental*, published in 1932 by Major Greenwood (1880–1949), who in 1929
became the first professor of Epidemiology and Vital Statistics at the London School

of Hygiene and Tropical Medicine (Greenwood, 1932). Since then, U. S. and European epidemiology textbooks understandably—albeit misleadingly—have routinely traced the origins of contemporary epidemiologic thinking to the Hippocratic text "Airs, Waters, Places," as if a direct link existed—when, in fact, the actual pathways of knowledge transmission are much more circuitous, rich, and indicative of the ways in which scientific knowledge depends on historical context.

Although cognizant of the benefits of self-rule, the focus of the Hippocratic corpus nevertheless was on the lives of the minority of men who enjoyed the democratic rights of citizens, coupled with discussion of the reproductive health of the women who bore them children (Pomeroy, 1975; Lloyd, 1983b; King, 1998; Jouanna, 1999; Nutton, 2004; King in King, 2005). Emphasizing diet, exercise, and rest for those who had the leisure and means to afford a healthy regimen, the texts included scant mention of the impact of work on humoral balance, whether it be the work of the women and men slaves engaged in producing food, staffing households, or laboring in the treasury-filling and deathly Athenian silver mines, let alone the work performed by the metics whose trading enabled Athens to flourish (Rosen, 1958 [1993]; Sigerist, 1961; Nutton, 1992; Nutton, 2004; Wilkins, 2005). That such work might be harmful to well-being was evidently known at the time, as revealed by Socrates' comment that "the trades of the artisans are decried and with good reason are held in low esteem in the cities" because "they disfigure the bodies of those who practice and pursue them" [(Austin & Vidal-Naquet, 1977, p. 169). But, despite slavery and manual work being even more ubiquitous than the seasonal recurrent fevers that garnered so much attention—the latter of which tellingly affected the powerful citizens (along with everyone else)—neither work nor hardship notably featured among the range of factors affecting humoral balance.

Not that the Hippocratic texts were alone in these omissions: it would not be for another 2000 years that the question of how work affects health would gain serious attention in European medical texts and nearly another five centuries thereafter before discussion of women's health would attend to more than just reproductive health (Rosen, 1958 [1993]; Porter, 1999; Krieger, 2000). The point is not that the authors of the Hippocratic texts should have been more "enlightened" than they were. Rather, understanding what is and is not addressed by Greek humoral theory requires considering who its authors and audience were, in their time and place; neither theory nor "balance" exists in a vacuum.

Hierarchy, Flux, Frequency, and Health: Balance and Theories of Disease Distribution in Context

I have considered the Greek humoral theory at some length because of the central place "Airs, Waters, Places" occupies in epidemiologists' accounts of the origins of the field (Greenwood, 1932; Buck et al., 1988; Schneider et al., 2008; Susser & Stein, 2009). But I could just as easily have chosen many other equally compelling and complex ancient and traditional theories of disease distribution to make two points about common features integral to all of these theories—and relevant to contemporary epidemiologic theories as well. The first is that all of these theories employ metaphors and mechanisms involving balance, ecology, and politics to bridge between the visible world outside the human body and its inner workings. The second is that all are cognizant of frequency and distinguish between causes of disease that affect many people simultaneously versus those that variously afflict diverse individuals or are uncommon.

Nevertheless, the ways in which these theoretical features play out is contingent and varies by time, place, and society: what is considered self-evident in one context is immaterial in another. To provide more critical insight into the kinds of assumptions that pervade etiologic and epidemiologic theorizing, the next section briefly highlights selected aspects of three very different theories of disease distribution: those of text-based ancient Chinese medicine, and those of the oral traditions of the Kallawaya in the Bolivian Andes and the Ogori in Nigeria. In all three cases, as with the discussion of Hippocratic texts, I draw on the research and translations of other scholars, whose efforts to analyze the etiologic ideas of diverse societies, past and present, can usefully inform epidemiologic thinking.

China, Hierarchy, and Health. Scholarly analyses emphasize there is no one single system of "traditional Chinese medicine," but rather a syncretic amalgam forged over the course of millennia through the present day (Veith, 1966; Porkert, 1974; Pei, 1983; Unschuld, 1985; Zmiewski, 1985; Sivin, 1987; Hoizey & Hoizey, 1993; Kuriyama, 1999; Hsu, 2001; Unschuld, 2003). These complexities notwithstanding, its foundational texts, compiled roughly in the same time period as those of the ancient Greeks (c. 500–200 BCE), similarly treated health as the emotional and bodily manifestation of right living—that is, in accord with the natural and social order (Lloyd, 1990; Unschuld, 2003). Yet, whereas the Greek approach emphasized the equal balance of humors for health and deemed disease caused by the undue influence of any given humor, the Chinese approach highlighted the preservation of hierarchy for health and viewed disease as arising from a disturbance in ordered relationships.

Central to the Chinese system were elaborate systems of correspondence concerned with change, growth, and decay (Porkert, 1974; Unschuld, 1985; Sivin, 1987; Hoizey & Hoizey, 1993; Unschuld, 2003). As illustrated in **Figure 2–2a** and **2–2b**, one system involved the principles of *yin* and *yang*, interdependent dynamic constructs, each containing part of the other and always in transformation; the terms themselves initially denoted the sunny and shady side of the hill, symbolic of the ceaseless cycle from day to night back to day. The second system, referred to as the "Five Phases" (*wu-hsing*), employed tangible symbols—water, fire, metal, wood, and soil—to signify ordered and distinct phases of growth ("Mutual Production") and decay ("Mutual Conquest"). Together, these systems, in conjunction with *qi* (or *ch'i*)—a term simultaneously referring to processes and substances that can enable health or produce illness (Unschuld, 1985, pp. 2, 72; Sivin, 1987, pp. 46–53; Hoizey & Hoizey, 1993, p. 23; Unschuld, 2003, pp. 144–146) and literally translated as meaning the "finest matter (forming the entire world and circulating in the body)" (Unschuld, 2005, p. 23)—were systematically connected through complex sets of correspondences, as shown in **Table 2–1** (Wong & Lien-Teh, 1932, p. 11; Veith, 1966, p. 21; Needham, 1969, pp. 262–263; Sivin, 1987, pp. 77, 208; Unschuld, 2003, pp. 393–488). Linking geography, climate, seasons, planets, diet, senses, emotions, and organ systems, these correspondences were used to explain both disease etiology and disease distribution. For example, according to classic text the *Huang Di nei jing* (typically referred to in English as the "Yellow Emperor's Classic of Internal Medicine," and likely initially compiled between 400 and 200 BCE and then subject to commentary for millennia thereafter) (Veith, 1966, pp. 6–9; Unschuld, 1985, pp. 56–58; Hoizey & Hoizey, 1993, pp. 27–28; Unschuld, 2003, pp. 1–7, 22–75), "The wise man will nourish himself in the spring and summer with yang influences but in the autumn and winter with yin influences" [Unschuld, 1985, p. 283]. The implication was that those who did not heed this advice would become ill, so as to account for why, despite common seasonal, geographic, and astronomic influences, some people stayed healthy and others did not.

(a)

Qualities of *Yin* and *Yang*		Visual symbol of flow and interpenetration of *yin* and *yang*
Yin	**Yang**	
dark	bright	
night	day	
cold	heat	
contracting	expanding	
responsive	active	
feminine	masculine	
interior	exterior	
exhaustion	repletion	
quiesence	movement	
lower	upper	
right	left	

(b)

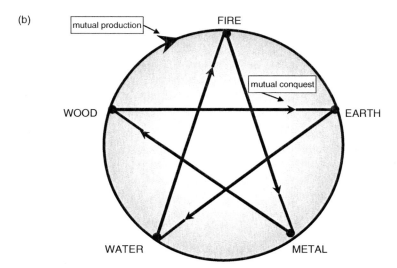

Figure 2–2. (**a**)*Yin/Yang* and (**b**) Relationship of the Mutual Production (circle) and Mutual Conquest (star) sequences of the Five phases.

Beyond differences in the types of correspondences considered, the Chinese approach also included bodily components and metaphors the Greek did not (Lloyd, 1990; Kuriyama, 1999; Unschuld, 2003, pp. 332–339). For example, in the Chinese schema, to circulate *qi*, the body contained "conduit vessels" (*ching-mo*, a word also used to refer to agricultural irrigation channels [Unschuld, 1985, pp. 74–78]), theorized to connect the body's *yin* and *yang* organ networks, with proper flow key for health and blockage posited to produce illness (Veith, 1966; Porkert, 1974; Gwei-Djen & Needham, 1980; Unschuld, 1985; Sivin, 1987; Hoizey & Hoizey, 1993; Unschuld, 2003). Also unlike the Greeks, the Chinese theories likened health to a well-ordered kingdom and disease to rebellion (Sivin, 1987, pp. 57–59; Unschuld, 1985, pp. 79–83, 99–100, 106–108; Machle, 1993, p. 81]; linguistically aiding this metaphors, words such as *zhi* could refer to not only "good government" but also "healing," and *luan* could mean not only social "chaos" and "disorder" but also

Table 2–1. Systems of Correspondence: (a) yin/yang, the Five Phases, and Other Phenomena* and (b) Text from the *Huáng dì nèi jīn* Describing These Relationships**.

(a) Systems of correspondence

Phenomenon	Five phases				
	Wood	**Fire**	**Earth**	**Metal**	**Water**
Yin/Yang	Immature *yang*	Mature *yang*	Harmony	Immature *yin*	Mature *yin*
Planet	Jupiter	Mars	Saturn	Venus	Mercury
Season	Spring	Summer	(Sixth month)	Autumn	Winter
Climate	Windy	Hot	Moist	Dry	Cool
Color	Green	Red	Yellow	White	Black
Direction	East	South	Center	West	North
Dynasties	Hsia	Chou	Huang Ti	Shang	Ch'i
Style of government	Relaxed	Enlightened	Careful	Energetic	Quiet
Stage of development	Birth	Growth	Transformation	Harvest	Storage
Number	Eight	Seven	Five	Nine	Six
Taste	Sour	Bitter	Sweet	Pungent	Salty
Odor	Rancid	Scorched	Fragrant	Rotten	Putrid
Emotion	Anger	Joy	Desire	Grief	Fear
Organ network	Liver	Heart	Spleen	Lungs	Kidney
Sense organs	Eye	Tongue	Mouth	Nose	Ear
Bowels	Gall bladder	Small intestine	Stomach	Large intestine	Bladder
Tissues	Muscles	Blood	Flesh	Skin and Hair	Bones
Animal class	Scaly (fish)	Feathered (birds)	Naked	Hairy (mammals)	Shell-covered (invertebrates)

(b) "Comprehensive Treatise on the Regulation of the Spirit in Accord with the Four Seasons," *Huáng dì nèi jīn, Sù wèn* 2

The three months of spring, they denote effusion and spreading. In heaven and earth everything comes to life; the myriad beings flourish. Go to rest late at night and rise early. Move through the courtyard in long strides. Dishevel the hair and relax the physical appearance, thereby cause the mind to come to life. Generate and do not kill. Reward and do not punish. This is the correspondence with the qi of spring and it is the Way to nourish life. Opposing it harms the liver. In summer, this causes changes to cold, and there is little to support growth.

The three months of summer, they denote opulence and blossoming. The qi of heaven and earth interact and the myriad beings bloom and bear fruit. Go to rest late at night and rise early. Never get enough of the sun. Let the mind have no anger. Stimulate beauty and have your elegance perfected. Cause the qi to flow away, as if that what you loved were located outside. This is correspondence with the qi of summer and it is the Way to nourish growth. Opposing it harms the heart. In autumn this causes *jie* and *malaria* and there is little to support gathering. Multiple diseases [develop] at winter solstice.

The three months of autumn, they denote harvest and balance. The qi of heaven becomes tense. The qi of the earth becomes clear. Go to rest early and rise early, get up together with the chicken. Let the mind be peaceful and tranquil, so as to temper the punishment carried out in the autumn.

Collect the spirit qi and cause the autumn qi to be balanced. Do not direct your mind to the outside and cause the lung qi to be clear. This is correspondence with the qi of autumn and it is the Way to nourish gathering. Opposing it harms the lungs. In winter this causes outflow of [undigested] food and there is little to support storage.

The three months of winter, they denote securing and storage. The water is frozen and the earth breaks open. Do no disturb the yang [qi]! Go to rest early and rise late. You must wait for the sun to shine. Let the mind enter a state as if hidden, as if shut in, as if you had secret intentions; as if you already had made a gain. Avoid cold and seek warmth and do not [allow sweat] to flow away through the skin. This would cause the qi to be carried away quickly. This is correspondence with the qi of winter and it is the Way of nourishing storage. Opposing it harms the kidneys. In spring this causes limpness with receding [qi], and there is little to support generation.

---

* (Wong & Lien-The, 1932, p. 11; Veith, 1966, p. 21; Needham, 1969, pp. 262–263; Sivin, 1987, pp. 77, 208)
**(Unschuld, 2005, pp. 101–102)

"sickness" (Machle, 1993, p. 81). Linking these themes together is a well-known passage in the *Huang Di nei jing* (Unschuld, 1985, p. 100):

The heart is the ruler. Spirit and enlightenment have their origin here. The lung is the minister; the order of life's rhythms has its origins here. The liver is the general; planning and deliberation have their origin here. The gall is the official whose duty it is to maintain the [golden] mean and what is proper; decisions and judgments have their origin here. The heart-enclosing network is the emissary; good fortune and happiness have their origin here. The spleen and the stomach are officials in charge of storing provisions; the distribution of food has its origins here. The kidneys are officials for employment and forced labor; technical skills and expertise have their origins here. The triple burner is the official in charge of transportation conduits; water channels have their origins here. The urinary bladder is the provincial magistrate and stores body fluids; once the influences [of the latter are exhausted through] transformation, they may leave the bladder.

If the ruler is enlightened, peace reigns for his subjects. He who carries out his life on these principles is assured of longevity; he will never be in danger. He who rules the empire in accordance with these principles will bring forth a golden age. If, however, the ruler is not enlightened, the twelve officials are endangered; streets shall be closed and all traffic interrupted. Form will suffer great harm. He who carries out his life on these principles will bring down misfortune. He who rules the empire on such principles shall endanger his clan.

Likening treatment of disease to "an attempt to restore order only after unrest has broken out," the text accordingly admonished that the reason "the sages do not treat those who have already fallen ill, but rather those who are not yet ill" is because "they do not put [their state] in order when revolt [is underway], but before an insurrection occurs" (Unschuld, 1985, p. 282).

The variance in the ecological and political metaphors embedded in the ancient Greek and Chinese medical systems should not be surprising. Hippocratic texts were written by physicians and elite citizens who lived in relatively small city-states, with some of these city-states practicing an Athenian version of democracy, and all of them located amidst ancient Greece's compact coastal and mountainous topography, rendering irrelevant the possibility of any major irrigation systems for growing crops. By contrast, the core texts of Chinese medicine, although likewise written by a literate minority, were formulated during the course of sprawling Chou dynasty (1122–256 BCE), rife with disputes between warring feudal lords, who not only ruled their peasants (who were bound to the land they farmed) but also, at their discretion, supported various scholars in their courts and with all of these groups—the Emperor, the imperial court, feudal lords, peasants, and scholars alike—dependent on the Yellow River for irrigation, transport, and trade (Wilbur, 1943; Needham, 1954; Unschuld, 1985; Lloyd, 1990; Bodde, 1991; Fairbank, 1992; Hoizey & Hoizey, 1993; Lloyd & Sivin, 2002). Concerns about maintenance of the irrigation channels, and prevention of flooding and drought resulting from their blockage and disrepair, were of paramount importance; so, too, was preservation of the feudal and bureaucratic order. Had each system not resonated with "obvious" features of the societal and ecological context of their authors and audience, it is unlikely either the Greek or Chinese disease theories would have been so widely adopted in their respective societies.

It would be misleading to think, however, that connections between the worlds inside and outside of people's bodies, and between disease distribution and etiology, were drawn only by literate scholars and their patrons. When it comes to matters of life and death, there is plentiful evidence that people in all societies have scrutinized their environs, whether their focus be on the stars and planets, to plan for planting or navigate routes, or on the "airs, waters, places" and biota, to determine what is harmful versus salubrious; they also unsurprisingly have developed diverse meaningful narratives linking human existence to the broader world or cosmos in which we live—and of which we are a part (Ackerknecht, 1946; Sigerist, 1951; Rosen, 1958 [1993]; Hughes, 1963; Unschuld, 2003, pp. 319–349). Two examples of such oral traditions—one from the Andes, the other from sub-Saharan Africa—make this point and make vividly clear the context-dependent meaning of "balance" for conceptualizing the determinants and meaning of the people's health.

Oscillatory Balance: the Kallawaya in the Andes. First, the understandings of health offered by the Kallawaya (Bastien, 1985; Bastien, 1989; Fernández Juárez, 1998; Loza, 2004), a lineage of healers among the Aymara, an Indigenous people living high in the altiplano of Bolivia, north of Lake Titicaca, and surrounded by the towering snow-capped mountains of the Andes (Bastien, 1985; Cusicanqui, 1987; Bastien, 1989; Crandon-Malamud, 1991; van Lindert & Verkoren, 1994; Llanque et al., 1994; Fernández Juárez, 1998; Loza, 2004). Their theories and practices, preserved by memory and ritual rather than by text, live on in oral tradition because of their continued salience in everyday life. Recognition of their contemporary as well as historical importance was bestowed in 2003, when the United Nations Educational, Scientific, and Cultural Organization (UNESCO) declared the "Andean cosmovision of the Kallaway" to be one of the "masterpieces of the oral and intangible heritage of humanity" (UNESCO, 2003; Loza, 2004), an honor accorded between 2001 and 2005 to only 90 such masterpieces worldwide.

As documented by the anthropologist Joseph W. Bastien (1985;1989;1992) and others (de Tichaer, 1973; LLanque et al., 1994; Loza, 2004), the Kallawayan "topological-hydraulic" understanding of the body, health, and illness (**Figure 2–3**) is grounded in the *ayllu* in which they live (Lehman, 1982; Bastien, 1985; van Lindert & Verkoren, 1994). These *ayllu*, each comprised of mountainous regions whose boundaries are defined geographically, socially, and spiritually, span a mountainside's lower, central, and upper regions, on which live communities integrated by trade and united by marriage (Lehman, 1982; Bastien, 1985; Bastien, 1989; Schull & Rothhammer, 1990; Fernández Juárez, 1998; Klein, 2003). Daily fluctuations in temperature—from freezing cold of night to scorching heat of day—often exceed differences between winter and summer in North America. Moisture-laden trade winds continually collide with mountain peaks, precipitating endless cycles of fog and mist cascading down ravines; during the rainy season, powerful storms replete with hail and lightning are an almost daily occurrence. Their downpours (which are crucial for crops) collect at the summit, disappear into subterranean streams, surface in pools at natural terraces on

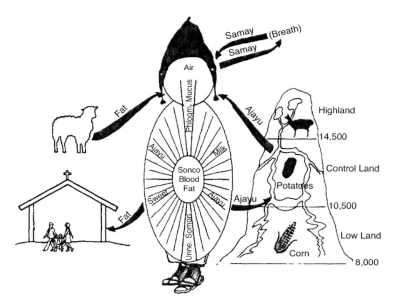

Figure 2–3. Topographical-hydraulic model of Kallaway body concept, as depicted by Bastien. (Bastien, 1989, p. 46). (©1989 Elsevier, Inc. Reprinted with permission.)

the mountain's slopes, and surge forth as streams and rivers, eventually feeding the Amazon and the Atlantic beyond. Not only do the mountains shape life and death: they are themselves sacred and alive.

Mountains, flow, and flux figure prominently in Kallawaya notions of well-being (Bastien, 1985; van den Berg & Schiffers, 1992; Kolata, 1995; Fernández Juárez, 1998; Loza, 2004). Of central importance is the metaphor of the mountain/body (Bastien, 1989). Mountains are understood in terms of people's bodies, and their bodies in terms of mountains. Both have a head, trunks, and legs, each with different functions and together forming an interdependent organic whole. Moreover, just as mountains have inner streams through which life-giving water flows and valleys through which winds pass, so too do people—by analogy and observation—have inner conduits transporting the body's three primary media: air, blood, and fat (Bastien, 1989; Crandon-Malamud, 1991; Loza, 2004). In both cases, dependable cycles of flow are vital, because blocked or flooded passageways can cause serious damage (an observation akin to those of the Chinese concepts concerning the health implications of blocking the flow of *c'hi*). The body is thus comprehended as "a vertically layered axis with a system of ducts through which air, blood, fat and water flow to and from the sonco (heart)… in a hydraulic cycle of centripetal and centrifugal motion" (Bastien, 1989, p. 47), which, like the weather, routinely encompasses "pendulum-like swings" (Bastien, 1989, p. 48). In this system, too little fat leads to wasting diseases, such as tuberculosis, whereas too much fat clogs the ducts and prevents nourishment from reaching the muscles; one telling hallmark symptom of late-stage endemic Chagas disease, endemic to this region of the world, is a swollen abdomen caused by congestion of feces and fluids (Bastien, 1989; Schull & Rothhammer, 1990; Llanque et al., 1994).

Construing healthy balance as oscillation, and healthy exchange as reciprocal, the Kallawayan schema, rooted in its particular ecologic and societal context, at once resembles and differs sharply from the Greek and Chinese approaches.

In summary, in the Kallawayan system, mountains, and people together are part of endless cycles of life, death, and transformation, sometimes disintegrating rapidly (as with a landslide or sudden illness) and sometimes eroding slowly, exhibiting the wear of time. Preservation of health hence requires attention not only to people but also to the mountains (via ritual), as harm to the mountains can damage health. Attesting to the literal meaning of this linkage between people's health and that of the mountains is the continued health impact of the colonial and post-colonial ravaging of the Bolivian silver and then tins mine, located on the Andean peaks. For centuries, the adjacent Indigenous populations have lived amidst the mines' toxic detritus and for centuries were also coerced—first by law, then by poverty—into working in the unsafe conditions of these unforgiving mines, with the consequent social, cultural, economic, and ecologic degradation all taking a huge toll on their health (Galeano, 1973; Taussig, 1980; Cusicanqui, 1987; van Lindert & Verkoren, 1994; Klein, 2003). In other words, break the mountain and you break the people; Kallawayan theory would predict no less.

Normal is Natural: the Nigerian Ogori. Finally, to underscore how causal reasoning about disease frequency, a hallmark of twentieth and twenty-first century CE epidemiologic and medical theorizing (Greenwood, 1932; Canguilhelm, 1991), has longstanding roots in not only ancient text-based theories but also oral traditions, consider the thinking about disease occurrence evident in the theories of the Ogori (Gillies, 1976), a Yoruban-descent population currently living in the southwestern part of Nigeria (Akerejola, 1973; Osheidu, 1980; Faolola & Heaon, 2008). Behind this particular case lies a contentious debate in the anthropological literature over whether traditional theories of disease causation overwhelmingly favor magical as opposed to natural explanations of illness (Ackerknecht, 1946; Loudon, 1976; Iwu, 1986; Ranger, 1988; Vaughan, 1991; Feierman & Janzen, 1992; Vaughan, 1994; Baer et al., 1997; Green, 1999). Exemplifying the former stance is the classic 1937 text *Witchcraft, Oracles, and Magic among the Azandes* (Evans-Pritchard, 1937; Evans-Pritchard, 1976) (a group residing in north-central Africa), in which the author, Sir Edwards Evans-Pritchard (1902–1973), a leading British anthropologist, famously asserted, "[The] Azande attribute sickness, whatever its nature, to witchcraft and sorcery" (1937, p. 479; Gilles, 1976, p. 385). To test the validity and universality of Evans-Pritchard's conclusion, another anthropologist, Eva Gilles, conducted a study among the Ogori (Gillies, 1976) with her research taking place from 1965 to 1966, in the brief window between independence (won in 1960 from the British) and the onset of military rule (1966–1979) (Akerejola, 1973; Osheidu, 1980; Isichei, 1983; Curtin et al., 1995; Davidson, 1998; Falola & Heaton, 2008).

What Gilles found was that far from attributing all diseases to magic, the Ogori invoked natural explanations for the vast majority of health problems, including both common, expected events (such as deaths among old persons) and trivial or common diseases (such as colds, malaria, upset stomachs, and infestation by guinea worms), and treated the latter with natural substances, including herbal remedies. By contrast, only events that were either very rare (e.g., death of a young adult), very serious (e.g., leprosy), or very widespread but sporadic (e.g., an epidemic of small pox) elicited explanations involving malevolent humans, spirits, or deities. Thus, although not quantitatively measured, prevalence and severity of illness or cause of death affected causal attribution, premised upon a sense of the common, uncommon, and customary. The Ogori thus categorized the bulk of health problems—that is, frequent and expected diseases and deaths—as naturally caused and reserved non-naturalistic explanations only for those maladies or deaths that were rare, unexpected, or unusually grave.

In considering why Evans-Pritchard may have overlooked naturalistic approaches to etiologic explanation in African oral traditions, Gillies called attention (1976, p. 386) to a passage in his 1937 book, in which he stated (Evans-Pritchard, 1937, p. 481):

> Knowing nothing at all of pathology, physiology, botany and chemistry, I soon tired of the fruit-less labor of collecting the names of innumerable diseases and medicinal plants, few of which I could render either into the English language or into scientific terminology and which remained therefore useless and unintelligible.

The net result was to remove from discussion the myriad diseases attributed to natural causes and treated by natural remedies, an omission paralleled by the Greek humoral theory's inattention to links between work and health. The broader implication is that critical evaluation of theories of disease distribution requires considering what might be missing as well as what is included. At issue is how analytic and etiologic inferences can be affected by seemingly "self-evident" assumptions as to what constitutes "balance"—and also who or what matters as possible determinants of individual's health and the patterns of health exhibited in their societies. On that note, we can shift to examine whether these concerns, revealed by analysis of ancient text-based and oral traditional theories, are relevant to more familiar early modern and contemporary epidemiologic theories of disease tradition.

3

Epidemiology Emerges

Early Theories and Debating Determinants of Disease Distribution—Poison, Filth, Class, & Race (1600–1900)

Bodies Count: Epidemiology Emerges as a Self-Defined Scientific Discipline

The development of epidemiology as a self-defined scientific discipline—with its concomitant theories of disease distribution expressly intended to explain empirical data on the patterning and determinants of population rates of morbidity and mortality—had its origins in Europe in the seventeenth century. The term *epidemiology*—literally the science and study of epidemics—apparently was coined in 1802, when Don Joaquin Villalba published *Epidemiología Española*, a chronicle of epidemics in Spain (Villalba, 1803). By the 1830s, epidemiology had emerged as a self-designated field of inquiry. Its focus, as expansively enumerated in 1839 by William Guy (1810–1885; a Professor of Forensic Medicine at the University of London and early member of both the London Statistical Society, founded in 1834, and the London Epidemiological Society, founded in 1850; Guy, 1865; Rosen, 1958 [1993], pp. 235–238) was none other than [Guy, 1839, p. 35]:

> Man (*sic*), considered as a social being, is its object; the mean duration of his life, and the probable period of his death; the circumstances which preserve or destroy the health of his body, or affect the culture of his mind; the wealth which he amasses, the crimes which he commits, and the punishments which he incurs—all these are weighed, compared, and calculated; and nothing which can affect the welfare of the society of which he is a member, or the glory and prosperity of the country to which he belongs, is excluded from its grand and comprehensive survey.

To Guy, the goal was to establish a new "science of statistics," by which he meant "the application of the numerical method to living beings in all their social relations" (Guy, 1839, p. 39).

Indeed, a social orientation was built into the very terminology used. The word *statistic*, after all, was derived from the term *state* and was coined in 1749 by Gottfried Achenwall (1719–1772) as a term of statecraft referring to systematic methods of summarizing, in words, a nation's strength, in terms of its natural, economic, military, and human resources (Koren, 1918; Shaw & Miles, 1981; Donnelly, 1998). Entering the English language in 1791 in the title of John Sinclair's (1754–1835) massive 21-volume *Statistical Account of Scotland* (Sinclair, 1791–1799), *statistics* did not acquire its subsequent meaning as a branch of mathematics concerned with probability and causal inference until the early twentieth century (Shaw & Miles, 1981; Desrosières, 1998). A similar breadth of concerns was evident in the 1865 founding statement of the American Social Science Association, whose first meeting was called to order by Dr. Edmund Jarvis, an expert in vital statistics, advisor to the U.S. census, and one of the founders of the American Statistical Association (Koren, 1918; Haskell, 1977; Ross, 1991; Silverberg, 1998).

As with any scientific discipline, epidemiology's emergence built on prior conceptual, technical, and logistical developments. One core precondition was acceptance of the new and controversial belief that people and societies could be meaningfully studied using the same kinds of numerical methods deployed in the "natural sciences." This stance, treated as commonplace if not common sense in modern epidemiology (Rothman, 1988, p. 3), was in fact very far from intuitive, as it countered then (and perhaps still) prevalent views about the role of inscrutable divine will and free choice in determining individuals' fates. To many, it was heretical and outrageous to suggest that peoples' behaviors and social phenomena were "governed" by "laws," whether they be impersonal universal "laws," akin to Newton's law of gravitation, or the then new-fangled type of statistical "laws," still being discovered and elucidated by that era's mathematicians (Hacking, 1975; Hacking, 1981; Stigler, 1986; Daston, 1987; Hacking, 1990; Porter, 1995; Desrosières, 1998; Burton, 1999). How could, after all, free will, not to mention moral responsibility, be compatible with regularities in rates—that is, group properties? (This is a question that still gives many in the population sciences grounds for pause.)

To tackle these novel, truly never-before-asked questions—and to develop this new approach to studying people—a new conceptual orientation was needed. Expressing this new outlook was the coining of *social science*, a quickly adopted term that first appeared (as *la science sociale*) in a 1789 revolutionary pamphlet written in the thick of the French Revolution by the influential mathematician-turned-political-philosopher, the Marquis de Condorcet (1743–1794) (Baker, 1969; Baker, 1975; Cohen, 1994a; Walker, 1998). Further making the links between the natural and social science, shortly thereafter, the first French medical school chartered after the revolution created the first-ever chair of "medical physics and hygiene"; its faculty member was required to possess "A knowledge of man as an individual (private hygiene) and of man as a member of society (public hygiene)" (Ackerknecht, 1948a; Coleman, 1982, pp. 16–17; La Berge 1992), thereby establishing the idea of "public health."

Soon thereafter, the Belgian astronomer-turned-statistician-turned-sociologist-turned-nosologist Adolphe Quetelet (1796–1874) (Quetelet, 1842; Hankins, 1968; Eknoyan, 2008) followed suit, arguing for a "social physics" in the very title of his widely read 1835 opus, *Sur l'homme et le développement de ses facultés, ou Essai de physique sociale* (Quetelet, 1835). In this volume, Quetelet introduced the idea of *l'homme moyenne*—the *average man*. Inverting the approach taken in astronomy to fix the location of stars, whereby results of observations from multiple observatories (each with some degree of error) were combined to determine a star's most likely celestial coordinates, Quetelet ingeniously (if erroneously) argued that the distribution of a population's characteristics (such as height) served as a guide to its true (inherent) value, one obscured by the "deviations" of "errors" expressed in the imperfect variations of individuals (each counting as an "observation-with-error" akin to the data produced by each observatory) (Hankins, 1908 [1968]; Stigler, 1986; Desrosières, 1998). For Quetelet, this understanding of "means" meant that population averages could be meaningfully compared, revealing important fundamental differences (or similarities) between groups.

Only: was the observed difference truly "real," representing the true effects of a constant cause (Quetelet, 1835; Cole, 2000)? Or was the "mean" instead something illusory that diverted attention from the phenomena it summarized? For example, did it obscure who was (within any given population) hardest hit by cholera?—or by crime rates? (Desrosières, 1998, pp. 76, 85). And who—and what—determined which groups comprised "populations" or groups that merited comparison? Were boundaries between groups literally set solely by geography? By ostensibly innate features (such as age, sex, "race," and, as argued at the time, "nationality")? Or by acquired characteristics (such as occupation)? Far from being only academic questions, these questions of: (*1*) who meaningfully comprised a "group," and (*2*) whether an "average" (or "central tendency") conveyed profound information about a population group's intrinsic properties (including disease rates) versus simply was an arithmetic contrivance, had important scientific, political, and economic stakes, ones both understood and argued at the time (Stigler, 1986; Daston, 1987; Hacking, 1987; Porter, 1995; Desrosières, 1998; Cole, 2000).

In addition to this major conceptual reorientation that made statistical study of humanity make sense, several other essential preconditions for having the data and mathematical tools required to conduct epidemiologic research included:

- the rise of the modern state in the seventeenth century, with its administrative needs for data on population, commerce, and natural resources (Hobsbawm, 1992; Porter, 1995; Rueschemery & Skocpol, 1996; Heilbron et al., 1998; Cole, 2000);
- the creation of calculus and development of probability theory in the seventeenth century (Hacking, 1975; Burton, 1999);
- the upsurge of new classification systems for taxonomies of plants, animals, and diseases in the mid-eighteenth century (Mayr, 1988; Martin, 1990; Porter, 1997; Bynum, 2008);
- novel investigations of human anatomy, starting in the mid-sixteenth century, augmented by use of microscopes and new research on animal (including human) physiology in the seventeenth century (Wear et al., 1985; French & Wear, 1989; Porter, 1997; Bynum, 2008); and
- a rise in scientific societies and scientific journals, especially in the eighteenth century, promoting greater exchange of ideas within and across scientific disciplines (Cohen, 1985; Cunningham & French, 1990).

Still another impetus, discussed below and perhaps most galvanizing of all, was provided by:

- new patterns of living and dying ushered in by the Industrial Revolution, commencing in England in the latter part of the eighteenth century, along with Europeans' encounters with what to them were new diseases in tropical colonies and the New World (Crosby, 1986; Hobsbawm, 1996a; Hays, 1998).

Together, these varied components spurred novel efforts to describe and explain different societies' patterning of overall and specific types of morbidity and mortality—in other words, the very stuff of the new discipline of "epidemiology." Keeping in mind the distinguishing features of scientific disciplines (*see* **Chapter 1, Textbox 1–1**), what sharply demarcated these new efforts to explain the people's health from the older text-based and oral traditions discussed in **Chapter 2** was not simply their quantitative empirical approach but also the new substantive concepts—especially about disease specificity—that made the counting of cases (numerators) and the population (denominators) feasible, along with the novel metaphors invoked and mechanisms proposed to make sense of the newly observed patterns of health, disease, and death.

Quantifying Patterns of Life, Death, and Disease: Life Tables and Epidemic Constitutions.
Among the precursors to epidemiology's self-designated appearance in the early nineteenth
century, two seventeenth century efforts merit mention because of what they reveal about
the ingredients needed for epidemiologic evidence and for devising and testing epidemiologic theories. At issue are: (*1*) the development of quantitative approaches to tabulating
and comparing population health data, and (*2*) a growing appreciation for conceptualizing
and treating diseases as separate nosological entities, defined in relation to the specificity
of symptoms and causes.

The first effort concerns the pathbreaking work by William Petty (1623–1687), an
English physician, anatomist, and economist and John Graunt (1620–1674), a London
merchant, to tally the features of—and links between—human life, health, and wealth
(Greenwood, 1948; Hull, 1963; Roncaglia, 1985; Olson, 1993). In the 1670s, Petty argued,
in his classic works *Political Arithmetick* (Petty, 1676, in Hull, 1963, pp. 233–313) and
Political Anatomy of Ireland (Petty 1672 [1690], in Hull, 1963, pp. 121–231), the new idea
that society—like any organism—could be studied numerically and objectively (*see*
Textbox 3–1 for how Petty expressed these ideas, using the available language and concepts of his day).

Informing Petty's approach was the parallel of the "body natural" and the "body politic"
that featured widely in the bodily metaphors favored by mercantilists of his era (Roncaglia,
1985, p. 29; Magnusson, 1998). Just as each "body" had a guiding intellect (head; king),
division of labor (the "hands" serve the "head"; the people serve the king), appetite
(for food; for resources), and need to circulate nourishment (by organ systems; via commercial transactions and trade routes), so too did each "body" exhibit "disease" if the
relationship between its respective parts was in any way disrupted. Also relevant to Petty's
work were his experiences in the 1650s of organizing, on behalf of the English army, a massive survey of Ireland to adjudicate redistribution of its conquered territory, including to
Petty himself (Hull, 1963; Roncaglia, 1986; Olson, 1993; Poovey, 1998, pp. 120–142).
Together, Petty's volumes helped establish the conceptual and empirical foundations for the

---

Textbox 3–1. William Petty (1623–1687) on "Political Arithmetik" and
"Political Anatomy"

"Sir Francis Bacon, in his Advancement of Learning, hath made a judicious parallel in
many particulars, between the Body Natural, and Body Politick, and between the Arts
of preserving both in Health and Strength; And it is as reasonable, that as Anatomy
is the best foundation of one, so also of the other... I therefore, who profess no
politicks, have, for my curiosity at large attempted the first Essay of Political Anatomy."
(Preface to *Political Anatomy of Ireland* (written in 1672; published in 1690) (Petty,
1963, p. 129)).

"The method I take to do this is not yet very usual; for instead of using only comparative and superlative words, and intellectual arguments, I have taken the course
(as a specimen of the Political Arithmetik I have long aimed at) to express myself
in terms of number, weight, or measure; to use only Arguments of sense, and to
consider only such causes as have visible Foundations in Nature; leaving those that
depend upon the mutable Minds, Opinions, Appetites and Passions of particular Men,
to the consideration of others." (Preface to *Political Arithmetick* (written in 1676; published in 1690) (Petty, 1963, p. 244)).

quantitative study of people. Also critical was Petty's claim that "evidence" speaks unbiasedly for itself (Poovey, 1998), a politically expedient stance likewise taken by one of the world's first national scientific societies—the English Royal Society (founded in 1662), which included Petty among its original charter members of 119 learned men (no women were included) (Cohen, 1994b). Without this profession of neutrality, it would have been unlikely for the head of state to grant the society its charter (Cohen, 1994b; Poovey, 1998).

Inspired by Petty's approach—and likely assisted directly by Petty himself—Graunt calculated the world's first documented life table. It appeared in 1662 in Graunt's tract *Natural and Political Observations Made upon the Bills of Mortality* (Graunt, 1662), for which Petty wrote the introduction. Based on London Bills of Mortality for 1604 to 1661, Graunt's tables newly showed how many members of a given birth cohort survived in each successive decade (as based on imperfect data and assuming a stationary population, limitations imposed by the available records [Greenwood, 1948, pp. 28–32; Burton, 1999, pp. 402–404]). Among Graunt's many striking findings (*see* examples in **Textbox 3–2**), his analyses revealed that more than one-third of the population died by age 6 years, only 10% survived to the age of 46 years, the number dying each year from non-epidemic disease was fairly constant, and women on average lived longer than men (Graunt, 1662).

Graunt's calculations were soon found to be highly useful to governments, who until then had sold annuities (a widely used method of raising money without raising taxes, typically to defray costs of waging war) on the wager that more people would buy the annuities to guarantee a pension for a set number of years than would live to collect them. Specifically, the use of lifetables suddenly made much more profitable a practice that previously had led to some costly mistakes, as earlier approaches to issuing annuities typically had not taken into account differential risks of dying at a given age (Buck, 1982, p. 30).

Textbox 3–2. John Graunt (1620–1674): Assorted "Natural and Political Observations Made upon the Bills of Mortality" (Graunt, 1662 [1939], pp. 4–16) (italics in original)

- "*A true Accompt of the* Plague *cannot be kept, without the Accompt of other Diseases*"
- "That two parts of nine die of Acute, and seventy of two hundred twenty nine of Chronical Diseases, and four of two hundred twenty nine of outward Griefs"
- "*That the* Rickets *is a new disease, both as to name, and thing*"
- "*There hath been in* London *within this Age four times of great* Mortality, *viz. Anno* 1592, 1603, 1625, *and* 1636, *wherof that of* 1603 *was the greatest*"
- "*The more* sickly *the year is, the less* fertile *of Births*"
- "*There are about* 24000 Teeming women (of fertile age).... . *in, and about* London"
- "*That there be... near* 70000 Fighting Men, *that is Men between the Ages of 16, and 56*"
- "*There come yearly to dwell at* London *about 6000 strangers out of the Country, which swells the Burials about 200 per Annum*"
- "*In the Country but about one of fifty dies yearly, but at* London, *one of thirty, over and above the Plague... It is doubted whether* encrease *of People, or the* burning *of Sea-coal were the cause, or both*"
- "That *London, the Metropolis of England, is perhaps a Head too big for the Body, and possibly too strong: That this Head grows three times as fast as the Body unto which it belongs, that is, It doubles its People in a third part of the time*"

Building on Graunt's success, in 1683 Petty published *Observations upon the Dublin Bills of Mortality*, followed by *Further Observations on the Dublin Bills* in 1687 (Roncaglia, 1985, p. 14). In 1693, the astronomer Edmond Halley (1656–1742) (Halley, 1693)—who gave the famed Halley comet its name—further improved on these early efforts by calculating a lifetable for Breslaw, the capital of the province of Silesia, a site Halley chose because, unlike London and Dublin, it had an essentially stationary population (i.e., virtually no immigrants or emigrants, who could alter the population's "natural" age and mortality structure). Aware of the utility of his work for business and governance alike, Halley noted his results could be used not only to regulate the valuation of annuities and price of life insurance ("it being 100 to 1 that a man of 20 dies not in a year, and only 38 to 1 for a man of 50 years of age") but also to determine the number of "fencible men" (i.e., eligible for induction into military service) (Halley, 1693, p. 483). Finding regularities in patterns of death just as astronomers found regularities in the motions of planets, Halley—along with Petty and Graunt—brought human experience into the orbit of numerical analysis (Krieger, 2000).

It was in medicine, however, that the second effort crucial to epidemiology's emerged occurred, one that enabled the counting of "cases" for disease-specific morbidity and mortality rates. At issue was the shift:

- *from* the Hippocratic conception of disease as unique person-specific humoral imbalances (as expounded in European medical texts during the prior half-millenia; *see* **Chapter 2, Textbox 2–1**),
- *to* disease as a distinct pathological entity, each with its own specific causes and treatments (Guerrini, 1989; Martin, 1990; Porter, 1997; Bynum, 2008).

Critical to this conceptual change was the work of the physician Thomas Sydenham (1624–1689), a contemporary of Petty and Graunt, who—despite ultimately challenging the basis of Hippocratic etiologic thought—was called the "English Hippocrates" by his contemporaries because of his insistence that physicians directly and meticulously observe their patients rather than rely on text-based dogma (Sydenham, 1922; Dewhurst, 1966; Cunningham, 1989; Porter, 1997; Bynum, 2008).

Sydenham's shift in the 1660s and 1670s to the view that, in his words, "all disease be reduced to definite and certain species… with the same care which we see exhibited by botanists in their phytologies" (Dewhurst, 1966, p. 60) was informed by three experiences. The first was his semi-quantitative analysis (*see* **Textbox 3–3** for a description) of 14 years' worth of London data on epidemic disease (1661–1675). Observing that different febrile diseases clustered together in different years, a phenomenon that only made sense if fevers were distinct entities, Sydenham coined the term *epidemic constitution* and sought to understand why distinct fevers did or did not exhibit the same temporal patterns (Sydenham, 1922; Dewhurst, 1966, pp. 60–61). A second experience solidifying his new disease-specific view was Sydenham's convincing demonstration that cinchona bark (a source of quinine) was successfully and uniquely suited to treating the ague (as malaria was then termed) (Dewhurst, 1966; Cunningham, 1989; Bynum, 2008). This finding challenged the idea that one type of fever could simply morph into another, because disease-specific cures implied disease-specific etiologies.

The third experience that affected Sydenham's scope of observation, however, was decidedly more social in nature and consisted of his forced change, in the 1660s, from treating more affluent to predominantly poorer patients. Precipitating this shift was the 1660 Restoration to the throne of Charles II (1630–1685), ending Oliver Cromwell's

Textbox 3–3. The Shift to Quantifying Population Rates of Disease
and Death: Reflections of William Farr (1807–1883),
the First Compiler of Medical Statistics for Newly
Established United Kingdom General Registrar's Office
(Founded in 1836), on: (a) Sydenham's Late
Seventeenth Century Efforts to Describe Disease
Occurrence in Quantitative Terms, and (b) the Study
of Disease as a Mass Phenomenon

(a) on Sydenham (Farr, 1885 [1975], p. 214):

"… Sydenham, one of the most accurate of medical writers, in speaking of small-pox, employed such terms as these: (1661) "It prevailed a little, but disappeared again."— (1667–9) "The small-pox was more prevalent in town for the first two years of this constitution than I ever remember it to have been."—(1670–2) "The small-pox arose; yielded to the dysentery; returned," &c., &c. These terms admit of no strict comparison with each other; for it is difficult to say in which year the small-pox was the most fatal, and impossible to compare Sydenham's experience thus expressed with the experience of other writers in other places and other ages; for "prevailed a little," "raged with violence," and similar terms, may imply either that small-pox destroyed, 1, or 2, or 5 or 10 per cent. of the population. The superior precision of numerical expressions is illustrated by a comparison of Sydenham's phrases with the London bills of mortality in the same years.

Deaths from small-pox in London

Years	Deaths	Years	Deaths	Years	Deaths	Years	Deaths
1661	1,246	1666	38	1671	1,465	1676	359
1662	768	1667	1,196	1672	696	1677	1,678
1663	411	1668	1,987	1673	1,116	1678	1,798
1664	1,233	1669	951	1674	853	1679	1,967
1665	655	1670	1,465	1675	2,507	1680	689

The 1,987 deaths from small-pox in 1668, and the 951 deaths from that disease in the year following, express the relative intensity of small-pox in distinct terms. The method of the parish clerks, although imperfectly carried out, was the best. Sydenham guessed the quantity with sagacity, and called it great or small; the parish clerks measured it, and stated the results in figures. The present Registrars will furnish medical science with an unbroken series of observations expressed numerically."

(b) on the study of disease as a mass phenomenon (Farr, 1837):

"Like the universe, mankind may be studied in individuals or in masses. The physiologist may take the body to pieces, separate every bone, muscle, nerve, vessel, and pursue these to their last globules, or decompose them into their elementary principles; and in every step of the analysis discover interesting facts: or he may study the successive generations of men in nations, the great results of their organization, the general laws which regulate their evolution, the modifications wrought on them by the earth, the atmosphere and the arts of civilization. Both kinds of investigations are

> necessary, but the latter invites especial attention at the present time. A stone falling to the earth, and the planets in their revolutions, obey the same law; but this law was first demonstrated in the larger masses; so in like manner it may be anticipated that the researches into the history of man, individually and collectively, will throw mutual light on each other, but that the great laws of vitality will be first discovered by observations extending over entire nations."

(1599–1658) Commonwealth, which cut Sydenham off from London's more privileged society. This was because Sydenham and his family had been supporters of Cromwell, who had, in the 1640s, led the civil war against (and ultimately executed) Charles I (1600–1649). Dissolving Parliament and declaring England to be Commonwealth, Cromwell served as its Lord Protector until his death in 1658, after which the royalist opposition gained the upper hand and successfully re-installed the monarchy in 1660 (Hill, 1972; Gaunt, 1996; Sherwood, 1997; Wilson, 1999). With this change in political fortunate, Sydenham was no longer physician to those in power but instead began treating more impoverished patients, thereby immersing him in observation of the latter's more prevalent and varied illnesses and fevers (Sydenham, 1922; Dewhurst, 1966; Cunningham, 1989). His capacity for nuanced observation, along with his openness to considering diseases to be specific, not just person-bound humoral disturbances, together informed his new nosological orientation to disease specificity, a conceptual shift essential for epidemiologists to "count cases."

Nevertheless, indicative of the profound change Sydenham's views meant for etiologic understanding and disease classification, the shift to a "universal" nomenclature for specific causes of death and disease took a full two centuries. Thus, building on various country-specific efforts that commenced in the late 1700s, it was only in 1853 that First International Statistics Congress, organized by Quetelet, hammered out the first attempt to establish a "uniform nomenclature of causes of death applicable to all countries," with its work the direct forerunner to what in 1948 officially became termed the "International Classification of Disease", under the aegis of the newly created World Health Organization (WHO; Rosen, 1958 [1993]; Eyler, 1979; Desrosières, 1998; Eknoyan, 2008; WHO, 2009).

Changing Patterns of Life, Death, and Disease: Revolutionizing Population Health.
Also contributing to growing Western European and North American interest in the contours and causes of population health were marked changes in people's ways of living and dying. One spur to the era's new quantitative health investigations were mounting outbreaks of deadly new epidemic diseases—especially yellow fever and cholera, never before encountered in Europe or the Americas. These terrifying and rapidly fatal ailments burned through fast-growing and increasingly congested cities, home to commercial ports and to squalid neighborhoods barely housing the multitudes of laborers employed in the new factories of what was dubbed, by as early as the 1820s, the "Industrial Revolution" (Smillie, 1952; Rosen, 1958 [1993]; Lilienfeld & Lilienfeld, 1977; Lilienfeld, 1980; Lilienfeld & Lilienfeld, 1982; Delaporte, 1986; Terris, 1987; Hobsbawm, 1996a; Steckel & Floud, 1997; Porter, 1999). Granted, outbreaks of assorted epidemic disease certainly had caused much misery and mortality long before the industrial era and the rural poor had long endured hardships and poor health (Rosen, 1958 [1993]; Porter, 1999). Nevertheless, the unprecedented urban concentration of people and deaths, including the appearance of new, awful, and highly fatal diseases, along with rising social unrest, further heightened levels of fear, concern, and action.

Two classic descriptions (one from the late eighteenth century, the other approaching the mid-nineteenth century) provide a vivid sense of the disease-related fears engendered in the new urban context. The first of these chronicled the United States' first major yellow fever outbreak, which occurred in 1793 in Philadelphia, then the largest city in the United States and seat of its capital (which did not move to Washington, D.C., until 1800) (Powell, 1993). As detailed by Benjamin Rush (1745–1813) (Runes, 1947; Winslow, 1952; Brock, 1990), a prominent U.S. physician and signatory of the Declaration of Independence, Philadelphia's epidemic was fierce and terrifying (Runes, 1947, pp. 404, 406, 409):

> The disease is violent and of short duration… Many people are flying from the city… You can recollect how much the loss of a single patient used to affect me. Judge then how I must feel, in hearing every morning of the death of three or four!…Thirty-eight persons have died in eleven families in nine days in Water Street, and many more in different parts of the city… Our city is a great mass of contagion….

Notably, in the course of the epidemic, Rush not only lost his sister to the disease but was himself stricken yet managed to recover.

A half-century later, the best-selling and unprecedented 1840 exposé *Promenades dans Londres* (translated as *London Journal: A Survey of London Life in the 1830s*), written by Flora Tristan (1803–1844) (Beik & Beik, 1993), reported on the stricken health-status, workplaces, neighborhoods, and homes of the new generation of factory workers and city-dwellers. Recounting the arduous work, low pay, and inadequate diet they endured, and detailing the stinking slums in which they resided, Tristan reported, "the wretches are all sickly, rachitic, debilitated; they are thin and stooped, with weak limbs, pale complexions and lifeless eyes" (Tristan, 1840 [1986], pp. 62–63). Moreover, among the 100,000 or so London women estimated to be ensnared in the city's explosive growth of exploitative prostitution, she recorded that nearly 20,000 were believed to die each year, some "in hospitals from shameful disease or pneumonia;" others, "who cannot be admitted," "die in their frightful hovels, deprived of food, medicine, care, and everything else" (Tristan, 1840 [1986], p. 79). Summing up her impressions, including the sharp contrast between the enormous power of the new industrialists and their political supporters versus the plight of the many, Tristan wrote: "In 1839 I encountered extreme poverty in the London populace; passions were high and dissatisfaction widespread" (Tristan, 1840 [1986], p. xix).

Simultaneously, the epochs' signal revolutions—the American revolution in 1776, the French revolution in 1789, the Haitian revolution of 1791—augured a turning point for Western states and their colonial possessions, rulers, and inhabitants who would be citizens, not subjects—or slaves (James, 1938 [1989]; Hobsbawm, 1996a; Krieger, 2000). To count, for purposes of representation—let alone taxation—one must be counted, and the U.S. Constitution, adopted in 1790, became the first anywhere to mandate a full and public census of population, to be held every 10 years—albeit in language that codified inequality, setting slaves equal to only three-fifths of a free person and excluding counts of American Indians (Buck, 1982; Anderson, 1988). Census data, along with vital statistics, become essential instruments for states to understand their assets and deficits, their growth and changes, variously reckoned in human, economic, and military terms (Koren, 1918; Glass, 1973; Rosen, 1974; Shaw & Miles, 1981; Cole, 2000). To facilitate computation of population statistics, governments devoted new resources to consolidate the registration of births and death and to analyze them in conjunction with the newly available census denominator data (Rosen, 1958 [1993]; Desrosières, 1998; Porter, 1999).

In other words, coincident with—if not constitutive of—the birth of epidemiology as a discipline was a profound interest—by investigators, physicians, statesman, military officers, and the broader polity alike—in connections between bodies and the body politic (Baecque, 1997; Krieger, 2000). Clearly articulating these connections was the famous essay authored in 1790 by Johann Peter Frank (1745–1821), a leading architect of European health systems and public health advisor to monarchs (Rosen, 1974; Lesky, 1976), titled "The People's Misery: The Mother of Diseases" (Frank, 1790). Delivered as a commencement speech to a class of graduating physicians, Franks' address appeared 1 year after the French Revolution of 1789. In this essay, Frank not only described in detail the disease and suffering of the rural poor (*see* excerpts in **Textbox 3–4**) but also duly warned rulers of the need for enlightened policies to prevent worsening conditions from provoking revolutionary ardor. Inadequate attention to the "body natural," in other words, could threaten the "body politick."

Debating the Determinants of Disease Distribution: Nineteenth Century Arguments

Not that an interest in links between society and health automatically translated to any single etiologic perspective. Instead, underscoring the importance of theory, the same facts of disease distribution could lend themselves to differing interpretations, whether about disease mechanisms or determinants of the population patterning of health. Illustrating this fundamental point are three pertinent parallel and interwoven critical debates that I will now briefly review—all well-known to public health historians, albeit with only the first typically receiving any mention in epidemiology textbooks. These etiologic controversies concern: (*1*) contagion versus miasma versus poverty as the cause of epidemic disease, and hence quarantine versus sanitation versus social reform as a solution; (*2*) liberal versus radical explanations of links between social class, work, economics, and disease; and (*3*) climate versus innate constitution versus colonialism versus slavery as explanations for links between race/ethnicity and health.

Poison or Filth, Contagion or Miasma, and "Predisposing" Conditions: Places, People, Polemics, Poverty, and Politics. One core etiologic debate dominating the early days of epidemiology—and a discipline-defining dispute still analyzed to this day (La Berge, 1992; Hamlin, 1998; Baldwin, 1999; Aisenberg, 1999; Bynum, 2008)—was whether "contagion" versus "miasma" explained that era's novel and horrific outbreaks of cholera and yellow fever (Hirsch, 1886; Allen, 1947; Smillie, 1952; Coleman, 1987; Rosenberg, 1987; Humphreys, 1992), along with the occurrence of those more familiar but still dreaded mass killers, such as typhus, typhoid, and scarlet fever (Hirsch, 1886; Smillie, 1955; Hays, 1998). At one extreme, the contagionists (from the Latin "con" and "tangere," to "touch together" [OED]), who were ascendant at the start of the nineteenth century, argued that epidemics resulted from direct person-to-person contact that spread invisible poisons (conceptualized as non-living, non-reproducing toxins) (Ackerknecht, 1948b; Pelling, 1978; Bynum, 2008). Citing centuries of experience with leprosy and plague as well as smallpox and syphilis (which all sides agreed were contagious), along with evidence of epidemics following military and trade routes, the contagionists sought to prevent the importation of epidemic disease. Their primary strategy was to restrict contact via quarantining ships (including their crews and cargo) and sealing off affected neighborhoods, cities, and even borders behind *cordons sanitaires* enforced by military troops. At the other extreme, proponents of miasma held that putrid organic matter arising from locally generated decaying filth (e.g., excrement, rotting food) corrupted the air, making it noxious (or "stained," per the Greek root of "miasm," "to stain or defile" (OED)), and further argued that this miasm of

Textbox 3–4. Confronting the "Misery of the People": the Compassionate Paternalism of Johann Peter Frank (1745–1821), Advisor to Eighteenth Century "Enlightened Rulers"

In "The People's Misery: Mother of Diseases," an oration Frank gave in 1790, he argued that benevolent rulers must look after the health of their population, because a sick and discontent population worn down by poverty and strenuous labor is ultimately unproductive and susceptible to disloyalty (Frank, 1790; Sigerist, 1941). Far from being a revolutionary call to arms, it is at once a cautionary, compassionate, and paternalistic text, revealing both a deep concern about the extreme deprivations and daily miseries endured by the rural poor and a fear for fate of rulers and countries that allowed such privations to endure.

Accepting that "every social class must have its own diseases determined by the different mode of living" (Frank, 1790, p. 93) and that inequalities in wealth are inevitable, Frank nevertheless disputed the fatalistic view that the poor must suffer so badly. His central thesis was that unrelenting arduous labor, combined with woefully inadequate diets and shelter, were the root causes of their high infant mortality, maternal mortality, premature aging, and early death. To Frank, it was obvious that "the human machine must break down in a very short time if food of the right kind and quantity does not replace what labor has used up every day and sweats have consumed" (p. 97).The cycle started at conception (pp. 93–94):

> Sowed in exhausted soil, the fetus has hardly drawn the first juices through the animal roots of the placenta when, without resistance, it already is shaken and torn as a result of the awful physical labor imposed upon the ill-nourished mother... How often does it not happen that the dire necessity of supporting the family compels pregnant women to undertake work that far exceeds their strength! Bent to the earth, they dig the soil relentlessly, make ditches, cut the grain under the burning rays of the southern sun, and are crushed by the enormous weights they carry with their arms and head... And yet pregnant animals are kept away from hard work entirely, lest the horses bring forth the foals and the cows the calf prematurely, to the detriment of the owner. The human females, however, who carry the germ of a citizen must die from gruesome starvation or submit their fertile bodies to the yoke... [and] often undergo childbirth in a very cold and almost open place or among the cattle.

Were the infant to survive, its health was next imperiled by poverty forcing the mother to hire themselves out as wet-nurses for wealthier women, which they did at the cost of weaning their own children too soon, feeding them instead on coarse gruel. Whatever children survived were then "compelled by their parents' poverty to get ready for too hard labors" (p. 94), with both child and parents predisposed to catch "any matter of diseases," including ailments arising "from insufficient clothing, lack of fuel, bitter frost, sooty and unclean habitations, or the filthy skin diseases due to neglect of cleanliness of the body" (p. 98). In Frank's view, their suffering ended only when their "shrunken body breaks down under the weight of so much misery" (p. 99).

Alarmed by both the health and social implications of the "misery of the common people" (p. 91), Frank warned, writing in the wake of the French Revolution, that if immiseration became too great, it "makes people ready for any vile action... extinguishes the mutual love of parents to children and children to parents... [and] destroys and throttles respect for the Ruler, for the law and even for religion" (p. 92). To "drive away the causes of disease"—"just as the sun drives away the rain" (p. 91)—rulers, acting in enlightened self-interest, must evince a "fatherly affection for even the lowest class of his subjects" (p. 91), abolish servitude, and "not let prices of vital commodities rise beyond what labor and sweat can pay" (p. 99). Frank's conclusion? (p. 90):

> Let the rulers, if they can, keep away from the borders the deadly contagion of threatening diseases! Let them place all over the provinces men distinguished in the science of medicine and surgery! Let them build hospitals and administer them more auspiciously! Let them pass regulations for the inspection of pharmacies and let them apply many other measures for the citizens' health—but let them overlook only one thing, namely, the necessity of removing or of making more tolerable the richest source of diseases, *the extreme misery of the people*, and you will hardly see any benefits from public health legislation.

unsalubrious air would, under the right atmospheric conditions, provoke epidemic disease. To the anti-contagionists, the "obvious" solution was not quarantine but rather to clean up filth. In the middle, unconvinced by the arguments and evidence of either side, were promoters of "contingent contagionism," which held that an individual's contagiousness depended on factors ranging from climate to personal predisposition (Ackerknecht, 1948b; Pelling, 1978; Delaporte, 1986; Hamlin, 1998). Still another alternative explanation, termed the *zymotic* theory, held that epidemics were caused not by general filth but rather by specific airborne non-living poisons released by the exhalations and skin of the ill (Pelling, 1978; Eyler, 1979; Porter, 1999).

Feeding the debate's fury were the myriad observations unexplained by each side's hypotheses (*see* **Textbox 3–5** for a century's worth of debate over yellow fever, as but one example) (Ackerknecht, 1948b; Pelling, 1978; Rosenberg, 1987; Delaporte, 1986; Hamlin, 1995; Hamlin, 1998; Aisenberg, 1999; Baldwin, 1999). For example, contagion could not account either for the failure of quarantine to stop the spread of yellow fever or cholera or for the simultaneous eruption of cases in different neighborhoods in a given city or different locales. Conversely, miasma left unexplained why disease migrated with sick people, why outbreaks typically started in port towns, and why persistently filthy neighborhoods only sporadically experienced epidemics. No one, moreover, had a good explanation for why only some people—not everyone—became sick during an epidemic; the general consensus was that an individual's risk reflected an interplay of exposure to "exciting causes" (i.e., whether the miasma or a specific disease-produced contagious poison) and "predisposing conditions" (e.g., pre-existing health status), which differentially rendered individuals more or less susceptible to the "exciting cause."

Indicative of how these various hypotheses were invoked to address the confusing and mixed nature of the evidence was an ingenious study conducted in 1848 by the aforementioned William Guy, in which he compared attacks of fever among different groups of workers in London. Guy's hypothesis was that workers most exposed to noxious smells would be at highest risk. His results, however, indicated that not only "the bricklayers' labourer is more than four times, and the brickmaker nearly three times as liable as to fever as the scavenger" (who collected, sorted, and disposed of street trash) but also that all three groups were at higher risk than the nightmen who removed nightsoil (i.e., excrement) from public privies and who cleaned sewers, with the respective percentages attacked by fever being 35.5%, 21.5%, 8%, and 4% (Guy, 1848). To try to make sense of these data, Guy discussed not only the occupational exposures but also who was in the different occupations, noting that bricklayers were the most poorly paid, least well-nourished, and most likely to live in the most wretched neighborhoods (in which they were exposed to foul air day and night, not just on the job).

Textbox 3–5. A Century of Miasma-Contagion Polemics: the Case of Yellow Fever, Europe, and the United States

1790s: In the United States, the 1793 Philadelphia yellow fever epidemic sparked fierce debates, affecting state politics and policy, over whether it resulted from "local origins"—that is, filth, as argued by Benjamin Rush (1746–1813) (Rush, 1809) versus imported from overseas, as argued by William Currie (1754–1828) (Currie, 1794). In response to these disputes, Noah Webster (1758–1843), the prominent intellectual of dictionary fame, researched and published, by act of Congress, an original and massive two-volume report: *A brief history of epidemic and pestilential diseases; with the principal phenomena of the physical world, which precede and accompany them, and observations deduced from the facts stated* (1799) (Webster, 1799). Preceding Villalba's *Epidemiología Española* (Villalba, 1803) by four years, the text offered one of the first systematic historical reviews of epidemic disease (Spector, 1947); in it, Webster declared he was "*convinced...* of the fallacy of the vulgar opinion, respecting the origin of the yellow fever in the United States, from imported sources" (Webster, 1799, pp. vii–viii).

1807: Struck by the spotty and seasonal distribution of the disease, a small minority of physicians, such as John Crawford (1746–1813) of Baltimore, speculated that insects, such as the mosquito, might somehow transmit the disease (Mitchell, 1948[1977]; Allen, 1947).

1819: The eminent British naval physician, Sir Gilbert Blane (1749–1834) published a major text presenting "a statement of the evidence respecting the contagious nature of the yellow-fever" (Blane, 1819), in which he argued that outbreaks always originated in port towns, could be traced to the arrival of specific ships, and could be deterred by quarantine.

1820: New York City's appointed resident physician, David Hosack, argued filth was not a necessary or sufficient cause of yellow fever, but nevertheless recommended sanitary measures because filth could increase vulnerability to contagion (Hosack, 1820). Noting that yellow-fever broke out in clean ships carrying only loads of salt and yet often was absent among horrendously filthy boats, Hosack indignantly asked: "Are the investigations and accumulated experience of Huxham, Haygarth, Currie, Gregory, Ferriar, Percival, Blane, Chisholm, M'Gregor, Pym, Gilpin, Wright, and a host of others, to be prostrated by the arrogant assertions, the overweening conceits, and flippant remarks of those juniors in knowledge and in years, who have lately obtruded themselves upon the public attention?" (Hosack, 1820, p. 9).

1822: The first serious threat to Europe by yellow fever, following a major outbreak of yellow fever in Barcelona that killed between 5,000 to 20,000 of the city's 100,000 inhabitants (Coleman, 1987, pp. 25–27); this outbreak led the French government to enact, on March 3, 1822, its first comprehensive quarantine law to defend the nation's boundaries from imported contagious disease; the penalty for transgressing this law was death (Aisenberg, 1999; Delaporte, 1986).

1827: Nicholas Chervin (1783–1843), a prominent French physician, submitted a massive report, containing 602 supporting documents, to the French Académie de Médicine, in which he argued that a miasmatic hypothesis fit the facts best (Académié de Médicine, 1828); the evidence he presented and the ensuing debate (Chervin, 1827; Chervin, 1828) led the Académie to concur with Chervin and to recommend the repeal of France's quarantine legislation (Académié de Médicine, 1828).

1828: The French government repealed quarantine, paving the way for other states to do likewise; the Académie awarded Chervin the Grand Prix de Médicine for his work (Ackerknecht, 1948b).

1851: The world's first international sanitary conference was held in Paris; working under a miasmatic framework, its participants advocated sanitary reform and developed a new international sanitary code free of what they deemed to be obsolete and irrelevant quarantine laws (Rosen, 1958 [1993], pp. 268–269).

1880s: The Cuban physician Carlos Finlay (1833–1915) produced empirical and experimental evidence favoring the mosquito transmission hypothesis, which addressed such puzzles as the disease's climatic affinities and patchy pattern of spread (Finlay, 1881, in Buck et al., 1988, pp. 60–66).

1890s: Building on Finlay's work, the U.S. physician Walter Reed (1851–1902), as part of his investigations of high yellow fever mortality among U.S. troops stationed in Cuba during the 1898 Spanish-American war, conclusively demonstrated the role of the mosquito in transmitting yellow fever and also hypothesized that the presumed microbial cause was in fact a virus (one that was eventually isolated in the late 1920s) (Porter, 1997, pp. 472–475; Coleman, 1987, pp. 1–24).

Adding to the intensity of the miasma-contagion debate were its social, political, and economic ramifications, as argued and recognized at the time (Ackerknecht, 1948b; Pelling, 1978; Delaporte, 1986; Rosenberg, 1987; Hamlin, 1995; Hamlin, 1998; Aisenberg, 1999; Baldwin, 1999). "Contagion," invoking the metaphor of invasion, implied the need for a strong military, regulated trade, and quarantine—the last of which imposed costs on commerce and invited riots when forced on restive working class neighborhoods (McDonald, 1951; Delaporte, 1986; Rosenberg, 1987; Porter, 1999; Aisenberg, 1999). "Miasma," by contrast, pointed to a local disturbance resulting from local filth and corruption (literally, of the air; metaphorically, of politics) and called for installing sewage systems, relocating slaughterhouses outside of cities, preventing goods from accumulating and rotting at wharves, improving ventilation in people's homes, and encouraging higher standards for personal hygiene (Ackerknecht, 1948b; Pelling, 1978; Delaporte, 1986; Rosenberg, 1987; Hamlin, 1995; Hamlin, 1998; Aisenberg, 1999; Baldwin, 1999). Moreover, within both camps, sharp divisions existed over whether it was sufficient to tackle the "exciting causes" versus also being necessary to reckon with the "predisposing conditions" that respectively weakened bodily "defenses" and "integrity." Vehement arguments likewise existed over whether the poor's greater susceptibility to epidemic disease resulted from individual immorality or social injustice (Ackerknecht, 1948b; Delaporte, 1986; Rosenberg, 1987; Hamlin, 1998).

Exemplifying the economic case against contagion was the 1824 tome, *Evils of Quarantine Laws, and Non-Existence of Pestilential Contagion; Deduced from the Phaenomena of the Plague of the Levant, the Yellow Fever of Spain, and the Cholera Morbus of Asia* (Maclean, 1824), written by the anti-contagionist English physician Charles Maclean (1788–1824) (Pelling, 1978). Arguing "There is not upon record a single instance of sanitary regulations having, even in appearance, proved efficient for their proposed ends," he chastised the English government for quarantining on average 700 boats per year between 1815 and 1823, resulting in what he deemed a needless loss of more than 100,000 pounds annually (caused by "tear and wear of ships, cordage, and rigging, wages and maintenance of crews, damage, deterioration and pilferage of cargoes, &c."). Maclean's blunt conclusion?—"SANITARY LAWS ARE A SOURCE OF GRATUITOUS EXPENSE AND VEXATION TO AN ENORMOUS AMOUNT" and "OUGHT TO BE FORTHWITH ABOLISHED" (Maclean, 1824, pp. 253–259; uppercase in the original). So explicit were these economic arguments that John Snow (1813–1858), in an 1853 pamphlet elaborating his then-new (1849) theory of cholera being a water-borne disease transmitted by a parasitic micro-organism present in the feces of infected persons (Snow, 1853; Frost, 1936; Lillienfeld, 2000), was compelled to observe (Snow, 1853, pp. 173–174):

> The question of contagion in various diseases has often been discussed with a degree of acrimony that is unusual in medical or other scientific inquiries... The cause of the warmth of feeling... is the great pecuniary interests involved in the question, on account of its connection with quarantine [and the millions of pounds] jeopardised by quarantine.

Taking the anti-contagionist economic logic one step farther, Edwin Chadwick (1800–1890) (Lewis, 1952; Rosen, 1958 [1993]; Porter, 1999), author of Great Britain's draconian 1834 Poor Law (Englander, 1998) (whose wretched workhouses were immortalized in Charles Dickens' *Oliver Twist*), argued in his extraordinarily influential 1842 *Report on the Sanitary Condition of the Labouring Population of Great Britain* (Flinn, 1965) that the sanitary approach could even end up reducing government costs in the long-term. To Chadwick, the excess disease and death resulting from filth-related disease imposed shocking costs—on government and business (the foci of his concerns). Tallying the impact of illness on both poor relief and workers' productivity, he wrote (Flinn, 1965, p. 223):

> It is an appalling fact that, of all who are born of the labouring classes in Manchester, more than 57 per cent die before they attain five years of age; that is, before they can be engaged in factory labour, or in any other labour whatsoever.

Chadwick's central premise was that filth breeds sickness, sickness breeds unemployment, and unemployment breeds poverty. Two corollaries were: (*1*) poverty was not a cause of disease (but instead was at best a correlate, if not an outcome, of poor health), and (*2*) abolishing filth through adequate sewage systems should simultaneously reduce sickness and the number of impoverished and their dependence on state-administered relief and charity; no other anti-poverty measures were needed (Hamlin, 1998). Linking his economic liberalism (i.e., belief in the free market and limited government regulation) to social conservativism, Chadwick further believed, as did many of his contemporaries, that immorality was antecedent to both filth and poverty. Capturing this view were the comments Chadwick included in his report, from one Reverend Whitewell Elwin of Bath, who, describing an 1837 smallpox outbreak that "carried off upwards of 300 persons," observed (Flinn 1965, pp. 234–235):

> ... yet of all this number I do not think there was a single gentleman, and not above two or three tradesmen. The residences of the labouring classes were pretty equally visited, disease showing here and there a predilection for particular spots, with full virulence in Avon-street... the very place which every person acquainted with Bath would have predicted... Everything vile and offensive is congregated there. All the scum of Bath—its low prostitutes, its thieves, its beggars... this mass of physical and moral evils... whatever contagious or epidemic disease prevailed,— fever, small-pox, influenza—this (Avon-street) was the scene of its principal ravages...

Lemuel Shattuck's (1793–1859) classic *Report of a General Plan for the Promotion of Public and Personal Health... Relating to a Sanitary Survey of the State; The Shattuck Report* (1850), the United States' first comprehensive public health report (Shattuck, 1850 [1948]), likewise linked immorality, filth, and disease (Rosenkrantz, 1972). Like Chadwick, Shattuck's argument was that both sanitation and moral instruction were required to prevent the filth and epidemics arising from "an adult population, short-lived, improvident, reckless, intemperate, immoral, and with excessive desires for sensuous gratification" (Shattuck, 1850 [1948], p. 48).

The view that moral depravity drove risk of disease, however, was not unique to anti-contagionists; contagionists shared it too. Writing in 1833, the contagionist U.S. physician Bernard Byrne (1807–1860) commented, "it is scarcely necessary to observe, that intemperance in drinking is another very general, and very powerful exciting cause of cholera" (Byrne, 1833, p. 129). His stance was indistinguishable from that of the anti-contagionist French physician Henry Boulay de la Meurthe (1797–1858) (Delaporte, 1986), who during the 1832 Parisian cholera epidemic posited its greater toll on the poor resulted from their excessive drinking (Boulay de La Meurthe, 1832, p. 78). Thus, according to de la Meurthe, cholera principally afflicted "individuals subject to bad habits or ways of living, who cannot or will not take advantage of the sound advice being offered them" (Boulay de la Meurthe, 1832, p. 116).

By contrast, other investigators of more socially liberal or even radical persuasion—mainly miasmatists but also some contagionists—respectively held that that filth and contagion mattered, but only as one step in a causal pathway leading from economic exploitation to ill health (Delaporte, 1986; Hamlin, 1995; Hamlin, 1998). Pointing to the primacy of economic conditions in the timing of epidemic outbreaks, for example, in 1839 Somerville Scott Alison (1813–1877), an anti-contagionist physician who attended poor miners and their families in a small Scottish mining town (Alison, 1839; Alison, 1840a; Hamlin, 1995), reasoned (Alison, 1839, p. 142):

> The occurrence of typhus fever among the labouring classes of this country, which is observed every winter, but more especially on those occasions when provisions, the necessaries of life, are high in price, when employment is with difficulty obtained, and when the wages are low, sufficiently attests to the fact that scanty food is a powerful cause of disease, and one of a widely extended range of action.

Notably, his views on the importance of poverty were shared by one of his contagionist contemporaries, the Edinburgh physician William Pulteney Alison (1790–1859) (Alison, 1844; Stephen & Lee, 1921–22; Pelling, 1978; Hamlin, 1995). Based on his experiences taking care of working class patients, Alison (the contagionist) held that his patients' impoverishment was not chiefly a result of "misconduct" (i.e., immoral behavior, as invoked by Chadwick, Shattuck, and others) but rather "misfortune" (e.g., factories precipitously closing), and he likewise challenged Chadwick's view that sanitation alone would end epidemic disease (or poverty). Instead, viewing impoverishment as a correctable factor that facilitated transmission of and susceptibility to contagious disease, in 1840 Alison (the contagonist) wrote (Alison 1840b, p. 12):

> I have had many opportunities observing that, among the most destitute of the people in Edinburg, fever often spreads rapidly in situations as well ventilated and as far removed from any filth, external to the inhabited rooms, as can be desired. For example, in the highest stories of some of the highest houses in the vicinity of the High-street (particularly at Covenant-close, Dickson's-close, and Skinner's-close), I have seen numerous and rapid successions of fever cases originating from individual patients; while even at the same time, in the lower parts of the common stairs, worse ventilated and nearer to the collections of filth to be founds in the closets, but which are inhabited by people better employed and in more comfortable circumstances, fever has not appeared nor has it spread.

Indeed, because of his overall concern about the deplorable conditions in which the poor were forced to live, Alison, despite being a staunch contagionist, supported removal of filth. Why? To Alison, one Dr. Bancroft (whom he quoted approvingly), said it well: "I hope that we shall always find it within ourselves sufficient motives to remove or avoid filthiness, even when convinced that it does not produce contagious fever" (Alison, 1840b, p. 3).

Calling for even more radical steps, in 1848 the radical anti-contagionist Rudolf Virchow (1821–1902), a founder of both "social medicine" and cellular pathology—to which he brought the powerful and novel metaphor of the body as a "republic of cells" (Ackerknecht 1953; Rosen 1974; Waitzkin, 1981; Rather, 1985)—published his classic analysis of a typhus epidemic then devastating Upper Silesia, an extremely poor and Polish-speaking province of Germany (Virchow 1848a). Deeming typhus a filth-generated and non-contagious disease (Virchow, 1848a, p. 278), Virchow vividly described the afflicted population's destitution, illiteracy, and political disenfranchisement. Concluding that the immiseration of the Upper Silesian populace simultaneously was imposed by and enriched the region's small but wealthy and powerful landed gentry, Virchow polemically asked (Ackerknecht 1953, p. 126):

> Don't crowd diseases point everywhere to deficiencies of society? One may adduce atmospheric or cosmic conditions or similar factors. But never do they alone make epidemics. They produce them only where due to bad social conditions people have lived for some time in abnormal conditions.

To Virchow, solving the epidemic and preventing future ones required no less than establishing "full and unlimited democracy" (Virchow, 1848a, p. 307).

Nevertheless, 35 years later, the eminent epidemiologist August Hirsch (1817–1894)—whose magnum opus, the encyclopedic *Handbook of Geographical and Historical Pathology* (Hirsch, 1883), presented exhaustive evidence on how disease rates varied by "time and place," as influenced by differences in climate, soil, animal and plant life, and "the vicissitudes of politics, of social affairs, of the food-supply, and of mental training" (Hirsch, 1883, p. 2) (*see* excerpt in **Textbox 3–6**)—although sympathetic to Virchow's analysis, held that typhus was clearly a contagious disease. Totally agreeing that typhus epidemics were occasioned by "*the state of want brought about by the failure of the crops, commercial crisis, war, and other far-reaching calamities*" (italics in original) (Hirsch, 1883, p. 578), and even citing Virchow's analysis of the "typhus epidemic of 1847–48 in Upper Silesia" (Hirsch, 1883, p. 579), Hirsch simultaneously declared that "(t)here can be no question, on the part of anyone, that the typhus counts among the exquisitely contagious diseases" (Hirsch, 1883, p. 591). To Hirsch, there was no contradiction between stating, on the one hand, that "the specific poison of the disease reproduces itself within the sick body, and is eliminated therefrom in a perfect state of potency" (Hirsch, 1883, p. 591) and, on the other, that "(i)t is always and everywhere the wretched conditions of living, which spring from poverty and are fostered by ignorance, laziness, and helplessness, in which typhus takes root and finds nourishment; and it is above all in *the want of cleanliness, and in the overcrowding of dwellings, that are ventilated badly or not at all and tainted with corrupt effluvia of every kind*" (italics in the original) (Hirsch, 1883, p. 581) (*see* excerpt in **Textbox 3–6**).

In other words, as highlighted in **Textbox 3–7**, support for a specific disease mechanism—whether contagion or miasma—did not by itself dictate the approach taken to analyzing disease distribution or explanations offered for the disproportionate burden on the poor. As the physician-historian Erwin H. Ackernecht famously first argued in 1948 (Ackerknecht, 1948b) and others have elaborated since (Pelling, 1978; Coleman, 1987;

Textbox 3–6. August Hirsch's (1817–1894) Magnum Opus: *Handbook of Geographical and Historical Pathology. Volume I.* Translated from the second German edition by Charles Creighton, M.D. London: The New Sydenham Society, 1883—general framework and specific analysis of typhus.

General Framework

pp. 1–2: "The life of the organic world is the expression of a process called forth and sustained, in organisms that are capable of life, by the sum of all the influences which act upon them from without. The form and fashion of this process, accordingly, are determined by the kind of individuality and by the character of the environment. Each of those two factors shows many differences in time and space. As regards the human species, the differences are expressed, for the first factor, in the distinctive qualities of generations separated by the years, and of races and nationalities scattered over the globe; for the second factor, they are expressed in peculiarities of the climate and the soil, and of the animal and vegetable kingdoms in so far as these are brought into direct relation with man, and further, in the vicissitudes of politics, of social affairs, of the food-supply, and of mental training.

In these considerations lie the germs of a science, which, in an ideally complete form, would furnish a *medical history of mankind* [*sic*](italics in the original)... And this science I have named, from the dominating point of view, the science of *geographical and historical pathology* (italics in the original)."

p. 6: "In arranging the subjects treated of in this work I have followed the order at present in general use of classification of disease. I accordingly distinguish: (1) Acute infective diseases; (2) Chronic infective and constitutional diseases; (3) Diseases of organs."

Analysis of typhus:

p. 545: "The *history of typhus* is written in those dark pages of the world's story, which tell of the grievous visitations of mankind by war, famine, and misery of every kind."

pp. 547–574: summary of typhus occurrence, as epidemic and endemic disease in every nation for which data was available, from 16th through 19th century, and associations with poverty, war, and famine.

pp. 574–578: summary of data on typhus occurrence in relation to climate and soil, noting that although it has been documented more in temperate versus tropical countries, and in colder versus warmer months, nevertheless "typhus is quite independent of *season* and *weather* in its development and epidemic diffusion" (p. 577), with the text cautioning "It follows from the prevalence of the disease in Persia, and the epidemics that have been observed in Tunis, Algiers, and Nicaragua–to mention only well-established facts–that the doctrine which used to be held, of the palm-zone and regions with an isotherm of 68°F. (20°C.) and upwards enjoying a complete immunity from typhus, is not universally applicable" (p. 575).

pp. 578–589: text summarizing the associations between epidemic typhus with "a time of want" (p. 578), noting that "When we inquire into the influence exerted by the state of social well-being on the production of typhus, there is always one fact forcing itself into the foreground, which has arrested the chief attention of observers at every period, viz. *the coincidence in time between epidemics of typhus and the state of want brought about by failure of the crops, commercial crisis, war, and other far-reaching calamities* (original in italics) (p. 578). Noting, however, that '[f]amine and typhus... have no necessary connexion as cause and effect, as Virchow has already pointed out in his history of the typhus epidemic of 1847–48 in Upper Silesia,' nevertheless '[t]he typhus poison... finds a particularly suitable soil wherein to develop and acquire potency in a populace reduced by hunger; but that detriment only amounts to a material predisposing factor of disease, and will make itself felt all the more where other lowering causes have been reducing the power of resistance in the individual at the same time (pp. 580–581).

p. 581: "It is always and everywhere the wretched conditions of living, which spring from poverty and are fostered by ignorance, laziness, and helplessness, in which typhus takes root and finds nourishment; and it is above all in *the want of cleanliness, and in the overcrowding of dwellings, that are ventilated badly or not at all and tainted with corrupt effluvia of every kind*" (italics in the original).

p. 591: "There can be no question, on the part of anyone, that typhus counts among the exquisitely contagious diseases, or, in other words, that the specific poison of the disease reproduces itself within the sick body, and is eliminated therefrom in a perfect state of potency."

Hamlin, 1998; Aisenberg, 1999; Baldwin, 1999; Rosenberg, 2009), the triumph of anti-contagionism by the mid-nineteenth century (shortly before its overthrow by germ theory) had less to do with undisputable evidence than it did with the impact of liberal economic and political opposition to quarantine, along with reformist responses to the deepening immiseration and rising agitation of the growing urban working class and slum-dwellers. The debate accordingly was never just solely about the etiologic mechanisms of epidemic disease. After all, as contemporary research on molecular microbial pathogenesis makes clear (Pier, 2008), both sides partially had it "right" but for the wrong reasons. Thus, depending on the actual infectious agent at issue (whether a self-replicating bacteria, virus, parasite, or prion, as opposed to inert poison) and its specific mode of transmission (e.g., by air [inhalation], water or food [ingestion], or direct contact of skin or mucosal mem-branes with the excrement, saliva, or genital secretions of symptomatic or asymptomatic infectious persons [including "carriers"]), or via skin injury and injection [e.g., by animal vectors such as mosquito and lice, or by animal bite or needle stick])—sometimes cleaning up "filth" would have been effective, sometimes quarantine would have helped, and some-times neither measure would have been of any use. Rather, the dispute's core debates about disease distribution—as a function of individual versus societal defects—extended to all maladies, not just epidemic disease.

Liberal Versus Radical Explanations of Links Between Social Class, Work, Economics and Disease: Explaining Broader Health Inequities. As a parallel example, consider the simultaneous debates over whether the new political economy of the factory system—and its working conditions—threatened health and, if so, whether these new hazards could be averted within or only outside of a laissez-faire free market system. At issue were the causes and distributions of non-epidemic diseases, which, along with injuries and violence, constituted the bulk of conditions producing morbidity and death—and additionally and unduly burdened the poor, both working and unemployed (Rosen, 1958 [1993]; Porter, 1999). Once again, different theories of disease distribution entailed different approaches to and understandings of the data. Continuing the shift from natural to social metaphors, and from naturally-produced to socially-produced disease mechanisms, these investiga-tors sought to understand how the changing nature of work, poverty, and human-made environs affected health (Krieger & Birn, 1998). Just as factories produced goods, and

Textbox 3–7. An Example of When Social Analyses of Disease Distribution do not Map Precisely onto Postulated Disease Mechanisms: the Heterogeneous Political Affinities of the Supporters of Both the Miasma and Contagionist Hypotheses—and Also the Prevailing Common Sense...

Social group	Miasma	Contagion
Health professionals	Liberal epidemiologists who saw themselves as enlightened researchers using the best evidence available, open to shedding outmoded ideas and their unnecessary restrictions on individual liberties.	Seasoned civilian and military physicians who believed the evidence (let alone common sense) showed that epidemic diseases were spread by direct person-to-person contact, with epidemics migrating along trade routes and with war.
Economic and political elites	The new class of industrial capitalists, who called for abolition of quarantine under the banner of unrestricted free trade and commerce.	Political conservatives who supported governmental authority to institute quarantine, regulate commerce, and constrain individual liberties.
Advocates of the poor and working class	Advocates of the poor, including physicians, researchers, reformers, and the newly organizing urban working class, who campaigned against wretched working conditions and abysmal and filthy living conditions, including lack of sanitation, reflecting immiseration due to starvation wages and exorbitant rents, plus government incompetence and corruption for not removing waste.	A handful of proponents of the poor, who argued—like the liberal and radical advocates of miasma theory—that greed of factory owners (via low pay) and of landlords (via high rents) combined to produce a destitute, hungry, and weakened population living in overcrowded abysmal lodgings, overripe for passing along and succumbing to contagious disease.
Social conservatives	Social conservatives who viewed immorality as the chief cause of filth and poverty, with filth being the cause of epidemic disease and poverty its non-causal correlate.	Conservative moralists who believed that innate immorality is the reason why the poor are poor and live in crowded unsanitary households conducive to passing disease by direct transmission.

Prevailing common sense: From the perspective of the general public, these learned disputes over corrupted air vs contagious poison and exciting vs predisposing causes nevertheless boiled down to one logical response: when epidemic disease hits, flee town (noting that, typically, only the affluent had the means to do so).

Note: for examples of historians' changing views of and analyses about the miasma-contagion debates and their complex relationships to political perspectives and economic interests, *see* Ackerknecht, 1948a and 1948b, Richmond, 1954, Rosenberg, 1962 [1987], Hamlin, 1995, Tomes, 1997, Hamlin, 1998, Porter, 1999, and Rosenberg, 2009.

politicians produced policies, so too did society produce health—and disease. Increasing mechanization invited thinking about disease mechanisms in increasingly human-made, and not just natural, terms. Transforming societal conditions and economic policies from "predisposing conditions" into "causes," a new raft of investigators brought into play a key new etiologic actor: society itself. Part and parcel of epidemiology's emergence was the birth of what would now be termed *social epidemiology*, whose various and competing schools of thought explored the promising realm of *political arithmetik* that Petty had first glimpsed a century and a half before.

Among the earliest and foremost investigators linking population health to political economy was Louis René Villermé (1782–1863), a French physician and liberal supporter of the free market who, in the post-Napoleonic period between 1820 and 1840, published landmark studies on wealth, work, and health—and who, in 1829, co-founded one of the world's first public health journals, *Annales d'hygiène publique et de médecine légale* (Ackerknecht, 1948b; Coleman, 1982; La Berge, 1992; Weir, 1997; Cole, 2000). Representing the dominant view in the field, his myriad pathbreaking investigations influenced science and policy alike (*see* selected examples in **Textbox 3–8**). From the standpoint of epidemiologic theory, two particularly stand out for their original theorizing and novel data: an 1826 study on neighborhoods, wealth, and mortality (Villermé, 1826) and an 1840 landmark volume on the health of factory workers, the first of its kind (Villermé, 1840).

Villermé's 1826 study innovatively combined recently amassed and unprecedented Parisian census data with 1817 to 1821 mortality data to demonstrate empirically, for the first time for any city anywhere, the surprising and novel finding that variations in annual mortality rates across neighborhoods (even in non-epidemic years) were patterned not by the "natural environment" of Hippocratic doctrine but instead by poverty and wealth (*see* data excerpted from the study in **Table 3–1**) (Villermé, 1826; Coleman, 1982, pp. 149–163). His discovery was that death rates were highest among areas whose residents paid the least in "untaxed rents," a type of tax paid only by the wealthy (**Table 3–1**) and exhibited a continuous socioeconomic gradient (one rediscovered with some fanfare 170 years later [Krieger, 2001a]). Three years later, Villermé found similar results for short stature (including relative leg length), illness, and deformities (**Table 3–1**) (Villermé 1829). His interpretation? Body size, body proportions, and longevity, far from being fixed or shaped only by natural environs, instead bore the imprint of economic conditions and could be affected by government policies (Coleman, 1982; Krieger & Davey Smith, 2004). No longer could the causes of disease or their distribution be found solely in the natural world; the social world also profoundly mattered.

Villermé's 1840 two-volume 850-plus page opus, *Tableau de l'état physique et moral des ouvriers employés dans les manufactures de coton, de laine et de soie* ("A description of the physical and moral state of workers employed in cotton, wool, and silk mills") (Villermé, 1840) in turn took on the fiercely debated question as to whether factory workers' poor health (which no one disputed) was caused by factory work *per se* or by a low standard of living. Marveling at mechanization (Villermé, 1840, Tome I, pp. 2–3), Villermé ultimately exonerated workplace hazards, including dust, air, noise, temperature, and type of physical labor. He instead attributed workers' poor health to "forced labor, lack of rest, carelessness, inadequate food of poor quality, and habits of improvidence, drunkenness, and debauchery; to put it all in a single phrase, by salaries below the real needs [of life]" (Villermé, 1840, Tome II, p. 209; Coleman, 1982, p. 230). To Villermé, neither the factory system nor factory work were inherently "insalubrious"—at least not any more so than other essential yet unhealthy occupations (such as mining, cleaning sewers, or skinning and pelting rabbits). Indeed, in Villermé's view, the factory jobs constituted a marked improvement over the grim lot of poor rural laborers so vividly described by Frank (*see* **Textbox 3–4**) and others

Textbox 3–8. Early Liberal Social Epidemiology: Selected Studies of—and Theoretical Arguments Explored by—Louis René Villermé (1782–1863)

Date	Study
1826	Villermé's pathbreaking study, innovatively linked newly amassed Parisian census data and mortality data to show, for the first time ever, that neighborhood mortality rates varied by wealth and poverty (**Table 3–1**), and not by the "airs, waters, places" predicted by Hippocratic hypotheses (such as exposure to sunlight (or lack thereof), proximity to the Seine, wind patterns, and presence of trees and parks, none of which were correlated with neighborhood mortality rates) (Villermé, 1826; Coleman, 1982, pp. 149–163). Villermé noted that future research would need to determine if the observed socioeconomic differentials in mortality rates were caused by standard of living, type of work, dissolute behavior, or all three combined (Villermé, 1826, p. 235).
1828	In the first issue of a new journal published by France's newly founded Royal Academy of Medicine, *Mémoires de l'Académie royale de medicine*, Villermé presented one of the world's first life expectancy tables that explicitly compared longevity in economically poor vs rich administrative regions (Villermé, 1828). The data conclusively demonstrated that the poor die younger, a fact Villermé attributed to their lacking the necessities of life; he conducted this study to address a contemporary debate over who dies sooner: the poor, because of deprivation, or the rich, because of dissipation.
1829	In the first issue of *Annales d'hygiène publique et de médicine légale*, which Villermé helped found (Coleman, 1982, p. 20), he published one of the first studies showing associations between short height and economic deprivation, in which he creatively employed data from military records never before used for empirical research (Villermé, 1829); based on these data, Villermé inferred that economic deprivation and inadequate nutrition in childhood led to both short height and poor health as an adult.
1833	In one of the first-ever published reviews on socioeconomic inequalities in health, Villermé summarized available evidence on secular trends in frequency of epidemics, mortality from epidemics, and mortality during non-epidemic years, and concluded that those with the best health had the highest standard of living, for both between- and within-country comparisons (Villermé, 1833). Villermé interpreted these findings as refuting the still-influential beliefs of the Enlightenment philosopher Jean Jacques Rousseau (1712–1778), who had argued that "civilization" harmed health (Rousseau, 1755; Rosenberg, 1998); to Villermé, the data made clear that health derived from a "state of civilization" and disease from "barbarism" and want (Villermé, 1833, p. 55).
1840	Villermé published the world's first comprehensive study of factory workers: *Tableau de l'état physique et moral des ouvriers employés dans les manufactures de coton, de laine et de soie* ("A description of the physical and moral state of workers employed in cotton, wool, and silk mills") (Villermé, 1840; Coleman, 1982, pp. 205–238), in which he attributed workers' poor health to low wages and "improvident" habits, rather than to factory work *per se*; his conclusion was that economic growth unleashed by an unregulated free market was the best route for improving workers' health.

Table 3–1. Villermé's Data on Socioeconomic Gradients in Paris for Average Annual Mortality Among the Total Population (1817–1821) and for Height Among Military Recruits (1816–1823), by a Neighborhood Measure of Wealth (Percent Untaxed Rents, With Taxed Rents Paid Only by the Wealthy)

Arrondisement (neighborhood)	Population in 1817	% untaxed rents	Average annual mortality: total population		Average height (m): military conscripts (young men, 18–21 y)
			proportion	rate per 100,000*	
2 (wealthiest)	65,623	7	1 in 62	1612.9	1.688
3	44,932	11	1 in 60	1666.7	1.690
1	52,421	11	1 in 60	1666.7	1.690
4	46,624	15	1 in 58	1724.1	1.680
11	51,766	19	1 in 51	1960.8	1.678
6	72,682	21	1 in 54	1851.8	1.678
5	56,871	22	1 in 53	1785.7	1.681
7	56,245	22	1 in 52	1923.1	1.683
10	81,133	23	1 in 50	2000.0	1.689
9	42,932	31	1 in 44	2272.7	1.680
8	62,758	32	1 in 43	2325.6	1.681
12 (poorest)	80,079	38	1 in 43	2325.6	1.679

* In original table: presented only as a proportion
Villermé, 1826; Villermé, 1829; Krieger & Davey Smith, 2004

(Villermé, 1840, Tome I, pp. 1–33, Tome II, pp. 342–354). In accord with his liberal beliefs, Villermé's solution to factory workers' poor health was improved morals and higher wages, which he held would result from the economic growth uniquely afforded by a flourishing private sector free from government interference (Villermé, 1840, Tome II, pp. 355–373). Villermé nevertheless did part company with his liberal laissez-faire contemporaries on one issue: He strongly supported government prohibition of child labor. His argument was that schooling enhanced children's moral instruction and physical development, thereby leading to a healthier and more sober workface; moreover, without a government ban, economic competition would ruin those benevolent employers who expended more to improve children's working conditions (Coleman, 1982; Weissbach, 1989; Nardinelli, 1990). Villermé's work, in conjunction with other reformers, led to France passing its first comprehensive child labor legislation in 1841, which banned employment of children under age 8 years, regulated work hours and work conditions for children ages 8 through 16 years, and required proof that working children under 12 years were enrolled in school (Coleman, 1982; Weissbach, 1989).

The alternative competing view, labeled in the language of the day as *radical* or *proletarian* (OED; Williams, 1985), both re-interpreted and supplemented the kinds of data that economic liberals, like Villermé and also Chadwick, presented in their reports. Rejecting static and moralistic analyses, they posited that the poorer health of the urban and rural poor was the outcome of unjust class relations, whereby the new and rapidly expanding system of industrial capitalism, as it was then termed (Williams, 1985; Hobsbawm, 1996b), inherently produced great wealth for the few at the cost of impoverishing and destroying the health of the many (noting that recent late twentieth century analyses support the claim that the first generation of industrial workers, in the 1840s, did experience a decline in standard of living that was reflected in both a reduction of height and a stagnation of mortality rates (Steckel & Floud, 1997; Szreter, 1997)).

One classic work articulating the radical perspective is *The Condition of the Working Class in England*, written in 1844 by Friedrich Engels (1820–1895) and published 1 year later, first in Germany, then in England (Engels, 1845 [1958]; Marcus, 1974; Wheen, 1999). Focused on "how industralisation has affected their [the workers'] bodily, intellectual, and moral conditions" (Engels, 1845 [1958], p. 108), Engels drew not only on official government health reports and scientific studies but also on information about workers' wages and expenditures, industrialists' profits, "the attitude of the bourgeoisie" (including their contempt for workers and the poor), and "working-class movements," supplemented by observations he made during his time in England, "seeing for myself how the proletariat lives" (Engels, 1845 [1958], pp. 3–4). More than half the book focused on the health of workers' and their families.

Throughout, the text employed an historical perspective, from its opening pages, which traced the origins of the "English working classes" to the mid-eighteenth century rise of the "Industrial Revolution" (Engels, 1845 [1958], pp. 9–26), on through Engels' observation that "the sufferings of children are indelibly stamped on the adults," leaving "traces that are never wholly removed" (Engels, 1845 [1958], p. 115). Not only the facts of deprivation but also their underlying class dynamics were of concern. For example, in addition to documenting workers' wretched and inadequate diet, Engels investigated the realities of food shopping, finding that (Engels 1845(1958), p. 80):

> ... Most workers can only get to the market on Saturdays at four, five or even 7 o'clock in the evening, and by that time the best food has been purchased in the morning by the middle classes. When the market opens, there is an ample supply of good food, but by the time the worker arrives the best has gone. But even if it were still there, he probably could not afford to buy it. The potatoes purchased by the workers are generally bad, the vegetables shriveled, the cheese stale and of poor quality, the bacon rancid. The meat is lean, old, tough and partially tainted...

Observing that in Manchester, "the premature ageing of the working-class population is so universal that practically all operatives in their forties look between ten and fifteen years older than this" (Engels, 1845 [1958], p. 180), he systematically compiled evidence on the exposures and policies that would yield these bodily effects.

Unlike Chadwick's and Villermé's reports, which respectively ignored or downplayed workplace hazards, Engels provided vivid descriptions of myriad illnesses and early deaths resulting from dangerous conditions at work (*see* **Textbox 3–9**). Recognizing that workers were impelled to compete constantly for poorly paying jobs, given the continual threats of unemployment and starvation (Engels, 1845 [1958], pp. 88–103), he delineated specific hazards affecting workers in a variety of trades, ranging from textile workers to potters to miners and metal grinders (Engels, 1848 [1958], pp. 184–185, 223–234, 275–284). He also described particular hazards harming children and pregnant women (Engels, 1845 [1958], pp. 169, 182–183, 237–238) and more general hazards resulting from shift work (Engels, 1845 [1958], p. 170), standing on one's feet all day (Engels, 1845 [1958], pp. 174, 181–182), and boredom coupled with the noise inherent in operating machinery (Engels, 1845 [1958], pp. 199–200). To Engels, it was no surprise that workers turned to alcohol and other stimulants in response the degrading, demoralizing, and disgusting conditions they endured at

Textbox 3–9. Observations, Inference, and Verdict: the Radical Perspective of *The Condition of the Working Class in England* (1845) (Engels, 1845 [1958]).

Observations:

Enduring effects of childhood deprivation: "Common observation shows how the sufferings of childhood are indelibly stamped on the adults. The vast mass of the workers' children are neglected; this leaves traces which are never wholly removed and leads to the weakening of a whole generation of workers." (p. 115)

Premature aging: In Manchester, "the premature ageing of the working-class population is so universal that practically all operatives in their forties look between ten and fifteen years older than this." (p. 180)

Mortality rates: Cited evidence from Chadwick's *Report on the Sanitary Conditions of the Labouring Population,* showing that "In 1840 in Liverpool the average age of death of the 'gentry and professional persons' was 35 years, of 'tradesmen and their families' 22 years, and 'labourers, mechanics and servants' was actually only 15 years... The main reason for the high death rate is the heavy mortality among infants and small children... If both parents go out to work for their living, or if either parent is dead, the child is so neglected that its health inevitably suffers... it is not surprising to learn from the report that we have just cited that in Manchester, for example, nearly 54 percent of the workers' children die before attaining their fifth birthday. On the other hand only 20 percent of the children of the middle classes die before they are five." (p. 121)

Textile workers: "In the cotton and flax spinning mills there are many rooms in which the air is filled with fluff and dust. This leads to chest and bronchial complaints, particularly among the workers in the carding and combing rooms... The usual consequences of inhaling factory dust are the spitting of blood, heavy, noisy breathing, pains in the chest, coughing and sleeplessness–in short, all the symptoms of asthma, which, in the worst cases, culminates in consumption" (p. 184).... "The runners are engaged in the most unhealthy occupation of all... Their work consists in keeping track of a solitary thread which is picked out from a complicated pattern by means of a needle. This work is very damaging to the eyesight, particularly when, as is usual, fourteen to sixteen hours is the usual length of the spell of duty." (p. 217)

Potters and lead poisoning: "The most scandalous way in which the health of the workers is undermined is when they have to handle pottery which has been dipped in a fluid [glaze] which contains large quantities of lead and also arsenic. Some workers actually have to put their hands into the liquid. Both men and boys do this work. Their hands and clothes are consequently always wet... These workers suffer from violent pains, serious stomach and intestinal complaints, severe constipation, colic, and, in some cases, tuberculosis... The men usually suffer the partial loss of the use of the muscles of the hands, painter's colic, and total paralysis of the limbs." (p. 234)

Miner's disease: "A disease which is largely confined to miners is 'black spittle.' It arises because the lungs become impregnated with fine coal dust and this leads to general debility, headaches, constriction of the chest and the expectoration of black mucus." (p. 281)

Pregnancy and childbirth: "If a pregnant operative left work too early she would be afraid of dismissal and of finding her place taken by another when she wished to return to work. In addition, absence from work means loss of wages. It is quite common for women to be working in the evening and for the child to be delivered the following morning, and it is by no means uncommon for babies to be born in the factory itself among the machinery." (p. 182)

Sleep deprivation, commenting on night-shift workers: "These workers were permanently deprived of their sleep at night, and this can never be replaced by sleeping during the day... The inevitable consequences were the appearance of nervous disorders, and a general lassitude and bodily weakness." (p. 170)

Health-destructive effects of intolerable boredom: "To tend machinery—for example, to be continually tying broken threads—is an activity demanding the full attention of the worker. It is, however, at the same time a type of work which does not allow his mind to be occupied with anything else... This is really no work at all, but just excessive boredom. It is impossible to imagine a more tedious or wearisome existence. The factory worker is condemned to allow his physical and mental powers to be atrophied... And if they are workers who are not inspired to a fury of indignation against their oppressors, then they sink into drunkenness and all other forms of demoralising vice." (p. 200)

Street, market, and housing conditions: "The streets themselves are usually unpaved and full of holes. They are filthy and strewn with animal and vegetable refuse. Since they have neither gutters nor drains the refuse accumulates in stagnant, stinking puddles... The narrowness of the roads is accentuated by the presence of streetmarkets in which baskets of rotting and virtually uneatable vegetables and fruit are exposed for sale. The smell from these and the butchers' stalls are appalling. The houses are packed from cellar to attic and they are as dirty inside as outside. No human being would willingly inhabit such dens." (pp. 33–34)

Neighborhood contextual effects   Data showing mortality rates varied by both class [quality] of street and class of house, for Chorlton-on-Medlock, a suburb of Manchester, United Kingdom, 1844. (pp. 120–121)

				Class of Houses	Proportion	Mortality* Rate per 100,000
Class of Streets						
1st	...	...	...	1st	1 in 51	1960.8
				2nd	1 in 45	2222.2
				3rd	1 in 36	2777.8
2nd	...	...	...	1st	1 in 55	1818.2
				2nd	1 in 38	2631.6
				3rd	1 in 35	2857.1
3rd	...	...	...	1st	(not given)	——
				2nd	1 in 35	2857.1
				3rd	1 in 25	4000.0

*in original table: presented only as a proportion

Overall impact of adverse living and working conditions: "All of these adverse factors combine to undermine the health of the workers. Very few strong, well-built, healthy people are to be found among them—at any rate in the industrial towns, where they generally work indoors. And it is with the factory workers that we are concerned here. They are for the most part, weak, thin and pale. The bone structure is prominent but gives no evidence of strength. All their muscles are flabby, except for those which may have been abnormally developed because of the nature of their work. Nearly all suffer from digestive troubles, and consequently they suffer from more or less permanent mental depression and general irritability, so that their outlook on life is a gloomy one. Their weakened bodies are in no condition to withstand illness and whenever infection is abroad they fall victims to it. Consequently they age prematurely and die young. This is proved by the available statistics of death rates." (pp. 118–119)

Verdict: "social murder" "... An illness from which a well-fed person would speedily recover soon carries off those who are hopelessly undernourished. The English workers call this 'social murder' and denounce a society which permits the perpetration of this crime. Is not their protest justified?" (p. 32)

"If one individual inflicts a bodily injury upon another which leads to the death of the person attacked we call it manslaughter; on the other hand, if the attacker knows beforehand that the blow will be fatal we call it murder. Murder has also been committed if society places hundreds of workers in such a position that they inevitably come to premature and unnatural ends. Their death is as violent as if they had been stabbed or shot. Murder has been committed if the workers have been forced by the strong arm of the law to go on living under such conditions until death inevitably releases them. Murder has been committed if society knows perfectly well that thousands of workers cannot avoid being sacrificed so long as these conditions are allowed to continue... At first sight it does not

> appear to be murder at all, because responsibility for the death of the victim cannot be pinned on any individual assailant… But it is murder all the same… evidence concerning the deaths of workers from such unimpeachable sources as official documents, Parliamentary papers and Government reports… proves conclusively that society is aware of the fact that its policy results not just in manslaughter but murder." (pp. 108–109)

work and in the slums where their low pay forced them to reside (Engels, 1845 [1958]), pp. 115–119, 200). Considering their lot, he exclaimed (Engels 1845[1958], p. 188):

> Simply in order to fill the pockets of the bourgeoisie, women are rendered unfit to bear children, children are crippled, while grown men are stunted and maimed. The health of whole generations of workers is undermined, and they are racked with diseases and infirmities.

Affixing blame on "the revolting greed of the middle classes" (Engels, 1845 [1958], p. 188) and the manufacturers, landlords, land owners, and politicians who represented them, Engels provocatively charged English society using a phrase he said he learned from the English workers: "social murder" (Engels, 1845 [1958], p. 32). To Engels, it was clear: When considering "the condition of the English industrial proletariat," "[e]verywhere we find permanent or temporary suffering, sickness and demoralization all spring either from the nature of the work or from the circumstances under which they are forced to live" (Engels, 1845 [1958], p. 240). In other words, disease and its distribution were socially caused and could no longer be conceptualized as only natural phenomena.

It was an indictment Virchow repeated 4 years later, in 1848, in his essay on "Public Health Service," in which he condemned a system in which "thousands must always miserably die, so that a few hundred may live well" (Virchow, 1848c, p. 24). From their radical perspective, any real solution would require wholesale social transformation, not simply more economic growth or piecemeal reform—a stance that, in the politically turbulent mid-1840s, likely seemed a plausible proposition (Hobsbawm, 1996a), perhaps especially to two young authors then only in their mid-20s. Although the rapid suppression of the 1848 revolutions quickly squelched overt articulation of any such radical perspectives, the ideas developed nevertheless later seeded the development of kindred analyses proposed in the twentieth century (Waitzkin, 1981; Krieger, 2000; Krieger, 2001b), as discussed in **Chapter 6**.

Much as the liberal and proletarian perspectives might disagree on their political and economic analyses and on their appraisal of the hazards associated with the labor process itself, they nevertheless concurred that poverty and other political, economic, and social conditions caused—and were not merely correlates (or consequences) of—diseases and their distributions. The nature of society and of work, and not just nature itself, became etiologic agents. Demonstrating the impact of their ideas—and the evidence they marshaled to support and test them—is a statement made by Farr, the previously mentioned eminent and iconic Victorian public health official, who in 1866, towards the end of his career, matter-of-factly observed, as a self-evident fact and not a controversial pronouncement: "No variation in the health of the states of Europe is a result of chance; it is the direct result of the physical and political conditions in which nations live" (Eyler, 1979, p. 199).

Theorizing Racial/Ethnic Differences in Disease Distribution: Colonialism, Slavery, and Climate Versus Innate Constitution. Concerns about nature, however, did not disappear from the roster of arguments about causes of disease and disease distribution. Far from it: even in an increasingly mechanized and de-naturalized age, the new field of epidemiology was deeply embroiled in contentious debates over the natural versus social causes of racial/ethnic patterning of disease and death (Krieger, 1987). As contact between Europeans and people from other continents intensified because of seventeenth century growth in the African slave trade, other commercial trade, and the expansion of European countries' colonial reach, a combination of new health data and increased social conflict fueled new controversies about connections between complexion, country of origin, and health (Arnold, 1988; Harrison, 1996; Saakwa-Mante, 1999). In the Americas, comparisons focused on physical appearance and diseases of American Indians and enslaved Africans versus the free White population; in Europe, treatises addressed global varieties of "mankind" while stressing comparisons of "native" populations with their European conquerors. As with class inequalities in health, European and North American physicians and scientists were positioned, like every other sector of society, on both sides of a fundamental divide. The crux of the argument was whether people from around the globe constituted one or several "races," endowed with innately equal versus unequal mental, moral, and physical capacity—and rights (Haller, 1971; Takaki, 1993; Harding, 1993; Augstein, 1996; Gould, 1996; Banton, 1998; Ernst & Harris, 1999; Desmond & Moore, 2009). Translated to health, the question became: Were the causes of differential health status by race/ethnicity to be found in climate, innate constitution, or society? (Krieger, 1987; Ernst & Harris, 1999; Harrison, 2002).

Initial explanations of "racial" distinctions in physique and health, propounded in the seventeenth century by European natural philosophers and physicians alike, drew inspiration from Hippocratic environmental doctrines combined with Christian theology, whereby observed differences were theorized to reflect effects of variable climates on a single human race, divinely created only once by God (Stanton, 1960; Haller, 1971; Stepan, 1982; Augstein, 1996; Goodman, 1998; Banton, 1998; Ernst & Harris, 1999; Desmond & Moore, 2009, Painter 2010). Exemplifying this "environmental" approach to understanding human diversity was the 1775 opus *On the Natural Variety of Mankind* (Blumenbach, 1865, pp. 65–145), among the most influential late eighteenth century scientific efforts to systematize the categorizing of human "varieties." Authored by Johann Friedrich Blumenbach (1752–1840), a German anatomist deemed even in his lifetime to be a founder of the new discipline of anthropology (Floures, 1865; Stanton, 1960; Haller, 1971; Stepan, 1982; Gould, 1996; Baer et al., 1997; Augstein, 1999; Baker, 1998), Blumenbach's quickly and widely adopted typology divided humanity into five "varieties": *Caucasian, Mongolian, Ethiopian, American,* and the *Malay.* According to Blumenbach, these five groups all belonged, co-equally, to one species; even so, he nevertheless set the *Caucasians* (a term he invented) as constituting the archetypal variety, and termed the other four varieties *degenerations* brought about by climate and other external influences (Blumenbach, 1865, pp. 146–276) (*see* **Textbox 3–10** for excerpts of Blumenbach's description and reasoning).

Two epidemiological corollaries stemmed from the "environmental" thesis of racial difference:

1. New locales were likely to pose new disease risks to new arrivals, because new "airs, waters, and places" and new diets were expected to cause different ailments. (Sheridan, 1985; Curtin, 1989; Harrison, 1996)
2. Newcomers could nevertheless "acclimate" to their new environs by adopting a suitable diet, dress, and mode of living, with "acclimation" considered to be a bodily

Textbox 3–10. The Enduring Impact of Johann Friedrich Blumenbach (1752–1840): From Human "Varieties" to Human "Races"—and the Invention of "Caucasians"

Blumenbach's On the Natural Variety of Mankind (1775) (Blumenbach, 1865):

- Central question: "*Are men, and have the men of all times and of every race been of one and the same, or clearly of more than one species?*" (italics in original) (pp. 97–98).
- Answer, presented in the chapter "Five principal varieties of mankind, one species" (p. 264):

a. the "*[i]nnumerable varieties of mankind run into each other by insensible degrees*" (p. 264), and
b. "As, however, even among these arbitrary kinds of divisions, one is said to be better and preferable to another; after a long and attentive consideration, all mankind, as far as it is at present known to us, seems to me as if it may best, according to natural truth, be divided into the five following varieties; which may be designated and distinguished from each other by the names Caucasian, Mongolian, Ethiopian, American, and the Malay"(p. 264), whereby
c. the "Caucasian," the "primeval" variety, "degenerated"–to use Blumenbach's language–in one direction into "Mongolian," by way of the intermediate "American" variety; in the other, it degenerated into the "Ethiopian," by way of the "Malay" variety (pp. 264–246); the net total was 5 "varieties" of human kind–all equally members of humanity—with "Caucasian" at the center.

- Why *Caucasian*?

a. In Blumenbach's words (p. 269):
"I have taken the name of this variety from Mount Caucasus, both because its neighbourhood, and especially its southern slope, produce the most beautiful race of men, I mean the Georgian; and because all physiological reasons converge to this, that in that region, if anywhere, it seems we ought with the greatest probability to place the autochthones of mankind… Beside, [their skin] is white in colour, which we may fairly assume to have been the primitive colour of mankind, since, as we have shown above (s. 45), it is very easy for that to degenerate into brown, but very much more difficult for dark to become white, when the secretion and precipitation of this carbonaceous pigment (s. 44) has once deeply struck root."
The footnote he offered to justify his choice was as follows (p. 269):
"From a cloud of eye witnesses it is enough to quote one classical one, Jo. Chardin, T.l.p.m. 171. 'The blood of Georgia is the best of the East, and perhaps in the world. I have not observed a single ugly face in that country, in either sex; but I have seen angelical ones. Nature there has lavished upon the women beauties which are not to be seen elsewhere. I consider it to be impossible to look at them without loving them. It would be impossible to paint more charming visages, or better figures, than those of the Georgians.'
On this basis, 'Caucasian' became a scientific term (Scheibinger, 1993, pp. 115–142; Augstein 1999; Krieger, 2005, Painter 2010).

b. As other analysts have pointed out, however, Blumenbach choice of "Caucasian" reflected not only racially and sexually influenced "aesthetics" (as articulated by European White men) but also national politics and religious beliefs (Scheibinger, 1993, pp. 115–142; Augstein, 1999; Krieger, 2005, Painter 2010). The Caucasus mountain range, located between the Black Sea and the Caspian Sea in a region bordering Europe, Asia, and the Middle East, included Mount Ararat—of Biblical fame for being the peak on which Noah's ark rested to survive the Deluge—and also was legendary in Greek myths (Augstein, 1999). Amidst its summits and shores, homeland to the Amazons, Zeus seduced Europa, Jason sought the Golden Fleece, and the Greek gods chained Prometheus to a mountain peak as punishment for giving humanity fire (Hamilton, 1942; D'Aulaire & D'Aularie, 1962). In the late eighteenth century, the Caucasus region was also a still mysterious region under Russian rule, relatively unknown to Western Europeans; its name, of mythic character, consequently was free of the stamp of "nationality." Serving well as "the neverland of myth-making" (Augstein, 1999, p. 69), the Caucusus region thus constituted as a safe place on which to project back a common European ancestry without getting embroiled in nationalist politics. Having attained acceptance as a "scientific term," the word "Caucasian" has remained entrenched in the scientific literature–despite its fundamentally flawed premise that that humanity originated in the Caucuses, and not, as contemporary research demonstrates, in Africa (Cavilli-Sforza et al., 1996; AAA, 1999; AAPA, 1999; Cavilli-Sforza, 2000). Adherence to scientific evidence accordingly would suggest that "Caucasian" should no longer be employed and instead should be replaced by the term "White," which more accurately reflects the social realities of the "color line" that simultaneously create and justify "race"-based inequity (Kaplan & Bennett, 2003; Krieger, 2005).

Blumenbach's *Contributions to Natural History* (1806) (Blumenbach, 1865)

- From "variety" to "race": still asserting the "identity of mankind in general" whose extremes "join unobservedly into each other" (p. 300), Blumenbach nevertheless shifted to a discussion of "race," rather than "varieties," as reflected in his statement: "Then also as evidence of the natural division of the whole species into the five principal races of which I shall speak in the next section" (p. 300).
- But still challenging ideas of racial inequality: Concomitantly, aware of—and seeking to counter—invidious theories of racial distinction, Blumenbach included a section titled "Of the Negro in particular," in which he praised their abilities, temperament, and beauty (pp. 305–312).

The enduring impact of Blumenbach's work, melding "race" with "racial inequality":

Preface to the 1865 collection of Blumenbach's work, appearing as a special volume published by the British Anthropological Society (Bendsyhe 1865, p. x):

"Of the five races there are three which he considers above all as the principal races; and therefore he deals with those first. These are the Caucasian, which is not only for Blumenbach the most beautiful, and that to which pre-eminence belongs, but the primitive race; then, the Mongolian and Ethiopian, in which the author sees the extreme degeneration of the human species. As to the other races, they are only for Blumenbach, transitional: that is the American is the passage from the Caucasian to the Mongolian; and the Malay, from the Caucasian to the Ethiopian... Thus it has happened that these races, after having been once introduced into science by Blumenbach, have been retained there; and we may assert that they will always be retained, with some rectifications in their characteristics and in their several boundaries."

Reflecting on "the five races of Blumenbach," "considered as natural groups," the editor asked "is it proper to place them in the same rank, and allow them all the same zoological value?"–to which his scientific answer was unequivocally: "no" (Bendsyhe, 1865; p. x).

process that typically was accompanied by a bout of "seasoning sickness" and, if survived, augured resistance to future local scourges. (Curtin, 1989; Harrison, 1996; Harrison, 2002)

Medical and military texts, for example, advised Europeans to acclimate to tropical climes by eating lighter food, wearing lighter fabrics, and avoiding the mid-day sun (Curtin, 1989; Harrison, 1996). Other texts discussed acclimation for non-Europeans: a 1764 medical tract by the Scottish physician John Grainger (1721?–1766) (Gilmore, 1999), one of the first "purposely written on the method of seasoning new Negroes" in the West Indies (Grainger, 1764), declared that "no Negroe can be said to be seasoned to a West India climate, till he has resided therein for at least twelvemonth" (Grainger, 1764, p. 11). Assuming the Hippocratic hypothesis was correct, the presumption was that colonists, imported slaves, and "natives" alike could be expected increasingly to resemble each other in both disease and physical appearance.

By the early nineteenth century, however, the medical and theological consensus on single creation and single species shattered. One contributing reason was that despite lengthening colonial cohabitation in similar climes, "natives" and slaves still looked different— and ailed differently—from their conquerors and masters (Crosby, 1986; Kunitz, 1994; Augstein, 1996; Harrison, 1996; Curtin, 1998; Hays, 1998; Augstein, 1999; Saakwa-Mante, 1999; Ernst & Harris, 1999; Harrison, 2002). Smallpox offered one horrific example: although deadly to and feared by Europeans, its introduction to the "new world" of the Americas by Europeans in 1518 was singularly catastrophic to the Indigenous populations (Hopkins, 1983; Sheridan, 1985; Crosby, 1986; Cook, 1997a; Boyd, 1999; Mann, 2005). Current estimates suggest smallpox likely killed upward of 50% of the Amerindians in the Caribbean, Mexico, and South America (Thorton, 1987; Young, 1994; Waldram et al., 1995; Cook, 1997a; Cook, 1997b; Duffy, 1997; Boyd, 1999; Mann, 2005); entering the North American colonies in the 1630s, it destroyed half the Huron and Iroquois confederations, a calamity deemed a blessing by the first governor of the Massachusetts Bay Colony, John Winthrop, who declared: "For the natives, they are neere all dead of small Poxe, so as the Lord hathe cleared our title to what we possess" (Crosby, 1986, p. 208). Similarly, with yellow fever, eighteenth century beliefs that "seasoned" Europeans and Africans in the Caribbean and North America could become equally resistant gave way to the nineteenth century views that Europeans were inherently more susceptible to the disease (for examples of changing and conflicting views, *see* **Textbox 3–11**) (Nott, 1856; Fenner, 1858; Curtin, 1998; Harrison, 2002). During this same time period, a parallel shift from optimism to pessimism regarding the possibility of British troops acclimating to the Indian subcontinent likewise occurred (Harrison, 1996; Harrison, 2002). In this pre-germ theory era with no recourse to the idea of acquired immunity, only differences in "innate constitution," rather than environmental context, would seem to account for the observed "racial" variations in epidemic and endemic diseases (Sheridan, 1985; Crosby, 1986; Coleman, 1987; Young, 1994; Curtin, 1998; Harrison, 2002).

Reflecting what the public health historian Harrison has termed the *hardening* of *racial categories* (Harrison, 1996; Harrison, 2002), by the early nineteenth century the scientific discourse about human "variety" had morphed into discussion of human "races," ordered by superiority (Stanton, 1960; Augstein, 1996; Gould, 1996; Banton, 1998; Ernst & Harris, 1999; Desmond & Moore, 2009, Painter 2010). In this schema, "race" simultaneously and tautologically became a category defined by—and used to explain—"racial" differentials in morbidity and mortality. In other words, contemporaneous with the emergence of epidemiology as a population science, "race" science came into its own. Consequently, "racial" categories become so entrenched and "naturalized" in scientific thought that, by the early-to-mid

Textbox 3–11. Changing Views on "Seasoning" and Yellow Fever: From the Affirmative Views in 1773 of the Abolitionist U.S. Physician Benjamin Rush (1746–1813) to the More Dubious Perspective in 1806 of the English Physician George Pinckard, (1768–1835), Deputy Inspector-General of Hospitals to his Majesty's Forces

Benjamin Rush: *An Address on the Slavery of the Negroes in America* (1773) (Rush, 1773 [1969])

- on the feasibility of "seasoning": discounting the then prevalent view that Africans were singularly suited to work in the "excessive heat and labor of the West-India islands," Rush instead stated that Europeans who survived "the first or second year, will do twice the work, and live twice the number of years than an ordinary Negro man." (p. 8)
- on the role of climate and slavery in shaping "Negro" characteristics: "... when we allow for the diversity of temper and genius which is occasioned by climate," Africans in their own countries are "equal to the Europeans" in "their ingenuity, humanity, and strong attachments to their parents, relations, friends, and country" (p. 2); the implications: under similar circumstances they will have similar diseases and "All the vices which are charged upon the Negroes in the southern colonies and the West-Indies, such as Idleness, Treachery, Theft, and the like, are the genuine offspring of slavery." (p. 2)

Pinckard G. *Notes on the West Indies, Written During the Expedition under the Command of the Late General Sir Ralph Abercromby: Including Observations on the Island of Barbadoes, and the Settlements Captured by the British Troops, upon the Coast of Guiana; Likewise Remarks Relating to the Creoles and Slaves of the Western Colonies and the Indians of South America: with Occasional Hints, Regarding The Seasoning, or Yellow Fever, of Hot Climates. In Three Volumes.* London: Printed for Longman, Hurst, Rees, and Orme, Paternoster-row, 1806. (Pinckard, 1806)

- in a section titled "Concerning the seasoning, or yellow fever," Pinckard drew on his years of experience in the West Indes to address why "this fever attack[s] Europeans, newly arrived in the West Indies, in preference to creoles, negroes, and those who, by a long-continued residence, have become acclimatés" (pp. 418–419). His explanation (pp. 418–419):

"To the inhabitants of different regions is given something of a constitutional difference, which it were difficult precisely to define: but it belongs to a certain original conformation, creating a difference of fibre or stamina, which more particularly befits the body for the specific region, in which it is designed to move. Yet, while much is attributed to our parent Nature, it ought not to be forgotten that habit is our foster-mother, and that she follows nature very closely, in her influence upon the human frame; and hence it is that by long residence, and similarity of pursuit, so near an approach to this specific and original structure may be acquired, as to promote healthy action, and even to an ungenial climate: still, this is only the yielding of a body originally different; for the assimilation is never so complete as to be in all respects the same. The constitution of a negro from Africa, or the West Indies, never becomes

> entirely British, although he reside in England the greater part of his days: and however much an European, by long residence in the West Indies, be brought to resemble a creole, he can never acquire, precisely, the constitution of a native: some marks of original conformation will remain, and a something, even in his general appearance, to distinguish him."

nineteenth century, medical discussion about populations—and research on their health status—without "racial" categories became virtually unimaginable.

Emblematic of the new racialized typology was one proposed by George Cuvier (1769–1832), the renowned French paleontologist and comparative anatomist, whose 1812 schema, modified in 1817, emphasized "racial" distinctions over common humanity. Following Blumenbach, Cuvier placed *Caucasians* at the top, superior to both *Mongols* and *Negroes*, but further dividing *Caucasians* into superior (Germanic, Greek, and Indian) and inferior (Semetic) stocks (Cuvier, 1863 [1969]; Augstein, 1999; Banton, 1998). A small but influential group of physicians and scientists, including Dr. Samuel George Morton (1799–1851) and the internationally esteemed biologist Louis Agassiz (1807–1873), went further and argued, contrary to Blumenbach and religious conventions, that God had created people not once (monogenesis) but multiple times (polygenesis), divinely making unique and innately unequal "races" of "mankind," each with their own distinctive anatomies and disease patterns—and with "superior" "races" destined to rule and to be served by their "inferior" counterparts (Morton, 1839; Agassiz, 1850; Nott & Glidon, 1854 [1969]); Lurie, 1954; Stanton, 1960; Desmond & Moore, 2009). In the United States, a veritable cottage-industry of scientific papers routinely reported on what were then termed the *peculiarities* of the American "*Negro*," ranging from anatomic features to mental abilities to disease susceptibility (Tidyman, 1826; Rossingnol, 1848; Pendelton, 1849; Krieger, 1987; Ernst & Harris, 1999). One especially prominent and prolific pro-slavery physician, Dr. Samuel A. Cartwright (1793–1863), for example, wrote streams of widely-cited articles on "negro" inferiority and disease (Cartwright, 1850; Cartwright, 1851; Cartwright, 1853a; Cartwright, 1853b; Cartwright, 1855; Cartwright, 1858; Cartwright, 1860 [1969]). In 1850, he went so far as to announce he had discovered two new diseases unique to Blacks: "drapetomania, or the disease causing slaves to run away" and "dysesthesia Ethiopia, or hebetude of mind and obtuse sensibility of body—a disease peculiar to negroes—called by overseers, 'rascality'" (Cartwright, 1850), a claim so remarkable as to have elicited two critiques in Southern medical journals (Smith, 1851; Anon, 1851–1852).

Further underscoring the centrality of debates over differential disease rates among Blacks versus Whites to both U.S. national politics and population data (and also epidemiological arguments) was an infamous dispute that lasted from 1843 to 1850, reaching well into the halls of Congress, regarding the results of the 1840 Census, which seemingly indicated that rates of insanity were higher among Blacks in the U.S. north versus south (Deutsch, 1944; Stanton, 1960; Grob, 1976; Cohen, 1982; Anderson, 1988). Proponents of slavery claimed these findings proved freedom drove Blacks mad; skeptics, including members of the newly formed American Statistical Association (founded in 1839) (Jarvis, 1842; Forry, 1843; Forry, 1844; Jarvis, 1844; Jarvis, 1852) eventually proved that the 1840 census data on which these claims were based were seriously flawed, with egregious errors affecting counts in both the numerators and denominators (*see* **Textbox 3–12** for the chronology of this highly contentious and nationally prominent debate).

Textbox 3–12. The Infamous U.S. Debate Over the (Fallacious) 1840 Census Results Indicating Higher Insanity Rates Among Blacks in Free Versus Slave States

Perhaps the era's most prominent battle over Black/White disparities in health, attracting national attention from 1842 through 1850 and occasioning debate within Congress itself, involved returns from the U.S. census of 1840 (Deutsch, 1944; Grob, 1976; Cohen, 1982; Anderson, 1988). On their face, the returns, released after considerable delay only in 1842, indicated that rates of insanity among Blacks were highest in the North (1-in-162) and lowest in the South (1-in-1558). Seizing upon these results, the powerful pro-slavery Southern Senator John C. Calhoun (1782-1850) and twice former Vice President of the United States (under Presidents John Quincy Adams and Andrew Jackson) declared "the African is incapable of self-care and sinks into lunacy under the burden of freedom" (Deutsch 1944, p. 473)—and then used this argument to justify the annexation of Texas as a slave state in 1844.

Careful and well-publicized research by Dr. Edmund Jarvis, a specialist in medical disorders and co-founder of the American Statistical Association in 1839, however, revealed—as early as 1843—that the census data were erroneous (Jarvis, 1842; Jarvis, 1844; Jarvis, 1852). Specifically, because of transposed columns of numbers, many Northern towns which had no Black population were nevertheless listed as having "insane and idiot" Blacks, thereby grossly inflating the Northern rate of Black insanity (Jarvis, 1844; Cohen, 1982). Additional problems artificially reduced rates of Black insanity in the South (e.g., the practice of treating Black insanity as insubordination and also the exclusion of Blacks from insane asylums, both of which led to undercounting of the Black insane) (Jarvis 1844; Forry 1844). Together, the Northern overcount and Southern undercount of cases led to the alarming but false findings of higher Black insanity rates in the free states. The exposé of the erroneous data not only provided a critical challenge to the erroneous "race" science of the day but also led to increased efforts to professionalize the U.S. census and improve the quality of vital statistics. In other words, debates about Black/White health status were central, not ancillary, to the content, conduct, and validity of the U.S. census, U.S. health data, and U.S. health research.

In opposition to the dominant view, a minority of health professionals, including U.S. physicians concerned with the poorer health of Blacks versus Whites, turned from increasingly discredited climatic explanations of racial differences to newer social explanations of the observed disparities (Krieger, 1987). As with the parallel debates, discussed above, regarding societal versus innate individual explanations of poverty and the greater disease burden of the poor, proponents of this alternative view sought to locate the source of Blacks' poorer health in their societal context, as opposed to their innate constitutions.

Prominent in the ranks of those emphasizing social conditions was the first generation of credentialed Black physicians, who had only just won the right to attend medical school (Bousfield, 1944; Link, 1967; Morais, 1978; Falk, 1980; Levesque, 1980). Featured among them were: Dr. James McCune Smith (1811–1865), who in 1837 became the first African-American to receive a medical degree (from the University of Glasgow, in Scotland, as no U.S. medical school at that time would admit Blacks [Bousfield, 1945; Falk, 1980]); Dr. John S. Rock (1825–1866) (Rock, 1858; Levesque, 1980), who received his medical degree in the United States in 1852, then studied law and in 1861 was admitted to the Massachusetts Bar, and 4 years later, in 1865, became the first African-American authorized to argue cases before the U.S. Supreme Court; and Dr. Rebecca Lee, who in 1864 became the first credentialed African-American woman physician (Crumpler, 1883; Sterling, 1994; National Library of Medicine, 2008). Countering mainstream accounts that denigrated the biology, morality, and health of Black Americans, these physicians used irony as well as evidence to make their case, as illustrated by **Textbox 3–13**, which includes an excerpt from one of Rock's rebuttals to then conventional racially biased explanations of Black/White disparities in health.

Demonstrating the difference a divergent theoretical perspective can make, in 1859 McCune Smith took the unprecedented step of comparing the health of Blacks to poor

---

Textbox 3–13. **Opposing Descriptions of Racial Appearance and Implications for Health and Well-Being Offered by Two Prominent U.S. Physicians: the Pro-Slavery Dr. Josiah C. Nott (1804–1873) and the Abolitionist Dr. John S. Rock (1825–1866)**

Description and Inferences by Josiah C. Nott (1843) (Nott, 1843):

Stated seriously: "The Caucasian, Ethiopian, Mongol, and Malay may have been distinct creations, or may be mere varieties of the same species produced by external causes acting through many thousand years: but this I do believe, *that at the present day the Anglo-Saxon and the Negro races are, according to the common acceptation of the terms distinct species, and that the offspring of the two is a hybrid* (italics in the original). Look first upon the Caucasian female with her rose and lily skin, silky hair, Venus form, and well-chiseled features—and then upon the African wench, with her black and odorous skin, woolly head, and animal features—next compare their whole anatomical structure, and say whether they do not differ as much as the swan and the goose, the horse and the ass, or the apple and the pear tree." (p. 30)

Inference: According to Nott, mulattoes are "less capable of endurance and shorter lived," "less prolific," and more likely to be insane than either Blacks or Whites.

Description and Inferences by John S. Rock (1858) (Levesque, 1980; Rock, 1858)

Stated tongue-in-cheek: "I will not deny that I admire the talents and noble character of many white men. But I cannot say I am particularly pleased with their physical appearance. If old mother nature had held out as well as she had commenced, we should, probably, have had fewer varieties in the races. When I contrast the fine, tough, muscular system, the beautiful, rich color, the full broad features and the gracefully frizzled hair of the Negro with the delicate physical organization, wan color, sharp features and lank hair of the Caucasian, I am inclined to believe that when the White man was created, nature was pretty well exhausted. But, determined to keep up appearances, she pinched up the features and did the best she could under the circumstances."

Inference: First, contrary to Cartwright's assertion that Black resistance to slavery is a disease and Black submission results from the "the spiritual force of the white man's will" (Cartwright, 1858, p. 162), Rock argued that resisting slavery is healthy and that continued servitude reflects being outnumbered by White men and their guns. Second, he predicted: "[w]hen the avenues to wealth are opened to us, we will then become educated and wealthy, and then the roughest looking colored man that you ever saw, or ever will see, will be pleasanter than the harmonies of Orpheus, and black will be a very pretty color."

Whites, rather than to Whites overall. He opened up this new avenue of inquiry in his influential pamphlet, *On the Fourteenth Query of Thomas Jefferson's Notes on Virginia* (Smith, 1859), which addressed Jefferson's famous query whether Blacks and Whites could ever live together as equals, given their physical differences. Focusing on bone deformities resulting from rickets (a condition he attributed to poor diet), Smith observed that rickets was common among not only among slaves but also "the inhabitants of a portion of the western coast of Ireland, a people who submit to the same low diet, and other privations analogous to those endured by a portion of natives of the African coast" (Smith, 1859, p. 230). Noting that "as much difference is found to exist between the forms of the bones of different individuals, who are undoubtedly [W]hite, as are said to exist between the [B]lacks and the [W]hites" (Smith, 1859, p. 227), McCune Smith accordingly argued that high rates of rickets occurred among Blacks not because they were biologically "[B]lack," but because they were poor—and they were poor because they lived in a society that condemned them to slavery in the South and to a marginal existence as poorly paid workers in the North. Turning "race" science on its head, McCune Smith re-conceived racial disparities in health as an *effect* of racism, not caused by "race." Viewing the "same" data from a completely different perspective, to McCune Smith it was evident that the existence of differential rates of disease did not automatically provide "proof" of innate biological inferiority (or superiority) but instead could diagnose the existence of social injustice (Krieger, 1987). These were uncommon views, but then, 1859 was an uncommon year (Krieger, 1987), in which John Brown's abolitionist raid at Harper's Ferry unleashed the U.S. Civil War (Zinn, 2003) and Charles Darwin published *On the Origin of Species* (Darwin, 1859 [2004]; *see also* Desmond & Moore, 2009). Opening up new conceptions of both society and biology, these epoch-changing developments would reverberate through and transform epidemiologic theories of disease distribution during the second half of the nineteenth century.

4

Epidemiology Expands

Germs, Genes, and the (Social) Environment (1900–1950)

Miasma. Contagion. Epidemics. Heredity. Evolution. Environment. Survival of the fittest. Race. Sex. Age. Communicable disease. Tropical disease. Endemic disease.

To an epidemiologist at the start of the twentieth century CE—or in the latter part of the nineteenth century—all of these terms would have been well-known. By the early twentieth century, however, two of them would have been deemed totally discredited—*miasma* and *contagion*—and two seen as glaringly missing—*germ* and *gene*. Linking these latter two terms both conceptually and etymologically was their shared emphasis on biological transmission as key to disease causation. In the case of *germs* ("referred by some to the root *gen- of gign re to beget and by others to the root ges- of ger re to bear," Oxford English Dictionary (OED)), at issue was the replication and dispersion of living microbes (not the non-living poisons of *contagia*); in the case of *genes* ("ancient Greek γεν-, stem of γενος race, offspring" (OED)), the focus was on the fundamental information passed from one generation to the next that made an organism what it is. In both cases, the mysteries of disease etiology were to be revealed by delving ever more deeply into the microscopic world within—and surrounding—people's bodies. Basic science, applied to humanity at large, offered new hope for both understanding disease causation and preventing disease occurrence.

Yet, as the epidemiologic research of the early twentieth century was also to reveal, not only was there a major change in the substantive concepts used to explain disease etiology, there was also a major shift in disease types and rates—that is, a profound alteration of disease distribution (*see* **Table 4–1**), the very phenomenon that theories of disease distribution are intended to explain. As observed in the article "Public Health at the Crossroads" (Winslow 1926; quote: pp. 1077–1078), written in 1926 by Charles-Edward Amory Winslow (1877–1957), an internationally renowned U.S. public health leader during the first half of the twentieth century (American Association of Public Health, 1957; Acheson, 1970; Viseltear, 1982a, 1982b; Terris, 1998; Rosner, 1998; Markowitz, 1998):

> … the major problems of public health have fundamentally changed in fifty years. In 1875 the outstanding causes of death were pulmonary tuberculosis, acute respiratory diseases, infant diarrhea and diphtheria and croup in the order named. During the half-century that has passed

Table 4–1. Early Twentieth Century Declining U.S. Mortality Rates and Changing Leading Causes of Death, as Reported in 1926 and in 1943 by the U.S. Public Health Leader C-EA Winslow (1877–1957)

a) Winslow C-EA. Public health at the crossroads. *Am J Public Health* 1926; 16:1075–1085. (data from p. 1077): "Mortality from certain specified causes and from all causes per 100,000 population"

	Manhattan and Bronx 1873–1875	Greater New York 1923–1925	Percent change
Scarlet fever	80	1	−99
Diphtheria and croup	235	11	−95
Diarrhea under 5 years	335	22	−93
Diseases of the nervous system	252	39	−85
Pulmonary tuberculosis	404	84	−79
All other causes not listed	874	316	−64
Acute respiratory diseases	352	164	−53
All causes	*2,890*	*1,220*	*−42*
Bright's disease and nephritis	100	69	−31
Violence	120	85	−27
Cancer	41	113	+176
Heart disease	89	255	+187
Diseases of the arteries	8	61	+650

b) Winslow C-EA. *The Conquest of Epidemic Disease: A Chapter in the History of Ideas.* Princeton, NJ: Princeton University Press, 1943. (data from p. 379): Comparison of U.S. Death Rates in 1935 versus 1900

Causes of death	Actual deaths 1935	Number of deaths which would have occurred in 1935 on the basis of the 1900 rates	Number of lives saved	Percent reduction
Tuberculosis, all forms	51,269	224,384	173,115	77
Influenza and pneumonia	110,191	232,187	121,996	53
Diarrhea and enteritis	17,018	125,448	108,430	86
Communicable diseases of childhood*	13,182	72,127	58,945	82
Typhoid and paratyphoid	2,386	35,652	33,266	93
All other causes	1,103,313	1,285,963	272,650	21

*Measles, scarlet fever, whooping cough, diphtheria
Source: Winslow, 1926; Winslow, 1943

the communicable and environmental diseases have been so substantially reduced that the problems of the future are heart disease, the acute respiratory diseases and cancer. We face a new situation and we must adopt new methods if we are to meet it with any measure of success.

Early twentieth century epidemiologic theorizing can thus be characterized as a dialogue and debate over whether and how changing patterns of disease occurrence, including racial/ethnic and socioeconomic differences in health status, were caused by germs, genes, evolution, and the environment, however defined.

Germ Theory: Epidemiologic Evidence—and Questions

By the early twentieth century CE, epidemiologic theorizing about disease causation had been thoroughly transformed by the scientific embrace of the germ theory—in the basic sciences, clinical medicine, and public health alike (Winslow, 1923; Winslow, 1926; Greenwood, 1935; Frost, 1936; Winslow, 1943; Winslow et al., 1952; Rosen, 1958 (1993); Tomes, 1997; Rosenberg, 1987; Porter, 1997; Porter, 1999; Bynum, 2008). This theory, worked out and tested during the latter part of the nineteenth and early twentieth centuries (*see* selected chronology in **Table 4–2**), primarily through laboratory research but also through clinical use of vaccines, epidemiologic research, and public health interventions, offered a fundamentally new way of understanding the causes and spread of infectious disease. Its ability to newly organize and clarify the welter of epidemiologic, clinical, and laboratory evidence about infectious disease, and to provide new grounds for preventing disease, led many late nineteenth- and early twentieth century scientists and health professionals, as well as the general public, to hail germ theory as nothing short of revolutionary and transformative (*see* **Textbox 4–1**) (Maclagan, 1876; Gradle, 1883; Chapin, 1885; Chapin, 1928; Winslow, 1923; Greenwood, 1935; Frost, 1936; Doull, 1952; Rosen, 1958 (1993); Evans, 1980; Tomes, 1997; Bynum, 2008). Resolving many of the unexplained observations about the propagation of communicable disease that neither miasmatic or contagionist theories could explain, germ theory not only superseded these prior theories but also raised new questions for epidemiologists and others to address.

The Generative Germ: Key Concepts, Mechanisms, and Metaphors of Germ Theory. In brief, germ theory posited that infectious diseases were caused by a "contagium vivum"—that is, a living micro-organism (the "germ")—something entirely different than the contagionists' postulated inanimate poisons (Maclagan, 1876; Gradle, 1883; Chapin, 1885; Winslow, 1923; Frost, 1936; Doull, 1952; Evans, 1980; Tomes, 1997). Moreover, each specific disease was caused by its unique germ. Two corollaries were that: (*1*) each germ had its own particular mode of transmission, and (2) infection by any given germ produced the range of symptoms characteristic of and specific to its associated disease. Or, as clearly stated in 1876 by Dr. T. J. Maclagan (1838–1903) in his pathbreaking text, *The Germ Theory: Applied to the Explanation of the Phenomena of Disease: The Specific Fevers* (Maclagan, 1876), one of the first book-length treatments of the theory (Maclagan, p. 39):

Each contagium has its own definite and specific action–its own disease, which it alone produces. Each, too, produces its symptoms in so regular a manner, that seeing a patient for the first time in the middle of any one of these fevers, the physician can not only tell the symptoms which have presented themselves in the past but can prognosticate, with more or less certainty, the future course and duration of the malady.

Table 4–2. Selected Notable Events in the Nineteenth and Early Twentieth Century Development and Acceptance of Germ Theory

Year	Selected notable events relevant to germ theory
Precursors	
1546	Publication of *De Contagionibus* by Hieronymus Fracastorius (1478–1553), which proposed the idea of "seminaria" of contagion, which, like seeds, had the ability to multiply and propagate their kind .
1796–1801	Successful trials of smallpox vaccine by Edward Jenner (1749–1823).
Mid-Nineteenth century	
1840	Essay by Jacob Henle (1809–1885) on "On Miasma and Contagion," which established the principles that living organisms caused contagious and infectious diseases and offered proposals for how to test them.
1844	Agostino Bassi (1773–1856) demonstrated a fungus was associated with the muscardine disease of silkworms.
1850	Casimir Davaine (1812–1882) caused anthrax in sheep by inoculating them with diluted blood of sheep sick with anthrax.
1865–1870	Research by Louis Pasteur (1822–1895) showed that contagious microbes caused silkworm disease and that the disease could be controlled by isolation and quarantine.
1865	Joseph Lister (1827–1912) applied Pasteur's theory to control of disease, using antiseptics in surgery. Jean-Antoine Villemin (1827–1892) demonstrated tuberculosis could be transmitted by inoculation from one infected animal to another.
1873	G.H. Armauer Hansen (1841–1912) demonstrated the presence of *Mycobacterium leprae* in the tissue of all persons ill with leprosy.
1876–1877	Pasteur and Robert Koch (1843–1910) independently demonstrated the anthrax germ caused anthrax.
1880–1884	Pasteur's work on creating vaccines by attenuating the germs, as applied to chicken cholera, anthrax, and rabies.
1881	Dr. Carlos J. Finlay (1833–1915) proposed that yellow fever was transmitted by mosquitoes.
1882–1884	Koch described the germs for tuberculosis (1882), cholera (1883), and typhoid (1884).
1884	Edwin Klebs (1834–1913) and Friedrich Loeffler (1852–1915) isolated the typhoid bacillus, and Loeffler identified the presence of virulent diphtheria bacilli in the throats of healthy individuals.
1889	Theobold Smith (1859–1934) and F.L. Kilbourne identified the protozoan parasite, *Piroplasma bigeminum*, that caused Texas fever in cattle and described its tick-borne dissemination, demonstrating the importance of animal carriers.
1893	Koch demonstrated the importance of healthy carriers for cholera.
1894	William Hallock Parke (1863–1939) and colleagues demonstrated the importance of healthy carriers for diphtheria. Alexandre Yersin (1863–1943) and Shibasabura Kitasato (1853–1931) independently identified the plague bacillus.

Year	Selected notable events relevant to germ theory
1897	Ronald Ross (1857–1932) demonstrated the bird malaria parasite in the stomach of a mosquito and that mosquito bites were capable of transmitting the parasite.
1898	G.B. Grassi (1854–1925) and colleagues identified the human malaria parasite in the Anopheles mosquito.
Early twentieth century	
1900	Proof from the Walter Reed (1851–1902) Commission that yellow fever was spread by the mosquito.
1906	Howard Ricketts (1871–1910) demonstrated the tick-borne transmission of Rocky Mountain spotted fever. The English Plague Commission experiments demonstrating that the plague bacillus was transmitted by fleas.
1909	Charlos Chagas (1879–1934) demonstrated the transmission of South American trypanosomiasis (now called Chagas disease) by the infected *Triatoma megista*. Milton Rosenau (1871–1940) and colleagues demonstrated the existence of healthy carriers for typhoid.
1910	Publication of Charles V. Chapin's (1856–1951) *The Sources and Mode of Infection* (New York: J. Wiley), which advocated focusing on disease carriers and quarantine of individuals, rather than mass sanitary campaigns.

Sources: Winslow, 1923; Doull, 1952; Rosen, 1938; Rosen, 1993

As Maclagan also clearly acknowledged, "The idea that many of the diseases to which man and the lower animals are subject, result from the presence in the system of minute organisms, is not a new one" (Maclagan, 1876, p. 1). Nevertheless, the crystallization of germ theory, as such, constituted something new; in Maclagan's words, "But only of late years have the vague hypotheses to which this idea has from time to time given rise, assumed definite shape and form" (Maclagan, 1876, p. 1). Maclagan accordingly defined "The Germ Theory of Disease" as positing "that many disease are due to the presence and propagation in the system, of minute organisms having no part or share in its normal economy" (Maclagan, 1876, p. 1).

Investigation and analysis of the distribution and spread of infectious disease accordingly required obtaining empirical information about a range of germ-specific characteristics. These attributes included:

1. the incubation period (the time between infection and the appearance of symptoms);
2. the timing and mode of shedding the replicated germ (the infectious period, during which time the germ exited the body—for example, via saliva, mucus, vomit, feces, genital secretions, blood, or other bodily media);
3. how long the germ could survive outside the body (and under what conditions);
4. whether the germ was transported from an infectious person to another via air, water, skin-to-skin contact, skin contact with a germ-contaminated surface, ingestion of germ-contaminated food or dirt, or by an insect or animal vector;
5. whether infection by the germ, among those who survived, resulted in immunity to subsequent infections by that particular germ;
6. whether a person could be infected and not only be symptom-free but infectious (i.e., a healthy carrier) or else have a dormant chronic infection that at some future point could reactivate as virulent disease; and

7. the germ's "reservoir" (e.g., in humans or other species, or in other parts of the ecosystem)—that is, where it resided when not manifested as an epidemic outbreak among people.

The presumption was that knowledge about each of these germ characteristics would enable understanding of the course of disease within both individuals and populations.

To convey these novel ideas, the scientific and popular literature employed two instantly understandable metaphors. One had its roots in agriculture, the second in war. The first was the well-known "seed and soil" metaphor (Tomes, 1997), long used to explain why only some individuals—not everyone—became sick during epidemics. It was, after all, well-known that not all seeds necessarily sprouted, whether because the seed was somehow defective or the soil was somehow inhospitable. Thus, as argued in 1876 by Maclagan (Maclagan, 1876, pp. 172–174):

> The comparative rarity of the eruptive fevers, need no more be matter of surprise, than the rarity of oak trees as compared with the number of acorns which are annually produced, or the disproportion which exists between the frequency of tapeworm and the number of ova which each worm produces.
>
> Theoretically, there is no reason why each oak tree should not give rise to hundreds of similar trees, and each tapeworm to thousands of its kind: in each case the requisite number of acorns and ova are produced. Practically, we find that, of the acorns produced, not one in a thousand develops into an oak, and that, of the ova of tapeworm, not one in a million come to maturity.
>
> Theoretically, there is no reason why each case of each of the eruptive fevers should not give rise to thousands of others: the requisite number of germs is certainly produced. Practically, we find that only a few of the germs which are given off from the body during the course of the eruptive fevers, comes to maturity: the vast majority perish and undeveloped and inoperative...
>
> ... it follows that the number of persons attacked by any of the eruptive fevers must represent but a fractional portion of the number of germs which were produced at the same time as those which ultimately reached their nidus in the persons of those so attacked.
>
> The comparative rarity of the eruptive fevers we, therefore, regard, as an argument not against, but in favor of, the view which attributes them to the propagation of an organism in the system.

Hence, germ theory could readily encompass a scenario whereby exposure to a germ was widespread but not everyone became ill. The "seed and soil" metaphor additionally abetted the acceptance of germ theory in two other ways. One was that it helped to underscore disease specificity, as it was common knowledge that particular seeds produced only particular plants. Second, because seeds obviously took time to sprout, the metaphor also helped capture the time dimensions of infectious diseases, including the time period when people were infected and infectious yet not obviously manifesting any disease symptoms.

What the "seed and soil" metaphor missed, however, was the potentially antagonistic nature of the relationship between the germ and the organism, to the point where the germ could not simply sicken but could outright kill the infected organism. After all, a plant growing in soil did not destroy the soil *per se* (even as too many plants growing in one place could perhaps exhaust the soil as a base for future plants). Accordingly, the second major metaphor for germ theory drew on military language. Scientists, health professionals, and others thus routinely declared bacteria to be "mortal enemies of men" and "invisible enemies in the air" that "invaded" people's bodies, and hence needed to be fought off with both defensive (e.g., sanitary) and offensive (e.g., disinfectant) measures (Gradman, 2000).

Despite their seeming difference, the two metaphors—one pastoral, one pugilistic—nevertheless were also linked by the nascent ideas of evolutionary theory, albeit as reduced to the simplified idea of "survival of the fittest" (Tomes, 1977). In the case of "seed and soil," as per the Maclagan excerpt above, the metaphor facilitated conceptualizing the importance of individual variation for population phenomena, by virtue of the differential likelihood of specific individuals (whether germs, acorns, or the ova of tapeworms) surviving in any given context. And, with reference to the "war" metaphor, the first U.S. book-length treatise on the germ theory, *Bacteria and the Germ Theory of Disease* (published in 1883 by Dr. Henry Gradle [1855–1911]), commenced by declaring (Gradle, 1883, p. 2):

> In the light of the germ theory, diseases are to be considered as *a struggle between the organism and the parasites invading it*. As far as the germ theory is applicable, it eliminates the factor "accident" from the consideration of disease, and assigns disease a place in the Darwinian programme of nature. (italics in the original)

The embrace of germ theory by epidemiologists thus involved more than solely a critical appraisal of the empirical evidence tracing the many steps from exposure to germs to the population patterns of both epidemic and endemic infectious disease. Also key was its use of powerful metaphors that readily linked well-understood ideas—about "seed and soil," about war—to the new phenomena being explained.

Once articulated, germ theory's simultaneously universal, yet germ-specific, principles regarding infectious disease enabled epidemiologists and others to make sense of the previously puzzling population data on the incidence and spread of acute and chronic infectious diseases (Maclagan, 1876; Gradle, 1883; Chapin, 1885; Winslow, 1923; Greenwood, 1935; Frost, 1936; Winslow, 1943; Doull, 1952; Rosen, 1958 [1993]; Evans, 1980; Tomes, 1997; Bynum, 2008). The theory clarified, for example, why quarantining ships was not effective in blocking transmission of yellow fever (as the mosquito vectors were not stopped by the quarantine measures imposed) but could work for other diseases (if the germs were not vector-borne, and if the quarantine period exceeded the incubation and infectious period). It illuminated why sanitary measures involving sewage and water supply were key to curbing cholera (given its fecal-oral transmission, especially by contaminated water), whereas cleaning streets and fumigating houses had little effect for this disease; conversely, it explained why removing "filth" mattered for others (e.g., by curtailing the population of rats and other germ-carrying rodents and insects). Revelation of the role of insect vectors and the importance of temperature for the viability of shed germs helped explain the seasonal nature of malaria and other infectious diseases. Variable lengths of incubation and infectious periods, along with the discovery of "healthy carriers," in turn offered new insights into the origins of disease outbreaks, because disease could be spread by non-symptomatic yet still infectious individuals. Evidence of acquired immunity (attained by then unknown biological mechanisms) added yet another reason why not everyone exposed at a given time was stricken, because some fraction of those not affected presumably had been previously infected and survived. None of these ideas had existed—or else had not been integrated into a coherent account—in either the previous "miasma" or "contagion" theories.

As with other theories informed by evolutionary concepts (Mayr, 1982; Gould, 2002), germ theory's dual engagement with broad biological principles and germ-specific characteristics encouraged conceptualization and testing of myriad new hypotheses concerning any given germ's type, mode of transmission, incubation and infectious period, and human and non-human "reservoirs." Perhaps most important, the theory afforded new possibilities for improving disease prevention via three different strategies (Winslow, 1923; Winslow, 1946). The first was by clarifying what sewage treatment and water filtration needed to purify and what preventing food contamination entailed. As summarized by Winslow (1923, p. 37):

> The first result of the new science of bacteriology was to make precise and definite the shotgun methods of the empirical sanitation and the empirical isolation of an earlier day. The pythogenic theory, erroneous though it was, had yielded substantial results because, as has been said, 'filth if not the mother, is at least the nurse of disease.' Yet a scientific comprehension of the real elements of contagion made possible advances of a far-reaching kind, as may be illustrated by tracing its influence upon the control of three great groups of diseases, spread respectively by water supplies, by insects, and by direct contact.

The second strategy for improving disease prevention was to identify those diseases for which isolation of infectious individuals (as opposed to mass quarantine) might prove useful. The third was to encourage development of vaccines, which Winslow hypothesized would win "some of the most signal victories of the coming generation" (1923, p. 48), as well as drugs to inhibit or kill germs, including antiseptic measures taken before, during, and after surgery. Summarizing—and expressing the profound appreciation for—how germ theory's etiologic insights readily translated to effective preventive action, Winslow wrote (1923, pp. 64–65):

> In the Registration Area of the United States, the reduction in the death rate from four diseases only, typhoid fever, tuberculosis, diphtheria and the diarrheal diseases of infancy between 1900 and 1920 amounts to a savings of 230,00 lives a year... If we had but the gift of sight to transmute abstract figures into flesh and blood, so that as we walk along the street we could say 'That man would be dead of typhoid fever,' 'That woman would have succumbed to tuberculosis,' 'That rosy infant would be in its coffin,'–then only should we have a faint conception of the meaning of the silent victories of public health.

But Are Germs Sufficient to Explain Epidemic Disease? Yet, even as many appreciated the potency of germ theory, it was not without its critics. Numerous accounts of its rise to the dominant disease theory framework by the late nineteenth century emphasize the fierce and protracted intellectual battles between the theory's adherents and skeptics (Winslow, 1923; Winslow, 1943; Doull, 1952; Richmond, 1954; Rosen, 1958 (1993); Rosenberg, 1987; Porter, 1997; Tomes, 1997; Bynum, 2008). Among the latter were many who held to the miasmatic idea that disease was produced by chemical poisons and who argued that the ubiquity of bacteria and the episodic nature of epidemic outbreaks undermined the case that germs were causal agents—otherwise, why wouldn't there be mass occurrence of infectious disease all the time? Refuting these non-trivial objections took decades, requiring a mix of basic science, clinical, and epidemiological research. Examples include the painstaking work to differentiate distinct types of bacteria, viruses, and other microbes; the research leading to discovery of immunity resulting from subclinical infections; and intensive work on mathematical modeling of the epidemic dynamics in relation to contact rate and the exhaustion and addition of susceptibles to the population (Chapin, 1928; Frost, 1928 [1976]; Doull, 1952; Richmond, 1958; Rosen, 1958 [1993]; Tomes, 1997). As discussed in **Chapter 1**, the work to build confidence in—or undermine—scientific theories, especially those pertaining to probabilistic phenomena, is far from a simple process, and it should not be surprising that it took decades to address the many objections to the idea of living germs, comprising a microcosm of myriad unique microbes, acting as disease-specific etiologic agents.

A different type of challenge was posed by the concerns raised by scientists and others who accepted the idea that germs caused disease and readily embraced the new insights and interventions germ theory afforded—yet were still skeptical that a focus on germs alone was sufficient to explain the onset of epidemics and distribution of infectious disease. Among the ranks of these supportive critics were several leading epidemiologists, including Wade Hampton Frost (1880–1938), who in 1921 was appointed in as the first-ever Professor of Epidemiology in the United States at the recently founded Johns Hopkins School of Hygiene and Public Health (Daniel, 2004; Fee, 1987), and Major Greenwood (1880–1949), who in 1928 was appointed as the first-ever Professor of Epidemiology and Vital Statistics at the London School of Hygiene and Tropical Medicine (ABH & Butler, 1949). Even as both relied on germ theory for explicating epidemiologic evidence and to guide their own research on communicable disease, both Frost and Greenwood nevertheless held that a focus only on the germs was inadequate to explain the actual epidemiology—that is, the spatiotemporal population distribution—of epidemic and endemic infectious diseases.

For example, as argued by Frost in 1928 in his review on "Some conceptions of epidemics in general" (Frost 1928 [1976]), the characteristics of not only the microbial "agent" but also the "host" and "environment" mattered (*see* excerpts in **Textbox 4–2**). That Frost felt compelled to call attention to these latter two factors was indicative of how, by the early 1920s, research was increasingly focusing on only the germs themselves, contrary even to the earliest articulations of germ theory, which viewed infectious disease as the outcome of a "struggle" between, minimally, the "germ" and the "organism," as attested to by Maclagan's 1876 and Gradle's 1883 presentations of the theory, described above (*see also* **Textbox 4–1**). Highlighting the depth of the problem were the second thoughts articulated by Dr. Charles V. Chapin (1856–1941), whose 1910 landmark book on *The Sources and Modes of Infection* [1910] played a major role in reorienting public health practice away from general approaches to addressing environmental conditions to instead emphasizing "the search for carriers, the quarantine of contacts and the prompt isolation of early cases of disease" [Winslow, 1923, p. 45]. In 1928, he nevertheless felt compelled to state: "Since the development of bacteriology, many have been inclined to forget that, as it takes two to make a quarrel, so it takes two to make a disease, the microbe and the host" (Chapin 1928, p. 196). Even so, in making this comment, Chapin notably left out any notion of the "environment" (as underscored by the additional text excerpt provided in **Textbox 4–2**).

As observed by Greenwood, there was no "logical reason why identification of contagia viva should lead us to disregard general epidemiological principles"—including the importance of addressing, in Hirsch's famous words, issues of "geographical and historical pathology" (Hirsch, 1883, p. 2) (*see* **Textbox 3–6** in **Chapter 3**)—but this nevertheless "was the practical effect of the discovery" (Greenwood, 1935, p. 60). As an alternative, Greenwood offered an expansion of the bacteriological metaphor of "seed and soil" to bring in social agency, writing (1935, p. 359):

> One may perhaps sum up in this way. The genesis of active tubercular disease involves three factors: (1) a seed; (2) a soil; and (3) some methods of husbandry. Of these three, only the first is essential. Given a sufficiency of seed, the plant will grow in any soil and without any gardener's attention. In actual life, variations of the two non-essential factors are of great importance.

To Greenwood and other epidemiologists concerned about not only disease causation but also disease distribution, explaining the actual epidemiology of even infectious disease

Textbox 4–1. Selected examples of texts contemporaneous with the advent and consolidation of germ theory, emphasizing its scope and implications.

Maclagan TJ. *The Germ Theory: Applied to the Explanation of the Phenomena of Disease: The Specific Fevers.* London: Macmillan, 1876.

p. i: "A sound pathology is the basis of all rational medicine: a correct knowledge of the mode of production of diseased processes, the surest means of finding out how these processes may be prevented and checked. Bearing as The Germ Theory of Disease does, on the pathology of the most important ailments to which man [*sic*] is liable, the establishment, or the refutation of this theory, is a matter of importance not only to medical science, but to mankind... The diseases to the explanation of whose causation this theory is applicable, are so numerous and varied, that their separate consideration would have prolonged by labours indefinitely..."

p. 169: "The facts to which we now direct attention are: (1) that each animal has its own special parasites; (2) that each parasite has its own special nidus, out of which it is not propagated; (3) that each animal has its own peculiar contagious and specific diseases; and (4) that each contagious disease has, as a rule, its own peculiar local lesion. The juxtaposition of these facts cannot fail to indicate an analogy between ordinary parasites and contagia... Contagia, then, we regard as minute parasitic organisms, all of which, organism-like, exercise a definite action on their environment; and each of which, parasite-like, requires a special nidus for its development."

p. 222: "The immunity from a second attack, enjoyed by those who have once suffered from the eruptive fevers, is one of the most remarkable features in the history of these maladies... [and] can only be explained on the supposition that, by the action of the contagium, there is produced some peculiar and indelible impression on the system, as a consequence of which the body no longer presents to the contagium all the elements requisite to its propagation."

pp. 257–258: "We have now considered all the phenomena of the common specific fevers, and have found them to be such as may be explained by the growth and propagation of an organism in the system.

The theory as to the causation of the specific fevers, to which we must give our adherence, is that which explains this or that phenomenon, or even this or that fever, but that which best explains the whole of the phenomena which present themselves for our consideration.

We think we may claim for the theory advanced in these pages of being the only one which fulfills this condition.

Of the phenomena presented by the contagium out of the body, of the phenomena to which its reception into the system gives rise, of those which accompany its reproduction in the system, as well as those which follow such reproduction, it leaves not one unexplained.

That it should be so competent to explain the occurrence of phenomena so numerous, so varied, and sometimes to apparently contradictory, may be regarded as the crowning argument in favor of that theory which attributes these phenomena to the growth and propagation in the system of minute parasitic organisms."

Gradle H. *Bacteria and the Germ Theory of Disease: Eight Lectures Delivered at the Chicago Medical College.* Chicago, ILL: W.T. Keener, 1883.

p. 2: "Without underrating the earnest work done by medical men [*sic*] of a former period, it is evident that the causes of diseases, with the exception of some of the more patent instances, escaped them. it is only within the last twenty years, or less, that evidence is accumulating showing that many ailments to which flesh is heir, are due to the invasion of the organisms by microscopic parasites or their germs. Daily, almost, new facts are discovered, which substantiate more and more this *germ theory of disease*." (italics in the original)

p. 65: "The study of contagious diseases leads to the inference that disease germs are distinct and separate species, but that their virulence can vary. The infection from a small-pox patient, or a case of scarlet fever, or measles, produces only the original infection and never any other disease, but the severity of an epidemic varies a great deal in different years."

p. 211: "The study, which promises the greatest immediate benefits to mankind [*sic*], is that of the nature of the resistance of the tissues to the parasites. An insight into this will probably give us the clue to the immunity against a second invasion of the parasites, for which the tissues have just vanquished. For it is only a complete analysis of this process, that will enable us to aid the tissues in their struggle, i.e., to cure the disease, especially since the hope of finding some remedy, which kills bacteria, but is harmless to animal tissues, has never been realized. Whether the artificial production of immunity by vaccination with mitigated parasites will ever become practical in many diseases, can of course not be foretold."

p. 212: "But it is narrow-minded to think, that the detection of parasites explains everything. The question of predisposition, obscure as it is, cannot be ignored. It shows more sagacity to investigate, why the bacillus tuberculosis does not attack all beings, exposed to it, than to scoff at its significance, because many can resist its attacks. Moreover we are not to forget that the parasites are not the disease, but only its cause. The disease itself is an alteration of the physiological processes, as a response to some unwonted influence. Of course it may and it often does happen, that the reaction of the tissues is the same to different forms of irritation, be they living parasites or other agencies. Hence a symptom or a lesion may by itself not always have the same mode of origin in different instances."

pp. 75–216: range of disease discussed under rubric of "germ theory" (in order presented): (1) chicken-cholera, (2) surgical infection, (3) osteomyelitis, (4) pyæmia, (5) septicæmia, (6) erysipelas, (7) progressive gangrene, (8) tuberculosis, (9) glanders, (10) typhoid fever, (11) relapsing fever, (12) small-pox, (13) cow-pox, (14) sheep-pox, (15) measles, (16) malaria, (17) diphtheria, (18) leprosy, (19) syphilis, (20) milk-fever, (21) gonnorrhœa, (22) trachoma, (23) croupous pneumonia, (24) endocarditis, (25) whooping-cough, (26) rhinoscleroma, (27) pterygium, and (28) carious teeth.

Chapin CV. *The Present State of the Germ-Theory of Disease.* Providence, RI: Kellogg Printing Co., 1885.

p. 4: "Twenty-five years ago very little attention was paid to the micro-organisms now generally known by the name of bacteria, but the labors of Pasteur in 1861–62, and the discovery a little later, of the anthrax bacillus by Davaine, drew the attention of chemists and pathologists to these forms of life which had hitherto interested only a few botanists... Meanwhile, Lister, without waiting for the complete proof of the theory in which he had so much faith, developed and gave to the world his famous system of antiseptic surgery. Ever since then the 'germ-theory' has occupied a great share of the attention of the medical profession.

This theory maintains that many pathological conditions are cause by the presence of the body of certain micro-organisms..."

pp. 5–43: diseases discussed through the unifying lens of the germ-theory of disease (presented in the text in alphabetical order): (1) anthrax; (2) cattle plague (rinderpest); (3) chicken cholera; (4) cholera; (5) diphtheria; (6) erypsipelas; (7) glanders; (8) gonorrhea; (9) hydrophobia (rabies); (10) leprosy; (11) malarial disease; (12) measles; (13) milk sickness; (14) osteomyelitis; (15) pleuro-pneumonia (of cattle); (16) pneumonia; (17) relapsing fever; (18) silk-worm disease; (19) scarlet fever; (20) pyæmia; (21) scepticæmia; (22) surgical lesions; (23) swine-plague; (24) syphilis; (25) tuberculosis; (26) typhoid fever; (27) ulcerative-endocarditis; (28) ulcerative-stomatitis (in the calf); (29) variola; (30) vaccine; (31) Welbeck meat poisoning; (32) whooping-cough; and (33) yellow-fever.

Winslow C-EA. *The Evolution and Significance of the Modern Public Health Campaign.* **New Haven, CT: Yale University Press, 1923.**

pp. 36–37: "The two decades between 1890 and 1910 formed in a sense the golden age of public health. The germ theory was now thoroughly established and its applications went forward by leaps and bounds. No previous period of twenty years had ever seen equal progress in the application of sanitary science and it is doubtful if any similar period in the future will ever witness quite such phenomenal achievements."

required attention to not only the characteristics of germs, individuals ("host factors"), and populations (e.g., the proportion of susceptibles, or conversely, the extent of "herd immunity") but also to the human shaping ("husbandry") of the context—social, physical, and geographical—in which people lived (Mendelsohn, 1998). Epidemiology, in other words, was more than bacteriology.

In a complementary attack on germ theory's other military metaphor, the British epidemiologist F.G. Crookshank (1873–1933) in 1920 chastised colleagues for failing to distinguish between the armaments used in war (i.e., the germs) and the causes of war itself (i.e., determinants of epidemic outbreaks). To make his case, he elaborated an allegorical "fable" involving a stubborn police surgeon who insisted there was no causal difference—for either etiology or prevention—in conceptualizing a single bullet as causing a murder and multiple bullets as causing war (Crookshank, 1919–1920) (*see* **Textbox 4–2**). By the early twentieth century, however, such broader epidemiologic questions and principles—the very stuff of epidemiologic theory—had become increasingly uninteresting because, as Greenwood observed, "the bacteriological school had become psychologically omnipotent" (1935, p. 60).

Eugenics: The Seed Within–Genetic Determinism, Innate Inferiority and Superiority, and Disease Rates

Good Breeding, Good Blood, Good Health. Germs, however, were not the only microscopic entity to eclipse the study of macroscopic determinants of population health: genes mattered too. Indeed, highly germane to development of twentieth century epidemiologic theories—and methods—was the late nineteenth century rise of eugenic thinking among scientists and health professionals. Together with its popular analog of Social Darwinism, the science of eugenics—which occupied the mainstream, not fringe, of late nineteenth and early twentieth century scientific discourse—powerfully influenced health sciences, social sciences, and social policy in the early twentieth century (Davenport, 1911; Chase, 1977;

Textbox 4–2 . Early Twentieth Epidemiologic Arguments for Considering Not Only "Germs" But Also Population Dynamics and Characteristics of the "Host" and "Environment."

Crookshank FG. First principles: and epidemiology. *Proc Roy Soc Med* 1919–1920; Sect Epidem, 13:159–184. (italics in the original)

pp. 178–179: "May I conclude by the brief narration of a fable? Several years ago, an ingenuous police surgeon, investigating what he was told was a case of murder, found a bullet in a heart. This he decided, and so told the coroner, was the *causa vera*, the *causa causans*, of the symptoms in this case of murder. Shortly after he went abroad to a war, and, honestly believing that war is but murder on a large scale, he investigated the appearances of many bodies; again finding bullets, he declared that bullets are the cause of war, as of murder. But, in not every fatal case was the bullet of the same kind. Moreover, the occasional absence of bullets disconcerted him until he realized that he had once found gas poisoning the *causa vera*, in a case of murder, and he therefore came to the conclusion that several wars here existed, side by side; each one *sui generis*, and boasting a different *causa vera*. He then proposed to end war by discharging other and like bullets and gases in a contrary direction, and found many who approved his plan as sensible. However, some pestilent and philosophic person told him that war was not the mere numerical exaggeration of cases of murder, brought about either by an exaltation in the virulence of bullets or gas, or by a diminution in resistance to these agencies: it was our name for a state of affairs that we conceive as brought about by the play and interplay of racial, economic, and other factors. He was told, moreover, that while undoubtedly various kinds of killing are elements of war as, conceived by the historian and statesman, wars are not to be prevented, as he hoped, by avoiding persons who, in tramcars and in cinemas, carry bullets, or who project poisonous gas in public places. He was, however, unconvinced, and returned to England more settled than ever that the causal agents of war are bullets (of various kinds, no doubt) and gases (of various toxicities, certainly), while the best hope of preventing war in future lies, not in talk about vague racial, economic, or political conditions (which can only, he thought, at most be predisposing), but in devising some means of circumventing the *causae causantes*, bullets and gas!"

Frost WH. Some conceptions of epidemics in general. Presented as the first of two Cutter lectures at Harvard University on February 2, 1928. Reprinted in: *Am J Epidemiol* 1976; 103:141–151.

pp. 143–144: "Now the continued existence of an obligate parasite requires an unbroken series of transfers from host to host, hence we are dealing with a reaction between host and parasite which is continuous, and, being continuous this reaction must be constantly tending to establish an equilibrium...

The factors concerned in keeping up this equilibrium and bringing about the changes from one level of prevalence to another are:

A specific microorganism capable of producing the infection and the disease. As this organism is present not singly, but in numbers, we may refer to it as a microbial population.

A host population (man [sic] being usually the host to which we refer) containing susceptible individuals in sufficient numbers to keep up the infection.

Such conditions of the environment as are necessary for bringing the specific microorganism into potentially effective contact with infectible hosts."

pp. 150–151: "In conclusion it seems to me that, considering all kinds of epidemics, the regularly recurrent waves of endemic prevalence, local outbreaks, and the rare wide-spreading epidemics in history, we may reasonably believe they are governed *to some extent* by the general law that infection tends to increase progressively, due to multiplication of foci; and that it is progressively checked by the resultant decrease in susceptibles, due to specific immunizations and deaths in the host population. But I do not think we need to suppose that these are the sole forces, or that they are necessarily the principal ones, or that they are of the same relative importance in all diseases, or in all times and places. On the contrary, I think we are obliged to recognize as possible and probable influences, changes in the habits affecting rates of exposure, perhaps seasonal and other variations in host susceptibility, and in certain cases, quite important variations in the properties of specific microorganisms... we can hardly expect to discover any simple and general law which will take into account all these variables."

Chapin CV. The principles of epidemiology (1928). In: Gorham FP (ed).
Papers of Charles V. Chapin, M.D. A Review of Public Health Realities.
New York: The Commonwealth Fund, 1934; pp. 172–216. (originally
published as: Chapin CV. The science of epidemic diseases. *The Scientific*
Monthly **1928; 26:481–493)**

p. 196: "Since the development of bacteriology, many have been inclined to forget that, as it takes two to make a quarrel, so it takes two to make a disease, the microbe and its host. There is a constant struggle between disease germs and the bodies of animals and of the human beings they invade. There is also a tendency for an equilibrium to become established. The germs kill off the most susceptible and immunize the more resistant. In some of the resistant individuals, the germs become more or less firmly established, thus producing carriers, which carry over the virus until more susceptible material is available. This group of experiments has forcibly called attention to this tendency to equilibrium, and to the importance of carriers and of herd immunity in the rise and fall of outbreaks of infectious disease. Much light is also thrown on changes in the virulence of the germs, and on the effects of the dosage of the germs, and on the diet of animals."

Kevels, 1985; Gould, 1996; Porter, 1999; Carlson, 2001; Stern, 2005a; Stern, 2005b, Painter 2010). The central tenets of these two related frameworks were:

1. the vast majority of human traits (including intelligence, behavior, disease susceptibility, and longevity) were primarily determined by heredity rather than social context;
2. the distribution of resources in a society and its social order reflected the "survival of the fittest," especially in relation to class, racial/ethnic, and national hierarchies; and
3. "society" had interest in supporting the breeding of the "fit" and suppressing that of the "unfit."

Textbox 4–3 provides excerpts from key eugenic works stating these arguments in their own terms.

Coined in 1883 by Sir Francis Galton (1822–1911), the term *eugenics* (linking the Greek roots "eu-" ["good"] and "gene") literally meant "to produce" the "good"—that is, the

Textbox 4–3. Mainstream Eugenic Explanations of and Solutions to Public Health Problems, Including Metaphorical and Actual Links to Germ Theory, and as Applied to Racial/Ethnic Health Disparities

Eugenics: Overall Theoretical Stance and Policies

Davenport CB. *Heredity in Relation to Eugenics.* New York: Henry Holt and Company, 1911.

p. 4: "It is a reproach to our intelligence that we as a people, proud in other respects of our control of nature, should have to support about half a million insane, feeble-minded, epileptic, blind and deaf, 80,000 prisoners and 100,000 paupers at a cost of over 100 million dollars per year. A new plague that rendered four per cent of our population, chiefly at the most productive age, not merely incompetent but a burden costing 100 million dollars yearly to support, would instantly attract universal attention."

pp. 164–165: "Of the diseases of the lungs the most fatal is tuberculosis. We know that it is induced by a germ and that if there is no germ there will be no tuberculosis in the lungs. The first impulse of the modern sanitarian is to eliminate the germ. But this is a supraherculean task; for germs of tuberculosis are found in all cities and in the country amongst most domesticated animals. The germs are ubiquitous; how then shall any escape? Why do only 10 per cent die from the attacks of this parasite?... It seems perfectly plain that death from tuberculosis is the resultant of infection added to natural and acquired non-resistance. It is, then, highly undesirable that two persons with weak resistance should marry, lest their children all call this weakness."

pp. 255–256: "The practical question in eugenics is this: What can be done to reduce the frequency of the undesirable mental and bodily traits which are so large a burden to our population? There is, first, the method of surgical operation. This prevents reproduction either by destroying or locking up germ cells."

1927 US Supreme Court Decision for *Buck v. Bell,* written by Justice Oliver Wendell Holmes (Buck vs. Bell, 1927):

"We have seen more than once that the public welfare may call upon the best citizens for their lives. It would be strange if it could not also call upon those who already sap the strength of the State for these lesser sacrifices, often not felt to be such by those concerned, in order to prevent our being swamped with incompetence. It is better for all the world, if instead of waiting to execute degenerate offspring for crime, or to let them starve for their imbecility, society can prevent those who are manifestly unfit from continuing their kind. The principle that sustains compulsory vaccination is broad enough to cover cutting the Fallopian tubes. *Jacobson v. Massachusetts,* 197. U.S. 11. Three generations of imbeciles is enough."

As Applied to Race/Ethnicity:

Hoffman FL. Race *Traits and Tendencies of the American Negro.* New York: Macmillan, for the American Economic Association, 1896.

p. 95: "For the root of the evil lies in the fact of an immense amount of immorality, which is a race trait, and of which scrofula, syphilis, and even consumption are the inevitable consequences. So long as more than one-fourth (26.5 per cent. in 1894) of the births of the colored population of Washington are illegitimate,—a city in which we should expect to meet with the least amount of immorality and vice, in which at the same time only 2.6 per cent of births among the whites are illegitimate,—it is plain why we should meet with a mortality from scrofula and syphilis so largely in excess of that of the whites. And it is also plain now, that we have reached the underlying causes of the excessive mortality from consumption and the enormous waste of child life. It is not in the *conditions of life*, but in the *race trace and tendencies* that we find the causes of excessive mortality (italics in the original). So long as these tendencies are persisted in, so long as immorality and vice are a habit of the life of the vast majority of the colored population, the effect will be to increase the mortality by hereditary transmission of weak constitutions, and to lower still further the rate of natural increase, until the births fall below deaths, and gradual extinction results."

p. 148: "The general conclusion is that the negro is subject to a higher mortality at all ages, but especially so at the early age periods... Its extreme liability to consumption alone would suffice to seal its fate as a race. That alone would suffice to make impossible numerical supremacy in the southern states. 'Sufferers from phthisis,' writes Mr. Haycraft, 'are prone to other diseases such as pulmonary and bronchial attacks, so that over and above the vulnerability to the one form of microbe, they are to be looked upon as unsuited not only for the battle of life but especially for parentage and for the multiplications of the conditions for which they themselves suffer.'"

Brunner WF. The Negro health problem in southern cities. *Am J Public Health* 1915; 5:183–190.

pp. 188–189: "A people, or that portion where the negro blood predominates over the white blood, depends absolutely upon the white race for everything that makes up a civilization. If he [*sic*] is allowed to remain here, as he is, he will be a menace to himself and to us... we are faced with the evidence of our neglect to safeguard the white race by disinclination to recognize the negro as a potent factor in the transmission of disease. If you continue to allow him to be herded in the basements of houses and to be colonized in colored districts, you will suffer. The negro of the lower class is thrown into domestic contact with you and he furnishes 80 per cent of your household help."

p. 190: "There is in Savannah a condition which is interesting to the sanitary observer. I refer to a section of the city where dwell two races of people, differing widely in every respect save one thing, which they possess in common–their dirt. A narrow street divides these people, the Russian Jew from the negro. The first named have the lowest death-rate of the city, while the death-rate of the other is five times as great as that of his neighbor. The one, the hardiest race of city dwellers in the whole world, the other but a comparatively short time from the jungle... The Southern man is the negro's best friend, but they do not realize the line of sanitary endeavor necessary for the care of the negro..."

Allen LC. The Negro health problem. *Am J Public Health* 1915; 5:194–203.

p. 194: "The negro health problem is one of the 'white man's burdens'... Disease germs are the most democratic creatures in the world; they know no distinction of 'race, color, or previous condition of servitude'... From dirty homes, in these disease-infested sections, negro people come into intimate contact with white people every day that passes. We meet them in our homes, offices, stores, in street cars, and almost everywhere we go... Various diseases are often spread this way."

p. 195: "When freedom came, and all restraints removed, the negro began to indulge in all kinds of dissipation... To make bad matters worse, his unwise friends rashly gave him the ballot before he was sufficiently intelligent to use it properly... All this was bad for Cuffy–dreadfully bad... Disease began to prey upon him..."

p. 198: "A noticeable defect in the negro character is the want of initiative. He waits to be told... Habitually careless about most things, the negro is especially careless about caring for the sick..."

p. 201: "A good friend of mine, a physician, says: 'You might as well try to teach sanitation to mules as to try to teach it to negroes.' With this opinion I do not fully agree. I agree the task is a hard one. Progress will necessarily be slow. But the negro is not incapable of learning..."

"well-born" (OED). In the United States, one of eugenic's leading proponents was Charles B. Davenport (1866–1944), a professor of evolutionary biology at Harvard (Chase, 1977; Kevels, 1985; Carlson, 2001). In 1910, Davenport became director of the Cold Spring Harbor Laboratory, funded by the Carnegie Institute and one of the first institutions in the world to specialize in genetics research. While there, he founded the highly influential Eugenic Record Office (Chase, 1977; Kevels, 1985; Carlson, 2001), an entity curiously not mentioned in the brief online history included in the Laboratory's website (Cold Spring Harbor Laboratory, 2009).

As Davenport explained in 1911 in the opening pages of his landmark book, *Heredity in Relation to Eugenics* (1911, p. 1):

Eugenics is the science of the improvement of the human race by better breeding, or, as the late Sir Francis Galton expressed it: 'The science which deals with all influences that improve the inborn qualities of a race.' The eugenical standpoint is that of the agriculturalist who, while recognizing the value of culture, believes that permanent advance is to be made only by securing the best 'blood.'

Davenport's metaphoric use of "blood" is telling for what it reveals about how the early twentieth century scientific understanding of what constituted a "gene"—and what made for "good breeding"—was every bit as "fuzzy" (Keller, 2000; Gould, 2002) as had been the case for *miasma, contagion*, and *germs* in the mid-nineteenth century (Tomes, 1997); limited scientific precision once again left much room for debate.

The first major articulation of Galton's eugenic views appeared in 1869 in his ground-breaking and highly praised work *Hereditary Genius: An Inquiry into its Laws and Consequences* (Galton, 1869). In this book, Galton argued it was both conceivable—and desirable—"to produce a highly-gifted race of men (*sic*) by judicious marriages during several consecutive generations" (Galton, 1869, p. 1). The idea of inborn superiority, as might be expected, was held to operate both within and between "races," with Galton ranking ancient Athenians highest, the English somewhat lower, and "negroes" and the "Australian type"—that is, aboriginal peoples—the lowest (Galton, 1869, pp. 336–350). Thus, although every group might be expected to have its talented members and its "imbeciles," such that there could be exceptional "negroes" who were superior to the average English person, some populations, by virtue of better breeding, were concentrated at the top rank and others, as a result of inborn inferiority, were at the bottom.

To Galton, Davenport, and other eugenicists, it was a scientifically self-evident fact that "good breeding" was, literally, a matter of heredity rather than upbringing. To test these ideas (and presumably lend them scientific support), Galton invented new statistical methods to analyze correlations and conduct linear regression, so as to quantify the contribution of heredity to such outcomes as longevity, intelligence, and also the variation of other traits within and between groups (MacKenzie, 1979; MacKenzie, 1981; Porter, 1986; Desrosières, 1998). Galton's intellectual stamp on the nascent field of biostatistics was strong. As is well-documented, an explicit eugenics agenda motivated the early twentieth century biometrical research on correlation coefficients, analysis of variance, regression, and randomized trials conducted by both Sir Karl Pearson (1837–1936), the first holder of the Galton Chair of Eugenics at the University of London, and R. A. Fisher (1890–1962), the second holder of this chair (MacKenzie, 1979; MacKenzie, 1981; Porter, 1986; Desrosières, 1998). These widely applicable statistical techniques, along with their inbuilt assumptions about correlation and variance of traits, continue to inform epidemiologic research to this day.

Bad Blood and Bad Genes As a Threat to Health and a Menace to Society. Eugenics, however, was not only framed as a "positive" science encouraging procreation among the "fit"; it also had an explicit "negative" side dedicated to "weeding out" the "unfit" (Chase, 1977; Kevels, 1985; Gould, 1996; Carlson, 2001; Stern, 2005a; Stern, 2005b, Painter 2010). As early as 1869, Galton argued that "[i]t may be monstrous that the weak should be crowded out by the strong, but it is still more monstrous that the races best fitted to play their part on the stage of life, should be crowded out by the incompetent, the ailing, and the desponding" (Galton, 1869, p. 357). Four decades later, in 1911, Davenport bluntly stated the eugenic solution to the problem Galton posed and its social justification (Davenport, 1911, pp. 267–268):

> The commonwealth is greater than any individual in it. Hence the rights of society over the life, the reproduction, the behavior and the traits of the individuals that compose it are, in all matters that concern the life and proper progress of society, limitless, and society may take life, may sterilize, may segregate so as to prevent marriage, may restrict liberty in a hundred of ways.
> Society has not only the right, but upon it devolves the profound duty, to know the nature of the germ plasm upon which, in the last analysis, the life and progress of the state depend… It may and should locate antisocial traits such as feeble-mindedness, epilepsy, delusions, melancholia, mental deterioration, craving for narcotics, lack of more sense and self-control, tendency to wander, to steal, to assault and to commit wanton cruelties upon children and animals. It may and should locate strains with an inherent tendency to certain diseases such as tuberculosis, rickets, cancer, chronic rheumatitis, gout, diabetes insipidus, goiter, luechemia, chlorosis, hemophilia, eye and ear defects and the scores of other diseases that have a hereditary factor. It should know where the traits are, how they are being reproduced, and how to eliminate them.

For society not to act on the scientific evidence linking heredity to health was, in the eyes of the eugenicists, profoundly shortsighted—and immoral.

At the broadest public health level, the late nineteenth and early twentieth century eugenic hereditarian postulates of inborn deficiencies—deemed also the basis of innate class and racial inferiority—reinforced epidemiologic explanations of class, racial/ethnic, and international health disparities as a consequence of "nature," rather than "nurture" (Chase, 1977; Kevels, 1985; Gould, 1996; Pernick, 1997; Porter, 1999; Ernst & Harris, 1999; Stern, 2005a; Stern, 2005b; Duster, 2006). At once competing with and complementing germ theory (Pernick, 1997), eugenic thinking blamed medicine for hindering the "weeding out" of the "unfit" and castigated the late nineteenth and early twentieth century hygienic and bacteriological triumphs of public health and epidemiology as self-defeating interventions (Davenport, 1911; Weingart, 1995; *see* **Textbox 4–3**); in Davenport's words (1911, p. iv):

Modern medicine is responsible for the loss of appreciation of the power of heredity. It has had its attention too exclusively focused on germs and conditions of life. It has neglected the personal element that help determines the course of every disease. It has begotten a wholly impersonal hygiene whose teachings are false in so far as they are laid down as universally applicable. It has forgotten the fundamental fact that all men are created *bound* by their protoplasmic makeup and *unequal* in their powers and responsibilities.

From a eugenic perspective, the population distribution of disease clearly mirrored the distribution of "negative and positive traits," passed on from parents to their offspring (Davenport, 1911, pp. 181–182); inborn "host factors" decisively trumped exogenous exposures, be they germs or the "environment."

Together, eugenics and germ theory provided mutually reinforcing ways to define groups deemed to pose a threat to the public's well-being (Pernick, 1997)—and became a staple of mainstream scientific thinking and both public health and policy discourse (Chase, 1977; Kevels, 1985; Gould, 1996; Stern, 2005a; Stern, 2005b; Duster, 2006). Bad "genes" joined dangerous "germs" as a key menace to civilization—and woe to any population deemed to harbor both.

During the era of these theories' joint ascendance, it accordingly should not be surprising that in the early twentieth century United States, "[B]lacks were," in the words of historian Vanessa Northington Gamble, "depicted more as public health pests than as the hapless victims of disease" (Gamble, 1989, p. iii). Exemplifying this tendency, in 1915 the *American Journal of the Public Health* published a special issue (volume 5, no. 3; *see* Allen, 1915; Brunner, 1915; Fort, 1915; Graves, 1915; Hindman, 1915; Lee, 1915) focused on the "Negro health problem"—and in it portrayed Black Americans as an inherently inferior, germ-infested population, whose existence posed a threat to White population's well-being: "a menace to himself and to us" (Brunner, 1915, p. 188; *see* excerpts in **Textbox 4–3**). Published in the era's pre-eminent public health journal, these views closely echoed the arguments presented in the highly influential 1896 treatise on *Race Traits and Tendencies of the American Negro* by Frederick Hoffman (1865–1946), a text widely read and cited by scientists, health professionals, and politicians alike (Wolff, 2006) (*see* excerpts in **Textbox 4–3**). Deeming his position scientific, objective, and supported by the evidence, Hoffman argued (1896, p. 310):

In marked contrast with the frequent assertions, such as that of Mill, that race is not important and that environment or conditions of life are the most important factors in the final result of the struggle for life, we have here abundant evidence that we find in race and heredity the determining factors in the upward or downward course of mankind.

In the field of statistical research, sentiment, prejudice, or the influence of pre-conceived ideas have no place. The data which have been brought here together in a convenient form speak for themselves. From the standpoint of the impartial investigator, no difference of interpretation of their meaning seems possible. The decrease in the rate of increase in the colored population has been traced first to excessive mortality, which in turn has been traced to an inferior vital capacity. The mixture of the African with the white race has been shown to have seriously affected the longevity of the former and left as a heritage to future generations the poison of scrofula, tuberculosis and most of all syphilis.

Going further, he declared: "It is not in the conditions of life, but in race and heredity that we find the explanation of the fact to be observed in all parts of the globe, in all times and among all people, namely, the superiority of one race over another, and of the Aryan race

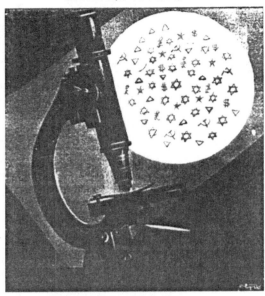

Figure 4–1. Nazi cartoon depicting, through the lens of a microscope, the Jewish star (and Communist sickle) as lethal bacteria; originally published in *Der Stürmer* in 1943 (Gradman, 2000, p. 25).

Translation of the poem accompanying the cartoon:

By means of his poison the Jew corrupts
The sluggish blood of weak nations,
And thus, a syndrome is produced
That has a rapid downward trend.
With us, however, the report is this:
The blood is pure. We are sound.

over all" (Hoffman, 1896, p. 312). It should likewise not be surprising, then, that German Nazi racial ideology similarly identified Jews not only as biologically degenerate but also as pests, parasites, and germs (Proctor, 1988; Gradman, 2000), with this linkage well-captured by a famous 1943 cartoon that depicted, magnified under a microscope, the Jewish star (and Communist sickle) as lethal bacteria (Gradman, 2000; **Figure 4–1**).

Translated into public health policy, eugenic beliefs set the basis for state-mandated sterilization laws, which had the dual purpose of reducing the number of the "unfit" and reducing state welfare expenditures (Chase, 1977; Kevels, 1985; Pernick, 1997; Ladd-Taylor, 1997; Carlson, 2001; Stern, 2005a; Stern, 2005b). The first such law anywhere in the world was enacted in the United States in 1907 (in Indiana) and was upheld by the U.S. Supreme Court decision *Buck* v. *Bell* in 1927 (*see* excerpt in **Textbox 4–3**). By 1932,

27 U.S. states had passed these laws, and in that year alone, an estimated 3,900 women were sterilized—predominantly poor, of color, and foreign-born (Stern, 2005a; Stern, 2005b; Proctor, 1988; Duster, 2006). One year later, in 1933, the Nazi regime in Germany passed its first eugenic sterilization laws, directly drawing on U.S. laws and eugenic expertise (Chase, 1977; Kevels, 1985; Proctor, 1988). By 1939, more than 40,000 such sterilizations had been performed in the United States (Proctor, 1988, p. 97); other countries that adopted eugenic sterilization programs in the early twentieth century included Canada, Sweden, Switzerland, Norway, Iceland, and Finland (Wahlsten, 1997; Zylberman, 2004; Hansen et al., 2008). Consistent with Galton's reasoning in 1869 (Galton, 1869), and Davenport's policy prescription in 1911 (Davenport, 1911), the basic premises were: (*1*) a clear biological distinction existed between the "fit" and "unfit" (Hansen et al., 2008), and (*2*) eliminating poverty, degeneracy, and their affiliated diseases required preventing the literal reproduction of people whose inborn traits, rather than societal context, were posited to be the source of these afflictions.

The (Social) Environment: Beyond "Germs" and "Genes"

Not surprisingly, sharp opposition to the views of the eugenicists existed within the many disciplines in public health, in medicine, in the social sciences, and in the broader civil society as well (Sydenstricker, 1933; Greenwood, 1935; Rosen, 1958 [1993]; Chase, 1977; Kevels, 1985; Porter, 1999). In the case of epidemiology, the early twentieth century theoretical and empirical work countering not only the eugenic argument but also, as noted above, the overly narrow framing of germ theory explicitly brought attention to the causal role of social and environmental conditions in shaping disease distribution—of both infectious and non-infectious disease alike (Sydenstricker, 1933; Greenwood, 1935). Motivating this work were not only social concerns but also, as noted previously, the growing awareness—as morbidity and mortality caused by infectious disease was on the decline (*see* **Table 4–1**)— that new thinking and new efforts were needed to address the rising toll of chronic and non-communicable diseases. The ensuing discussion and debate underscore that epidemiologic theorizing was not deterministically constrained to develop on only one track; the availability of different ways of thinking was a contemporaneous fact.

Occupational, Class, and Racial/Ethnic Health Disparities. One illustration of new (or renewed) twentieth century epidemiologic orientation to investigating factors other than germs and genes was research in the nascent field of occupational health epidemiology (Weindling, 1985). A leader in this work was Dr. Alice Hamilton (1869–1970) (1943; Sicherman, 1984; Sellars, 1997), whose 1925 book, *Industrial Poisons in the United States* (Hamilton, 1925), constituted the first such textbook in the field.

Commencing with her first investigation in 1911, which focused on lead poisoning (Hamilton, 1911), Hamilton encountered obstacles caused both by a lack of data and by attitudes that held workers responsible for their own illness; in the preface to her 1925 textbook, she ruefully noted (Hamilton, 1925, pp. v–vi):

> ...If the recording intern would only treat the poison from which the man is suffering with as much interest as he gives to the coffee the patient has drunk and the tobacco he has smoked, if he would ask as carefully about the length of time he was exposed to the poison as about the age at which he had measles, the task of the searcher for truth about industrial poisons would be so very much easier....

Apparently it is impossible for some physicians to treat industrial diseases with the detachment and impartiality with which they approach those diseases which are not confined to the working classes. For a striking example of this, the reader is referred to a bulletin issued by the Bureau of Labor Statistics on a trade disease—not an intoxicant—in stonecutters. The evidence is given from a doctor who worked for the stonecutters' union and from two who were brought in by the employers. Not only is there the widest divergence of views presented, but the physician who was retained by the men shows so strong a sympathy for them as to quite dull his critical sense, and the physicians for the company accept evidence which on the face of it is one-sided and then indulge in moral observations on the character of the workingmen and the evils of trade-unionism.

Also troubling to Hamilton was the lack of acceptance of the principles of differential susceptibility so routinely invoked for infectious disease, with variation instead typically attributed by physicians, researchers, and employers to workers' improvident—if not immoral—behavior (Hamilton, 1925, pp. 15–16):

> ... Among 167 smelter workers who had plumbism, were 18 who came down with lead poisoning in less than three weeks, the rest averaged more than three months... It is safe to say that there is no feature of industrial poisoning so troublesome to the physician as this difference in susceptibility... It will be very hard for him to get his employer to see this, for the practical layman believes what is dangerous for one man will be dangerous for all. He knows that a spurt of molten metal will burn any man it strikes; a falling scaffold, a current of electricity, a bursting fly wheel, these do not injure one and spare another. The damage is in direct proportion to the exposure. Why then, he argues, should one man get lead poisoning from work over a melting pot when twenty men in the same room do not show the slightest sign of ill-health? Yet this same employer recognizes the everyday fact than in any epidemic of any kind a large proportion of the population is not taken sick. Even at the height of the great influenza visitation the victims were always in the minority. If a village with 500 inhabitants has its water supply infected with typhoid bacilli, there will not be 500 cases of typhoid, there may not be 50. But if there are no more than five, the infected water is responsible and not some depravity of the five individuals. Even animals show a great variation in their susceptibility to poisons, yet they cannot be accused of alcoholism, or dyspepsia from eating pie, or late hours and excessive dancing, or any of the other sins against personal hygiene so comforting to the worried employer ...

At the same time, Hamilton was cognizant that notions of differential susceptibility could be—and were—erroneously invoked when it came to explaining racial/ethnic and gender disparities in occupational disease, and in her textbook she provided examples (*see* excerpts in **Textbox 4–4**) showing that Black and White workers, and also women and men workers, could have similar rates of occupational disease if they worked under the same conditions (which, given occupational employment patterns, they almost never did) (Hamilton, 1925, pp. 6–9). At once hearkening back to the more radical socially oriented epidemiologic theories of the prior century, including their emphasis on employers' responsibility for workplace exposures (Hamilton, 1925, pp. 541–542), while also engaging with the newer ideas about exposure and susceptibility at play in germ theory (and, in a different way, eugenics), Hamilton's conceptual approach to investigating occupational disease accordingly opened new possibilities for integrating biological and social concepts into epidemiologic theories of disease distribution.

Equally groundbreaking was new epidemiologic research broadly reframing U.S. Black/White health inequities in economic and social terms (Gamble, 1989; Krieger & Fee, 1996). Exemplifying this new work were two texts prepared by the eminent U.S. scholar W.E.B. Du Bois (1868–1963), the first Black American ever to be awarded a Ph.D. by Harvard University (Marable, 2005). The first was his 1899 pathbreaking analysis of "The Health of

Textbox 4–4 . Early Twentieth Century Examples of U.S. Epidemiologic Analyses Reframing Occupational and Black/White Health Disparities in Social and Environmental Terms

Hamilton A. *Industrial Poisons in the United States.* **New York: Macmillan, 1925.**

p. v: "The sources of our knowledge of industrial poisoning in the United States are neither full nor, for the most part, accurate. We lack the sickness insurance system which obtains in all industrial countries in Europe and which brings to light the incidence of illness of all kinds in all groups of workers... Not one [US] hospital in twenty has records which yield the sort of information which the student of industrial toxicology craves and yet this is not elaborate"

pp. 6–7: *Influence of Race* (italics in original)–Experienced foremen and employers of labor believe there is a difference between colored and white men with regard to their susceptibility to certain industrial poisons... [in] a shell-loading plant in Virginia, Te Linde found no case of TNT sickness among the Negroes... On the other hand, Herman and Putnam, working in a nitration plant in Pennsylvania, found no difference in the susceptibility of the two races... These observations were of more value than those made in the shell-loading plants, because in the latter the Negroes and whites were in only rare instances employed in the same department, while in the nitration plant they worked together. Besides this, the Negroes in the Virginia plant lived in their own cabins, the whites in company barracks with the company canteen, and the Negroes were much more cleanly in their habits, more willing to take baths than were the mountain whites. In the Pennsylvania plant the two races lived and worked under the same conditions. This disappearance of the apparent difference in susceptibility between the two races when they are placed under the same conditions was found by the French also in munitions plants during the war... At first it seemed that the yellow race [*sic*], the Annamites, were decidedly the most resistant, and the whites the least so, with blacks occupying the middle place. Later on, however, the French concluded that the differences between the yellow race and the white could be accounted for on grounds other than that of racial susceptibility. The white men were more intemperate, more uncleanly in their habits, and less obedient to shop discipline than were the yellow men (*sic*), and in addition the most expert medical supervision was given to the white men, resulting in a more careful diagnosis and the detection of earlier cases."

pp. 8–9: *Influence of Sex* (italics in original)–It is to the literature on lead poisoning that one must turn for material on the question of sex as a factor in industrial poisoning. British observers who have had much experience with women exposed to lead in the white lead industry and also in the glazing, finishing, and decorating of pottery and tiles, hold that women not only succumb more quickly to lead but suffer more severely from its effects...

... an investigation of lead poisoning in potteries made by me in Trenton, New Jersey and in the East Liverpool and Zanesville regions of Ohio in 1912, and it brought to light a high rate of lead poisoning among the women as compared with the men, but a closer analysis threw doubt upon the part played by sex in this difference.

The pottery industry in the United States falls into two divisions: the so-called white-ware potteries which are organized in a strong trade union, and the art and utility potteries and tile which are unorganized. The women are entirely unorganized in both fields. In the white-ware potteries, the contrast between the two sexes was striking. There were only 39 cases of lead poisoning among 796 men, or 4.89 per hundred, and 29 cases among 150 women, or 19.3 per hundred, but the women had many handicaps aside from that of sex idiosyncrasy. They were unorganized, under-paid, poorly housed, poorly fed, subject to the worry and strain of supporting dependents on a low wage, while the men made high wages, were sure of their jobs, and lived comfortably. In the unorganized pottery fields, however, in the tile works and arts and utility potteries, the men and women were in the same economic class, all making low wages with everything that that implies, and no appreciable difference was found there between the two sexes with regard to susceptibility to lead. Among 304 men there were 48 cases of lead poisoning, or 15.78 per hundred, and among 243 women there were 28 cases or 11.52 per hundred, a slightly lower rate, but then the women averaged a shorter period of employment than the men."

pp. 541–542: "A sanitary engineer may be told by a city council that it cannot afford a pure water supply and he may have no choice but to accept the verdict. But he would be greatly at fault if he allowed the city fathers to believe that the half-way measures they plan will safeguard the community against typhoid fever. In the same way the industrial physician may be obliged to abandon his plan for protecting his charges against poisoning because the expense is greater than management will allow or because a change in the method may make the product less perfect. But in so yielding let him be careful never to sacrifice his own intellectual integrity nor adopt the standards of the non-medical man to whom the proper working of the plant is of first importance. His task is to safeguard the health of the patients who are entrusted to him, often without any volition of their own."

Du Bois WEB (ed). *Health and Physique of the Negro American.* **Atlanta, GA: The Atlanta University Press, 1906.**

p. 89: "If the population were divided as to social and economic condition the matter of race would be almost entirely eliminated. Poverty's death rate in Russia shows a much greater divergence from the rate among the well-to-do than the difference between Negroes and white Americans. In England, according to Mulhall, the poor have a rate twice as high as the rich, and the well-to-do are between the two. The same is true in Sweden, Germany and other countries. In Chicago the death rate among whites of the stock yards district is higher than the Negroes of that city and further away from the death rate of the Hyde Park district of that city than the Negroes are from the whites in Philadelphia.

Even in consumption all the evidence goes to show that it is not a racial disease but a social disease. The rate in certain sections among whites in New York and Chicago is higher than the Negroes of some cities. But as yet no careful study of consumption has been made in order to see whether or not the race factor can be eliminated, and if not, what part it plays."

Trask JW. The significance of the mortality rates of the colored populations of the United States. *Am J Public Health* **1916; 6:254–260.**

p. 254: "To one interested in the public health the questions which will arise in connec-tion with this difference between the white and colored death-rates are (1) the reason for the difference; (2) whether the cause is an essential one, inherent in one element of the population and not in the other, and finally (3) whether the factors which produce the difference in the death-rates can be removed and the colored death-rate lowered until it approximates that of the white element of the population."

p. 257: "A study of the colored mortality rates of cities and of the urban and rural populations of states shows that the colored death-rate is subject to influences which produce variations and that the rate is by no means fixed."

> pp. 258–259: "In considering the separation of deaths into those of white and colored, one must bear in mind the possibility that in many communities such separation may amount to a classification according to the industrial or economic status, the colored deaths being those in households having smaller incomes. In this connection one is reminded that investigations into the rate of infant mortality and of the relative prevalence of certain diseases, such as tuberculosis, have revealed that the infant mortality rate varied usually with the incomes of the population groups and that the relative prevalence of tuberculosis seemed to be largely determined by the same factor. It may be that if in the average community deaths could be classified according to economic status, that is, according to the family or household income, a difference in mortality rates would be obtained approximately as great as that resulting from a white and colored classification."
>
> p. 259: "In conclusion, it is believed that the comparison of mortality rates previously discussed shows: (1) That the colored death-rates of most communities of the United States are not discouragingly high; (2) that they are undoubtedly lower than they have been in the past; (3) that they are as low as many white population groups possessed twenty or thirty years ago, and are in fact as low as some white populations possess at the present time; and (4) that with the economic and industrial progress of the colored population its death-rate will gradually approach nearer to that of the white population."

Negroes" appearing in Chapter 10 of *The Philadelphia Negro* (Du Bois, 1899), which was simultaneously the first in-depth comprehensive analysis of an urban African-American community and also a pathbreaking work in both sociology and public health (Nelson, 2004; Marable, 2005); the second was the 1906 volume Du Bois edited on the *Health and Physique of the Negro American* (Du Bois, 1906) (*see* excerpt in **Textbox 4–4**).

Following the same logic McCune Smith had employed over a half-century before when comparing the health status of then enslaved Blacks to poor Whites (*see* **Chapter 3**), Du Bois held that Black/White health disparities were not fixed, but instead depended on economic and social conditions. Explicitly taking on Hoffman's racial inferiority thesis, he argued (Du Bois, 1906, p. 89):

> ... The undeniable fact is, then, that in certain diseases the Negroes have a much higher rate than the whites, and especially in consumption, pneumonia and infantile diseases.
>
> The question is: Is this racial? Mr. Hoffman would lead us to say yes, and to infer that it means that Negroes are inherently inferior in physique to whites.
>
> But the difference in Philadelphia can be explained on other grounds than upon race. The high death rate of Philadelphia Negroes is yet lower than the whites of Savannah, Charleston, New Orleans and Atlanta ...

To buttress his case, Du Bois drew on admittedly limited empirical data to demonstrate that not only could rates of disease be higher among poor Whites compared to the Black population but also that class gaps in health often exceeded those observed for race/ethnicity. He realized, however, that a true testing of this hypothesis would require more complete data, and he acccordingly called for more research jointly employing racial/ethnic and socioeconomic data to "see whether or not the race factor can be eliminated, and, if not, what part it plays" (Du Bois, 1906, p. 89).

Others soon followed Du Bois' lead, as illustrated by an article on "The Significance of the mortality rates of the colored populations of the United States" (Trask, 1916), written by John William Trask (1877-?), Assistant Surgeon General in the United States Public Health Service, and published in 1916 in the *American Journal of Public Health*. Appearing 1 year after this same journal's 1915 special issue on "the health of the Negro," Trask's paper offered an analysis diametrically opposed to those proffered in the previous year. Reviewing the evidence on mortality rates in relation to both race/ethnicity and "industrial or economic status," Trask reported that not only had Black rates declined substantially and varied by economic level but were sometimes even lower than White rates—and he predicted that "with the economic and industrial progress of the colored population its death-rate will gradually approach nearer to that of the white population" (Trask, 1916, p. 259) (*see* excerpt in **Textbox 4–4**).

Subsequent U.S. epidemiologic research conducted in the 1930s jointly addressing race/ethnicity and socioeconomic position—as done in 1933 in New York City (Holland & Perrott, 1938a) and in the 1935–1936 National Health Survey (Holland & Perrott, 1938b)—likewise found: (*1*) an association between poor health and poverty among both Blacks and Whites, and (*2*) Black/White differences in health largely resulted from higher poverty rates among the Black compared to White population. As summarized in a 1937 review article titled "The Socio-Economic Background of Negro Health Status" written by Clark Tibbitts (1903–1985), the U.S. Public Health Service researcher in charge of the 1935–1936 National Health Survey, "[i]t seems safe to state the hypothesis that environmental conditions are important in determining Negro health status" (Tibbitts, 1937, p. 428). Effectively refuting Hoffman's claim that "(t)he data… speak for themselves" (Hoffman, 1896, p. 310), these contemporaneous analyses instead clarified epidemiologic theory's vital role for hypotheses about population distributions of health.

Theorizing the Role of Environments—Social and Biophysical—in Shaping Population Rates of Disease, Disability, Death, and Health. One of the first early twentieth century comprehensive English-language texts to articulate and start to cohere a broader epidemiologic framework that encompassed but was not restricted to "germs" and "genes" was the landmark volume *Health and Environment*, written by Edgar Sydenstricker (1881–1936), one of the era's leading public health researchers (Wiehl, 1974; Krieger & Fee, 1996; Krieger, 2000). Having joined the U.S. Public Health Service shortly after its founding in 1912, where he served as its first statistician (with a prior training in economics), Sydenstricker quickly moved into investigating associations between economic conditions and health status. His research spanned from the effects of income on New York City garment workers' health in 1916 (Warren & Sydenstricker, 1916), to the classic studies in the 1920s establishing pellagra as a dietary deficiency disease linked to low income (Goldberger, Wheeler, & Sydenstricker, 1920; Sydenstricker & King, 1920; Terris, 1964; Etheridge, 1972), to the establishment of the first U.S. population-based surveys in the 1920s to study morbidity, including in relation to income (Sydenstricker, 1925), on through designing multi-city surveys to examine the effects of the Great Depression on illness (Sydenstricker, 1934; Perrott & Collins, 1934; Perrott & Sydenstricker, 1935); he died in 1936, shortly after having written much of the legislation that became the Social Security Act of 1935 (Wiehl, 1974; Krieger & Fee, 1996).

Sydenstricker prepared *Health and Environment* as a monograph for the U.S. President's Research Committee on Social Trends, which was established in 1929 in the wake of the stock market crash and the onset of the Great Depression (Sydenstricker, 1933, p. v). The monograph not only grappled directly with eugenic arguments and evidence but also, as clearly delineated in the volume's table of content (*see* **Textbox 4–5**), it explicated the myriad ways in which "geographic," "urban and rural," "social," and "occupational" environments—in conjunction with people's "social heritage" (Sydenstricker, 1935, p. 13)—could influence rates of somatic and mental illness, physical disability, and death. To Sydenstricker,

Textbox 4–5. Edgar Sydenstricker's *Health and Environment*. (New York: McGraw-Hill, 1933): Table of Contents and Selected Excerpts

Table of Contents

Selected Excerpts

On Conceptualizing "The Environment":

a) *Scope of "Environment": Physical + Social + Their Dynamic Inter-relationship*

p. 13: "Environment is not merely the physical world upon which we live–the topography of its surface, the variety of climate, the kind of water, the fauna and flora. Nor does it include also only the physical changes that man [*sic*] has accomplished in adapting his [*sic*] physical habitat to himself [*sic*]—by houses, roads, agriculture, manufacture, use of electricity, radio, and the like. Our 'social heritage,' as Graham Wallas puts it, is also a very important part of our human environment."

b) *The Physical Environment and Population Health: Impact of Fixed Features, Features Changed by People, and the Process of Change*

pp. 14–15: "Not forgetting that our population is composed of individuals biologically diverse by reason of genetic processes, let us see what this concept of the environment implies.

In the first place there is a physical environment in which innumerable conditions and relations may affect, directly or indirectly, health. The more advanced the progress of civilization, the greater is the alteration of physical environment that man [*sic*] has accomplished. Climate, for example, in itself has not been changed by man, but he [*sic*] is modifying its effects by clothing, by the type of building, by supplying heat, and more recently, by overcoming heat. Soil is changed by cultivation, by use of chemical fertilizers, and by irrigation. Topography is changed by constructing roads; the obstacles it so presents may be so readily overcome by further development of aviation as to constitute no barrier to communication. Animals and plants are altered by breeding. Distance is overcome by telegraph, telephone, radio, and speed of travel. Physical materials are rearranged and changed in form so that an almost infinite variety of mechanical tools and instruments exists. Thus there are three important ways in which physical environment may affect the well-being of a population, namely, (a) by its unchangeable composition and form; (b) by its changed composition and form; and (c) by the process of changing it. Not only our physical surroundings but civilization in the making should be regarded as possible factors in a population's health."

c) *The Population as Part of the Environment: Health Influences of Social Structure, Social Relations, Social and Cultural Traditions, and Social Change*

p. 15: "In the second place the population itself constitutes a part of the total environment. We speak of this as a *social* environment, and the more we study it, the more we are impressed with its importance as a factor in determining the physical and mental well-being of the population and the rate at which the individual members survive. In every group of human beings there exist certain social relations and modes of social behavior. The community has not only a geographic habitat but also a social structure. The individuals composing the community are clustered in families; associated into overlapping groups for trade, occupation, religion, and amusement; separated into classes differentiated by caste and economic achievement; swayed as a mob from one course of social action to another; guided by newly acquired knowledge, such as inventions or discoveries of ways in which to escape or cure disease. Tradition, superstition, and mores; modes of living, fads, and fashions; standardization of ideas and attitudes by the press, movies, radio, and schools; cultural factors, such as the esthetic idea of posture or a religious regimen of diet or of personal cleanliness–these go to make up our social environment and constitute conditions that may influence health in an even greater degree than physical surroundings. Again, in considering social environment, not only the social surroundings that exist at a given instant in time but the process of change must be taken into account."

d) *Social, Economic, and Political Beliefs and Actions As Environmental Influences on Population Health*

p. 16: "In the third place the commonly held biological concept of adaptation of man [*sic*] to environment and of man's [*sic*] adaptation of environment to his [*sic*] needs is insufficient to account for all the genetic and environmental factors involved in his well-being. Man [*sic*] is a sentient being, possesses volition, and acts consciously, although some individuals of the species are less sentient, less capable of volition and of conscious action than others. But every human population, every cluster of individuals, is deliberately forming group attitudes, developing popular aims, and seeking to carry out these aims by group action. To deny this is to deny all civilization and culture.

This is not the place to discuss at length the sociological aspects of the relation of a people to its environment, but a few illustrations are pertinent. Economic factors in the conservation or waste of health, for example, are not merely the rate of wages; the hours of labor; the hazard of accident, of poisonous substances, or of deleterious dusts; they include also the attitude consciously taken with respect to the question of the relative importance of large capitalistic profits *versus* maintenance of the worker's welfare. Religious dogma or the expression of group volition in the form of laws may impose a behavior that is beneficial or harmful to physical well-being. The misuse of intoxicants is generally regarded as prejudicial to health, but the prohibition of all intoxicants has been found to result in other prejudicial conditions..."

On Elucidating the Pathways by Which Social and Economic Factors Affect Health:

pp. 109–110: "The fact that the incidence of illness and of death is relatively more frequent in the lower economic, occupational, and social strata of society than in the higher does not throw much light upon the specific reasons why this is so. It is confirmation by experience of the correctness of the thinking that leads us to expect this result; but it does not explain, nor is it of much practical value except as an argument against an economic system that is characterized by so much poverty.

What we need to understand are the precise ways in which various social and economic factors influence the prevalence of a given impairment, the incidence of a given disease, or the death rate from a given cause. To obtain this knowledge of the interaction of environment and health, thorough inquiries are necessary into the etiology of each disease and into the specific conditions that affect its prevalence. Epidemiology has been confined so far almost entirely to a few infectious diseases; untouched fields remain for exploration. The student in these fields should be trained not only in the etiology of disease and in human pathology but also in the social sciences. We know, for example, that typhoid fever is caused by the transmission, to susceptible persons, of a specific bacillus from the excreta of human beings who either are affected by the disease or are healthy carriers of it. Many carefully made observations have demonstrated that the bacilli may reach susceptible persons in sufficient quantities to cause an attack of the disease through water, milk, and food supplies and through carriage of excreta from infected persons by direct contact or by insects that have come into contact with infected excreta. We have not, however, troubled ourselves sufficiently to find out the extent to which, or the ways in which, social and economic factors may determine or influence any of these modes of transmission of the disease, and in what ways they operate."

the concept of the "environment" necessarily included "all of the external circumstances, both physical and social, which come into relation to the lives of human beings" (Sydenstricker, 1933, p. 206). At issue were dynamic interrelationships involving (*see* **Textbox 4–5**): (*1*) the health impacts of the physical environment, as mediated by its fixed features (geographical and climactic), those features changed by people, and the process of change itself; (*2*) the health influences of the population (itself construed as part of the environment), as mediated by social structure, social relations, social and cultural traditions, and social change; and (*3*) the role of social, economic, and political beliefs and actions as environmental influences on population health. In Sydenstricker's words (Sydenstricker, 1933, p. 206):

> "[E]conomic factors in the conservation or waste of health, for example, are not merely the rate of wages; the hours of labor; the hazard of accident, of poisonous substances, or of deleterious dusts; they include also the attitude consciously taken with respect to the question of the relative importance of large capitalistic profits *versus* maintenance of the workers' welfare." (Sydenstricker, 1933, p. 16)

Sydenstricker had no illusions that all of these aspects of the environment could be analyzed in any single study. Instead, in calling attention to complexity, Sydenstricker's intent was to urge "the student of the relation of environment to health," who although likely "to confine himself (*sic*) to some one phase of the environment, such as the economic, the occupational, or the geographic," of the necessity of being "aware of the fact that environment is not compassed by the specific condition upon which his (*sic*) interest is centered, as well as keep in mind the fact that the individuals composing his (*sic*) population group are differentiated by biological inheritance" (Sydenstricker, 1933, pp. 12–13). He further reassuringly explained, albeit with a critical caveat:

> Actually, however, there is no need for so complete an array of facts as the concept appears to imply. Data are relatively important in proportion to their relevancy. The search for knowledge cannot be carried on in all directions simultaneously by any one student. The most practicable procedure obviously is to arrive at a reasonably accurate understanding of one specific environmental factor at a time. If the student is in a position to collect the data that appear pertinent as the logic of the particular situation unfolds, he (*sic*) will be able to suggest conclusions that, if confirmed by other inquiries, will possess scientific value and ultimately social utility. All experience of an army of painstaking workers in scientific fields attests the soundness and the practicability of this method. Yet it is a dangerous procedure because the too cocksure are likely to overlook important factors other than the one which is the especial object of study for the moment. It is for this reason that so broad a concept of environment has been insisted upon and the perils of too narrow an outlook upon the complexities of the subject of environment and health have been so persistently emphasized in this monograph.

As the last two sentences sharply clarified, a comprehensive approach to conceptualizing the "environment" was critical for the valid design, conduct, and interpretation even of studies seemingly focused on "one" factor. In other words, epidemiologic research required epidemiologic theory.

To Sydenstricker, the epidemiologic challenge was twofold: both to elucidate how people's physical and sociological relationships to diverse aspects of the environment affected health and to assess the impact of "conscious social efforts to modify the environment for the purposes of preventing disease, promoting health, and prolonging life" (Sydenstricker, 1933, p. 17). By delineating multiple facets of the environment, their mutability over time, and the shared and different pathways by which they might affect different types of outcomes, Sydenstricker offered a glimpse of a simultaneously more expansive and systematic approach to epidemiologic theorizing than had previously existed.

Expanding Epidemiology's Scope—Including Its Scope of Theorizing. Indeed, as reflected by Sydenstricker's broad view, by the late 1920s and early 1930s it was clear to the era's leading epidemiologists that, in Sydenstricker's words, "Epidemiology has been confined so far almost entirely to a few infectious diseases; untouched fields remain for exploration" (Sydenstricker, 1933, p. 109). In 1927, Frost recognized that "usage has extended the meaning of epidemiology beyond its original limits, to denote not merely the doctrine of epidemics but a science of broader scope in relation to the mass-phenomena of diseases in their usual or endemic as well as their epidemic occurrences" (Frost, 1927, p. 493). In 1928, Chapin concurred, observing that "[r]ecently there has been a tendency to extend it (epidemiology) to include other diseases, such as cancer and the dietary disease, such as diabetes, pellagra, and beriberi"—with the latter two non-infectious ailments notably introducing the novel idea that disease could result from the absence of something good, rather than the presence of something bad. To Chapin, it was time to expand the definition to include more than infectious disease, and to affirm instead that: "The epidemiologist devotes himself (*sic*) chiefly to the study of disease as it actually occurs in human beings" (Chapin, 1928 7, p. 481).

Summing up the new orientation, Greenwood's 1935 book, *Epidemics and Crowd-Diseases: An Introduction to the Study of Epidemiology,* published 1 year after he became president of the U.K.'s Royal Statistical Society (ABH & Butler, 1949), urged that epidemiology be conceptualized as "the study of disease, any disease, as a mass phenomenon" (Greenwood, 1935, p. 15). The implication was that "a complete treatise would deal with *every* 'disease' from the point of view of the crowd" (Greenwood, 1935, p. 137; italics in the original). Recognizing that "crowd" characteristics themselves could affect the appearance and course of disease "as a mass phenomenon" (Greenwood, 1935, p. 15), Greenwood accordingly argued that epidemiologists needed to investigate more than just "essential" (i.e., specific) factors—hence his call to extend germ theory's "seed and soil" metaphor, as noted above, with "some form of husbandry" (Greenwood, 1935, p. 359). Epidemiologic theories pertaining to "germs" and "genes," although necessary, were insufficient for explaining the actual and changing distribution of disease broadly writ—a larger conceptual frame was needed.

5

Contemporary Mainstream Epidemiologic Theory

Biomedical and Lifestyle

Enter, mid-century, two new terms, not to be found in the vocabulary of an early twentieth century epidemiologist: *biomedical* and *lifestyle*. Quickly adopted, they soon became ubiquitous and remain so to this day.

Together, these two concepts capture what has been, since the mid-twentieth century, the dominant approach to epidemiologic theorizing—including its ostensibly "atheoretical" stance. Its hallmark? The tripartite view that: (*1*) the "real" causes of disease comprise biophysical agents, genes, and "risk factors," with exposure largely a consequence of individual characteristics and behaviors; (*2*) these "real" causes of disease in individuals are *the* causes of—and are sufficient to explain—population rates of disease; and (*3*) theorizing about disease occurrence is equivalent to theorizing about disease causation in relation to mechanisms occurring within biological organisms; by implication, population-level theorizing is largely, if not wholly, irrelevant.

Given the contemporary lack of explicitness about epidemiologic theory, however, as discussed in **Chapter 1**, it would be unreasonable to expect the mainstream conceptual approach to appear in tidy, clear-cut, and well-elaborated formulations. It doesn't.

A first step, then, toward understanding what is meant by a "biomedical" and "lifestyle" approach to theorizing about disease distribution—and why they travel together—is to consider the origins of these terms and the assumptions that inform them. This is because neither term is unique to, nor originated within, epidemiology. They instead entered into the epidemiologic discourse from other fields, carrying with them sets of ideas about "how the world works" (i.e., ways of being, or ontology) and how the workings of this world can best be studied (i.e., ways of knowing, or epistemology).

Biomedicine and the "Biomedical Model": Reducing Explanations of Disease Occurrence to Disease Mechanisms within Individual Organisms

The words *biomedicine* and *biomedical* would, at first glance, appear to be straightforward terms that simply conjoin biological and medical thinking and practices. After all, as defined by the Oxford English Dictionary (OED), *biomedicine* refers inclusively to "biology and medicine collectively" (OED) (*see* **Textbox 5–1**). The focus, understandably, is on elucidating knowledge relevant to clinical practice. Indeed, as stated in 1988 by the U.S. National Research Council, the objective of the *biomedical model* is "to understand normal and abnormal function from gene to phenotype and to provide a basis for preventive or therapeutic intervention in human disease" (National Research Council 1988, p. 10) (**Textbox 5–1**). Clear, direct, and purposive: what more could one want from a description?

And yet, there is more to these and the other brisk definitions provided in **Textbox 5–1** than meets the eye. As usual, what matters is not only what is included but what is missing. In the case of the biomedical approach—heir to germ theory, hereditarian thinking, and eugenics—what is absent are causes of disease occurrence that lie outside the domain of biophysical exposures and processes.

Origins of the Term **Biomedicine.** Providing further insight into the restricted focus of a biomedical approach is the history of the term's actual usage, one that varies by country context. The word, in English, first surfaced in United Kingdom in the early twentieth century, as indicated by its appearance in the name of the "Institute for Biomedical Sciences," founded in 1912 (IBMS). As used by this Institute, "biomedical" functioned as an adjective that distinguished (and grammatically modified) a particular type of science: the science of hospital-based laboratories—for example, pathology and bacteriology labs oriented toward medical diagnosis and treatment. The specific and unique responsibilities of these labs included designing and implementing appropriately sensitive and specific routine diagnostic tests that could be used on a mass basis (i.e., for many patients). This "applied" orientation distinguished the "biomedical" sciences from their more "basic" research brethren. Starting in 1943, the Institute began publishing the *British Journal of Biomedical Sciences*, whose current description states it is "a scientific journal containing authoritative papers and short reports on new laboratory techniques" (IBMS).

In the United States, by contrast, the term *biomedical* took on a broader meaning, one that included "basic" as well as "applied" science. As with the United Kingdom, the term emerged through the institutional linkage of biology and medicine. In the United States, this occurred through the federal establishment, in 1930, of what was then called the "National Institute of Health," whose enabling legislation newly provided funds for research on "basic biological and medical problems" (Harden, 2009a)—that is, not just on biology, not just on medicine, but on biology and medicine in relation to each other. The goal was to strengthen the scientific moorings of medicine, in keeping with the aspirations of what was called *scientific medicine* during the interwar years (i.e., between World War I and World War II) and its nineteenth century precursor, known as *experimental medicine* (Lawrence & Weisz, 1998; Bynum, 2008).

From its inception, the research portfolio of the National Institute of Health (NIH) spanned from infectious disease (including vaccine development) to the rising mortality resulting from cancer and cardiovascular disease (Swain, 1962; Harden, 1986; Strickland, 1972; Harden & Hannaway, 2001). Underscoring the agency's commitment to basic science, the section on cancer research in the 1933 *Annual Report of the Surgeon General of the Public Health Services of the United States* stated the goal was to obtain "fundamental knowledge concerning the chemical conditions which control the life, growth, and multiplication" of normal and abnormal cells (U.S. PHS, 1933, p. 7, as quoted in Swain, 1962). During World War II, the scope and funding of the NIH expanded considerably—and, relevant to use of the term *biomedicine*, one new war-related focus was the physiology of high-altitude flying for military pilots (Harden & Hannaway, 2001). Research in this area required a new type of collaboration involving an interdisciplinary team of clinicians, physiologists, and engineers and garnered a new designation: *biomedical engineering*.

Textbox 5–1. Definitions of "Biomedicine," "Biomedical," and "Biomedical Model": What's Included Are Biophysical Exposures and Processes—and What's Excluded: Everything Else

Oxford English Dictionary (OED)	**Biomedicine:** Biology and medicine collectively; the biomedical sciences. **1923** DORLAND *Med. Dict.* (ed. 12) 172/2 *Biomedicine*, clinical medicine based on the principles of physiology and biochemistry. **1956** P. E. KLOPSTEG *Instrumentation in Bio-Med. Res.* (U.S. Nat. Res. Council: Biol. Council) 1 A secondary consideration is the enlistment into bio-medicine of those who are already trained in physics and engineering. **1966** *Ann. N.Y. Acad. Sci.* CXXVIII. 721, I believe that the applications of computers in biomedicine are going through a number of stages. **1973** *Biomedicine* XVIII. 4/1 The new name of the journal, *Biomedicine*, is to underline once more that it is at the *crossroads* of biological and clinical investigation. **1986** *Social Sci. & Med.* XXII. 83/2 A woman who expects to attend college and wants to work in biomedicine selects training in pharmacy, nutrition or even dentistry. **Biomedical:** *a.,* pertaining or relating to both biology and medicine; *spec.* pertaining to the biological effects of space-travel **1955** *Bull. Atomic Sci.* May 200/2 The only biomedical data which remains classified is in piecemeal or incomplete form and therefore inadequate for use by the medical profession. **1962** S. CARPENTER in *Into Orbit* 160 Next, you run a check on the intercom and the bio-medical leads to make sure they are working. **1963** C. D. GREEN in J. H. U. Brown *Physiol. of Man in Space* 257 (*title*) Biomedical capsules.
Medline Plus Medical Dictionary (Medline Plus, 2009) (same as: *Webster's Third New International Dictionary*, Unabridged [Webster])	**Biomedicine:** medicine based on the application of the principles of the natural sciences and especially biology and biochemistry; *also*: a branch of medical science concerned especially with the capacity of human beings to survive and function in abnormally stressful environments and with the protective modification of such environments. **Biomedical:** 1 : of or relating to biomedicine 2 : of, relating to, or involving biological, medical, and physical science

WordNet (WordNet 2009)	**Biomedicine:** the branch of medical science that applies biological and physiological principles to clinical practice; the branch of medical science that studies the ability of organisms to withstand environmental stress (as in space travel) **Biomedical:** relating to the activities and applications of science to clinical medicine
U.S. National Institutes of Health (Harden 2009b)	**Biomedical research and development** is a continuing process. New knowledge yields new drugs, devices, and procedures; the study of how the products act yields more knowledge; refinements in knowledge then enable the development of even better therapies.
United Kingdom Institute of Biomedical Sciences (IBMS)	**Biomedical science** is the term for investigations carried out by biomedical scientists on samples of tissue and body fluids to diagnose disease and monitor the treatment of patients.
On-Line Medical Dictionary (OLMD)	**Biomedical model:** a conceptual model of illness that excludes psychological and social factors and includes only biological factors in an attempt to understand a person's medical illness or disorder.
National Research Council (NRC, 1998)	**Biomedical models** can be of many types—from animal models of human diseases to animal, in vitro, or modeling systems for studying any aspect of human biology or disease... A **biomedical model** is a surrogate for a human being, or a human biologic system, that can be used to understand normal and abnormal function from gene to phenotype and to provide a basis for preventive or therapeutic intervention in human diseases. (p. 10)

NB: Interestingly, the *Oxford Dictionary of Science* includes no entry for *biomedicine* or *biomedical*, even as it does include entries for *biochemistry*, *bioenergetics*, *bioengineering*, *biogeography*, *biology*, *biomechanics*, and *biophysics* (Daintith & Martin, 2005); perhaps this exclusion is because *biomedicine* is not one specific scientific discipline, or maybe because *medicine* is broader than strictly the "natural" sciences? (The dictionary contains no definition of *medicine* either.)

This phrase, once codified, constituted the first consistent use of the term *biomedical* in the NIH lexicon (Cambrosio & Keating, 2001; OED; Whitaker Foundation, 2008).

By the early 1950s, however, the term *biomedical* outstripped its initial meanings and became ubiquitous in the health sciences as a way of referring to any biologically-oriented "basic" or "applied" research deemed relevant to understanding, treating, or preventing disease. The Public Health Service Act of 1944 in turn spurred the broader use of this term. This Act not only transformed the "National Institute of Health" into the "National Institutes of Health" but also newly authorized the expanded NIH to conduct clinical, and not solely basic science, research—that is, its research portfolio could now include patients in hospitals (Swain, 1962; Strickland, 1972; Harden & Hannaway, 2001). Funding for the agency increased dramatically, with total appropriations for the NIH jumping from $2.5 million in 1944 to $8 million in 1947 to $24.6 million in 1948 to $52.7 million in 1950 to $210 million in 1958 on up to $339 million in 1960 (NIH Alamanac-appropriations). The rising prominence of NIH raised not only the profile of *biomedical science* but also use of the term *biomedical*, with the impact felt both in the United States and worldwide (Strickland, 1972; Harden & Hannaway, 2001).

Tenets of a Biomedical Approach. By the early 1960s, the terms *biomedical* and *biomedicine* no longer referred simply to an amorphous amalgam of biology and medicine. They instead became transformed into a widely accepted "shorthand" for a particular way of thinking about health and disease (Lock & Gordon, 1988; Lawrence & Weisz, 1998; Cambrosio, 2001). Yet, in contrast to "germ theory," whose proponents clearly spelled out the terms of their theorizing, the biomedical literature has been tellingly characterized by a lack of explicit discussion of its assumptions—precisely because of its underlying premises, as I shall explain. Consequently, the most explicit analyses of the biomedical approach have been written not by its proponents but rather by its critics (*see* **Textbox 5–2**) (Doyal, 1979; Mishler, 1981; Lewontin et al., 1984; Navarro, 1986; Lock & Gordon, 1988; Tesh, 1988; Breilh, 1988; Fee & Krieger, 1993; Krieger, 1994; Conrad & Kern, 1994; Cambrosio & Keating, 2001; Burri & Dumit, 2007; Bynum, 2008).

Among the many features of a biomedical perspective, three stand out as fundamental regarding its approach to investigating disease (Lock & Gordon, 1988; Fee & Krieger, 1993; Krieger, 1994; Lawrence & Weisz, 1998; Cambrosio & Keating, 2001; Bynum, 2008). They are:

- First, specific to biomedicine: the domain of disease and its causes is restricted to solely biological, chemical, and physical phenomena;
- Second, shared with many natural sciences: an emphasis on laboratory research and technology and, as translated to health research, a discounting of research questions that cannot be studied by randomized clinical trials (or their analogs, e.g., "natural experiments"); and
- Third: an embrace of "reductionism," a philosophical and methodological stance (discussed more fully below) that holds that phenomena are best explained by the properties of their parts.

Evidence of all three features is apparent in the 1965 Woolridge Committee report to the U.S. President on *Biomedical Science and its Administration: A Study of the National Institutes of Health* (NIH Study Committee, 1965), the first large-scale appraisal of the NIH after its enormous period of growth in the 1950s and early 1960s (Strickland, 1972, pp. 178–183). As stated in the report's introduction (NIH, 1965, p. 2):

> When a goal is a broad as that of a national health program covering a wide range of human illness and suffering there is adequate justification from the past history of science for an emphasis on basic research, supplemented of course by a sharp watch for and exploitation of those findings which are capable of leading to treatments, cures, and preventives.

In other words, according to a biomedical perspective, the best route for acquiring knowledge to understand, treat, and prevent disease is by adhering to a "basic"—that is, reductionist—orientation, focused on biophysical phenomena that can be studied experimentally, preferably in laboratories.

Textbox 5–2. Descriptions and Assumptions of "Biomedicine" and the "Biomedical Model" as Presented by its Proponents and Critics: Mid-to-Late Twentieth Century Views.

By Proponents: Primarily Focused on Biomedical Justification for Focus on Basic Science and Reductionist Approach

1960s: National Institutes of Health (NIH) Study Committee. *Biomedical Science and its Administration: A Study of the National Institutes of Health. Report to the President.* Washington, DC: The White House, 1965.

p. 2: "The activities and accomplishments of the National Institutes of Health, like those of any other organization, must be judged in terms of its mission. In general terms, the public funds that support NIH activities are intended to 'buy' for the American people a commensurate degree of relief from suffering and improvement of health. To achieve this goal, the NIH devotes its principal effort to a broad program of investigation of the life sciences, rather than to a search for direct cure or prevention of specific diseases. It employs this approach for a simple and valid reason: life science is so complex, and what is known about fundamental biological processes is so little, that the 'head-on' attack is today frequently the slowest and most expensive path to the cure and prevention of disease.... The 'long way around' is in this case likely to be the shortest path to useful results."

1970s   Thomas L. The future impact of science and technology on medicine. *BioScience* 1974; 24:99–105.

p. 101: "I simply cannot imagine any long persistence of our ignorance about disease mechanisms in the face of all that is being learned about normal cells and tissues. Our time for the application of science on a major scale is approaching rapidly, and medicine will be totally transformed when it happens... the major triumphs of medicine... exemplified best by methods for immunization against diphtheria, pertussis, and various virus diseases, and the contemporary use of antibiotics and chemo- therapy for bacterial infections... comes as the result of a genuine understanding of disease mechanisms and, when it becomes available, it is relatively inexpensive, relatively simple, and relatively easy to deliver."

1980s   Committee on Models for Biomedical Research, Board on Basic Biology, Commission on Life Sciences, National Research Council. *Models for Biomedical Research: A New Perspective.* Washington, DC: National Academy Press, 1985. (Included as Appendix C in: *Biomedical Models and Resources: Current Needs and Future Opportunities*, National Academy of Sciences, 1998.)

pp. 62–63: "Investigators studying a phenomenon may analyze its various components at the organ, tissue, cellular, or subcellular levels and seek models for its different parts from the entire corpus of biological knowledge. This then allows them to study one organism or system in terms of related features from a variety of other organisms and other systems.... The body of biological knowledge is beginning to form a coherent and interrelated structure, but it lacks the tight theoretical formulation of physical science. As noted by Baldwin (1938) at the biochemical level, a general biology is emerging from our understanding of the vast number of interrelationships and common features that arose through organic evolution."

p. 64: "The committee's workshops have led inexorably to the conclusion that a theoretical biology or, to use Claude Bernard's phrase, a 'theoretical medicine' is beginning to exist (Bernard, 1865). It is different from theoretical physics, which consists of a small number of postulates and the procedures and apparatus for deriving predictions from those postulates. But it is far more than just a collection of experimental observations. The vast array of information gains coherence when organized into a conceptual matrix through empirical generalizations and reductionist laws–a construct that permits a view of models far more comprehensive than the committee envisioned at the outset of the study."

1990s   Kornberg A. Support for basic biomedical research: how scientific breakthroughs occur. In: Barfield CE, Smith LBR. *The Future of Biomedical Research.* Washington, DC: The American Enterprise Institute and The Brookings Institute, 1997, pp. 35–41.

p. 35: "In reflecting on the history of biomedical science in this century, I often resort to a hunting metaphor. The microbe hunters in the early decades discovered the microbial sources of the major scourges: tuberculosis, plague, cholera. They were followed by the vitamin hunters, who discovered that other scourges–scurvy, rickets, .beri-beri–were caused by the lack of a dietary substance, named vitamins. In the fifth and sixth decades, the enzyme hunters occupied the stage, explaining how the enzyme machinery depends on vitamins to make cells grow and function. Now they have been eclipsed by the gene hunters, the genetic engineers, who use recombinant DNA technology to identify and clone genes, the blueprints for the enzymes, and introduce them into bacteria and plants to create factories for the massive production of hormones and vaccines for medicine and better crops for agriculture."

p. 36: "Yet even more revolutionary but generally unnoticed, even by scientists, is a development that lacks a name or obvious applications but will lead to even more remarkable and unanticipated practical applications. I refer to the coalescence of the numerous basic biological and medical sciences into a single, unified discipline, which has emerged because it is expressed in a single universal language, the language of chemistry.

Much of life can be understood in rational terms if expressed in the language of chemistry. It is an international language, a language without dialects, a language for all time, and a language that explains where we came from, what we are, and where the physical world will allow us to go. Chemical language has great aesthetic beauty and links the physical sciences to the biological sciences."

2000s   Sargent MG. *Biomedicine and the Human Condition: Challenges, Risks, and Rewards.* Cambridge: Cambridge University Press, 2005.

p. xi: "The history of our species is marked by technical solutions that have made... problems of human biology bearable.... The idea of this book is to examine some of these adventures through the lens of twentieth-century biomedicine and to identify the risks and rewards involved in each... a better understanding of the glorious mechanics of human biology [has] provided a framework in which the hitherto baffling and intractable mysteries of chronic disease and aging could be investigated."

By Critics: Primarily Focused on Critiquing Biomedicine's Reductionist Approach, Individualistic Focus, and Exclusion of Social Phenomena From the Explanation of Disease Etiology and Distribution.

1960s   Cassel J. Social science theory as a source of hypotheses in epidemiological research. *Am J Public Health* 1964; 54:1482–1488.

p. 1484: "For greater utility we need to modify the mono-etiological model to one which recognizes that factors which may be causal under certain circumstances may under other circumstances be neutral or perhaps even beneficial. Thus the pattern or configuration of factors becomes the crucial issue."

p. 1486: "... by studying those causes of disease which provide useful knowledge for therapeutic purposes and by expecting that these same factors will be responsible for the onset of conditions, we may be guilty of the logical fallacy of saying that because water quenches fire the cause of fire is therefore lack of water..."

1970s   Engel GL. The need for a new medical model: a challenge for biomedicine. *Science* 1977; 196:129–136.

p. 130: "The dominant model of disease today is biomedical, with molecular biology its basic scientific discipline. It assumes disease to be fully accounted for by deviations from the norm of measurable biological (somatic) variables. It leaves no room within its framework for the social, psychological, and behavioral dimensions of illness... the biomedical model embraces both reductionism, the philosophic view that complex phenomena are ultimately derived from a single unitary principle, and mind-body dualism, the doctrine that separates the mental from the somatic. Here the reductionist principle is physicalistic: that is, it assumes that the language of chemistry and biology will ultimately suffice to explain biological phenomena... The historical fact we have to face is that in modern Western society biomedicine not only has provided a basis for the scientific study of disease, it has also become our own culturally specific perspective about disease, that is, our folk model. Indeed the biomedical model is now the dominant folk model of disease in the Western world... The biomedical model has thus become a cultural imperative, its limitations easily overlooked. In brief, it now has acquired the status of dogma. In science, a model is revised or abandoned when it fails to account adequately for all the data. A dogma, on the other hand, requires that discrepant data be forced to fit the model or be excluded..."

p. 131: "The biomedical approach to disease has been successful beyond all expectations, but at a cost... concentration on the biomedical and exclusion of the psychosocial distorts perspectives and even interferes with patient care..."

1980s   Gordon DR. Tenacious assumptions in Western medicine. In: Lock M, Gordon DR (eds). *Biomedicine Examined*. Dordrecht: Kluwer Publishers, 1988, pp. 19–56.

p. 19: "While biomedicine has successfully created and hoarded a body of technical knowledge to call its own, its knowledge and practices draw upon a background of tacit understandings that extend far beyond medical boundaries. The biological reductionism by which modern medicine is frequently characterized is more theoretical than actual; in its effects, biomedicine speaks beyond its explicit reductionist reference through the implicit ways that it teaches us to interpret ourselves, our world, and the relationships between humans, nature, self, and society. It draws upon and projects *cosmology* (ways of ordering the world), *ontology* (assumptions about reality and being), *epistemology* (assumptions about knowledge and truth), understandings of *personhood, society, morality,* and *religion* (what is sacred and profane) [all italics in the original]. Although biomedicine both constitutes and is constituted by society, this interdependency is nevertheless denied by biomedical theory and ideology which claim neutrality and universality."

Examples of assumptions analyzed [all italics in the original]:

p. 24: 1. "*'Nature' is Distinct from the 'Supernatural'; Matter is Opposed to Spirit...* Medicine exemplifies materialism. 'Real' illness corresponds to the degree to which physical traces show up in the body...

p. 26: "*Atomism: The Part is Independent of and Primordial to the Whole...* That parts of nature are considered autonomous 'things-in-themselves' has three major consequences: (1) Relationships are derivative; the whole is determined by the sum of its parts, rather than the whole determining the parts; (2) Given that their identity if self-determined, the parts may be removed from their context without altering their identity. They may be 'decontextualized." (3) Relations between parts are 'external,' not 'internal,' since parts interact across their distinct boundaries... Atomism of many sorts prevails in medicine: diseases are considered to have an identity separate from their specific hosts and are located and treated in the 'atom' of society–the individual, his/her body divided into parts and parts which are approached as autonomous units."

p. 28: "*Nature is Autonomous from Society.* The natural order is also separate from the social order... To be sure, different social classes become sick more than others, and this can be explained by differences in personal hygiene or 'lifestyle.' Disease is essentially an individual problem and is systematically abstracts from a social context."

p. 42: "*The Non-Autonomy of Naturalism and Biomedicine...* we must consider whether the adamant and relatively successful denial of the social dimension in medicine and naturalism is not paradoxically the exact evidence of the power of social assumptions and practices. To sustain as tenable an ideal of the autonomous, cultureless man, when from our first moments of life we exist in a social context, requires tremendous cultural and social support. Biomedicine and naturalism provide much of it." (italics in original)

| 1990s | Fee E, Krieger N. Understanding AIDS: historical interpretations and the limits of biomedical individualism. *Am J Public Health* 1993; 83:1477–1486. |

p. 1481: "As several critics have argued, 20th-century biomedical models typically are reductionist; they put primacy on explanations of disease etiology that fall within the purview of medical intervention narrowly construed, focus on disease mechanisms, and view social factors leading to disease as being secondary if not irrelevant. Proponents of such models may even consider emphasis on societal factors such as poverty or discrimination to be unscientific and polemical. Despite lip service to multifactorial etiology, they seek parsimonious biomedical explanations highlighting the role of one or a few proximate agents, and they generally assume that biomedical interventions, operating on biological mechanisms, will be sufficient to control disease.

The biomedical model is also premised on the ideology of individualism. Adopting the notion of the abstract individual from liberal political and economic theory, it considers individuals 'free' to "choose" health behaviors. It treats people as consumers who make free choices in the marketplace of products and behaviors, and it generally ignores the role of industry, agribusiness, and government in structuring the array of risk factors that individuals are supposed to avoid. There is little place for understanding how behaviors are related to social conditions and constraints or how communities shape individuals' lives. From this perspective, populations and subgroups within populations-including "risk groups" consist merely of summed individuals who exist without culture or history. There is no acknowledgment of the fact that when "risk groups" succeed in identifying populations at risk of disease, it is because these risk groups typically overlap with real social groups possessing historically conditioned identities.

The problems with the biomedical model extend beyond its exclusive focus on biological and individual-level factors and concern fundamental issues of scientific objectivity and the production of scientific knowledge. The canons of scientific objectivity, as embraced by this model, tend to discount the views and experiences of patients, the "objects" of scientific research and medical practice. Only scientists and physicians are seen as possessing the expertise to define disease and frame research questions... Subjectivity and culture of the scientists and health care professionals as well as of their patients are deemed irrelevant to "truth"; scientific knowledge is held to be outside the bounds of social context."

2000s   **Lock M. The future is now: locating biomarkers for dementia. In: Burri RV, Dumit J (eds).** *Biomedicine as Culture: Instrumental Practices, Technoscientific Knowledge, and New Modes of Life.* **New York: Routledge, 2007, pp. 61–85.**

p. 61: "The molecular vision of life that predominated during the second half of the twentieth century, culminating recently in the mapping of the human genome, is grounded in a mechanistic biology, one primary objective of which is to enable the engineering of bodies and minds. This particular form of molecularization is deterministic, one assumption being that knowledge about specific genes makes possible reliable predictions about the occurrence of disease..."

p. 65: "The majority of researchers working in molecular genetics today acknowledge that the environment and social variables play crucial roles in modifying organisms; even so, these variables are black-boxed in preference for an approach that remains resolutely concerned with interactions internal to the material body. Most modeling continues, therefore, to be reductionist and deliberately oversimplified, but characterizations of this research as one of genetic determinism is no longer apt."

Biomedicine, however, did not "invent" a reductionist approach. Rather, this perspective was common to most natural and social sciences in the 1950s, when "biomedicine" emerged—and remains strong to this day (Lewontin et al., 1984; Poovey, 1998; Ziman, 2000; Ross, 2003).

Key to defining a "reductionist" approach is the postulate that "the parts" explain "the whole" (Irvine et al., 1979; Rose & Rose, 1980; Mayr, 1982; Lewontin et al., 1984; Sayer, 1984; Gordon, 1988; Lawrence & Weisz, 1998; Poovey, 1998; Ziman, 2000; Lewontin, 2000; Gould, 2002; Ross, 2003; Grene & Depew, 2004; Turner, 2005). This premise is simultaneously ontological and epistemological, as it makes claims about both how the world works and how it can be known. At an abstract level, a reductionist approach holds that the properties of phenomena at a "higher level" can be "reduced" to—and hence be solely determined and explained by—phenomena at a "lower level." Two corollaries are: (1) causal pathways run solely from the "lower" to "higher" levels, and (2) properties of "the whole" cannot not influence those of "the parts" of which it is composed. Translated into concrete terms, in the case of biomedicine, this reductionist premise holds that the features of a biological organism and its diseases (i.e., the "higher level") can be fully explained by genetics and molecular biology (i.e., the "lower level") —and hence ultimately by chemistry and physics (*see* excerpt from Kornberg, 1997 in **Textbox 5–2**). The operational implication is that research at the "lower levels" is not only essential but also *sufficient* to explain the phenomena at "higher" levels.

The implications of a biomedical orientation to understanding disease is clearly elaborated in the 1965 Woolridge Committee report, which argued that the NIH's "broad mission of improvement of virtually all aspects of the Nation's health requires NIH to concentrate most of its effort on basic research" (NIH Study Committee, 1965, p. 2). The "simple and valid reason" offered to support this approach was that "life science is so complex, and what is known about fundamental biological processes is so little, that the 'head-on' attack today is frequently the slowest and most expensive path to the cure and prevention of disease" (NIH Study Committee, 1965, p. 2). In a revealing metaphor, the report asserted (NIH Study Committee, 1965, p. 79):

> Research is a venture into the unknown and, therefore, a risk. There is no guarantee that any particular medical research will ever be of any economic benefit to the community. When one finds a new biomedical fact, he is looking into the face of a newborn babe with no way of knowing whether the baby will grow up to be a pillar of the community or the town bum. The most likely possibility is usually that the new fact will turn out to be like a musician, adding a good deal of interest to the world but contributing no great wealth.

The premium thus was on basic knowledge; it was a secondary consideration, at best, if this knowledge was useful or if there might be "social and economic factors that make the full application of a new procedure extremely difficult or unfeasible" (NIH Study Committee, 1965, p. 156). Instead, health research should focus on fundamental biological processes (the "parts") to yield knowledge relevant for understanding and altering the course of disease in individuals (the "whole") and hence society at large (an even bigger— or, more accurately, higher level—"whole").

The equation of basic research with health research has remained a constant in the biomedical model. Enthusiasm for this approach is well-conveyed in a 1997 book titled *The Future of Biomedical Research* (Barfield & Smith, 1997), in which the opening paragraph of the opening chapter by then director of the NIH, Harold E. Varmus stated (Varmus 1997, p. 9):

> This is a wonderful time for the National Institutes of Health, probably the most exciting time ever in the history of biology, with the exploration of the blueprints of life, the genomes of many organisms, including man [*sic*]; studies of neuroscience that are linking behavior to genetics; and the appreciation of life's images–from the three-dimensional structures of proteins and nucleic acids to pictures of organs that can be taken from outside the body.

To Varmus, the benefits of biomedical research were not simply the "ever-popular prospects of living longer and living healthier," or "saving costs through the prevention of illness or its complications or through cheaper treatment," but also "the national esteem that comes from our discoveries and from our world leadership in the area of biomedical research" (Varmus, 1997, p. 14).

In essence, then, the "biomedical model" is more than a mere "model." It instead has a core set of interlinked ideas that underlie its approach to explaining disease occurrence (*see* **Textbox 5–2**). As I have previously noted (Krieger, 1994), it emphasizes biological determinants of disease amenable to intervention through the health-care system, considers social determinants of disease to be at best secondary (if not irrelevant), and views populations simply as the sum of individuals and population patterns of disease as simply reflective of individual cases. In this view, disease in populations is reduced to a question of disease in individuals, which in turn is reduced to a question of biological malfunctioning. This biologic substrate, divorced from its societal context, thus becomes the optimal locale for interventions, which chiefly are medical in nature.

Expressing the premises of the biomedical perspective, and as delineated in **Table 5–1**, the key metaphor that animates the "biomedical model" is that of the body being a machine, one whose component parts are governed by the laws of physics and chemistry—and which, if malfunctioning, can be "fixed" by using the appropriate technology. The optimism of this approach was well-expressed in 1974, when the influential physician and essayist Dr. Lewis Thomas, then president of Memorial Sloan-Kettering Cancer Center, a leading biomedical research institution, declared (Thomas 1974, p. 100):

> My dogmas are as follows: I do not believe in the inevitability of disease. I concede the inevitability of the risk of disease, but I cannot imagine any category of human disease that we are precluded, by nature, from thinking our way around… Nature is inventive but not so inventive as to continue elaborating endless successions of new, impenetrable disease mechanisms. After we have learned enough to penetrate and control the mechanisms of today's disease, I believe we will be automatically well-equipped to deal with whatever new ones turn up. I do not say this in any arrogance; it just seems reasonable… I believe that the mechanisms of disease are quite open to intelligent intervention and reversal whenever we learn more about how they operate.

To understand disease is thus to understand disease mechanisms as they manifest biologically to the point where it is possible to alter and block these mechanisms—this is the claim of biomedicine.

Thus, as intended, biomedicine and biomedical research has yielded prodigious knowledge about basic biology, pathobiology, and clinical treatment (Thagard, 1999; Cambrosio & Keating, 2001; Sargent, 2005; Burri & Dumit, 2007; Bynum, 2008). As summarized in one of the first major historical analyses of the NIH, published by Strickland in 1972 (Strickland 1972, pp. 240–241):

> How close national medical research policy has brought us to the central goal of conquering disease is a more difficult matter to judge then whether a first-rate biomedical science system has

Table 5–1. Biomedical and Lifestyle Approaches to Analyzing Disease Distribution: Metaphors, Mechanisms, and Theoretical Assumptions Regarding Individualism and Reductionism

Framework	Metaphor	Mechanisms	Assumptions regarding individualism and reductionism
Biomedical model	Body = machine = molecules governed by the laws of physics and chemistry	Emphasis on molecular biology and disease mechanisms (endogenous processes of pathogenesis), with a focus on factors in biological pathways that can be clinically diagnosed (using relevant biological, chemical, or physical devices or procedures) and whose occurrence can be prevented, halted, or reversed through clinical treatment (e.g., vaccines, pharmacologic agents, surgery, etc.)	Individualistic: *(a)* individuals defined by innate characteristics *(b)* population = sum of individuals (with demarcations of populations established in relation to individual characteristics) *(c)* population rates = consequence of individual events within specified population
Lifestyle	Behavior = choice = fashion	Health behaviors = freely-chosen "risk factors" (e.g., involving diet, smoking, sleep, sex) that lead to exposures that are harmful or beneficial to health, via pathways ultimately involving molecular biology and endogenous processes of pathogenesis	Reductionist: *(a)* "parts" determine properties of the "whole," hence "bottom-up" causation *(b)* studying the "parts" and their causal relationships is sufficient to understand the "whole"
Web of causation: biomedical + lifestyle	Web (with no spider), with strands connecting "risk factors"	Biomedical + lifestyle, with emphasis on decontextualized "risk factors" most "proximate" to onset of pathogenesis (within the body)	

been created. Yet no one has been known to dispute the broad statement of Dr. John A. Cooper, president of the Association of American Medical Colleges, that knowledge accumulated over a twenty-year period has "revolutionized the range of diagnostic, therapeutic and preventive capabilities of medicine," and has made it possible for physicians to offer more favorable prognoses to patients suffering from many diseases.

The early twenty-first century appraisal of "NIH Successes," offered on the NIH website, concurs (Harden 2009c):

> It is impossible to list all of the discoveries made by NIH-supported investigators. More than eighty Nobel prizes have been awarded for NIH-supported research. Five of these prizes were awarded to investigators in the NIH intramural programs. The in-house discoveries have included breaking the genetic code that governs all life processes, demonstrating how chemicals act to transmit electrical signals between nerve cells, and describing the relationship between the chemical composition of proteins and how they fold into biologically active conformations. In turn, these basic research discoveries have led to greater understanding of genetically based diseases, to better antidepressants, and to drugs specially designed to target proteins involved in particular disease processes. Long-term research has dispelled preconceptions that morbidity and dementia are a normal part of the aging process. Some cancers have been cured and deaths from heart attack and stroke have been significantly lowered. Research has also revealed that preventive strategies such as a balanced diet, an exercise program, and not smoking can reduce the need for therapeutic interventions and thus save money otherwise expended for health care.

As is evident, even benefits are cast solely in clinical terms.

Ultimately, perhaps the most profound confirmation of the reductionist orientation of biomedicine as conceived in the twentieth century is, ironically, the challenges to its premises being raised in the twenty-first century by its very successes: rapid new developments in epigenetics, "evo-devo" biology (linking evolutionary and developmental processes), and systems biology (Keller, 2000; Keller, 2002; Kitano, 2002; van Speybroeck et al., 2002; Noble, 2006; Lock, 2007; Systems Biology Institute, 2009; Institute for Systems Biology, 2009). Although beyond the scope of this chapter to review in any depth, common to these new fields of inquiry is their unseating of the "central dogma" that knowledge about DNA is sufficient to understand (or "compute") the organism, let alone disease. Tackling the genome in context, this work is prompting a profound shift away from the idea of DNA as the "master programmer" to a view instead whereby both the organism and environment are understood as interactively playing decisive roles in gene regulation and expression. Consequently, as stated in a 2002 review article in *Science* (Kitano 2002, p. 1662):

> To understand biology at the system level, we must examine the structure and dynamics of cellular and organismal function, rather than the characteristics of isolated parts of a cell or organism. Properties of systems… emerge as central issues, and understanding these properties may have an impact on the future of medicine.

Whether or not the new systems biology actually augurs the death-knell of biomedical reductionism, its explicit self-juxtaposition against the reductionist stance of prior research only serves to underscore the profound impact of such thinking on twentieth century biomedical research.

"Lifestyle": Methodological Individualism Meets Behavioral Sciences Meets Health Behaviors

Not that a reductionist orientation is unique to the natural or, even more specifically, bio-medical sciences. During the twentieth century, a similar perspective increasingly held sway in the social sciences, especially in the behavioral sciences that emerged in the mid-twentieth century. Appearing under the rubric of "methodological individualism" (discussed below; *see* definitions in **Textbox 5–3**) (Udehn, 2000; Picavet, 2001; Ross, 2003; Morgan, 2003; Bannister, 2003; Subramanian et al., 2009), this orientation, like its biomedical counterpart, has influenced mid-to-late twentieth century epidemiologic think-ing about disease distribution and its causes. It has done so two ways: first, methodologi-cally, and second, substantively, through its impact on the construct of "lifestyle."

   Tenets of Twentieth Century Methodological Individualism—In Historical Context. Akin to biological reductionism, *methodological individualism* holds that societal phenomena are ultimately reducible to and explained by individual actions (Udehn, 2000; Picavet, 2001; Ross, 2003; Morgan, 2003; Bannister, 2003; Turner, 2005; Subramanian et al., 2009). Thus, as stated in the *International Encyclopedia of the Social and Behavioral Sciences* (Picavet, 2001, p. 9751): "social phenomena are viewed as the aggregate results of indi-vidual actions," with the latter having "explanatory primacy in relation to… society's prop-erties…" (*see* **Textbox 5–3**). Or, as summarized in the *Oxford Dictionary of Sociology* (Scott & Marshall, 2005, p. 298): "explanations of… social phenomena… must be formu-lated as, or reducible to, the characteristics of individuals" (*see* **Textbox 5–3**).

   Consequently, the appropriate unit of analysis for methodological individualism is the individual person: conceptually, analytically, and empirically. Also as in the biological sci-ences, the contrast is to alternative "holistic" frameworks that posit: (*1*) characteristics of individual persons (the "parts") are, in part, shaped by the society (i.e., the "whole") to which they inherently belong, and (*2*) societies have characteristics irreducible to the indi-vidual-level, some of which may affect individuals' characteristics (Udehn, 2000; Picavet, 2001; Ross, 2003; Turner, 2005). A powerful irony is that in its original meaning, the term *individual* referred to being "indivisible" from the group of which it is a part (Williams 1983, pp. 161–165; *see* etymologic explanation in **Textbox 5–3**); the corollary is that recognition of "individuality" does not require embracing the philosophical stance of "individualism" that underlies methodological individualism (Williams, 1983, pp. 161–165; Krieger, 2007; Subramanian et al., 2009).

   Debates over "individualism" vs "holism" within the social sciences during the mid-to-late twentieth century, although akin to those in the natural sciences, have differed in two ways. First, in contrast to the biomedical discourse—in which theoretical explicitness was more a hallmark of the critics than proponents—in the case of methodological individualism, proponents were as theoretically explicit as their opponents, reflecting their shared disci-plinary emphasis on social theory. Second, conflicts within the social sciences over these opposing ways of conceptualizing and investigating phenomena were more politically charged, given the manifestly social nature of the subject matter. As is well-recounted in the literature on changing ideas and ideologies in the social sciences in the post-World War II period (Ross, 2003; Morgan, 2003; Bannister, 2003), these academic disputes were deeply connected to larger geopolitical conflicts, most specifically the Cold War (Krieger, 2000; Isaac, 2007; Subramanian et al., 2009). Framed in terms of political econ-omy, the conflict was between the "ruling ideas" of what was then referred to as "capitalism" (led by the United States and its Western allies) versus "communism" (based in the Union of Soviet Socialist Republics and joined by China in 1949). Cast in ideological terms, the

Textbox 5–3. Definitions of "Individualism," "Methodological Individualism," and "Lifestyle"

Oxford English Dictionary (OED, 2009)

Individualism:
1. Self-centred feeling or conduct as a principle; a mode of life in which the individual pursues his own ends or follows out his own ideas; free and independent individual action or thought; egoism.
2. The social theory which advocates the free and independent action of the individual, as opposed to communistic methods of organization and state interference. Opposed to COLLECTIVISM and SOCIALISM.
3. *Metaph.* The doctrine that the individual is a self-determined whole, and that any larger whole is merely an aggregate of individuals, which, if they act upon each other at all do so only externally.

Lifestyle:
a. A term originally used by Alfred Adler (1870–1937) to denote a person's basic character as established early in childhood which governs his reactions and behaviour.
b. *gen.* A way or style of living.
ADDITIONS SERIES 1997
c. *attrib.* Of or relating to a particular way of living; *spec.* in *Marketing*, designed to appeal to a consumer by depicting a product in the context of a particular lifestyle.

International Encyclopedia of the Social & Behavioral Sciences (Smelser & Baltes, 2001)

Methodological individualism (p. 9751; Picavet, 2001):... the explanatory and modeling strategies in which human individuals (with their motivations) and human actions (with their causes or reasons) are given a prominent role in explanations and models. Social phenomena are viewed as the aggregate results of individual actions. Explanation thus proceeds from the parts to the whole: individual action has an explanatory primacy in relation to social facts, society's properties, and observed macroregularities.

Lifestyle: (not defined)

Oxford Dictionary of Sociology (Scott & Marshall, 2005)

Individualism (pp. 297–298): Broadly any set of ideas emphasizing the importance of the individual and the individual's interests, the term is used to characterize a range of ideas, philosophies, and doctrines.

Methodological individualism (p. 298):... refers to the position adopted by those who argue that, in studying society, sociologists must not only (inevitably) study individuals, but also that the explanations of the social phenomena they study—phenomena such as social classes, power, the educational system, or whatever—must be formulated as, or reducible to, the characteristics of individuals. This position stands in marked contrast to "methodological holism," the theoretical principle that each social entity (group, institution, society) has a totality that is distinct, and cannot be understood by studying merely its individual component elements. (An example would be Émile Durkheim's claim that social facts can be studied and explained independently of the individual). The debate over methodological individualism reflects an underlying tension about the relation between the society and the individual. This tension is, however, now more commonly analysed in terms of "structure" and "agency"; discussions of methodological individualism as such are less common.

Lifestyle (p. 365): A concept that refers to alternative ways of living, usually conspicuous through values and modes of consumption. Such differentials correspond to the concept of status groups identified by Max Weber... More generally, and rather loosely, it refers to contrasting ways of life found among different groups in society, such as the young, unemployed, or deviant.

New Keywords (Bennet et al., 2005)

Individual (pp. 183–184; Parekh, 2005): **Individual** comes from L *individuum*, meaning that which is indivisible or cannot be broken up further... From the C17, however, a new and more atomizing conception of **the individual** emerges as a necessary singular entity...The modern conception of the person gave rise to two new words in the C19. **Individuality** refers to what distinguishes individuals and marks them out from others... **Individualism** refers to the view that individuals alone are the ultimate social reality... Society is nothing more than its members and their pattern of relationship.
Lifestyle: (not defined)

Oxford Dictionary of Public Health (ODPH, 2004)

Individualism and methodological individualism: (not defined)
Lifestyle (Green & Potvin, 2004).
p. 1: We use the term lifestyle to refer to any combination of specific practices and environmental conditions reflecting patterns of

living influenced by family and social history, culture, and socio-economic circumstances. pp. 13–14: Lifestyle has emerged as a concept in modern discourse to describe in shorthand what Madison Avenue advertising agencies call market segments—groups or types of people differentiated by a set of consumption and other living patterns related to their income, education, occupation, gender, residence, and geopolitical and ethnic identification. This commercialization of the term is not totally unrelated to the social science origins of the concept. In the health field, however, the term has been used more variously. At one extreme, it describes discrete narrowly defined behaviour related to chronic diseases or health enhancement. This usage is associated with elements of individualism. At the other extreme, *lifestyle* is used to describe the total social milieu including the *psycho-socio-economic environment* as well as personal health behaviors.

Annual Reviews:
Sociology, Public Health—definitions of *lifestyle*

Zablocki BD, Kanter RM. The differentiation of life-styles. *Annu Rev Sociol* 1976; 2:269–298.

p. 270: *Life-style* has been a term much used but poorly defined in contemporary social science writings. It has been confused with subculture, social movement, and status group. An ultimate goal should be to provide a distinct and analytically useful definition of life-style in terms of shared values or tastes as reflected primarily in consumption patterns but applicable also to the evaluation of intangible and/or public goods. A life-style might be defined over a given collectivity to the extent that the members are similar to one another and different from others both in the distribution of their disposable incomes and the motivations that underlie such distributions.

p. 271: Life-style is to be distinguished from culture and subculture. A given life-style may be characteristic of a specific social class, status group, or subculture; but since life-style is defined solely in terms of shared preferences, it is possible and indeed is often the case that a life-style may be defined over a collectivity that otherwise lacks social and cultural identity… Life-style is also to be distinguished from social class and social status, though it may stem from both.

p. 280: The emergence of the counterculture and life-style experimentation has taken place among people for whom occupational and economic role no longer provided a coherent set of values and for whom identity has come to be generated in the consumption rather than the production realm, and affluence has permitted a choice of goods from which to make up a life-style package

Green LW, Kreuter MW. Health promotion as a public health strategy for the 1990s. *Annu Rev Public Health* **1990; 11:319–334.**

p. 320: The debates surrounding these phrases often center on the sympathetic or pejorative uses of the word" lifestyle." As a target for health promotion policy and programs, lifestyle refers, for some, to the consciously chosen, personal behavior of individuals as it may relate to health. Others interpret lifestyle as a composite expression of the social and cultural circumstances that condition and constrain behavior, in addition to the personal decisions the individual might make in choosing one behavior over another. Both uses the term acknowledge that lifestyle is a more enduring (some would say habitual) *pattern* of behavior than is often connoted by the term behavior or action.

p. 323: Countries adopting health promotion as policy have directed it largely at primary prevention through modification of lifestyle factors that account for the largest numbers of deaths. These factors include patterns of food consumption, the misuse of potentially harmful substances, sedentary modes of work and recreation, and reckless, violent, or abusive interaction with others. In various combinations, these lifestyle patterns constitute the major risk.

A Dictionary of Epidemiology (Porta, 2008)

Individualism and methodological individualism: (not defined)

Lifestyle (p. 143): The set of habits and customs that is influenced, modified, encouraged or constrained by the lifelong process of socialization. These habits and customs include use of substances such as alcohol, tobacco, tea, coffee; dietary habits; exercise, etc., which have important implications for health and are often the subject of epidemiological investigations.

former ostensibly gave primacy to the individual (and hence political and civil rights); the latter, to the collectivity (and hence social and economic rights); these societies' actual observance and violation of these two sets of important rights is another story entirely (Wersky, 1988; Ross, 2003; Anderson, 2003; Isaac, 2007).

Within "the West," the individualist approach not surprisingly became dominant. Its power lay not simply in what proponents considered to be the persuasiveness of its ideas but also because of the frank exercise of political power (Fried, 1997; Shrecker, 1998; Isaac, 2007). In the case of the United States, for example, the year 1950 marked not only the start of the Korean War but also the rise of Senator Joseph M. McCarthy and the House Un-American Activities Committee (Fried, 1997; Shrecker, 1998; Isaac, 2007). During what has come to be known as the McCarthy era (Shrecker, 1998; Isaac, 2007), U.S. academics who seriously or publicly questioned the individualistic assumptions associated with free-market ideology found themselves variously marginalized, denied funding, or fired from their jobs (Schrecker, 1998, pp. 404–407; Isaac, 2007), including in economics (Morgan, 2003, pp. 296–297), sociology (Ross, 2003, pp. 230–232), and medicine and public health (Brickman, 1994; Derickson, 1997).

Moreover, following McCarthy's spurious claim in 1950 that "more than 500 of the 50,000 listed in American Men of Science had been openly associated with Communist Fronts" and that "the American Association for the Advancement of Science was dominated by a clique of fellow travelers" (Badash, 2000, p. 62), even scientists whose topic of study lay well outside the "suspect" social or public health sciences—for example, who did research in the more pristine fields of physics or chemistry—had their funding, careers, and lives derailed by allegations of political subversion (Badash, 2000). So, too, were certain lines of research proposed in the late 1940s and 1950s sidelined, as a result of the alleged "left-wing" origin of their ideas (Rose & Rose, 1980; Wersky, 1988). One classic case concerns the rejection of the U.K. biologist C.H. Waddington's (1905–1975) classic work, which he began in the 1940s, on what he called the *epigenetic landscape*, a term he coined to convey how an organism's biotic and abiotic context produced its phenotype by affecting gene expression (Waddington, 1940; Waddington, 1957; Waddington, 1975). Reclaimed if not "rediscovered" in the late twentieth century, Waddington's innovative ideas about "epigenetics" is now a major topic of study in twenty-first century biological research on context-dependent developmental biology (Gilbert, 2002; Goldberg et al., 2007).

The impact of these ideological battles, as noted by Ross, a leading historian of the social sciences, was felt not only in the United States but worldwide (Ross 2003, p. 230):

> As the strongest power to emerge from the war and a society that had escaped fascism and communism, the United States promoted its ideologies and cultural products around the world. United States government agencies, private foundations, universities and disciplinary organizations supported extensive exchange of social science faculty, students, and books. American models of social science were selectively imported into countries outside the Soviet sphere of influence, while the American model of graduate education that linked teaching and research was often emulated…

According to Ross, the theories that came to predominate in the United States and that were exported elsewhere in "the 1950s climate of Cold War scientism and burgeoning professional practice" retained "a basis in individualistic, voluntarist premises," whereby "[i]n line with the era's theories, behavioral social science methodologically endowed individuals with autonomy, while substantively enmeshing them in a world of increasing social complexity" (Ross, 2003, p. 231). These individualistically-oriented behavioral sciences in turn shaped the development of still one more construct relevant to understanding the dominant mid-to-late twentieth century epidemiologic theories of disease distribution: that of "lifestyle."

Lifestyle: A Long Strange Journey From Sociological Concepts of "Choice" Within "Constraint" to Individualistic Health Behaviors. From the vantage of early twenty-first century epidemiology, it would be difficult to imagine a time when "lifestyle" would be absent from epidemiologic articles or considered anything but a self-evident idea. Yet, not only is *lifestyle* a word whose meaning has changed considerably over the course of the twentieth century, but it is also a term effectively missing from the pre-1960 epidemiologic literature (*see* **Table 5–2**). Its current meanings in both the social and health sciences, discussed below (*see also* **Textbox 5–3**), reflect the enduring impact of methodological individualism on the rise of behavioral sciences in the mid-twentieth century (Sobel, 1981; Coreil et al., 1985; O'Brien, 1995; Krieger, 2000; Krieger, 2001; Slater, 2005; Hansen & Easthope, 2007).

Use of the term *lifestyle* in the early twentieth century, if not its emergence, is often traced to the renowned sociologist Max Weber (1864–1920) (Sobel, 1981; Coreil et al., 1985; Abel & Cockerham, 1993; Bogenhold, 2001). In his pathbreaking essay on "Class, Status, and Party" (contained within his magnum opus, *Economy and Society*, written around the time of World War I, shortly before his death, and published post-humously), Weber employed a term (*lebensführung*), which was first translated into English in 1944 as "lifestyle" but which subsequently, and more accurately, has been retranslated to mean "conduct of life" (Abel & Cockerham, 1993; Cockerham et al., 1997; Bogenhold, 2001; Swedberg, 2005, pp. 150–151). As employed by Weber, *lebensführung* referred to the ways in which groups and individuals consciously decided how to conduct their lives (including ethically) within what he termed their economic "class" (Swedberg, 2005, pp. 150–151). Weber added this latter stipulation because, in his view, "the possibility of status-specific life conduct is of course in part economically conditioned" (Swedberg, 2005, pp. 150–151). To the extent "choice" was operative in Weber's conceptualization of "lebensführung," it was "choice" made within the constraints and options of the economic realities afforded by different types of occupations and their income levels.

Table 5–2. Rise of Epidemiologic Literature Focused on "Lifestyle": Articles Indexed in Pubmed,1960–2008

Year	Number of articles indexed by terms and ratio compared to 1960–1969				Articles indexed by "lifestyle" also indexed by "epidemiology" (%)
	Lifestyle		Epidemiology AND lifestyle		
	N	ratio	N	ratio	
1960–1969	25	(1.0)	1	(1.0)	4.0
1970–1979	2822	113	288	288	10.2
1980–1989	8479	339	1180	1180	13.9
1990–1999	17077	683	4953	4953	29.0
2000–2008	36432	1457	13260	13260	36.4

Source: PubMed search Available at http://www.ncbi.nlm.nih.gov/sites/entrez (Accessed February 16, 2009).

Weber, however, was not the only prominent scholar in the early twentieth century to employ the idea of "lifestyle." Starting in the early 1930s, a different conception of "lifestyle"—termed *style of life*—was popularized by the psychologist Alfred Adler (1870–1937) (Adler, 1931 [1962]; Coreil et al., 1985). From his disciplinary stance, Adler redefined *style of life* to refer to how individuals, during their upbringing, developed "holistic" systems of emotions, values, aspirations, behaviors, and ways of being in their bodies, which—consistent with his socialist views—he held to be influenced by the larger societal (including economic), and not just familial, context in which they lived their lives (Adler, 1931 [1962]; Coreil et al., 1985). Arguing that each *style of life* had a "corresponding emotional and physical habitus" (Adler, 1931 [1962], p. 39), Adler rejected atomistic analysis of individuals' particular behaviors and emotions. Instead, they needed to be interpreted coherently, in relation to a fuller ensemble of the *style of life* that linked "the way the mind has interpreted its experiences, in the meaning it has given to life, and in the actions with which it has answered the impressions received from the body and the environment" (Adler, 1931 [1962], p. 40). Thus, Adler, like Weber, held that the "whole" (i.e., the societal economic context) shaped (albeit did not fully determine) the *style of life* or *lifestyle* of the "part" (i.e., both group and individual behavior).

Commencing in the 1950s, however, with the rise of mass consumer culture and the advertising industry (Sobel, 1981), on the one hand, and methodological individualism in the behavioral sciences (Ross, 2003) on the other, *lifestyle* took on a new meaning. No longer conceptualized as a property of groups defined by their role in the economy (i.e., what they produced, materially), lifestyle devolved to being a characteristic of individuals, who could then be aggregated into distinctive groups based on their patterns of consumption (Zablocki & Kanter, 1976; Coreil et al., 1985; Sobel, 1981; Tesh, 1988; Abel & Cockerham, 1993; O'Brien, 1995; Cockerham et al., 1997; Slater, 2005; Scott & Marshall, 2005). Thus, core to the construct of lifestyle are, as stated in the 2005 *Oxford Dictionary of Sociology*, "values and modes of consumption" (Scott & Marshall, 2005, p. 365). Premised on the notion of choice (as per the "tastes" and "preferences" of individuals as analyzed in micro-economics [Sobel, 1981]), lifestyle thus became equated with individuals' behaviors and consumption patterns, as linked to their values and "sense of identity," both viewed as independent from their occupations (*see* **Textbox 5–3**). In effect, as explicated in **Table 5–1**, the dominant metaphor for lifestyle analysis became that of "fashion"—and its central mechanism (whether for disease causation or any other outcome) was that of "consumer choice," once again as informed by individualistic and reductionist assumptions.

Consequently, when the lifestyle entered the public health and epidemiologic discourses in the mid-to-late twentieth century—with its first appearance in *Index Medicus* as a medical subject heading (MeSH) occurring in 1972 (Coreil et al., 1985, p. 427), it did so imbued with its consumer-oriented individualistic meaning (Terris, 1980; Coreil et al., 1985; Tesh, 1988; O'Brien, 1995; Hansen & Easthope, 2007). And once it appeared, it was rapidly adopted by epidemiologists, as revealed by the fast-rising number of articles indexed simultaneously by *epidemiology* and *lifestyle* in PubMed (the NIH website for citing biomedical literature [PubMed]) **(Table 5–2):** from one in 1960 through 1969 to 13,260 in 2000 through 2008. This proportionate increase is more than 1000 times that of the corresponding 12.7-fold increase in articles indexed just by the term *epidemiology* (from 42,605 in 1960–1969 to 540,796 in 2000–2008) **(Table 5–2)**. Even more tellingly, between 1960 and 2008, the proportion of articles in PubMed indexed by *lifestyle* (rising from 25 in 1960–1969 to 36,432 in 2000–2008) that were also indexed by *epidemiology* shot up from 4% to 36% **(Table 5–2)**.

As employed in the public health and epidemiologic literature, lifestyle accordingly has served as a term chiefly deployed to describe health behaviors, premised on (Coreil et al 1985, p. 428):

> ... the notion that personal habits are discrete and independently modifiable, and that individuals can voluntarily choose to alter such behaviors... What seems especially paradoxical is that the catch-phrase for this atomistic perspective–"life style"–grew out of a scholarly tradition which gave primacy to context and meaning. Current discussions of life style and health largely ignore systemic influences, and instead focus almost exclusively on individual responsibility.

Since this evaluation of the meaning of lifestyle, written by Coreil et al. in 1985, a lively and expanding literature within both sociology and health promotion has both critiqued and elaborated the consumer-oriented version of lifestyle theories (*see* **Textbox 5–3**) (Coreil et al., 1985; Green & Kreuter, 1990; Bunton et al., 1995; Davison & Davey Smith, 1995; Green & Potvin, 2004; Hansen & Easthope, 2007; Slater, 2005). For example, reflecting the term's still contested meaning, in 2004 the *Oxford Dictionary of Public Health* entry on "Education, health promotion, and social and lifestyle determinants of health and disease" noted that (Green & Potvin 2004, pp. 13–14):

> Lifestyle has emerged as a concept in modern discourse to describe in shorthand what Madison Avenue advertising agencies call market segments... In the health field, however, the term has been used more variously. At one extreme, it describes discrete narrowly defined behaviour related to chronic diseases or health enhancement. This usage is associated with elements of individualism. At the other extreme, 'lifestyle' is used to describe the total social milieu including the 'psycho-socio-economic environment' as well as personal health behaviours.

In other words, the conflicted conceptual history of *lifestyle* has yet to be resolved.

Despite the ongoing controversy, however, the 2008 5th edition of *A Dictionary of Epidemiology* opted to define *lifestyle* solely in relation to a "set of habits and customs" bearing the imprint of "the lifelong process of socialization"; the examples provided of such "habits and customs" tellingly referred only to "use of substances, such as alcohol, tobacco, tea, coffee; dietary habits; exercise, etc., which have important implication for health" (Porta, 2008, p. 143) (*see* **Textbox 5–3**). Thus, entering the twenty-first century, the dominant understanding of *lifestyle* within epidemiology continues to hold that *lifestyle* equals individual "choice" equals "health behavior" equals individual's exposure to "health behavior-related risk factors," chiefly involving smoking, alcohol, illicit drugs, food, exercise, and sexual behaviors (Green & Potvin, 2004; Aldana, 2005; Hansen & Easthope, 2007; Porta, 2008; Gluckman & Hanson, 2008; Leonard, 2008).

The Spiderless Web of Causation: Biomedical + Lifestyle Conjoined

In light of the past half-century's privileging of biomedical reductionism in the health sciences and methodological individualism and individualistic lifestyle analysis in the social sciences, it should come as no surprise that the biomedical and lifestyle orientation have synergistically dominated epidemiologic theories of disease distribution in the mid-to-late twentieth century. Indeed, it would be astonishing if they had not done so.

Equally unsurprising, and paralleling the discussion of the biomedical model itself (**Textbox 5–2**), explication of the premises of biomedical and lifestyle approaches in epidemiologic theorizing have been singularly absent in both twentieth century epidemiologic textbooks (as reviewed in **Chapter 1**) and the bulk of epidemiologic studies they have guided. Instead, analysis of their underlying assumptions has, as in the case of the biomedical model itself, been provided chiefly by these frameworks' critics (Crawford, 1977; Schnall, 1977; Navarro, 1977; Terris, 1980; Mishler, 1981; Waitzkin, 1981; Laurell, 1982; Tesh, 1988; Breilh, 1989; Breilh & Granda, 1989; de Almeida-Filho, 1992; Fee & Krieger, 1993; Krieger, 1994; Breilh, 1995; McMichael, 1995; Susser & Susser, 1996; McMichael, 1999; de Almeida-Filho, 2000; Krieger, 2000; Krieger, 2001; Krieger, 2008; Susser & Stein, 2009).

Nevertheless, the mainstream epidemiologic embrace, mid-twentieth century, of a jointly biomedical and lifestyle perspective was neither "unthinking" nor without its novelties. Instead, as discussed below, it represented a response to the increasing epidemiologic evidence—derived from population-based studies—that:

a. few if any of the rising non-infectious diseases had readily apparent "single" causes akin to disease-specific "germs";
b. the actual dynamics and distribution of infectious diseases were driven by more than just properties of these "germs" (whether bacterial, viral, or something else); and
c. for both types of the diseases, something about the characteristics of people had something to do with who was at risk of disease.

Thus, epidemiologists' supplementation of a biomedical approach with lifestyle analysis can be seen an attempt to increase the scope of epidemiologic theorizing.

The specific path taken, however, was not inevitable, as revealed by the contending social epidemiologic theories of disease distribution discussed in the next two chapters. The ready acceptance and dominance of individualistic and reductionist biomedical and lifestyle thinking was nonetheless assured by not only the entrenched modes of thought in mid-to late twentieth century health and social sciences but also by who could be a card-carrying epidemiologist in this era.

After all, prior to the 1970s, no matter what the country, people who obtained advanced degrees in epidemiology were, by academic preference (if not actual policy) either physicians or else had prior training in related biomedical fields (Buck et al., 1988, pp. 978–985; Greenhouse, 2003). Considering the case of the United States, data compiled by the American Public Health Association and the U.S. Association of Schools of Public Health, for example, reveal that in 1962 to 1963, fully 90% of U.S. graduate students in epidemiology had a prior medical degree (MD/DSS/DVM), and the remainder had "non-doctoral medical degrees or biological backgrounds–nurses, pharmacists, bacteriologists, biologists, etc." (Magee, 1983, p. 29). Moreover, the proportion with either prior medical degrees or a "biological background" still comprised about two-thirds of epidemiology graduate students well into the early 1980s (Magee, 1983, pp. 30–31). The net effect was to imbue the field's leaders, well into the 1990s, with a common prior exposure to a biomedical orientation—and little, if any, training in the social sciences and its explicit discussion of (and debates over) methodological individualism. Sydenstricker's 1933 plea that epidemiologists and other health researchers get training in the social as well as biological sciences (*see* **Textbox 4–5** in **Chapter 4**) (Sydenstricker, 1933, pp. 109–110) remained unheeded.

Why Combine Biomedicine With Lifestyle Analysis? Epidemiology's Mid-Twentieth Century Break From Mono-Causal Thinking. The consolidation of a biomedical and lifestyle perspective within mid-twentieth century epidemiologic thought accordingly represents what became the discipline's ascendant approach to grappling with the complexities of "multiple causation" (Gordon, 1950; Gordon, 1952; Dubos & Dubos, 1952; Gordon, 1953; Galdston, 1954; Morris, 1957; Dubos, 1959). As succinctly expressed in the title of a 1954 volume, it was time to move *Beyond the Germ Theory* (Galdston, 1954).

To advance their research on "multiple causation," epidemiologists in the 1950s both drew on existing ideas and developed new ones. Thus, on the one hand, they continued to expand the early twentieth century critique of "germ theory" by elaborating on how the occurrence of disease simultaneously depended on characteristics of what they then termed the *agent, host,* and *environment* (Gordon, 1950; Gordon, 1953). Prompted by their findings that many of these newly identified exposures increased risk but were themselves neither necessary nor sufficient to cause the occurrence of disease (Dawber et al., 1951; Morris, 1957; Dawber et al., 1959), epidemiologists were concomitantly also integral to advancing the still relatively novel ideas that not only could a given disease be caused by multiple *agents* or *factors* but also that a probabalistic—and not deterministic—orientation to understanding risk was required.

To express, conceptually, the idea of a non-necessary, non-sufficient, yet still important contributing cause, in 1961 investigators affiliated with the famous Framingham study on coronary heart disease—one of the world's first large population-based longitudinal epidemiologic cohort studies designed expressly to study multiple causes of disease—coined the term *risk factor*, (Dawber et al., 1951; Kannel et al., 1961; Rothstein, 2008; Framingham Heart Study, 2009). The first use of this phrase appeared in the following paragraph (italics added), in a paper titled: "Factors of Risk in Development of Coronary Heart Disease—Six-Year Follow-up Experience: the Framingham Study" (Kannel et al., 1961, p. 47):

> It thus appears that, in assessing the contribution to risk of developing CHD, of the three factors under consideration, hypertension represents a greater *risk factor* for women than for men, whereas for serum cholesterol levels the converse is true, cholesterol contributing only slightly to the increased risk among women. but very significantly increasing risk among men. Combinations of the three *risk factors* under consideration appear to augment further the risk of subsequent development of coronary heart disease. (italics added)

Within 3 years, the phrase secured its first-ever use in the title of a scientific study: "Risk Factors in Coronary Heart Disease: an Evaluation of Several Serum Lipids as Predictors of Coronary Heart Disease: the Framingham Study" (Kannel et al., 1964). As increasingly recognized in contemporary literature on causal inference, the epidemiologic shift to a "risk factor" orientation constituted a decisive break with purely deterministic accounts of causation—a shift impelled by the epidemiologic findings themselves (Susser, 1973; Thagard, 1999; Russo & Williamson, 2007; Brandt, 2007, pp. 131–157; Rothstein, 2008).

Contributing to epidemiologists' adoption of a "multiple cause" orientation (Morris, 1957; Taylor & Knowelden, 1957) was not, however, solely its conceptual plausibility: it also gained traction because, starting in the 1950s, it became technically more feasible to test "multifactorial" hypotheses (Susser, 1985; Krieger, 1994; Susser & Stein, 2009). Enabling this empirical advance was the advent of the computer age, whereby computers could both store large amounts of data and conduct "multivariate" analyses (Susser, 1985; Skeet, 1987). The first massive civilian demonstration of this new possibility involved the 1950 U.S. Census and employed the ENIAC computer, which had been built in the 1940s at the request of the U.S. War Department in World War II to compute missile trajectories (Anderson, 1988). In 1954, the computer language FORTRAN was developed, with the first introductory programmer manual published in 1957 (McJones, 2008); by the end of the decade, the potential of computers for epidemiologic analysis was clearly understood (Susser, 1985; Skeet, 1987; Krieger, 1994).

1960: Emergence of the Epidemiologic "Web of Causation." Although nothing about the idea of "multiple causes" inherently required adhering to a biomedical and lifestyle orientation to analyzing disease causation and distribution (**Chapter 6** describes markedly different approaches to grappling with "multiple causation" also advanced in the 1950s and thereafter, making clear alternatives were possible), this nonetheless occurred, precisely because of the overall dominance of biomedicine and methodological individualism. Cogently capturing its influence is the powerful metaphor and model of the "web of causation," introduced in 1960 in the first formal—and highly influential—epidemiologic textbook ever published in the United States (or anywhere): *Epidemiologic Methods*, by Brian MacMahon, Thomas F. Pugh, and Johannes Ipsen (**Figure 5–1a**; MacMahon et al., 1960). Widely adopted to orient epidemiologic research on the multifactorial etiology of disease (Stallones, 1980; Susser, 1985; Greenland, 1987; Buck et al., 1988, pp. 149–153; Krieger, 1994), the "web of causation" still appears in twenty-first century epidemiologic textbooks (e.g., Friedman 2004) published nearly 45 years later (**Figure 5–1b**).

As I have discussed previously (Krieger, 1994), MacMahon et al. intended their "web" to counter the then still-pervasive tendency of epidemiologists to think in terms of single agents causing discrete diseases via simple causal chains. Inviting epidemiologists to embrace a more sophisticated view of causality, conceptually their metaphor evoked the powerful image of a spider's web, an elegantly linked network of delicate strands, the multiple intersections representing specific risk factors or outcomes, and the strands symbolizing diverse causal pathways.

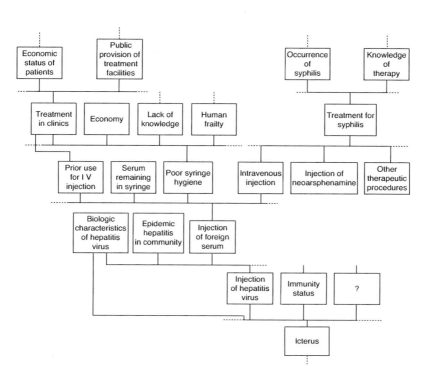

Figure 5–1a. The "web of causation" as introduced in the 1960 textbook *Epidemiologic Methods,* by MacMahon et al. (p. 18) (MacMahon et al., 1960, reprinted with permission from Lippincott, Williams, & Wilkins).

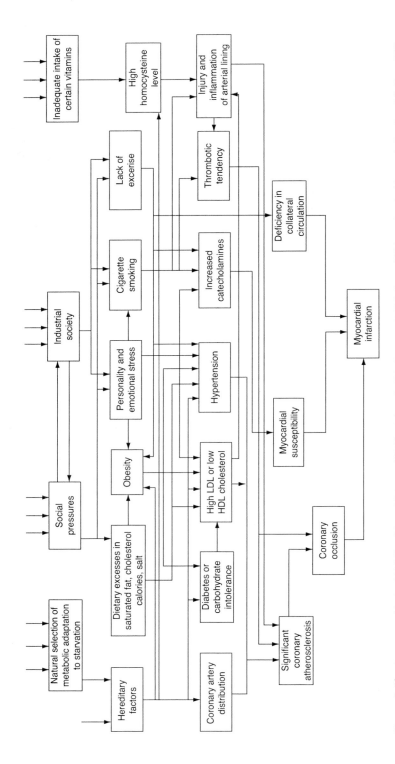

Figure 5–1b. As presented in the 2004 5th edition of *Primer of Epidemiology*, by Friedman (p. 4) (Friedman, 2004, reprinted with permission from McGraw-Hill)

Yet, woven into the very fabric of their "web" was its biomedical and lifestyle orientation. It was, by design, a "spiderless" web (Krieger, 1994). Deliberately unmoored from any discussion of what its strands included and excluded, MacMahon et al.'s web prioritized, from an etiologic standpoint, those factors closest to the onset of pathologic processes within the body, and, from a preventive standpoint, those strategies geared to cutting strands rather than attempting to identify and alter the source(s) of the web. Ignoring dimensions of both societal and historical context, and of time and place in the lives of individuals and populations, the web sans "spider" offered no ability to distinguish between factors that, in the trenchant formulation offered by the emininent UK epidemiologist Geoffrey Rose (1926–1993) (Rose, 1985; Rose, 1992) determined the occurrence of cases (chiefly with reference to disease mechanisms) versus determined population rates of disease. Unaddressed was why, given the identified constellation of risk factors, would the incidence (or prevalence) differ by social group and change over time? Instead, as noted by other critics (Tesh, 1988; Breilh, 1988), the web chiefly drew attention to static individual-level exposures and treated the individual-level parts as sufficient for explaining not only disease occurrence but also disease distribution in the whole.

Specifically, the "web" diagrammed by MacMahon et al. displayed "some components" of the relationship between two etiologically distinct diseases, syphilis and hepatitis, whose "causal chains" had no inherent reason to intersect (**Figure 5–1a**). Asserting that "the whole genealogy might be thought of more appropriately as a web, which in its complexity and origins lies quite beyond our understanding" (MacMahon et al., 1960, p. 18), they proffered a picture that simultaneously detailed how the hepatitis virus might get into syringe needles used to treat syphilis patients (in part by faulty behaviors), thereby producing an outbreak of jaundice (icterus), and yet left to the reader's imagination (as indicated by the suggestive dots trailing off the edge of the page) the determinants of other factors— including the "economic status of patients," "human frailty," the "public provision of treatment facilities," the "occurrence of syphilis," and "knowledge of therapy".

At no point did MacMahon et al. explain why they selected the components that appear in their web and left others out, nor did they offer any specific advice as to how others might elucidate the elements of other "webs." Instead, urging epidemiologists to abandon "semantic exercises aimed at hierarchic classification of causes" (MacMahon et al., 1960, p. 20), they in essence employed a type of weighting that leveled all distinctions (Breilh, 1988; Tesh, 1988; Krieger, 1994). Thus, in their web, "treatment in clinics" and the "economy" occupied the same level and rated the same kind of "box" as "injection of foreign serum" and "epidemic hepatitis in community" (**Figure 5–1**). Recommending a focus on the "necessary" (albeit rarely sufficient) causes most amenable to "practical" interventions and nearest (in terms of the web's configuration) to the specified outcome, MacMahon et al. argued that "to effect preventive measures, it is not necessary to understand causal mechanisms in their entirety," because "[e]ven knowledge of one small component may allow some degree of prevention," because "wherever the chain is broken the disease will be prevented" (MacMahon et al., 1960, p. 18).

Thus, in keeping with its underlying biomedical and lifestyle orientation, MacMahon et al.'s web focused on those risk factors most "proximate" to the "outcome" under investigation, and these in turn typically translated to the "direct" biologic causes of disease in individuals and/or to lifestyles and other risk factors that allegedly could be addressed at the individual level through education or medical intervention (Krieger, 1994). Concerned more with elucidating disease mechanisms than explanations for disease distribution, the web offered no guidance for conceptualizing broader societal determinants of population distributions of health and health inequities.

The Web Post-1960: Still Spinning. The endurance of the "web of causation" and its individualistic, biomedical, and lifestyle approach is underscored by a review article on environmental carcinogenesis, co-authored by MacMahon 20 years later (in 1980), that appeared in the second volume of the authoritative and then new journal *Epidemiologic Reviews* (Maclure & MacMahon, 1980). Biomedically defining the "environment" as "any influence other than that of the genetic material inherited from an individual's parents" (p. 19), the article additionally brought in a lifestyle perspective, whereby it "distinguished two basic categories of environmental agents; consumables, exposure to which is deliberate, and contaminants, exposure to which is inadvertent" (p. 21). Included among the former were "tobacco, alcoholic beverages, food, drugs, and cosmetics"; among the latter, "exposures in the workplace, pollutants outside the workplace, biologic contaminants, and radiation" (p. 21).

Inherent in the article's conceptualization of "environmental agents" thus were the twin biomedical and lifestyles premises that: (*1*) only individual-level decisions affected likelihood of exposure to the "consumables," and (*2*) exposure to "contaminants" was "inadvertent." Rendering these premises debatable, if not dubious, however, was then extant evidence that: (*1*) exposure to "consumables" was not necessarily "deliberate" or via "free choice" (e.g., already by the early 1970s scientific and public support led to laws banning exposure to secondhand cigarette smoke [Brandt, 2007, pp. 286–289]) and (*2*) exposure to "contaminants" was often not at all "inadvertent" (as demonstrated in 1970 by the establishment of both the U.S. Environmental Protection Agency and the Occupational Safety and Health Administration, created to address well-recognized problems posed by corporate opposition to, and willful neglect of, environmental and occupational safety regulations and standards [Berman, 1978; Markowitz & Rosner, 2002; Collins, 2006; Robbins & Landrigan, 2007]). The continued persistence of such biomedical and lifestyle approaches to analyzing disease risk, however, despite powerfully contradictory evidence, speaks to these frameworks enduring conceptual influence (if not ideological appeal).

The same biomedical and lifestyle emphasis is likewise visible in the 2004 "web of causation for myocardial infarction" (**Figure 5–1b**) appearing in the 5th edition of Friedman's *Primer of Epidemiology* (Friedman, 2004, p. 4). In the depicted web, 20 of the 23 boxes refer to discrete factors either measured within individuals' bodies (e.g., "hereditary factors," "obesity," "high HDL [high-density lipoprotein] or low HDL cholesterol," "coronary occlusion") or else involving individuals' health behaviors (e.g., "lack of exercise," "cigarette smoking"). Among the three exceptions, one refers to evolutionary processes ("natural selection of metabolic adaptation to starvation") and two to extremely broad nonspecific social "factors" ("industrial society," "social pressures"). As indicated by this twenty-first century example, the web endures—and continues to be used chiefly to array diverse individual-level risk factors identified by biomedical and lifestyle hypotheses and does so with scant attention to the larger societal and ecologic context in which these exposures are produced and distributed, let alone whether the depicted factors are sufficient to explain extant and changing population distribution of disease.

Contributions of Biomedical and Lifestyle Approaches on Epidemiology: Clear-Cut and Contested. Throughout the mid-twentieth to early twenty-first centuries, epidemiological research premised on a biomedical and lifestyle orientation has, like biomedical research more generally, generated enormous and valuable knowledge about specific factors linked to increased—and sometimes decreased—risk of disease (Ward & Warren, 2007). In doing so, this epidemiologic research has made important and unique contributions to the understanding of—and testing hypotheses about—mechanisms of disease causation. For example, continuing in the tradition of the Framingham Study, epidemiologic investigations, using apt comparison groups, have confirmed the importance of key factors implicated in cardiovascular disease, especially in relation to serum cholesterol, blood pressure, smoking, overweight and obesity, insulin resistance, adverse diets, and physical inactivity (a.k.a. "sedentary lifestyles") (Labarthe, 1998, pp. 17–26; Marmot & Elliott, 2005; Greenlund et al., 2007). Epidemiologic research on specific "risk factors" has likewise been instrumental to tracing the diverse and many adverse health outcomes attributable to specific exposures—for example, smoking (U.S. Department of Health and Human Services, Surgeon General's Reports on Smoking and Tobacco Use [1964–2006]; Brandt, 2007) and lead (Lansdown & Yule, 1986; ATSDR, 2007), to give but two well-documented and well-rehearsed examples.

Nevertheless, as also recognized in the field, not all biomedical- and lifestyle-oriented epidemiologic research on discrete risk factors has panned out, even on its own terms. Illustrating this point is the now well-known example of beta-carotene and the chemoprevention of lung cancer (Omenn, 1998; Forman et al., 2004; Nestle & Dixon, 2004). Building on a trend of nutritional research that took off during the 1950s, focused on specific nutrients as risk factors for common chronic diseases (as opposed diseases resulting from pathologic deficiencies of essential nutrients, such as beri-beri, kawashikor, or pellagra) (Greenwald et al., 1986; Graham, 1983; Willett, 2000; Forman et al., 2004), research suggested that higher levels of beta-carotene were protective against cancer (Greenwald et al., 1986; Omen, 1998; Forman et al., 2004). Support for this hypothesis was drawn from not only observational studies showing reduced risk of epithelial cancers among persons whose diets were rich in fruits and vegetables and who had elevated blood levels of beta-carotene but also animal studies and analysis of the chemistry and pharmacology of beta-carotene (Greenwald et al., 1986; Omenn, 1998; Forman et al., 2004). Based on this evidence, a famous 1981 review in *Nature* published by the epidemiologists Richard Peto (b. 1943), Sir Richard Doll (1912–2005), and co-authors, urged conduct of randomized clinical trials, which previously had not been done for nutritional supplements (Peto et al., 1981). Their argument? "[T]he possibility of discovering anticancer substances that can be prescribed rather than carcinogens that must be proscribed is attractive, for more people may be willing to accept prescription than proscription" (Peto et al., 1981, p. 201)—a quintessentially biomedical and lifestyle-oriented recommendation.

When the trials, however, revealed increased risk of not only cancer but also overall mortality among participants who had received the higher doses of beta-carotene, the resulting debates about the unexpected results were not only methodological but also substantive. Thus, above and beyond the many important methodological disputes about study design, including the respective strengths and limitations of observational versus experimental studies, the timing and size of the dose, and the problems posed by confounding and selection bias (Omenn, 1998; Forman et al., 2004), more basic questions were raised about the underlying reductionist premises of the initial hypothesis. Challenging the biomedical and lifestyle emphasis on isolated dietary supplements as pharmacologic agents that could be easily prescribed, these latter critiques called for renewed attention to people's real and complex diets in societal and cultural context (Omenn, 1998; Forman et al., 2004). Far from resolved, these different views are still in active debate in the nutritional literature today. At issue is whether epidemiologic research on nutrition should continue with a biomedical focus on single nutrients or supplements versus expanding the agenda to consider not only the heterogeneous biochemical composition of the food but also the economics and politics of food production, distribution, advertising, availability, and affordability (Kumanyika, 2000; Nestle & Dixon, 2004; Nestle, 2007; Garrety, 2007; Pollan, 2008).

Twenty-First Century Extensions of Biomedical and Lifestyle Approaches: "Gene–Environment Interaction," "Evolutionary Medicine," and the "Developmental Origins

of Health and Disease". As might be expected, the dominance of biomedical and lifestyle thinking in twenty-first century epidemiology remains strong. Three contemporary self-designated strands of theorizing that heavily bear their imprint are (*see* **Textbox 5–4**):

1. the widespread and highly influential "gene–environment interaction" (GEI) model (Wilson, 2002; Shostak, 2003; Maniolo et al., 2006; Vineis & Kriebel, 2006; Costa & Eaton, 2006; NIH/GEI, 2009), including as applied to epigenetic epidemiology (Jablonka, 2004; Waterland & Michaels, 2007; Sinclair et al., 2007; Foley et al., 2009);
2. the emerging perspective of "evolutionary medicine" (Eaton et al., 1988; Lappé, 1994; Nesse & Williams, 1994; Trevanthan et al., 1999; Stearns, 1999; Trevanthan, 2007; Trevanthan et al., 2007; Gluckman & Hanson, 2008; Stearns & Koella, 2008; Nesse, 2008); and
3. the increasingly ubiquitous "developmental origins of health and disease" (DOHaD) paradigm, emphasizing the importance of fetal programming to adult disease (Barker, 1986; Barker et al., 1989; Barker, 2004; Wintour & Owens, 2006; Gluckman & Hanson, 2006; Barker, 2007; Gluckman et al., 2007; Sinclair et al., 2007).

It is not my intent to review any of these three perspectives in depth; rather, the objective is to clarify how each continues to reveal the dominance of biomedical and lifestyle thinking in epidemiology while still cloaking key assumptions of these two underlying frameworks.

For both GEI and DOHaD, the research typically accords detailed attention to postulated mechanisms involving genes and other subcellular factors in the causal pathway to pathogenesis, with the latter focused especially on the impact of exposures occurring during the prenatal period (*see* **Textbox 5–4**) (Campbell, 1996; Wilson, 2002, pp. 2, 14; Shostak, 2003; Barker, 2004; Vineis, 2004; Corella & Ordovas, 2005; Hernandez & Blaser, 2006; Gluckman & Hanson, 2006; Sinclair et al., 2007; Wintour & Owens, 2006; Costa & Eaton, 2006; Barker, 2007; Gluckman et al., 2007). Moreover, like the "web of causation," both GEI and DOHaD offer scant theorizing about the nature of the "environment" and instead conceptualize it chiefly as anything that is not the "gene" or the "organism." The kinds of environmental "exposures" deemed to be relevant in turn are those that can be measured within individual bodies, with the entry of these factors into people's bodies deemed a consequence chiefly of people's diet and "lifestyle" and, to a lesser extent, exposure to other exogenous chemicals. Thus, in a 2002 Institute of Medicine report on *Cancer and the Environment: Gene-Environment Interactions* (Wilson, 2002), "environmental exposures" were "broadly defined here to include lifestyle factors, such as smoking, nutrition, and reproductive variables" (Fraumeni, 2002, p. 14). Similarly, a 2007 DOHaD review article defined the "environment" as that within which the organism "finds itself" and posited that "lifestyle disease in the human then occurs when the individual lives in an environment beyond their forecasted and induced physiological homeostatic range" (Gluckman et al., 2007). The imprint of biomedical and lifestyle theorizing is clear.

Similarly, a major theme in evolutionary medicine concerns the postulated "mismatch" between our biological bodies, held to have evolved to be adapted to Paleolithic "environmental" conditions and our modern "lifestyles" (Eaton et al., 1988; Nesse & Williams, 1994; Trevanthan, 2007; Trevanthan et al., 2007; Gluckman et al., 2007; Gluckman & Hanson, 2008; Stearns & Koella, 2008; Nesse, 2008). Extending the temporal frame to encompass a deeper sense of evolutionary time, as relevant to processes of selection, development, and adaptation, the primary thesis, referred to in a 1988 review article as "Stone Agers in the Fast Lane" (Eaton et al., 1988), is that chronic illnesses arise from the

Textbox 5–4. Biomedical and Lifestyle Influences in the Twenty-First Century: The "Gene–Environment Interaction (GEI)," "Evolutionary Medicine," and "Developmental Origins of Health and Disease" (DOHaD) Frameworks

"Gene–Environment Interaction" (GEI):
characterized by specificity about genes, an emphasis on lifestyle, and a broad, non-analytic definition of the "environment" as anything that is not a gene...

Fraumeni JF Jr. Genes and the environment in cancer etiology. In: Wilson SH, Institute of Medicine (U.S.) Roundtable on Environmental Health Sciences, Research, and Medicine, Institute of Medicine (U.S.), Board on Health Sciences Policy. *Cancer and the Environment: Gene-Environment Interaction.* Washington, DC: National Academy of Science Press, 2002, pp. 14–24.
p. 14: "For some time, the epidemiologic evidence has suggested that the bulk of cancer in the population is related to environmental exposures, which are broadly defined here to include lifestyle factors, such as smoking, nutrition, and reproductive variables. Although genetic mechanisms are fundamental to the development and progression of all forms of cancer, the actual role of inherited susceptibility as an etiologic factor has been very difficult to assess. The causes of cancer in the population can be assigned to one of four broad categories: (1) inherited susceptibility alone; (2) environment alone; (3) interactions between genes and the environment; or (4) a 'spontaneous' category of tumors that may arise randomly from the play of chance.'"

Corella D, Ordovas JM. Integration of environment and disease into "omics" analysis. *Curr Opinion Molecular Therapeutics* 2005; 7:569–576.
p. 570: "In the global framework of gene-environment interactions there are three relevant aspects that need careful definition for their successful integration into omics research; these are phenotype, genotype, and environment.... the environment is broadly defined to include all non-genetic factors, therefore, infectious, chemical, physical, nutritional, behavioral and social factors... Once scientists add the real world (environment) into the omics equation to solve the problem of complex diseases, the results from genomics, transcriptomics, proteomics, metabolomics and other omics will acquire the external validity needed to achieve practical solutions."
p. 571: "A complete mechanistic study of the environment-gene interactions in human disease is not yet technically possible. However, this is the

time to develop disease-specific environment-gene interaction models for future research. In the absence of such specific models, it is useful to remember the pragmatic general gene-environment interaction model proposed by Laframboise in the 1970s for public health policies. According to Laframboise, the interactive factors that influence health and disease, names "determinants of health," could be arranged into four major groups: human biology, lifestyle, environment and healthcare systems. Human biology (genetic inheritance) identified all aspects of health (physical and mental) developed within the human body as a result of organic make-up. Lifestyle included "the aggregation of personal decisions, over which the individual has control" (e.g., tobacco smoking, physical activity, dietary intake, consumption of alcohol and other non-prescribed drugs). Environment referred to "all matters related to health external to the human body and over which the individual has little or no control," and included the physical (e.g., air pollution, ionizing radiations, water contamination, electromagnetic fields, temperature, microorganisms and chemicals) and social environments. Finally, the healthcare organization included the quantity, quality, arrangement, nature and relationship of people and resources in the provision of healthcare (e.g., health technology, specialized units, diagnostics and treatments that include drugs prescribed by the physician)."

"Evolutionary Medicine":
characterized by specificity about genes and genetic selection and adaptation, an emphasis on lifestyle, and a broad, non-analytic definition of the "environment" as anything that is not a gene...

Eaton S, Konner M, Shotak M. Stone Agers in the fast lane: chronic degenerative diseases in evolutionary perspective. *Am J Med* **1988; 84:739–749.**
p. 739: From a genetic standpoint, humans living today are Stone Age hunter-gatherers displaced through time to a world that differs from that for which our genetic constitution was selected. Unlike evolutionary maladaptation, our current discordance has little effect on reproductive success; rather it acts as a potent promoter of chronic illnesses: atherosclerosis, essential hypertension, many cancers, diabetes mellitus, and obesity among others. These diseases are the results of interaction between genetically controlled biochemical processes and a myriad of biocultural influences–lifestyle factors–that include nutrition, exercise, and exposure to noxious substances. Although our genes have hardly changed, our culture has been transformed almost beyond recognition during the

past 10,000 years, especially since the industrial Revolution. There is increasing evidence that the resulting mismatch fosters "diseases of civilization" that together cause 75 percent of all deaths in Western nations, but that are rare among persons whose lifeways reflect those of our preagricultural ancestors."

Gluckman PD, Hanson M. *Mismatch: The Lifestyle Diseases Timebomb*. Oxford: Oxford University Press, 2008.

p. 133: "We have described in the first part of this book how we evolved to try to match our biology to our environment to live within a comfort zone. However we have intrinsic constraints on how far we can adapt... Our evolutionary past tries to match the range of phenotypes we can develop, using our repertoire of genes, to our environment–but that environment was largely determined more than 10,000 years ago. We have also been equipped through our evolution with the toolkit of developmental plasticity. This allows us to tune the degree of match with our environment further but there are limits imposed by our design... The greater the degree of mismatch, the greater the cost, and the more we need to understand it."

p. 205: "So what is to be done? A logical conclusion from this book is that to improve the human condition we must increase the degree of match between the biology of members of our species and their current and future environments... We live in an environment which in metabolic and other terms is well beyond the capacities that our biology has evolved to cope with over the last 150,000 years... We therefore need to change our environment again, to achieve a better match with our biology. This is not to say that we have to revert to some neo-Stone Age existence. But it does mean that we must now focus on how the built environment of our homes and workplaces can be modified to promote the amount of exercise we take every day. We must give far greater emphasis to promoting good nutrition and access to healthier foods to allow more people to eat a balanced diet better matched to their physiology. And because these lifestyle changes are much easier for the better-off members of society, we will have to give special attention to the poor, caught in a poverty trap–because the challenges of helping them to address problems of the metabolic mismatch are so much harder."

**Developmental origins of
health and disease (DOHaD)
paradigm:**
*characterized by specificity
about physiologic processes, an
emphasis on lifestyle, and a
broad, nonanalytic definition of
the "environment" as anything
that is not the organism...*

Leonard WR. Lifestyle, diet, and disease: comparative perspectives on the determinants of
chronic health risks. In: Stearns SC, Koella JC
(eds). *Evolution in Health and Disease.* 2nd ed.
Oxford: Oxford University Press, 2008, pp.
265–276.
p. 265: "Throughout most of our evolutionary
history, human lifestyle was characterized by
high levels of physical ac tivity and energy
expenditure, by seasonal fluctuations in food
availability, and by frequent periods of marginal
or negative energy balance. These conditions
selected for improvements in the energetic efficiency of human foraging strategies. Today, we
are in many respects victims of our own evolutionary success. Human populations of the
industrialized world live in 'obesogenic' environments with low levels of energy expenditure and
abundant food supplies contributing to strongly
positive energy balances and growing rates of
obesity and chronic, metabolic disorders."

Barker DJP. The developmental origins of
well-being. *Phil Trans R Soc Lond B* 2004;
359:1359–1366.
p. 1359: "The recent discovery that people who
develop chronic disease grow differently from
other people during foetal life and childhood
has led to a new 'developmental' model for a
group of disease including coronary heart disease, stroke, high blood pressure and type 2
(adult onset) diabetes... It has been argued,
however, that people whose growth was
impaired *in utero* and during infancy may continue to be exposed to an adverse environment
in childhood and adult life, and it is this later
environment that produces the effects attributed to intrauterine influences. There is not
strong evidence that this argument can be
sustained. The associations between low birthweight and later disease have been shown to be
independent of influences such as socioeconomic status and smoking, though adult lifestyle
adds to the effects of early life: for example, the
prevalence of type 2 diabetes is highest in
people who had a low birthweight and became
obese as adults."

Gluckman PD, Hanson MA, Beedle AS. Early
life events and their consequences for later
disease: a life history and evolutionary perspective. *Am J Human Biol* 2007; 19:1–19.
p. 2: "We suggest that the DOHaD phenomenon
represents the most visible manifestation of the
fundamental processes of developmental plasticity

by which mammals adjust their life history strategy in response to environmental cues during early development."

p. 7: "An important feature of such a model is that alternations in regulatory systems induced by the developmental cues may be subtle and not observable under basal conditions–they may affect the sensitivity of a physiological response underpinning a specific trait in the adult and thus make the organisms more or less susceptible to disease in an extreme postnatal environment. Lifestyle disease in the human then occurs when the individual lives in an environment beyond their forecasted and induced physiological homeostatic range... Implicit in this discussion is the view that the DOHaD phenomenon is underpinned by physiological mechanisms that have evolved in mammals to provide adaptive advantage..."

pp. 15–16: "Major research questions remain to be resolved: the genotypic determinants of environmental sensitivity during development, the identification of key regulatory genes, the fundamental epigenetic processes involved in phenotypic plasticity, the basis of the adjustment and integration of the various components of the life course strategy, and the complexities surrounding the role of the infant period in modifying earlier phenotypic choices... It shifts the disease paradigm from one of external causation to one of the match or mismatch between the evolutionary and developmentally defined constitution of the organism and the environment in which it finds itself."

interaction of genes "that have hardly changed" and "lifestyle factors—that include nutrition, exercise, and exposure to noxious substances," the latter of which no longer resemble what people were exposed to "10,000 years" ago (Eaton et al., 1988, p. 739). Or, as stated in a 2008 book tellingly titled *Mismatch: the Lifestyle Diseases Timebomb* (Gluckman & Hanson, 2008): "We live in an environment which in metabolic and other terms is well beyond the capacities that our biology has evolved to cope with over the last 150,000 years" (Gluckman & Hanson, 2008, p. 205). The conjoined lifestyle and biomedical orientation is clear, with the "environment" once again consigned to that which is external to the organism and its genes.

Thus, as with the "web," these three additional frameworks: (*1*) focus predominantly on the mechanisms of disease causation and (2) reduce variation in disease rates to being a consequence of: (*a*) genetic and epigenetic variation (involving both gene frequency and regulation), in conjunction with (*b*) behavioral "choices," together occurring (*c*) within a loosely defined "environment." None of the three frameworks offer any systematic analysis of the "environment," either overall or in relation to its societal aspects. Stated another way, the biomedical and lifestyle orientation not only lives on but actually thrives in the context of twenty-first century science. Whether this perspective constitutes the only—or best—way to approach questions of biology, behavior, and population distributions of disease is the question raised by less dominant alternative theoretical frameworks also present since the 1950s—and now gaining strength in the twenty-first century—as I next review.

6

Social Epidemiologic Alternatives

Sociopolitical and Psychosocial Frameworks

What might an epidemiologic alternative to biomedical and lifestyle theorizing about disease distribution encompass? During the mid-twentieth through early twenty-first centuries, a variety of epidemiologic schools of thought have constructively sought to answer this question (*see* **Figure 6–1**), all of which can be broadly encompassed within what is now termed *social epidemiology* (Berkman & Kawachi, 2000; Krieger, 2000; Krieger, 2001a; Porta, 2008, p. 231) (for a brief history of this term, starting with its English-language emergence in 1950, *see* **Textbox 6–1** [Krieger, 2001a]). Attesting to its growing influence, in 2009 the leading journal *Epidemiologic Reviews* devoted its first theme issue ever to "Epidemiologic Approaches to Health Disparities" (*Epidemiologic Reviews*, 2009)—the topic that lies at the heart of social epidemiologic inquiry.

Among the variants of extant social epidemiologic perspectives, I would argue three distinct theoretical trends exist—*sociopolitical, psychosocial, ecosocial*—each with myriad strands (*see* **Figure 6–2**). Of these, the first, *sociopolitical*, focuses principally on power, politics, economics, and rights as key societal determinants of health; the second, *psychosocial*, emphasizes psychologically-mediated social determinants of population health. Together, they comprise the main contemporary expressions of social epidemiologic theorizing. The third trend, which I discuss in the next chapter, is more nascent and is best represented by *ecosocial theory*, which builds on and extends these first two frameworks by analyzing both the embodied population distributions of disease and health *and* epidemiologic theories of disease distribution, each in relation to their societal, ecological, and historical context.

These three social epidemiologic alternative theoretical perspectives all share certain features in common. Three jointly held premises are:

1. the longstanding thesis that distributions of health and disease in human populations cannot be understood apart from—and necessarily occur in—their societal context;
2. the corollary that social processes causally (albeit probabilistically) determine any health or disease outcome that is socially patterned; and

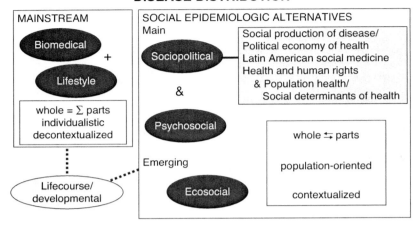

Figure 6–1. Mainstream biomedical and lifestyle versus alternative social epidemiologic theories of disease distribution.

3. the prediction that as societies change, whether in their social, economic, cultural, or technological features, so too will their population levels and distributions of health and disease.

Granted, these statements may seem obvious, yet they are nevertheless disregarded by the dominant decontextualized perspectives. In particular, the claim that societal processes drive the social patterning of population distributions of health and disease—within and between societies—far from being a tautology, runs diametrically opposed to the reductionist and individualistic biomedical and lifestyle assumptions that disease distributions arise from intrinsic characteristics of individuals, whether biological or behavioral.

Yet, despite these conceptual agreements and overlaps, these three theoretical perspectives differ in important ways. As I will discuss in this chapter and also **Chapters 7** and **8**, the distinctions matter: for the kinds of hypotheses they propose, the empirical research and data they generate, and their implications for efforts to change societal patterns of health.

Sociopolitical Frameworks: Searching for the Spider(s)—Power, Politics, Economics, Rights, & Health

What schools of thought comprise the *sociopolitical* epidemiologic theories of disease distribution? One listing, using terms self-designated by each variant, would include: *the social production of disease*; *the political economy of health*; *social determinants of health*;

Textbox 6–1. "Social Epidemiology" Gains a Name: Its Emergence in the Epidemiologic Literature and Text Books from 1950 to 2000 (Krieger, 2001a, pp. 668–669)

"Social Epidemiology" Gains a Name...

Building on holistic models of health developed between World War I and World War II (Lawrence & Weisz, 1998) and on the "social medicine" framework forged during the 1940s (Ryle, 1948; Galdston, 1949; Porter, 1997), it is in the mid-twentieth century that *social epidemiology* gains its name-as-such. The term apparently first appears in the title of an article published by Alfred Yankauer in the *American Sociological Review* in 1950: "The relationship of fetal and infant mortality to residential segregation: an inquiry into social epidemiology" (Yankaeur, 1950), a topic as timely now as it was then; Yankauer later becomes editor of the *American Journal of Public Health*. The term then reappears in the introduction to one of the first books pulling together the behavioral and medical sciences, edited by E. Gartly Jaco, published in 1958, *Patients, Physicians, and Illness: Sourcebook in Behavioral Science and Medicine* (Jaco, 1958), and is included in the title of Jaco's next book, *The Social Epidemiology of Mental Disorders; A Psychiatric Survey of Texas*, published in 1960 (Jaco, 1960). By 1969, enough familiarity with the field exists that Leo G. Reeder presents a major address to the American Sociological Association called "Social Epidemiology: An Appraisal" (Reeder, 1969 in Jaco, 1972). Defining *social epidemiology* as the "study of the role of social factors in the etiology of disease" (Reeder, 1969 in Jaco, 1972, p. 97), he asserts that "social epidemiology... seeks to extend the scope of investigation to include variables and concepts drawn from a theory" (Reeder, 1969 in Jaco, 1972, p. 97)—in effect, calling for a marriage of sociological frameworks to epidemiologic inquiry.

Soon thereafter, the phrase *social epidemiology* catches on in the epidemiologic literature. Articles appear with such titles as: "Contributions of Social Epidemiology to the Study of Medical Care Systems," published by S. Leonard Syme in 1971 (Syme, 1971), and "Social Epidemiology and the Prevention of Cancer," published by Saxon Graham et al. in 1972 (Graham & Schniederman, 1972). By the end of the century, the first textbook is published with the title *Social Epidemiology*, co-edited by Lisa Berkman and Ichiro Kawachi (Berkman & Kawachi, 2000).

---

population health; *fundamental cause*; *political epidemiology*; *Latin American Social Medicine*; and *health and human rights*. That these labels even exist is already one clue that the theoretical distinctions matter. Understanding the similarities and differences of these sociopolitical theories can thus provide insight into the data and explanations proffered by and debated within social epidemiologic research.

In brief, the common thread linking these different sociopolitical frameworks is their attention to analyzing patterns of disease distribution in relation to power, politics, economics, and rights (*see* **Figure 6–2**). Metaphorically, most—but not all—argue that "upstream" ("distal") social factors causally determine the array of "downstream" ("proximal") exposures that shape population and individual contexts and health (Krieger, 2008a). In doing so, they continue to accept the proximal/distal divide (Krieger, 2008a), one also embraced by the biomedical and lifestyle perspectives and woven deeply into the "web of causation," but reverse the direction of the causal arrows, pointing them instead from social conditions to disease occurrence.

SOCIAL EPIDEMIOLOGIC THEORIES: COMMONALITIES & CONTRASTS

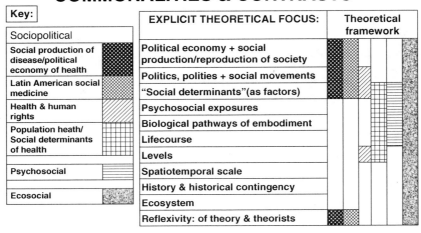

Figure 6–2. Social epidemiologic theories: commonalities and contrasts.

More literally, these sociopolitical theories of disease distribution all posit, to varying degrees, that societies' political and economic institutions and priorities together drive societal levels and distributions of disease and health. Relevant social determinants accordingly can include:

- a society's form(s) of governance;
- rules about property, ownership, and labor (including at what technological level);
- systems and sanctions about families, reproduction, and sexuality;
- upholding or denial of rights for specific groups (including in relation to cultural mores);
- economic and social policies (including in relation to health systems); and
- political and economic relationships with other societies and international or global institutions.

The emphasis of the theorizing is consequently on social conditions, social processes, and social relationships. The central concern is how characteristics of societal organization at different levels affect the social patterning of health. Receiving less or even no theoretical attention are the biological processes involved in embodying inequality, as ultimately manifested within individual bodies. Thus, even as all these alternative theories recognize the agency of individuals and also inter-individual social and biological variation (between persons both within and across diverse societally-defined groups), these individual-level phenomena are not the focus. At issue instead are how the societal processes creating the groups to which individuals belong—and delimiting their material and social conditions—powerfully shape the options and constraints that socially-determined membership in these groups affords for the possibility of living healthy and dignified lives.

Social Production of Disease/Political Economy of Health. The frameworks of the *social production of disease* (Doyal, 1979; Conrad & Kern, 1981; Smith, 1981) and *political economy of health* (Kelman, 1975; Flaherty et al., 1977; Doyal, 1979), which gained their names in the 1970s, are related—and some might argue identical—theories of disease distribution that focus on economic and political determinants of health and distributions of disease within and across societies (Krieger, 2001a; Krieger, 2001b). Highlighting structural barriers to people living healthy lives, a core postulate is that any given society's patterning of health and disease—including its social inequalities in health—is *produced by* the structure, values, and priorities of its political and economic systems, in conjunction with those of the political and economic systems of the other societies with which it interacts, and also the ensemble of available technologies (whether for producing food and material goods, building housing, enabling transportation, exchanging information, providing medical care, etc).

Conceptual Premises. Overall, the theorizing within these two sociopolitical frameworks has principally been concerned with economic and political systems, institutions, and decisions that create, enforce, and perpetuate economic and social privilege and inequality, globally to locally, thereby generating the social and material conditions under which people live and work—and hence *producing* both health inequities and overall population profiles of health and disease. Also encompassed is how political-economic systems and priorities that value social justice can produce health equity. In both cases, the issue of power is paramount—both power "to do" and power "over" (Giddens and Held 1982; McFarland, 2004; Clegg, 2004; McLennan, 2005; Krieger, 2008a; Beckfield & Krieger, 2009). The implication is that analyzing and altering population distributions of and inequities in health and disease necessitates engaging with, if not confronting, extant political and economic systems, priorities, policies, and programs.

The metaphorical and literal emphasis on *production* and *political economy* deliberately calls attention to societal processes and priorities (Krieger, 2001a; Krieger, 2001b). Designed to counter the biomedical view that disease rates and distributions in human societies are simply "natural" phenomena reflecting "adaptation" to any particular or changing "environment," the notion of *production* as linked to *political economy,* intrinsically mandates considering who is producing what, with what technologies, for whom, and why. Spanning multiple levels, the "who" in the first instance is abstractly conceptualized as political and economic systems operating within and across regions, countries, and localities, and the institutions and individuals who dominate them. Existing in historical context, these political-economic systems can include variants of capitalism, imperialism, communism, socialism, feudalism, and communalism, whose forms of governance in turn can encompass formal democratic, autocratic, dictatorial, monarchial, or communal rule.

In each case, the "what" these systems produce refers not only to their literal economic output (financially and in material goods), but also to:

1. their particular societal structure, including its constituent social and economic groups and their relationships with each other (whether adversarial or supportive);
2. the means and materials these social groups use to reinforce or challenge their social position and to sustain and reproduce themselves in the daily course of life (involving paid and unpaid labor outside and in the home; household, family, and childrearing structures; and access to and use of needed goods and services); and
3. the norms, values, and ideologies justifying—and challenging—their political and economic priorities.

Consequently, these frameworks conceptualize societies—and the relationships between them—not as intrinsically harmonious or static "wholes" but rather as dynamic entities comprised of often conflicting societal groups, whose between-group relationships of power and property define their social (and even spatial) boundaries and shape each group's characteristics, including their on-average health status. Examples of such groups, necessarily defined in relation to each other, include: employer/self-employed/employee; masculine/feminine; white/of color; straight (heterosexual)/LGBT (lesbian, gay, bisexual, transgender); colonizer/colonized; settler/Indigenous; occupier/occupied; and global North/global South.

It follows that institutions' and individuals' ability to act—including to protect or harm their health or that of others—necessarily depends on their location with the nexus of power relations and their corresponding options to exert influence, both on their own behalf and over others. By implication, analysis of causes of disease distribution requires attention to the political and economic structures, processes, and power relationships that *produce* societal patterns of health, disease, and well-being via shaping the conditions in which people live and work; a focus only on decontextualized "lifestyles," consumption, and exposures is incomplete and inadequate.

Historical Development. In one sense, the intellectual lineage of the theories of the *social production of disease* and the *political economy of health* extends back to the mid-nineteenth century emergence of the discipline of epidemiology, per the ideas and investigations of Rudolf Virchow (1821–1902), Louis René Villermé (1782–1863), and Friedrich Engels (1820–1895), as recounted in **Chapter 3**. Another antecedent was the early and mid-twentieth century European theorizing in "social medicine," concerned with social influences on the health of individuals, families, and communities (Ryle, 1944; Rosen, 1947; Ryle, 1948; Greenwood, 1948; Galdston, 1949; Stebbins, 1949; Sand, 1952; Rosen, 1974; Eisenberg, 1984; Porter, 1997; Porter, 2006; Stonington & Holmes, 2006), along with its U.S. counterparts, as per Sydenstricker's classic text on *Health and Environment* (Sydenstricker, 1933), discussed in **Chapter 4**.

Exemplifying this mid-twentieth century sociopolitical epidemiologic theorizing was the influential article on "Uses of Epidemiology" (Morris, 1955), published in 1955 in the *British Journal of Medicine* by Jerry Morris (1910–2009), one of the twentieth century's leading epidemiologists (Davey Smith, 2001; Krieger, 2007; Davey Smith, 2010; Oakley, 2010). Two years later, Morris expanded the ideas in his article into an acclaimed book by the same name (Morris, 1957), which to this day remains one of the classic texts of twentieth century epidemiology (Davey Smith, 2001; Krieger, 2007).

Among Morris' objectives were to delineate not only useful applications of epidemiology (**Textbox 6–2**) but also useful ways of epidemiologic theorizing. Portraying "epidemiology as a way of learning, of asking questions, and getting answers that raise further questions—that is, as a *method*" (italics in the original) for thinking (Morris, 1957, p. 3), Morris cautioned that: "epidemiology is the only way of asking some questions in medicine, one way of asking others (and no way at all to ask many)" (Morris, 1957, p. 96). The first step consequently was to get the questions right—after which it would of course be necessary to confront the "practical matters" and "kinds of difficulties that arise" when conducting epidemiologic research (Morris, 1957, p. 14). Doing so (**Textbox 6–3**) required engaging with epidemiology as an historical, population, and contextual science (Krieger, 2007), one that complemented but could not be reduced to either a clinical or laboratory science.

Morris dynamically integrated these ideas in his rich definition of epidemiology as a "mode of understanding of the changing picture of disease: study of changing people and

Textbox 6–2. Morris' Seven "Uses of Epidemiology" (Morris, 1957, p. 96)

1. In *historical study* of the health of the community and of the rise and fall of disease in the population; useful "projections" into the future may also be possible.
2. For *community diagnosis* of the presence, nature and distribution of health and disease among the population, and the dimensions of these in incidence, prevalence, and mortality, taking into account that society is changing and health problems are changing.
3. To study the *workings of health services*. This begins with the determination of needs and resources, proceeds to analysis of services in action and, finally, attempts to appraise. Such studies can be comparative between various populations.
4. To estimate, from the common experience, the *individual's chances* and risks of disease.
5. To *help complete the clinical picture* by including all types of cases in proportion; by relating clinical disease to the subclinical; by observing secular changes in the character of disease, and its picture in other countries.
6. In *identifying syndromes* from the distribution of clinical phenomena among sections of the population.
7. In the *search for causes* of health and disease, starting with the discovery of groups with high and low rates, studying these differences in relation to differences in ways of living, and, where possible, testing these notions in actual practice among populations.

their changing ways of living in changing environments; and the causes of disease that may be identified in these" (Morris, 1957, p. 120). To Morris, epidemiology's unique contribution lay in its dual engagement with studying "human biology" and "the social aspects of the disease" (Morris, 1957, p. 97), with the aim being to "*abolish the clinical picture*" (Morris, 1957, p. 98) and improve the "health of the community" (Morris, 1957, p. 96). This mission, as Morris forcefully pointed out a half-century later in a 2007 study on "Defining a Minimum Income for Healthy Living" (Morris et al., 2007), is "directly in the tradition since World War Two and the establishment of [World Health Organization] WHO for official acceptance of attainable levels of health as a human right and a prime goal of society" (Morris et al., 2007, p. 5).

Because of its premises—and despite its promise—during the 1950s and 1960s, social epidemiologic theorizing about disease distribution of the type that Morris proposed exerted relatively little influence in the field. Obstacles included the impact, as discussed in the previous chapter, of the post-World War II emphasis on methodological individualism, the chilling effect of the Cold War on progressive social analysis (sometimes by outright political censorship; more commonly by self-censorship [Porter, 1997; Schrecker, 1998; Badash, 2000; Isaac, 2007; Hobsbawm, 1994; Zinn, 2003]), along with difficulties in getting funding to develop and test—and find journals willing to publish—ideas that conflicted with the prevailing views (Fee, 1994).

Preventing the eclipse of the sociopolitical epidemiologic perspectives were developments not unique to epidemiology but instead linked to global changes in politics, ideas, and science. Impelled by the worldwide political, social, and intellectual ferment of the

Textbox 6–3. Historical, Population/Societal, and Contextual Approach to Epidemiologic Thinking in Morris' 1957 Classic Text *Uses of Epidemiology* (Morris, 1957; Krieger, 2007)

Historical approach

p. 1: the book opens with a review of the past century's trends, from 1850 to 1950, of mortality rates for women and men, 55–64 years old, in England and Wales, whereby rates for both groups began to drop in 1900, reflecting the impact of sanitary report, and fell until 1920, after which "rather abruptly there was a change," whereby:

> Female mortality kept its downward course, but the reduction of male mortality has slowed and almost stopped. As one result of this, the death rate among men aged 55 to 64 which was about 10 per cent higher than for women a hundred years ago, and about 33 percent higher after the first world war, is now approach about 90 percent higher... What has been happening?... The most important is the emergence of three diseases from obscurity to become exceedingly common, disease which particularly affect men and are very frequent in middle-age: duodenal ulcer, cancer of the bronchus and 'coronary thrombosis.', pp. 1–2

Reflecting on these trends, Morris asked: "What are the *social* changes that underlie the biological changes expressed"(p. 19) in the observed patterns?

p. 19, 22: In a section titled "Changing people in a changing society" Morris posed the following questions:

> What are the implications to Public Health of more married women going out to work? And less of the older men? Of still increasing urban—and surburbanisation? The rapid growth of new towns? Smokeless zones (still with sulphur)? The building of new power stations? Of less physical activity in work and more bodily sloth generally? Of the quickening transformations in industry? Of the prospect of an age of leisure? Or the growth of mass media and the use being made of these? Of the eleven-plus examination? Of the more than 1000 extra motor vehicles per day? Of the rising consumption of sugar; our astonishing taste for sweet–we eat more per head than any other population? Of the cheapening of fats? The multiplying interferences with food? The many physical and chemical exposures, known and potentially hazardous? More smoking in women? The prodigious increase of X-rays and antibiotics?

> Such questions (of contemporary history, it might be said) could readily be multiplied.

Population/ societal approach

p. 16: Morris defined epidemiology as "*the study of health and disease of populations and of groups in relation to their environment and ways of living.*"

p. 61: "The main use of epidemiology is to discover populations or groups with high rates of disease, and with low, in the hope that causes of disease and of freedom from disease can be postulated."

p. 51: Noting that population comparisons could give insight into what constituted both "disease" and what was "*healthy,* or '*normal*' (not just the common, or average), Morris observed:

> Thus, extending the customary picture obtained in any one country, population studies are beginning to make it clear that blood cholesterol levels may vary considerably from one country to another. Western populations may have higher levels than those in 'under-developed' countries, and may have different trends with age. The question at once arises: what are the *normal* ranges of blood cholesterol? May it be that most people in the West have *pathologically* high levels?... That is to say, it must now be considered what is the appropriate population or 'universe' for the study of physiological norms... My own first introduction to it was... when I was told of the laboratory technician in China who believed that what we call megloblastic degeneration of the bone marrow was 'normal.'

Contextual approach   p. 120: "'Organism-in-Environment' as unit of investigation of treatment," with an epidemiological approach being:

—"A mode of understanding of the changing picture of disease: studying of changing *people* and their changing *ways of living* in *changing* environments; and the causes of disease that may be identified in these," taking into account:

—"Groups have properties as such, e.g., herd immunity, morale of work group, rehabilitation unit, 'therapeutic community,'" Understanding of properties of *individuals* which they have in virtue of their *group* membership,"

while also recognizing, using the example of socioeconomic inequalities in reproductive outcomes:

p. 16: "Such demonstration of inequalities between groups is the standard function of epidemiology. Obviously there will be great and small individual differences *within* these social classes. But resolution of these differences, and summarising the group experiences as such, is also obviously useful."

p. 65: "The notion of 'pattern of causes' is a relatively modern restatement. With the glories of the bacteriological discovery, there was a period of emphasis on *the* 'germ theory' of disease and such formulations. Today the interest would not b e in *the cause* of syphilis by the (of course necessary) *treponema pallidum*. We would be concerned rather to understand the occurrence of syphilis among *causes* in host and environment as well: basic influences of race, of sex, and of age, and in such causes as the psychology of promiscuity, the economics of prostitution, the life of the merchant seaman, the horrors of war, the denial of family life in contract migrant labour, causes of which in one combination or another may produce a case of syphilis."

social change and revolutionary movements that erupted in the 1960s (Hobsbawm, 1994; Zinn, 2003), new possibilities arose to question the strictures and precepts of the entrenched Cold War dominance of individualistic ideologies and methodologies. More specifically, during this era, numerous scientists in many fields, including the health sciences, became influenced by the radical ideas of the period's many political and social movements, including national liberation movements and anti-dictatorship struggles in the Asian, African, and Latin American continents and the corresponding anti-war movements within the colonizing countries (in both Europe and the United States), along with movements calling for nuclear disarmament and for protecting the environment, and also movements for civil rights, women's rights, lesbian and gay rights, Indigenous rights, and workers' rights—all of which included health issues among their critical concerns (Rose & Rose, 1976a; Rose & Rose, 1976b; Arditti et al., 1980; Sanders, 1985; Jasanoff, 2004; Lefkowitz, 2007; Werskey, 2007). Questioning not only the application but the basic assumptions and theoretical orientation of mainstream science, these researchers called for creation of a "science for the people" (*Science for the People* magazine 1970–1989; Greeley & Tafler, 1980) to counter, intellectually and empirically, what they considered to be dehumanizing and destructive scientific priorities, ideas, and practices. Of particular concern were scientific activities that supported the "military–industrial complex," imperiled the planet, and, via the ideology and assumptions of biological determinism, "naturalized"—and hence justified or excused—social inequality, including social inequalities in health.

The gelling of the epidemiologic sociopolitical perspectives into the explicitly named *social production of disease* and *political economy of health* frameworks accordingly occurred in the 1970s, as progressive health researchers engaged in the radical critique of science extended their analysis to epidemiology. Not surprisingly, the early articles were not published in the mainstream epidemiologic literature but instead first appeared both in the "gray literature" and in non-epidemiologic journals that opened their pages to alternative perspectives (**Textbox 6–4**)— particularly the *International Journal of Health Services*, founded in 1971 by Dr. Vicente Navarro (Navarro, 1971), a leading Marxist analyst of medicine and health systems. Reflecting the impact of the Marxist frameworks of the time and especially the philosophical tenets of "dialectical historical materialism" (Rose & Rose, 1976a; Rose & Rose, 1976b; Arditti et al., 1980; Levins & Lewontin, 1985; Werskey, 2007), the initial epidemiologic forays in the English-language literature appeared under the rubric of "materialist epidemiology" (Gaynor & Eyer, 1976; Berliner, 1976) and "historical materialist epidemiology" (Schnall, 1977; Schnall & Kern, 1981).

Although it is beyond the scope of this chapter to delve into the complex and contested set of ideas called *dialectical historical materialism*, a small recap is warranted, given the salience of these concepts to the rise of the 1970s variants of sociopolitical epidemiologic theorizing. As encapsulated in *The Dialectical Biologist*, published in 1985 by two Harvard biologists, Richard Levins (b.1930) and Richard Lewontin (b.1929), and dedicated "To Frederick Engels, who got it wrong a lot of the time but who got it right where it counted" (Levins & Lewontin, 1985, p. v), several core dialectical principles exist, construed not as scientific laws but rather as "prior principles… analogous to Darwin's principles of variation, heritability, and section in that they create the terms of reference from which quantifications and predictions may be derived" (Levins & Lewontin, 1985, p. 268). Stated abstractly (Levins & Lewontin, 1985, pp. 273–274):

> The first principle of a dialectical view… is that the whole is a relation of heterogeneous parts that have no prior independent existence *as parts* (italics in original). The second principle, which flows from the first, is that, in general, the properties of the parts have no prior alienated existence

Textbox 6–4. "Political Economy of Health" and Its Application to Epidemiology: (a) Table of Contents of Two 1977 Publications Bringing Together a Critical Mass of Articles on the "Political Economy of Health", and (b) Excerpts From the First Book Titled *The Political Economy of Health*, Published in 1979 (Doyal, 1979)

(a) Table of Contents of Two 1977 Publications Bringing Together a Critical Mass of Articles on the "Political Economy of Health"

HMO Packets #2 (January 1977) and #3 (June 1977) on "historical materialist epidemiology," prepared by the Health Marxist Organization,* a "network for Marxist studies in health" (Schnall et al., 1977a; Schnall et al., 1977b)
The Social Etiology of Disease—Part I (Schnall et al., 1977a)
Table of Contents
Introduction by Evan Stark—pg. i

1. An introduction to Historical Materialist Epidemiology—Peter Schnall (p. 1)
2. Toward a historical materialist epidemiologic practice—Grace Ziem (p. 10)
3. Anxiety: the problem of change in capitalist society—Scotty Embree (p. 14)
4. Materialist epidemiology applied to occupational health and safety—David Gaynor (p. 23)
5. Toward a material epidemiology of dope—Don Goldmacher (p. 29)
6. Suicide—Kim Hopper and Sally Guttmacher (p. 32)
7. Notes toward a study of housewives' diseases—Carol Lopate (p. 57)
8. Economic and social causes of cancer—Peter Schnall (p. 61)
9. An analysis of coronary heart disease using historical materialist epidemiology—Peter Schnall (p. 73)
10. Hypertension—Hila Sherer (p. 83)
11. Accidents–towards a material analysis—Gel Stevenson (p. 91)
12. Society, "stress," and illness—Ingrid Waldron (p. 105)
13. Towards a historical materialist understanding of rheumatoid arthritis—Grace Ziem (p. 108)

Example of analysis

Schnall: "An introduction to historical materialist epidemiology" (Part I, pp. 1–9)
p. 2: "What differentiates materialist epidemiology from bourgeois social epidemiology is the attempt to relate the patterns of disease and illness in a society to the economic and social relations which are the determinants of the functioning of that society."
pp. 5–6: "Coronary heart disease is a disease of the 20th century...From whence arises this new disease? It is the combination of a series of technological developments combined with the new social relations surrounding the development of the mode of production that has come into existence. Cigarette smoking arose in the late 1890s with the development of the mass production of the cigarette. The cigarette was a unique product of capitalism; it involved a technology-intensive process which allowed a greater rate of exploitation. Its habituating properties ensured a continuing market; its improved storage allowed centralized production and less value loss during circulation... Technological developments of the late 19th and early 20th century make the food industry possible... all leading to supermarket sale of commodities and more consumption of lower quality food with decreased fiber content... The small grocery store which provides fresher produce and generally higher quality food is destroyed by the expansion of capital into the food industry..."

Gaynor: "Materialist epidemiology applied to occupational health and safety" (Part I, pp. 23–28)

The Social Etiology of Disease—Part II—Implications and Applications of HME (Schnall et al., 1977b)
Table of Contents
Introduction by Evan Stark—pg i

p. 23: "Occupational injury and disease statistics clearly indicate that these problems are of epidemic proportions. Among the 80 million workers in the United States, more than 14,000 deaths on the job are recorded annually, and about 2.2 million disabling injuries. Further, these estimates might be dramatically conservative figures. The actual numbers may run as high as 25,000 deaths and 20–25 million job-related injuries annually."

p. 25: "Peculiar to capitalist society is the central and largely autonomous process of capital accumulation... Given a society built on competition and the insecurity that develops as a result of competition, the following working conditions develop:

—Whenever workers demand safe working conditions, the employers charge that the expenses connected with safe working conditions would drive them out of business. That is, these costs would reduce profits to such an extent that the business can no longer accumulate enough capital to survive. With the threat of the loss of jobs, the workers' demands subside. Particularly now, in this period of economic crisis, occupational health and safety concerns have the lowest priority.

—In an economic system which not only accepts but maintains a high level of unemployment, there is always someone willing to take risks just to get work and there is always someone who is available to replace injured of (sic) killed workers. Historically, it has been cheaper for employers to absorb the costs of unsafe working conditions (turnover, Workers' Compensation, OSHA fines, etc.), than it is to provide safe working conditions."

p. 26: "Further we don't leave our work at the workplace. The boring mind-numbing routine of our jobs constitutes a high level of alienation..."

p. 27: "Until those who take the risk of job hazards can exercise control over their own working conditions, the possibility of truly healthy working conditions can never be realized."

The Review of Radical Political Economics (URPE), Spring 1977 (Flaherty et al., 1977)
Special issue: The Political Economy of Health
Table of Contents
Special Issue Editorial Collective (Evan Stark, Diane Flaherty, Sander Kelman, William Lazonick, Lee Price, Len Rodberg).
Introduction to the Special Issue on the Political Economy of Health (p. v)
Joseph Eyer and Peter Sterling
Stress-related mortality and social organization (p. 1)
Meredeth Turshen
The political ecology of disease (p. 45)
Vicente Navarro
Political power, the state, and their implications in medicine (p. 61)
Harry Cleaver
Malaria, the politics of public health, and the international crisis (p. 81)
Leonard Rodberg and Gelvin Stevenson
The health care industry in advance capitalism (p. 104)
Howard S. Berliner
Emerging ideologies in medicine (p. 116)
J. Warren Salmon
Monopoly capital and the reorganization of the health sector (p. 125)
Robert C. Hsu
The political economy of rural health care in China (p. 134)

Example of analysis
Eyer and Sterling: "Stress-related mortality and social organization" (pp. 1–44)
p. 2: "… a large component of adult physical pathology and death must be considered neither acts of God nor of our genes, but a measure of the misery caused by our present social and economic organization."
pp. 2–6: analysis of the "pathophysiology of stress," with emphasis on the "fight or flight" response to physical and psychological stress, the "acute and restorative changes" mediated by the autonomic and endocrine systems, and hypotheses regarding the impact of chronic stress on cardiovascular disease, diabetes, ulcers, immune system suppression, and cancer.
pp. 6–14: sources of stress mentioned in surveys: "family break-up, death of relatives, job insecurity and job changes, and migration" (p. 6) and distributions by age and income (in the United States)
pp. 14–16: "Cultural variation in stress," comparing "hunter-gatherers" and "agricultural societies."
pp. 16–34: "Sources of stress under capitalism": "The labor force: external controls"; "internal control of the work force," "capitalism and stress-related mortality," "rise of stress-related mortality with industrialization," "death rates and long economic-demographic cycles," "the impact of [economic] depression and recovery"
pp. 34–35: "How has medicine responded to these problems? So far, only superficial technical solutions…"
pp. 35–38: "New Directions": insufficient to rely on behavior modification or therapy; "the real problem clearly emerges: to initiate a successful community forming process which abolishes social hierarchy in the whole society and stops the capital accumulation process, with its attendant disruption and family structures aimed at socialization for high-pressure productivity…" (p. 37)

* **HMO** was an acronym deliberately chosen for its ironic humor, because "HMO" otherwise at the time referred to "health maintenance organization," a form of private-sector managed care being promoted in the United States in the early 1970s as an alternative to universal health care.

(b) Excerpts From the First Book Titled *The Political Economy of Health*, Written by Lesley Doyal (Doyal 1979).

pp. 24–25: "It is a commonplace of left wing rhetoric that 'capitalism causes disease,' but a generalized statement of this kind, uniformly applied to all ill health in all place and at all times has very little theoretical or political content... it is obviously important that we examine more concretely some of the ways in which the operation of a capitalist system creates contradictions between health and profit.

First, the physical processes of commodity production itself will affect health in a variety of ways. Clearly the imperatives of capital accumulation condition the nature of the labour process, and the need for shiftwork, de-skilling, overtime or the use of dangerous chemicals, will all be reflected in the health or ill-health of workers. They may suffer directly, either through industrial injuries and diseases, or in more diffuse ways with stress-related ill health, or psychosomatic problems. Yet commodity production also has more *indirect* (italics in the original) effects on health, and the physical effects of the production process extend beyond the workplace itself. Damage to the surrounding environment and pollution of various kinds are often the by-products of industrialized production..."

pp. 25–26: "But it is also characteristic of capitalist societies that everyone is not equally affected by these illness-producing processes. Class differences in morbidity and mortality are very pronounced. Working-class people die sooner, and generally suffer more ill health than do middle class people... The most obvious cause of class differences in morbidity and mortality will be the differential health risks of specific occupations... The distribution of ill health in capitalist societies broadly follows the distribution of income... In a capitalist society income is a major determinant of the standard of housing individuals and families can obtain, of where they live, of their diet, and of their ability to remain warm and well-clothed. All of these factors are significant for health... children of unskilled workers are likely to receive an inferior education and therefore go on to low paid and probably dangerous jobs themselves..."

p. 27: "It is, however, in underdeveloped countries that the extremes of ill health and premature death are to be found. Here, the major causes of death are not, as is often assumed, the endemic tropical diseases, but rather infectious diseases and malnutrition. These are not 'natural,' but arise in large part from the particular social and economic relationships characteristic of imperialism... Like urban and rural poverty, it (malnutrition) is often a direct result of the exploitative relationship between the metropolitan countries and the underdeveloped world, and the consequence uneven development and allocation of resources.

Ill health cannot, therefore, be attributed simply to capitalism in any crude sense. On the other hand, we cannot make sense of patterns of health and illness outside of the context of the mode of production in which they occur..."

p. 44: "As we have seen, patterns of health and illness are to a considerable extent determined by the existence of a particular mode of social and economic organization, and under capitalism there is often a contradiction between the pursuit of health and the pursuit of profits. Most attempts to control the social production of ill health would involved an unacceptable degree of interference with the process of capital accumulation, and, as a result, the emphasis in advanced capitalist societies has been on after-the-event curative medical intervention, rather than broadly-based preventive measures to conserve health."

p. 47: "The Social Production of Health and Illness"

"It has been suggested in Chapter one that the way health and illness are defined, as well as the material reality of disease and death, will vary according to the social and economic environment in which they occur. This is not to suggest that the physical and chemical laws governing disease mechanisms can simply be abandoned, but rather that they must be seen to operate within a social and economic context which is constantly changing. Thus, the historical development of the capitalist mode of production has had extremely far-reaching effects on health. On the one hand, the development of the productive forces on an unprecedented scale has meant that the standard of living of the entire population in developed capitalist countries has improved, with a consequent amelioration in standards of physical health. This same process however has simultaneously underdeveloped the health of many third world population. Moreover, new hazards to health have been created in the developed world by the large-scale economic, social and technological changes which were a necessary part of this development."

p. 295: "As we have already seen, bourgeois ideology offers two basic explanations of the generation of ill health. The first is that it is somehow 'natural,' resulting from a timeless set of biochemical processes which can rarely be interfered with, except after the event with curative medicine or, at best, with specific preventive measures such as vaccines... a second type of explanation–the 'life-style' approach–is becoming increasingly popular... Ironically, it is precisely the supposed achievement of widespread affluence in the developed countries which is said to be the problem..."

p. 296: "... It would be absurd to argue that individuals have *no* [italics in original] control over their lives—people make all kinds of real choices every day. What we do have to make clear however, is the nature of the social and economic context within which individual choices are made and the many limitations that are imposed on personal freedom. It is the detailed examination of how the power of capital structures the context in which personal choices are made that must lie at the heart of a marxist epidemiology. Only in this way can we make sense of the impact of living and working conditions, and pattern of social and economic relationships, on the health of individuals and groups, while at the same time creating the possibility of collective action to transform those conditions."

but are acquired by being parts of a particular whole... In the dialectical approach the "wholes" are not inherently balanced or harmonized, their identity is not fixed. They are the loci of internal opposing processes, and the outcome of these oppositions is balanced only temporarily...

A third dialectical principle... is that that the interpenetration of parts and wholes is a consequence of the interchangeability of the subject and object, of cause and effect... Organisms are both the subjects and objects of evolution. They both make and are made by the environment and thus are actors in their own evolutionary history.

As readily acknowledged by Levins and Lewontin, these principles—requiring thinking about history and about both variability and interactions (including conflict) within and across levels—had been "ignored and suppressed for political reasons, in no small part because of the tyrannical application of a mechanical and sterile Stalinist diamat," resulting in the term *dialectical* having "only negative connotations for most serious intellectuals, even those of the left" (Levins & Lewontin, 1985, p. vii).

By the late 1970s and early 1980s, the analytic work of this new round of social epidemiologic theorizing, moving away from the relatively abstruse terminology of *dialectical historical materialism*, coalesced into the more accessible self-designated frameworks of *social production of disease* and *political economy of health* (Doyal, 1979; Conrad & Kern, 1981; Tesh, 1988; Navarro, 1986a; Krieger, 2001a). In 1979, the first English-language book to be titled *The Political Economy of Health* was published, written by Lesley Doyal, which analyzed both "the social production of health and illness" and the "social production of medical care" in light of the routine functioning of capitalism and imperialism (Doyal, 1979) (*see* excerpts in **Textbox 6–4**). Although predominantly concerned with how capitalist political-economic systems' imperative to maximize profit harms health—especially that of people who are exploited and oppressed—the theory's intent was "to reinstate collective exploitation, alienation and struggle at the heart of the radical analysis of disease" (Stark, 1977, p. ii), whether in relation to capitalist or then extant "really existing" socialist and communist societies (Stark, 1977; Doyal, 1979). In other words, despite having been developed through a critique of the impact of capitalism and imperialism on people's health, the theory was meant to be applied to *any* society, no matter what it (or others) called its political-economic system. The larger claim was that understanding the population patterning of health requires analyzing who gains and who loses from the status quo and its structural inequities. A corollary was that active movements for social change, premised on principles of social justice, are key for advancing health equity.

Attesting to the global reach of these sociopolitical analyses of population health, not only in epidemiology but also public health and medicine more broadly (Navarro, 1971; Flaherty, 1977; Navarro, 1986a; Navarro, 1986b; Tesh, 1988; Birn et al., 2009), in 1978 they infused the Declaration of Alma-Ata, issued at the World Health Organization's landmark "International Conference on Primary Health Care" (Declaration of Alma-Ata, 1978). Offered "in the spirit of social justice" (Article V), the Declaration:

- in Article I, affirmed that "health, which is a state of complete physical, mental and social wellbeing, and not merely the absence of disease or infirmity, is a fundamental human right and that the attainment of the highest possible level of health is a most important world-wide social goal whose realization requires the action of many other social and economic sectors in addition to the health sector";
- in Article II, stated that "The existing gross inequality in the health status of the people particularly between developed and developing countries as well as within countries is politically, socially and economically unacceptable and is, therefore, of common concern to all countries"; and
- in Article X, concluded that : "An acceptable level of health for all the people of the world by the year 2000 can be attained through a fuller and better use of the world's resources, a considerable part of which is now spent on armaments and military conflicts. A genuine policy of independence, peace, détente and disarmament could and should release additional resources that could well be devoted to peaceful aims and in particular to the acceleration of social and economic development of which primary health care, as an essential part, should be allotted its proper share."

Explicitly underscoring the profound relationship between political and economic priorities with the status of population health, within and across countries, the Declaration offered hope that changing priorities would enable new possibilities for improving population health and mitigating health inequities. Undercutting its impact, however, the report was issued just 2 years before the 1980s advent of neoliberal policy regimes, which favored unfettered and deregulated free markets over state interventions to promote social, economic, and health equity (Birn et al., 2009; Stiglitz, 2009).

Etiologic Hypotheses and Empirical Investigation. Since the mid-1970s, epidemiologists have employed the theories of *social production of disease* and *political economy of health* in the English-language literature in the same way they have used other theories of disease distribution: to frame and interpret previously published data, to generate and guide the testing of new hypotheses, and to produce evidence relevant to improving the public's health, albeit with the added priority of reducing social inequalities in health. Typically, the focus has been on health inequities—that is, unfair, unjust, and ostensibly avoidable social inequalities in health (Dahlgren & Whitehead, 1993; Krieger, 2001b; Krieger, 2005; Braveman, 2006)—both within and across countries (Eyer & Sterling, 1977; Black et al., 1980; Turshen, 1984; Sanders, 1985; Packard, 1989; Townsend et al., 1990; Krieger et al., 1993; Amick et al., 1995; Krieger, 1999; Leon & Walt, 2001; Navarro, 2002; Davey Smith, 2003; Hofrichter, 2003; Krieger, 2004; Levy & Sidel, 2006; Schulz et al., 2006; Kunitz, 2007; Kawachi & Wamala, 2007; Graham, 2007; Birn et al., 2009).

To give but one example, the 1977 article by Joseph Eyer and Peter Sterling, on "Stress-Related Mortality and Social Organization," included in one of the earliest collection of papers on the *political economy of health* (**Textbox 6–4**), explicitly used this theory to guide their review of—and conceptually connect—evidence on the pathophysiology of chronic stress and the social epidemiology of what they deemed stress-related diseases. The causal link, they argued, involved specific "sources of stress under capitalism" (Eyer & Sterling, 1977, p. 16), which they characterized as "intensified, conflicted work and the destruction of cooperative, supportive forms of social community" (Eyer & Sterling, 1977, p. 1) Emblematic of their theoretical perspective, Eyer and Sterling's article further posited that social change tackling the systemic material and social conditions and inequities routinely produced by a capitalist economy, not just individual behavior modification or therapy, would be needed to improve population health overall as well as prevent social inequalities in health.

Recognition of the need to change relations between societal groups, and not just focus on remedial efforts to assuage the afflicted, is likewise evident in Peter Townsend's (1928–2009) classic 1986 article "Why Are the Many Poor?" (Townsend, 1986). Published 6 years after he co-authored the monumental and highly influential U.K. 1980 Black Report on *Inequalities in Health: A Report of a Research Working Group* (Black et al., 1980; Berridge & Blume, 2002), Townsend's essay deliberately resurrected the century-old Fabian argument that the problem is not just that there are more poor than rich but, rather, that the many are poor because the few are rich. In other words, economic immiseration of the many is the inevitable and unsurprising product of a political-economic system geared toward enriching the few, via their power over property, labor, and wages. Thus, to reduce health inequities, Townsend argued, based on a political economy of health perspective, "the only long-term remedy is to restrict the power and wealth of the rich, to dismantle the present structures of social privilege, and to build social institutions based on fair allocation of wealth and on social equality" (Townsend, 1986, p. 1). Attesting to this theory's continued salience, a 2009 textbook on international health likewise integrated discussion across three chapters regarding "the political economy of health and development," "epidemiologic profiles of global health and disease," and "societal determinants of health and social inequalities in health" (Birn et al., 2009).

Empirically, epidemiologic research based on the *social production of disease* and *political economy of health* theories has addressed a broad range of issues and hypotheses linking economic and political conditions to population health. Examples include research on the health impacts of: rising income inequality; structural adjustment programs imposed by the International Monetary Fund and the World Bank; neoliberal economic policies favoring dismantling of the welfare state; free-trade agreements imposed by the World Trade Organization; the collapse of the Soviet Union and related states in Eastern Europe; and the recent rise of more progressive governments in several Latin American countries (*see*, e.g., Lurie et al., 1995; Biljmakers et al., 1996; Wise et al., 1999; Leon & Walt, 2001; Franco-Giraldo et al., 2006; Moore et al., 2006; Oliver, 2006; Kunitz, 2007; Kawachi & Wamala, 2007; Navarro, 2007; Krieger et al., 2008a; Blakely et al., 2008; Beckfield & Krieger, 2009; Birn et al., 2009; Briggs & Mantini-Briggs, 2009; Armada et al., 2009).

Also addressed are social inequalities involving race/ethnicity, gender, and sexuality, as they play out within and across socioeconomic position, within and across diverse societies (Fee & Krieger, 1994; Doyal, 1995; Ruzek et al., 1997; LaVeist, 2002; Hofrichter, 2003; Krieger, 2004; Schulz et al., 2006; Meyer & Northridge, 2007; Birn et al., 2009). Relevant questions include asking what are the health consequences of: (*1*) experiencing economic and noneconomic forms of racial discrimination? (Krieger, 1990; Krieger et al., 1993; Krieger & Sidney, 1996; Krieger, 1999; Williams, 1999; Williams et al., 2003; Paradies, 2006; Mays et al., 2007; Williams & Mohammed, 2009); (*2*) men dominating and abusing women? (Stark & Flitcraft, 1995; Garcia-Moreno, 2000; Watts & Zimmerman, 2002; Campbell et al., 2003; Russo & Pirlott, 2006; Ellsberg et al., 2008; Krieger et al., 2008b); (*3*) discrimination and violence directed against LGBT people? (Meyer, 1995; Krieger & Sidney, 1997; Diaz et al., 2001; Mays & Cochran, 2001; Warner et al., 2004; Huebner et al., 2004; Huebner & Davis, 2007; Chae et al., 2010); and (*4*) historical trauma resulting from colonization, dispossession, resettlement, and cultural disruption imposed on Indigenous peoples? (Walters & Simoni, 2002; Walters et al., 2002; Whitbeck, 2004; Duran & Walters, 2004; Ferriera & Lang, 2006; Carson et al., 2007; Evans-Cambell, 2008; Kearns et al., 2009; Cunningham, 2009). Recently emerging environmental justice movements likewise have brought critical attention to corporate decisions and government complicity in transferring toxic waste to poor countries and to poor regions within wealthy countries—especially poor communities of color (Sexton et al., 1993; Committee on Environmental Justice, 1999; Malcoe et al., 2002; London, 2003; Morello-Frosch & Lopez, 2006; Maantay, 2007; Norton et al., 2007; Wing et al., 2008; Birn et al., 2009).

The call for action premised on this framework is thus, at the reform level, for "healthy public policies"—especially redistributive polices to reduce poverty and income inequality (Shaw et al., 1999; Whitehead et al., 1998; Dahlgren & Whitehead, 2006; WHO CSHD, 2008). More deeply, however, this school of thought holds that removing the structural political and economic barriers that hinder development of such policies requires engaging with, in the words of Doyal, "wider campaigns for sustainable development, political freedom, and economic and social justice" (Doyal 1995, p. 232).

Late Twentieth and Early Twenty-First Century De-Politicizing and Re-Politicizing of the Social Production of Disease/Political Economy of Health. A related body of important late twentieth and early twenty-first century epidemiologic theorizing and research has employed a subset of the core ideas included in the *social production of disease* and *political economy of health* frameworks. Although also raising serious concerns about distributions of power and resources, they nevertheless differ in their analysis of who loses—and who gains—from the status quo.

Among these subsidiary conceptual approaches, the two most widely referred to are:

1. the *social determinants of health* (Wilkinson & Marmot, 1998; Marmot & Wilkinson, 1999; Raphael, 2004; WHO Commission on the Social Determinants of Health [CSDH], 2008), a term apparently used as early as the mid-1970s (National Conference on Preventive Medicine, 1976) but not popularized—as a phrase or perspective—until the late 1990s, following the WHO's adoption of the phrase (Wilkinson & Marmot, 1998); and
2. *population health,* a term and perspective introduced in 1989 by the Canadian Institute for Advanced Research (CIFAR) (Evans & Stoddart, 1990) to guide resource allocation and policy development "to maximize overall health outcomes and minimize health inequities at the population level" (Kindig, 2007, p. 158) and which, by the mid 1990s, had gained considerable traction (Evans & Stoddart, 1990; Evans et al., 1994; Labonte, 1995; Frank, 1995; Kindig, 1997a; Kindig, 1997b; Young, 1998; Kawachi et al., 1999; Kindig & Stoddard, 2003; Szreter, 2003; Frolich et al., 2004; Heller, 2005; Labonte 2005; Etches et al., 2006), even as it also generated some controversy with regard to how it differed—or not—from existing conceptions of public health and determinants of disease distribution (Labonte, 1995; Frank, 1995).

Attesting to their global salience, these two frameworks—and phrases—feature prominently in the WHO's landmark 2008 report *Closing the Gap in a Generation: Health Equity Through Action on the Social Determinants of Health,* issued by the first-ever WHO Commission on the Social Determinants of Health (CSDH) (WHO CSDH, 2008).

A third related perspective is termed the *fundamental causes* thesis and was introduced into the U.S. social epidemiologic literature in the mid-1990s (Link & Phelan, 1995; Link & Phelan, 1996; Phelan et al., 2004; Phelan & Link, 2005; Ward, 2007; Link et al., 2008). Its name is derived from the sociological concept of *fundamental cause,* as articulated in 1985 by the U.S. sociologist Stanley Lieberson (b. 1933), to distinguish between what he termed *fundamental* or *basic* causes, arising from *fundamental* social processes (e.g., *de jure* and *de facto* racial discrimination), in contrast to the myriad specific *superficial causes* they caused and which, in turn, causally precipitated particular events (e.g., race riots) (Lieberson & Silverman, 1961; Lieberson, 1985). A central claim is that focusing only on *superficial causes* (e.g., in the case of epidemiology, *risk factors*) without addressing their underlying *fundamental causes* (e.g., social determinants) will lead to ineffective efforts to change conditions, as the fundamental causes, left intact, will continue to generate the myriad specific superficial causes (Link & Phelan, 1995; Link & Phelan, 1996; Phelan et al., 2004; Phelan & Link, 2005; Ward, 2007; Link et al., 2008).

In accord with aspects of the *social production of disease* thesis, all three of these perspectives posit that people's ability to live healthy lives is shaped by their socioeconomic position, race/ethnicity, and gender, in conjunction with the social and physical quality of their neighborhoods, schools, transportation, and workplaces and their access to affordable healthy food and affordable appropriate medical care. All three likewise emphasize what they deem to be the ubiquity of fine-grained socioeconomic gradients in health, which are postulated to reflect people's social standing in their society's "social hierarchy" and attendant resources (Link & Phelan, 1995; Wilkinson, 2001; Phelan et al., 2004; Marmot, 2004; Wilkinson, 2005; MacArthur Network, 2007; Adler & Rehkopf, 2008). Depicting this hierarchy metaphorically as a "ladder" (**Figure 6–3**) (Adler et al., 2000; Singh-Manoux et al., 2003; MacArthur Network, 2007; Ghaed & Gallo, 2007; Adler & Rehkopf, 2008), work within this perspective typically emphasizes the existence of ranked hierarchies (e.g., based on what is termed *dominance* or *status*) among not only people but also in various non-human primate species (Wilkinson, 2001; Marmot, 2004; Sapolsky, 2004; Wilkinson, 2005; Wilkinson & Pickett, 2009).

Despite their similarities, however, these three variants do have some noteworthy differences—both from *social production of disease* and *political economy of health* perspectives as well as with each other. For example, both the *social determinants of health* and *population health* perspectives, drawing upon the previously mentioned "developmental origins of disease and health" (DOHaD) framework, strongly emphasize the biological

a

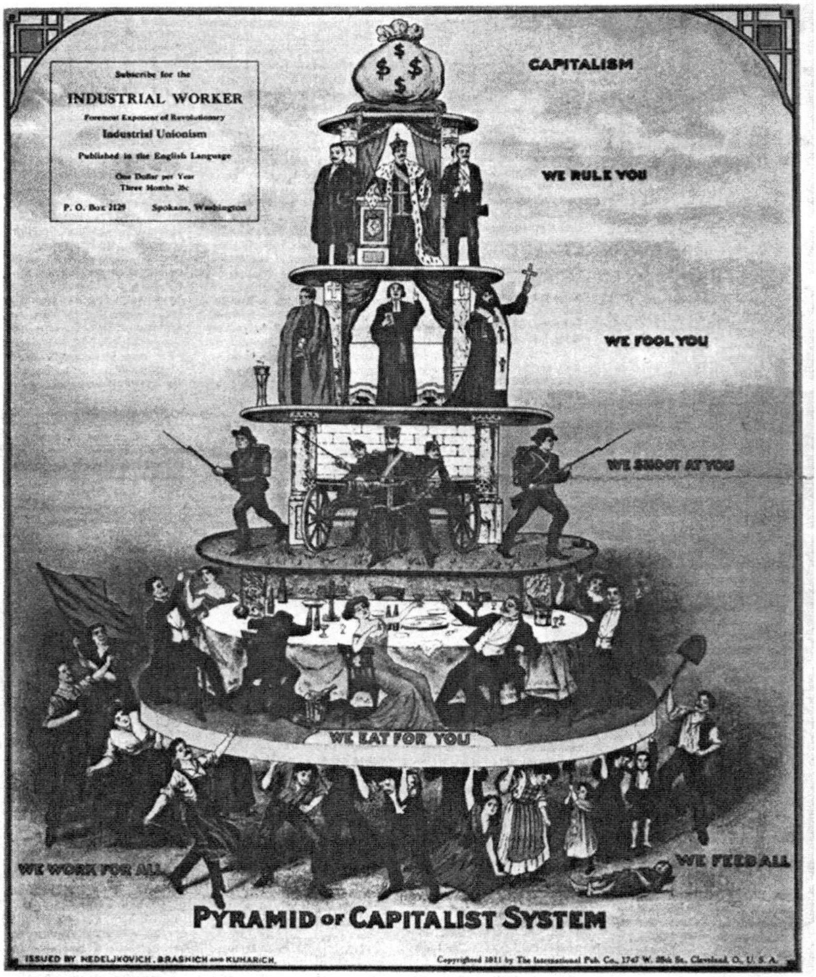

Figure 6–3. Contrasting depictions of societal structure, with and without political-economic relationships and conflict:

Figure 6–3a. Pyramid of capitalist system. Issued by Nedeljkovich, Brashick and Kuharich, for the International Workers of the World (IWW), 1913.

b   1a. Imagine that this ladder pictures
    how American society is set up.

    ♦   At the top of the ladder are the
        people who are the best off--they
        have the most money, the highest
        amount of schooling, and the jobs
        that bring the most respect.

    ♦   At the bottom are people who are the
        worst off--they have the least money,
        little or no education, no job or jobs
        that no one wants or respects.

    Now think about your family. Please
    tell us where you think your family
    would be on this ladder. Fill in the
    circle that best represents where your
    family would be on this ladder.

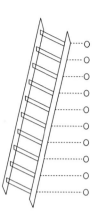

1b. Now assume that the ladder is a way
of picturing your school.

    ♦   At the top of the ladder are the
        people in your school with the most
        respect, the highest grades, and the
        hughest standing.

    ♦   At the bottom are the people who no
        one respects, no one wants to hang
        around with, and have the worst
        grades.

    Where would you place yourself on this
    ladder? Fill in the circle that best
    represents where you would be on this
    ladder.

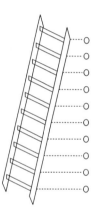

Figure 6–3b. "Society-as-a-ladder," per The MacArthur Scale of Subjective Social Status TK
(Goodman et al., 2001).

salience of early life conditions for both childhood and adult health and the biological
mechanisms by which these conditions exert these effects. This attention to biological
mechanisms notably distinguishes them from the less biologically oriented *social production of disease* and *political economy of health* theories. However, in contrast to the
DOHaD's focus on primarily the prenatal milieu in relation to people's—especially maternal—"lifestyles," the *social determinants* and *population health* approaches emphasize
both the broader societal context in which people have children and conceive fetuses and
also call attention to the roster of social conditions across the entire life-course, including
after one is born—that is, from post-natal early childhood development on up through
various phases of adulthood (Evans et al., 1994; Frank, 1995; Young, 1998; Wilkinson &
Marmot, 1998; Evans & Stoddardt, 2003; WHO CSDH, 2008; Marmot & Bell, 2009).
They thus are in accord with the burgeoning literature on socially oriented "life-course"
epidemiology, fast-growing since the late 1990s (Kuh & Davey Smith, 1997; Power &
Hertzman, 1997; Wadsworth, 1997; Hertzman, 1999; Ben-Shlomo & Kuh, 2002;
National Research Council and Institute of Medicine, 2002; Wise, 2003; Kuh et al., 2003;

Lynch & Davey Smith, 2005; Furumoto-Dawson et al., 2007; Blane et al., 2007), which is concerned with how social context can affect not only fetal programming but also the differential accumulation of exposures and health risks as linked to people's social trajectory over time.

A biological orientation likewise distinguishes the *social determinants of health* and *population health* perspectives from the more sociological *fundamental cause* thesis, which deliberately downplays the significance of specific exposures and specific diseases for explaining population patterns of health (Link & Phelan, 1995; Link & Phelan, 1996; Phelan et al., 2004; Phelan & Link, 2005; Ward, 2007; Link et al., 2008). Deeming specific risk factors to be in the category of *superficial causes*, it instead emphasizes, as fundamental causes, what are termed *flexible resources*, which are defined "broadly to include money, knowledge, power, prestige, and the kinds of interpersonal resources embodied in the concepts of social support and social networks" (Link & Phelan, 1995, p. 87). These types of fundamental causes are, in turn, posited to affect "access to resources that can be used to avoid risks or to minimize the consequences of disease once it occurs" (Link & Phelan, 1995, p. 87), thereby enabling persons with the most resources to avoid or mitigate illness (Phelan et al., 2004). Justifying the nonspecific etiologic orientation is the claim that "the persistence of the association" between "socioeconomic status" and health "over time and its generality across very different places suggests that no fixed set of intervening risk and protective factors can account for the connection" (Link et al., 2008, p. 72). Consequently, concerns about biological mechanisms—and also the question of why different diseases are more or less prevalent at a given point in time or over time, within and across countries—are outside of the purview of the *fundamental cause* explanatory schema.

Their different interest in biological mechanisms notwithstanding, these three subsidiary perspectives nevertheless are united by a core difference that demarcates them from the *social production of disease* and *political economy of health* theories: all three accord relatively little attention to the underlying political-economic systems and their varied structures, priorities, and conflicts that give rise to the material and social circumstances relabeled as "social determinants of health" (Poland et al., 1998; Raphael & Bryant, 2002; Coburn et al., 2003; Navarro & Muntaner, 2004; Labonte et al., 2005; Regidor, 2006; Graham, 2007; Schofield, 2007; Krieger, 2008b; Navarro, 2009; Birn et al., 2009; Birn, 2009). Of concern are the health consequences of, say, low income—but not why low income exists. The focus instead is chiefly on consumption and its relationship to people's relative social standing (a.k.a. "the ladder"), with little or no consideration of production— that is, who is producing, literally, what goods and services, for whom, for what reason, and at what cost to whom, not only monetarily but also in terms of impact on population and ecologic health.

Consequently, the arguments and evidence marshaled by these alternative frameworks to reduce or eliminate health inequities by improving social conditions and reducing social inequality (Link et al., 2008; WHO CSDH, 2008; Marmot & Bell, 2009; Woolf, 2009; Wilkinson & Pickett, 2009) typically do not embrace explicit political and economic analysis of whose interests are served by extant inequities (Navarro, 2009; Birn et al., 2009; Birn, 2009). Nor do they call attention to the considerable effort those benefiting from the status quo exert to ensure they continue to accrue their benefits and hold onto their wealth and privilege (Flaherty et al., 1977; Doyal, 1979; Hobsbawm, 1994; Grusky, 2001; Zinn, 2003; Anderson, 2003; Navarro & Muntaner, 2004; Levy & Sidel, 2006; Hobsbawm, 2008; Navarro, 2009; Birn et al., 2009). Profound sociopolitical obstacles to social change are thus unaddressed. Instead, the argument is framed: more equality is better for everyone (Marmot, 2004; Wilkinson, 2005; Wilkinson & Pickett, 2009).

Political Epidemiology and Societal Determinants of Health: Twenty-First Century Efforts to Repoliticize the Dominant Social Epidemiologic Frameworks. In response, seeking to bring back in the types of critical concerns central to a *political economy of health* framework, toward the end of the first decade of the twenty-first century, several epidemiologists have begun to call for supplementing social epidemiology with *political epidemiology* (Gil-González et al., 2006; Clarke et al., 2007; Gil-González et al., 2009). This latter term dates back in the English-language literature to at least 1981 (Brownlea, 1981) and refers to epidemiologic analyses of how population health is shaped by political systems and their economic priorities and conflicts. Types of political entities considered include capitalist countries, with their many varieties of welfare states and diverse histories as being colonizers versus colonized, and also currently or previously socialist and communist countries (Navarro & Shi, 2001; Navarro et al., 2003; Navarro et al., 2006; Gil-González et al., 2006; Clarke et al., 2007; Bambra et al., 2007; Eikemo & Bambra, 2008; Esplet et al., 2008; Gil-González et al., 2009). Empirically translating these ideas into testable hypotheses, a small but fast-growing body of work is investigating whether political-economic systems, priorities, and policies produce differentials in national and regional on-average health status—including overall mortality rates and life expectancy, disease-specific morbidity and mortality rates, and self-rated health—and also, within and across countries and regions, in the magnitude of health inequities (for a review, *see* Beckfield & Krieger, 2009).

Similarly, to counter the increasing tendency of epidemiologic research on the *social determinants of health* to focus solely on individuals' resources and to neglect societal-level conflictual political-structural determinants of health inequities, a new wave of public health scholars and some epidemiologists have begun to employ the more expansive term *societal determinants of health* to ensure that structural determinants, and not only social position, are addressed (Krieger et al., 2003; Raphael, 2003; Krieger, 2005; Starfield, 2007; Krieger, 2007; Krieger et al., 2008a; Krieger, 2008b; Krieger, 2009; Birn et al., 2009, p. 310; Birn, 2009; Krieger et al., 2010). The difference, broadly stated (Krieger et al., 2010), is between approaches that:

1. view *social determinants of health* as arising from a "social environment," structured by government policies and status hierarchies, with social inequalities in health resulting from diverse groups being differentially exposed to factors that influence health—hence, *social determinants* act as the *causes of causes* (WHO CSDH, 2008) versus

2. posit *societal determinants of health* as political-economic systems, whereby health inequities result from the promotion of the political and economic interests of those with power and privilege (within and across countries) against the rest, and whose wealth and better health is gained at the expense of those whom they subject to adverse living and working conditions; *societal determinants* thus become the *causes of causes of causes* (Birn, 2009).

The contrasts between these perspectives involve, at one level, differences in political analysis and, at another, theoretical understandings of societal structure. Related efforts distinguish, as I have argued in my analysis of the iconography of health inequities (Krieger, 2008b), between models of *determinants of health* versus *determinants of health inequities* (*see* **Figure 6–4**).

Suggesting these contrasts between critical versus depoliticized versions of sociopolitical epidemiologic theories of disease distribution will intensify are growing twenty-first

(a)

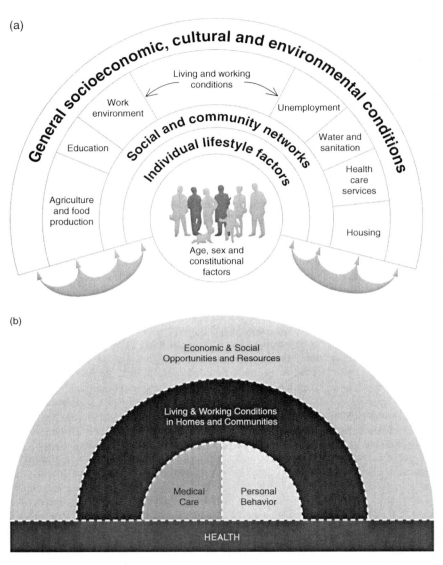

(b)

Figure 6–4. Contrasting models of "determinants of health" (Fig 6–4a. and 6–4b) versus "determinants of health inequity" (Fig 6–4c. and Fig 6–4d.).
Figure 6–4a. Dahlgren & Whitehead (1993)
Figure 6–4b. Robert Wood Johnson Foundation (2008) (Copyright 2008. Robert Wood Johnson Foundation Commission to Build a Healthier America. Used with permission from the Robert Wood Johnson Foundation).

(c)

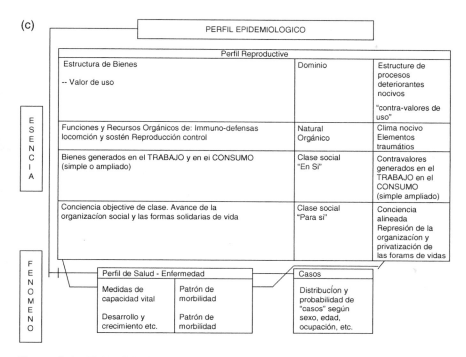

Figure 6–4c. Epidemiologic profile (Breilh, 1979, p. 217)

century critical discussions of and debates over the contemporary global political economy (Hobsbawm, 2008). In the early years of the twenty-first century, for example, the tenets of the dominant late twentieth century neoliberal policies, with their emphasis on deregulated free markets, have increasingly come under question, including by public health analysts (Navarro et al., 2006; Birn et al., 2009; Catalano, 2009). The near collapse of the U.S. banking industry in the fall of 2008 and the global economic recession it triggered, for example, both re-opened and, at least for a short while, intensified new and old questions about the relationship between public well-being and different political-economic variants of capitalism—and also what potential twenty-first century alternatives might exist (United Nations, 2009; Krugman, 2009; Stiglitz, 2009; Sen, 2009; Wainright, 2009). If the past is any guide, it is reasonable to conjecture that epidemiologic theorizing about societal and social determinants of health will be influenced by these new rounds of political and economic debate and continued changes in global, regional, and local economies.

Latin American Social Medicine/Collective Health. Further auguring the continued presence of structural critique in twenty-first century epidemiologic theorizing about political and economic determinants of societal patterns of disease and health is the growing influence of the varied perspectives termed *Latin American Social Medicine* and also, in Brazil, *collective health* (Waitzkin, 1981; Viniegra, 1985; Breilh, 1988 [1979]; Krieger, 1988; Laurell, 1989; Castellanos, 1990; Franco et al., 1991; Krieger, 1994; Morgan, 1998; Paim & Almeida-Filho, 1998; Almeida-Filho, 2000; Waitzkin et al., 2001a; Waitzkin et al., 2001b; Iriart et al., 2002; Krieger, 2003; Tajer, 2003; Laurell, 2003; Franco, 2003; Almeida-Filho et al., 2003; Eldredge et al., 2004; Solar & Irwin, 2006; Granda, 2008; Krieger et al., 2010).

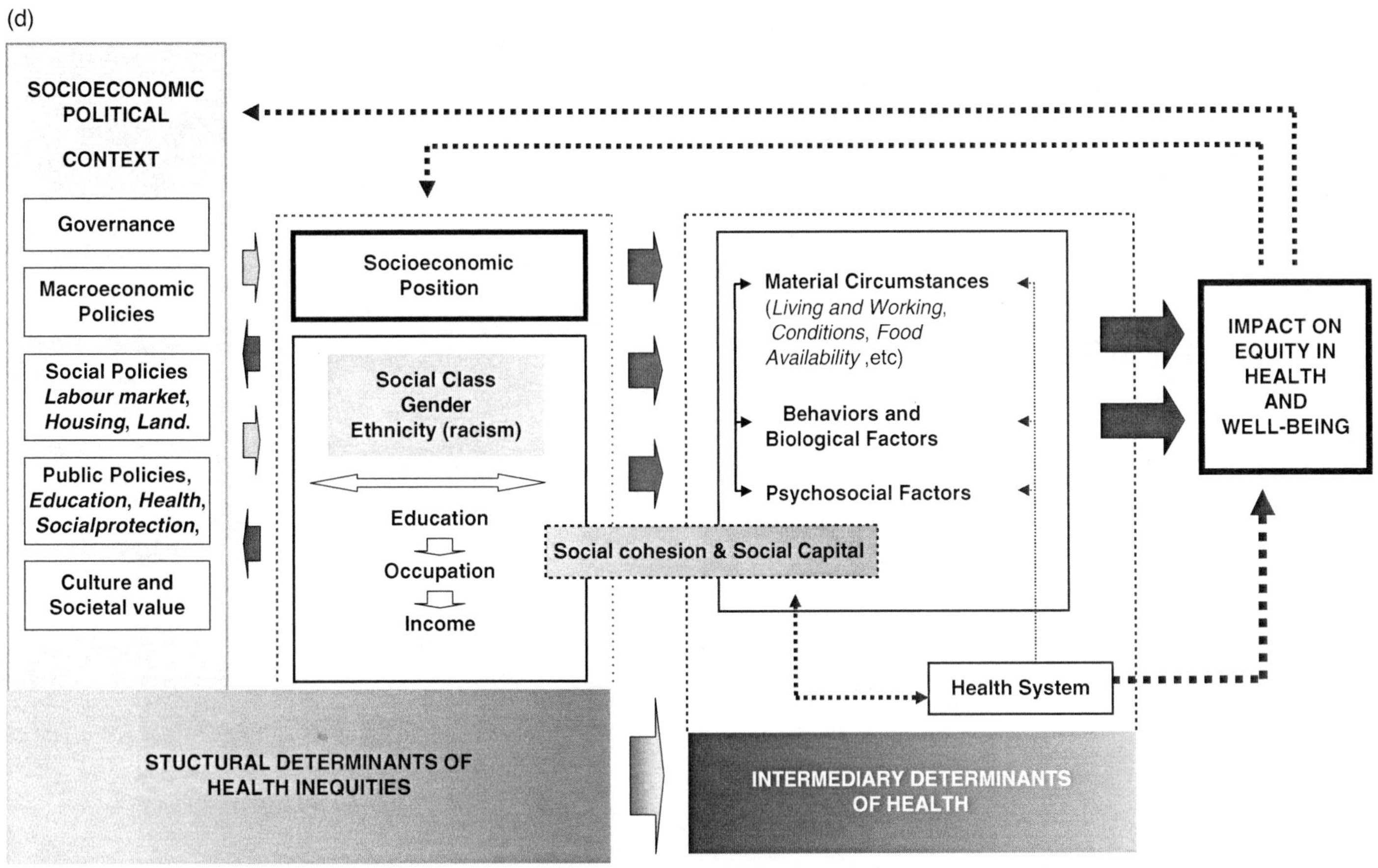

Figure 6-4d. The WHO Commission on the Social Determinants of Health (2007).

Akin to the *social production of disease/political economy of health* frameworks, these distinctive Latin American epidemiologic theories, like their North American and European counterparts, arose in the 1970s from kindred upswellings of popular and student movements in the 1960s, as informed by then prevalent Marxist intellectual traditions in the universities and their opposition to a succession of military regimes (Franco et al., 1991; Tajer, 2003; Laurell, 2003; Granda, 2008). Since 1984, with the founding of the Latin American Social Medicine Association (i.e., Asociación Latinoamericana de Medicina Social [ALAMES]), these frameworks have become increasingly visible as an explicit presence in Latin American epidemiologic theorizing, research, and pedagogy (XIV Conference, 1988; Franco et al., 1991; Granda, 2008).

Similarly grounded in an historical-structural analytic orientation, and likewise tracing their roots back to the nineteenth century ideas of Virchow and Engels and the early-to-mid twentieth century ideas of *social medicine*, including those advanced by Chilean physician-politician (and ultimately president) Salvador Allende (1908–1973) (Waitzkin, 1981; Birn et al., 2009), these Latin American schools of thought nevertheless have differed in several ways from their English-language analogs. Reflecting in part their different sociopolitical contexts, theoretical work from the *Latin American social medicine* framework has devoted more attention to the impact of capitalist development, imperialism, and politics on health; it likewise has more extensively critiqued the positivism and structural functionalism of dominant biomedical theories and has more strongly emphasized the importance of analyzing what was initially termed the *health–illness process*, and then later the *health–illness–care process*, as opposed to concentrating on static "outcomes" (Breilh, 1988 [1979]; Breilh & Granda, 1989; Laurell, 1989; Franco et al., 1991; Tajer, 2003; Granda, 2008). Moreover, given limits on the kinds of state-led public health action that could be expected and realized in the context of repressive governments whose regressive priorities were inimical to public health (in contrast to the greater possibilities for public health agencies and public sector action in "western democracies") (Almeida-Filho, 2000; Tajer, 2003; Granda, 2008; Birn et al., 2009), work within these frameworks has emphasized the critical importance of collective action by non-state actors—that is, *collectivities* and *social subjects*, such as social classes and popular movements—to shape and improve population health and health equity. More recent work has increasingly theorized and examined how diverse types of inequitable social relationships (e.g., involving gender, sexual, and racial inequality) act in concert with class relations to affect health (Almeida-Filho, 2000; Costa et al., 2000; Tajer, 2003; Granda, 2008).

Deeming social participation as essential for developing the knowledge and means to transform epidemiologic profiles, the epidemiologists engaged in developing these Latin American frameworks thus have conceived of both themselves and their frameworks as part of already existing and engaged social movements. In the words of one of the founders of ALAMES, Edmundo Granda (1946–2008), the point of epidemiologic and other health-related theorizing, research, policy, and action is to contribute to establishing a "**transformative political program that fights for the right to health, built with the support of different viewpoints and via consensual methods**" (bold in the original), one that conceptualizes "the fight for health as a *right* through the commitment and *empowerment* of the people" (italics in the original) (Granda, 2008).

To date, engagement between the social epidemiologic theories of Latin America and the global North has been hindered by the relative neglect of Latin American theorizing in the English-language epidemiologic literature. This situation is itself emblematic of the differentials in power, affecting both the production and dissemination of scientific knowledge, that these theories address (Waitzkin, 1981; Krieger, 1988; Franco et al., 1991; Waitzkin et al., 2001a; Waitzkin et al.,2001b; Iriart et al., 2002; Krieger, 2003;

Eldredge et al., 2004; Birn et al., 2009; Krieger et al., 2010). To address this problem, Latin and North American health professionals, including epidemiologists, have recently begun new collaborative initiatives, such as the "Latin American Social Medicine" database, which uses "Spanish, Portuguese, and English language trilingual structured abstracts to summarize classic and contemporary works" (Eldredge et al., 2004; Latin American Social Medicine, 2009). A similar effort, the "Virtual Health Library," implemented in 1998 by the Pan American Health Organization (Almeida-Filho et al., 2003; Bireme/PAHO/WHO, 2009), seeks to "to expand and strengthen the flow of scientific and technical information on health across Latin America and the Caribbean" (Bireme/PAHO/WHO, 2009).

Adding to the likely growing impact of Latin American theoretical and empirical epidemiologic literature are two additional trends. The first is rapidly rising interest in "global health" and "globalization" (Beaglehole, 2003; Kawachi & Wamala, 2007; Birn et al., 2009), potentially opening up new possibilities for more critical and equitable international scientific exchange. The second is changing Latin American economic and political circumstances, whereby the expanding number of newly elected twenty-first century center-left governments (Burns & Charlip, 2007; Barrett et al., 2009), including such emerging economic powers such as Brazil, are variously engaged in implementing policies and health practices based on the ideas of Latin American social medicine and collective health (Granda, 2008; Cohen, 2008; Alvarado et al., 2008; Borgia et al., 2008; Romero et al., 2008; Laurell, 2008; Briggs & Mantini-Briggs, 2009; Armada et al., 2009; Birn et al., 2009). A likely consequence is that Latin American theories will increasingly influence twenty-first century global epidemiologic theorizing and research.

Health and Human Rights. One additional framework, only just beginning to enter the social epidemiologic literature, is that of *"health and human rights,"* a field founded in the late twentieth century (Mann et al., 1994; Mann et al., 1999; Gruskin & Tarantola, 2001; Krieger & Gruskin, 2001; Gruskin et al., 2005; Gruskin et al., 2007; Beyrer & Pizer, 2007; Mullany et al., 2007; Birn et al., 2009). I mention it for two reasons: (*1*) its profoundly different basis, compared to the other sociopolitical epidemiologic theories, for theorizing links between individuals, societal structure, and population health and (*2*) its implications for not only government policies but also the work of epidemiologists employed by governmental agencies. In brief, human rights, as articulated in the "Universal Declaration of Human Rights" (UDHR) issued by the United Nations in 1948 in the aftermath of World War II, and with aspects subsequently codified in international human rights law (Mann et al., 1994; Mann et al., 1999; Gruskin & Tarantola, 2001; Glendon, 2001; Anderson, 2003; Gruskin et al., 2005; Gruskin et al., 2007), refer to a range of social, political, civil, economic, and cultural rights that are held to be universal (applicable to all individuals everywhere), inter-related, and indivisible. These rights inhere in all individuals by virtue of their being human—and simultaneously concern the relationship of individuals to the state.

Employing neither a purely individualistic nor structural analysis, the health and human rights framework focuses on government obligations to respect, protect, and fulfill human rights (Mann et al., 1994; Mann et al., 1999; Gruskin & Tarantola, 2001; Gruskin et al., 2005; Gruskin et al., 2007). These obligations include recognizing that "everyone is entitled to all the rights and freedoms set forth" in the 1948 UDHR, "without distinction of any kind, such as race, colour, sex, language, religion, political or other opinion, national or social origin, property, birth, or other status" (UDHR, 1948, Article 2). The health and human right framework accordingly lends itself to analysis of how both promotion and violation of human rights by governments and their policies—encompassing but not limited to health policies—can affect individual and population health. At issue not only are the actual health impacts but also the ability to analyze them, as related to the kinds of population data, including census and health data, that that government agencies do—or do not—collect and analyze.

Yet, despite its relevance to population-based research on the sociopolitical determinants of health, to date the bulk of work investigating links between health and human rights has been either policy-oriented or case-based, rather than epidemiologic (Mann et al., 1999; Gruskin & Tarantola, 2001; Gruskin et al., 2005; Gruskin et al., 2007; Beyrer & Pizer, 2007; Mullany et al., 2007; Birn et al., 2009). Suggesting this state of affairs will change is growing recognition globally of the utility of a rights-based approach to health both for holding governments' accountable for the health impacts of their policies and for assisting efforts to change inequitable policies (Gruskin et al., 2005; Gruskin et al., 2007; Gruskin & Ferguson, 2009; Birn et al., 2009). This is because evaluating the health impact of these policies requires engagement with measuring levels, distributions, and causes of health outcomes among populations—that is, the essential work of epidemiology. The added conceptualization of societal determinants of health in relation to human rights is thus also likely to be an increasingly prominent part of twenty-first century sociopolitical theories of disease distribution.

Psychosocial Determinants of Health: Stressed Minds, Sick Bodies, and Unhealthy Societies

A second major trend of mid/late-twentieth to early twenty-first century social epidemiologic theorizing, concerned with the psychosocial determinants of health, emphasizes individuals' perceptions of—and their health-damaging or health-enhancing responses to—social conditions, social interactions, and social status (Galdston, 1954a; Ahmed & Coelho, 1979; Elliott & Eisdorfer, 1982; Brunner, 1997; Marmot, 1988; McEwen & Stellar, 1993; McEwen, 1998a; Elstad, 1998; Adler, 1999; Brunner and Marmot, 1999; Krieger, 2001a; Wilkinson, 2001; Shulkin, 2004a; Sapolsky, 2004; Marmot, 2004; Wilkinson, 2005; McEwen, 2007; Wilkinson & Pickett, 2009). As stated by the internationally renowned epidemiologist Sir Michael Marmot (b. 1945), "psychosocial suggests that psychological factors of interest are related to the social environment" (Marmot, 1988, p. 639). At issue are individuals' appraisals of their socially-structured situation(s) (e.g., as threatening or rewarding, as fair or unfair, in relation to both immediate circumstances and anticipated scenarios) and how they respond, psychologically, biologically, and behaviorally, thereby affecting their health. Of interest are not only harms caused by adverse psychological stressors but also social phenomena hypothesized to buffer their impact (e.g., social support, social networks, social capital) (Elstad, 1998; Stansfield, 1999; Kawachi & Berkman, 2000; Sapolsky, 2004; McEwen, 2007). In both cases, whether the psychosocial stimuli are noxious or beneficial, a central interest, biologically, is how the brain perceives and responds to them (McEwen, 1998b; Marmot, 2004; Sapolsky, 2004; McEwen, 2007; McEwen, 2008), as graphically depicted in **Figure 6–5.**

Historical Development. Epidemiologic theorizing about and research on explicitly termed *psychosocial* exposures, including "stress," in relation to both somatic and mental disease, can readily be traced back to the 1940s (Halliday, 1946; Gordon, 1953; Kruse, 1954; Galdston, 1954b; King & Cobb, 1958; Chope, 1959). Informing its precepts were prior research in: (*1*) psychology (the field which originated the term *psychosocial* [OED, 2009]); (*2*) medicine (including *social medicine*, discussed above, and also *holistic medicine* [Lawrence & Weisz 1988] and *psychosomatic medicine*, with the first English-language journal by this name first published in 1939 [*Psychosomatic Medicine*, 2009]); and (*3*) physiology, and especially work on biology of "stress."

(a)

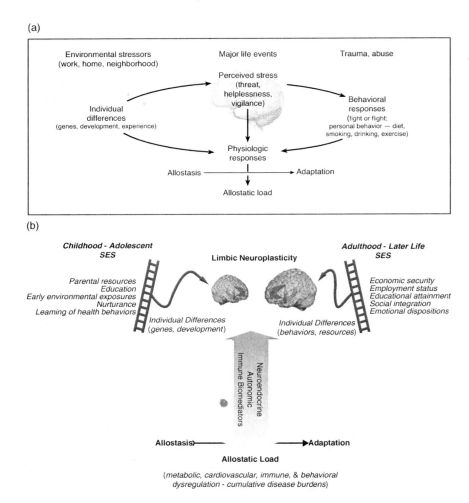

(b)

Figure 6–5. Psychosocial theory: stress, biology, and behavior: (a) "The stress response and the development of allostatic load". (McEwen, 1998) (Copyright © 1998 Massachusetts Medical Society. All rights reserved. Reproduced with permission) and (b) "Neurobiological pathways of SES and allostatic load." (McEwen, 2010) (Copyright © 2010 Wiley. Reproduced with permission.)

One key influence was the research of Walter B. Cannon (1871–1945), who in 1915 coined the phrase "fight or flight" to describe "bodily changes in pain, hunger, fear, and rage" (Cannon, 1915). Of particular relevance is his pathbreaking work, starting in the 1920s, both on the sympathetico-adrenal system and on *homeostasis*—a term he also coined, building on the renowned French physiologist Claude Bernard's (1813–1878) idea that living organisms need to keep a constant "internal milieu" to survive (Cannon, 1935; Galdston, 1954b; Wolfe et al., 2000, pp. 144–165; Shulkin, 2004b). Also salient was the work of Hans Seyle (1907–1982) (Galdston, 1954b; Selye, 1976; Elstad, 1998; Viner, 1999; Shulkin, 2004b), who in 1936 first described what he termed the *general adaptation syndrome* to describe organisms' "universal" response to stressors, a phenomena which he termed *stress* and which involved the stages of "alarm," "resistance," and "exhaustion" (Selye, 1936; Selye, 1946; Selye, 1976). By the mid-1950s, the ideas of "homeostasis," "stress," and "imbalance" in relation to what were explicitly termed *material deprivation,* and *psychological deprivation* became core concepts of psychosocial epidemiologic theorizing (Galdston, 1954b); by the mid-1960s, epidemiologic research increasingly investigated hypothesis linking the social patterning of psychological stressors to disease distribution (Henry & Cassel, 1969; **Textbox 6–5**).

During the latter part of the 1970s, psychosocial epidemiologic theorizing and research took off (Krieger, 2001a), as reflected in a series of seminal papers by such epidemiologists as John Cassel (1921–1976) (Cassel, 1974; Cassel, 1976) (**Textbox 6–5**) and S. Leonard Syme (b. 1932) and Lisa Berkman (b. 1950) (Syme & Berkman, 1976). Emphasizing the idea of "general susceptibility"—in contrast to "disease specificity" or specific exposures (Kunitz, 2007, pp. 27–42)—they argued that psychosocial stressors generated by human interaction, such as dominance hierarchies, social disorganization, marginal status, and rapid social change, acted as nonspecific exposures that altered neuroendocrine function. The net effect was that of "making subsets of people more or less susceptible" to what were claimed to be "ubiquitous agents in our environment" (Cassel, 1976, p. 108), conceived of as "direct noxious stimuli, i.e., disease agents" (Cassel, 1976, p. 109), thereby producing persistent "social class gradients of mortality and life expectancy" (Syme & Berkman, 1976, p. 1). Also in 1976, Selye published his 1256-page opus on *Stress in Health and Disease* (Selye, 1976), providing further evidence from both animal and human research linking stress and risk of disease. One year later, the physician George Engel (1913–1999) introduced his influential "biopsychosocial" model in the pages of *Science* (Engel, 1977; Frankel et al., 2003). That same year, Joseph Eyer and Peter Sterling published their critical article on "Stress-Related Mortality and Social Organization," discussed above, which brought a political economy perspective to the generation of psychosocial stressors under capitalism (Eyer & Sterling, 1977) and which advocated, as a solution, major sociopolitical change (**Textbox 6–4**).

Sterling and Eyer then subsequently, in 1988, advanced psychosocial theorizing by introducing a new concept: *allostasis* (Sterling & Eyer, 1988, p. 631). Challenging the idea of *homeostasis*, they coined their new term to refer to regulatory systems that achieve "stability through change," with two key premises about these systems being: "*parameters vary, and variation anticipates demand*" (italics in original) (Sterling, 2004, p. 21). Conceptually, the term *allostasis* helped clarify how pathophysiology could result from chronic overactivation of regulatory systems, in relation to both experienced and anticipated situations (Shulkin, 2004b; Sterling, 2004). One implication was that psychosocial stressors could be directly pathogenic, rather than alter only susceptibility; a second was that disease could arise from dysregulation of normal regulatory systems, as opposed to arising from some sort of intrinsic "defect" (whether genetic or otherwise) (Sterling & Eyer, 1981; Sterling, 2004).

A decade later, the term's successor, *allostatic load*, was introduced by Bruce S. McEwen (McEwen & Stellar, 1993; McEwen, 1998a; McEwen, 1998b). Explicitly drawing upon Sterling and Eyer's idea, McEwen's term referred to "wear-and-tear from chronic overactivity or underactivity" of systems "that protect the body by responding to internal and external stress," including "the autonomic nervous system, the hypothalamic-pituitary-adrenal (HPA) axis, and cardiovascular, metabolic, and immune systems" (McEwen, 1998a, p. 171). Elaborated since (Shulkin, 2004a; McEwen, 2004; McEwen, 2007; McEwen, 2008)—especially with reference to early life exposures, cumulative disadvantage across the lifecourse, and psychoneurobiology—the concepts of *allostasis, allostatic state*, and *allostatic overload* (Shulkin, 2004b, p. 7), along with their associated metaphors

Textbox 6–5. Psychosocial Theories of Disease Distribution (Mid-Twentieth to Early Twenty-First Century): "Stress," Biology, and Subjective Appraisal of—and Responses to—Social Circumstances

1950s   Galdston I (ed). *Beyond the Germ Theory: The Roles of Deprivation and Stress in Health and Disease.* New York: Health Education Council, New York Academy of Medicine, 1954.
a) Galdston I. Beyond the germ theory: the roles of deprivation and stress in health and disease, pp. 3–16.
p. 4: "To maintain homeostasis, i.e., the constancy of his internal milieu, man [*sic*] must have access to the balancing factors in the process. Unless man [*sic*] can obtain what is *required* (italics in original) and convert or eliminate what is *in excess* (italics in original) he cannot maintain *homeostasis* (italics in original)—or health.
This lays bare a new source of pathology, that of deprivation: disease due to a *lack* (italics in original) of essentials…
Deprivations are to be witnessed in the psychological, no less than in the material spheres of existence (italics in original).
More recently to the concept of homeostasis there has been added that of *stress* (italics in original). Even when given all the factors necessary for maintenance man [*sic*] can maintain homeostasis in the face of external variations, provided only that the external variations are not excessive in degree, nor too sudden in development… The critical factors are not alone the gravity of the stress but also the individual's tolerance…"
p. 12: "Thus we come upon a third source of morbidity different from the two I have already described. Thanks to Han Selye's eloquence and energy, it is popularly known under the name of the 'stress situation' and the 'stress syndrome.'"
b) Kruse HD. The interplay of noxious agents, stress, and deprivation in the etiology of disease, pp. 17–38.
p. 29: "Quite apart from the magnitude of the stress, the functional capacity of the regulatory system may vary over the life span under influences, both normal and pathogenic, that are accounted to ordinary vicissitudes and exigencies. Among the conditions that affect the regulatory processes which determine homeostasis are: infection, inactivity, worry, dissipation, loss of sleep."
p. 35: "From further observation Selye propounded the view that during the general adaptation syndrome some of the anterior pituitary and adreno-corticol hormones are produced in excess. This defensive endocrine response is useful since it raises resistance to stress. But the endogenous hormonal overproduction also has its harmful aspects since it can induce cardiovascular, renal, and joint diseases.
Thus the by-products of these excessive or abnormal adaptive reactions to stress are the so-called diseases of adaptation. They include some of the diseases that most frequently affect man [*sic*]."

1960s   Henry HP, Cassel JC. Psychosocial factors in essential hypertension: recent epidemiologic and animal experimental evidence. *Am J Epidemiol* 1969; 90;171–200.
p. 195: "Recent human and animal experimental studies of the role of psychosocial factors as determinants of disease increase the attractiveness of the view that the defense alarm reaction may be an important intervening neurohumoral link between unfulfilled social needs and the development of high blood pressure. The alarm response induces

modifications of the steady state condition which activate adaptive mechanisms. There is evidence that by acting repeatedly over the years, this defense reaction will lead to a chronic elevation of systolic arterial pressure in the majority of the members of a disturbed social group."

1970s   **Cassel J. The contribution of the social environment to host resistance. The fourth Wade Hampton Frost lecture.** *Am J Epidemiol* 1976; 104:107–123.

p. 108: "The question facing epidemiologic inquiry then is, are there categories or classes of environmental factors that are capable of changing human resistance in important ways and making subsets of people more or less susceptible to these ubiquitous agents in the environment? When we have thought of these questions at all, we have been accustomed to think in rather general terms of such things as nutritional status, fatigue, overwork or the like. I would suggest, however, that there is another category of environmental factors capable of producing profound effects on host susceptibility to environmental disease agents, and that is the presence of other members of the same species, or more generally, certain aspects of the social environment.

The problem is that as soon as one introduces the concept of the potential role of the social environment in disease etiology, the almost inevitable response is that this means stress and stress disease. I think the simple-minded invocation of the word stress in such thinking has done as much to retard research in this area as did the concepts of the miasma at the time of the discovery of microorganisms…"

p. 109: "… Stated in its most general terms, the formulation subscribed to (often implicitly) by most epidemiologists and social scientists working in this field is that the relationship between a stressor and disease outcome will be similar to the relationship between a microorganism and the disease outcome… The corollaries of such a formulation are that there will be etiologic specificity (each stressor leading to a specific stress disease) and there will be a dose-response relationship (the greater the stressor, the more likelihood of disease). There is serious doubt as to the utility or appropriateness of both of these notions."

p. 109: "A more reasonable formulation would hold that psychosocial processes acting as 'conditional' stressors will, by altering the endocrine balance in the body, increase the susceptibility of the organism to direct noxious stimuli, i.e., disease agents. The psychosocial processes thus can be envisaged as enhancing susceptibility to disease."

p. 110: "A remarkably similar set of social circumstances characterizes people who develop tuberculosis and schizophrenia, become alcoholics, are victims of multiple accidents, or commit suicide. Common to all these people is a marginal status in society. They are individuals who for a variety of reasons (e.g., ethnic minorities rejected by the dominant majority in their neighborhood; high sustained rates of residential and occupational mobility; broken homes or isolated living circumstances) have been deprived of meaningful social contact. It is perhaps surprising that this wide variety of disease outcomes associated with similar circumstance has generally escaped comment."

p. 113: "… a fuller explanation of the potential role of psychosocial factors in the genesis of disease requires the recognition of a second set of processes. These might be envisioned as the protective factors buffering

or cushioning the individual from the physiologic or psychologic consequences of exposure to the stressor situation. It is suggested that the
property common to these processes is the strength of the social supports
provided by the primary groups of most importance to the individual."

p. 121: "... Recognizing that throughout history, disease, with rare exceptions, has not been prevented by finding and treating sick individuals, but by
modifying those environmental factors facilitating its occurrence, this formulation would suggest that we should focus efforts more directly on attempts
at further identification and subsequent modification of these categories of
psychosocial factors rather than on screening and early detection.

Of the two sets of factors, it would seem more immediately feasible to
attempt to improve and strengthen the social supports rather than
reduce exposure to the stressors..."

1980s   **Elliott GR, Eisdorfer C (eds).** *Stress and Human Health: Analysis and*
Implications of research. A study by the Institute of Medicine/National
Academy of Sciences. **New York: Springer, 1982.**

p. 8: "A growing body of well-controlled studies document that disruptive life events are associated with an increased risk of a number of mild
and severe physical and mental disorders. For example, such life events
as job loss, bereavement, moving to a new location, or marriage have
been associated with increased likelihood of developing minor infections,
sudden cardiac death, cancer, and depression. At the same time, basic
scientists are measuring with increasing sensitivity the effects that severe
stressors can have on hormonal responses, on brain function, and on
cardiovascular, immune, and endocrine systems. Investigators have also
demonstrated the importance of psychosocial factors as mediators of
responses to stressors and are developing better methods for measuring
such effects. Factors such as the interpretation of an event or the availability of social supports may influence greatly how an individual responds
to a disruptive life event. Taken together, the evidence strongly supports
the conclusion that stress can affect physical and mental processes that
might alter an individual's susceptibility to disease,

with adverse health consequences for a large number of individuals
exposed to them."

1990s   **Brunner E. Stress and the biology of inequality.** *Br Med J* 1997; **314:**
1472–1476.

p. 1472: "It is well established that health depends on socioeconomic circumstances, but the biology of this relation is not well described.
Psychosocial factors operating throughout the life course, beginning in
early life, influence a variety of biological variables. Research with non-
human primates shows the effects of dominance hierarchy on biology, and
similar metabolic differentials are evident in a hierarchy of white collar civil
servants. The neuroendocrine 'fight or flight' response produces physiological and metabolic alterations which parallel those observed with lower
socioeconomic status. The biological effects of the psychosocial environment could explain health inequalities between relatively affluent groups."

2000s   **McEwen BS. Central effects of stress hormones in health and disease: understanding the protective and damaging effects of stress
and stress mediators.** *Eur J Pharmacol* 2008; **582:174–185.**

p. 174: "Stress begins in the brain and affects the brain, as well as the rest
of the body. Acute stress responses promote adaptation and survival via

responses of neural, cardiovascular, autonomic, immune and metabolic systems. Chronic stress can promote and exacerbate pathophysiology through the same systems that are dysregulated. The burden of chronic stress and accompanying changes in personal behaviors (smoking, eating too much, drinking, poor quality sleep; otherwise referred to as 'lifestyle') is called allostatic overload. Brain regions such as hippocampus, prefrontal cortex and amygdala respond to acute and chronic stress and show changes in morphology and chemistry that are largely reversible if the chronic stress lasts for weeks. However, it is not clear whether prolonged stress for many months or years may have irreversible effects on the brain. The adaptive plasticity of chronic stress involves many mediators, including glucocorticoids, excitatory amino acids, endogenous factors such as brain neurotrophic factor (BDNF), polysialated neural cell adhesion molecule (PSA-NCAM) and tissue plasminogen activator (tPA). The role of this stress-induced remodeling of neural circuitry is discussed in relation to psychiatric illnesses, as well as chronic stress and the concept of top-down regulation of cognitive, autonomic and neuroendocrine function. This concept leads to a different way of regarding more holistic manipulations, such as physical activity and social support as an important complement to pharmaceutical therapy in treatment of the common phenomenon of being 'stressed out.' Policies of government and the private sector play an important role in this top-down view of minimizing the burden of chronic stress and related lifestyle (i.e., allostatic overload)."

of imbalance, have become central to late twentieth and early twenty-first century epidemiologic psychosocial ideas and research.

Core Tenets. Building on this history, three basic postulates of contemporary psychosocial epidemiologic theorizing about disease distribution can be discerned. These are:

1. the distribution of adverse psychological stressors (and their buffers) is socially patterned, as linked to people's social position, living conditions (e.g., at home, in their neighborhood), and, if employed, workplace conditions;
2. relative rank in social hierarchies is a—if not *the*—major adverse psychological stressor; and
3. adverse psychological stress, especially if chronic, can harm somatic and mental health via pathways that can, independently and synergistically, involve the central nervous system, regulatory physiology, behavior, and illness itself.

Postulated mechanisms include:

1. most commonly: brain-mediated allostatic overload, resulting in physiological damage that can potentially lead directly to disease (e.g., sustained hypertension) and also to increased susceptibility to other exposures (e.g., infectious agents, via immune system suppression) (McEwen & Stellar, 1993; McEwen, 1998b; Kubzansky & Kawachi, 2000; Brunner, 2000; Sapolsky, 2004; Sterling, 2004; McEwen, 2007; McEwen, 2008);

2. the triggering of health-damaging behaviors, whether by elevating core obligate daily activities (e.g., sleeping, eating) to unhealthy levels (i.e., sleep deprivation, excessive eating) (McEwen & Stellar, 1993; Sterling, 2004; Sapolsky, 2004; McEwen, 2007; Wilkinson & Pickett, 2009) or by increasing the likelihood of people of employing nonobligate psychoactive substances (e.g., tobacco, alcohol, and other licit and illicit substances) to alleviate their distress and which, if used in excess (acutely or over the long-term), can harm their somatic and mental health (McEwen & Stellar, 1993; Emmons, 2000; Sterling, 2004; Sapolsky, 2004; Koob & Le Moal, 2004; McEwen, 2008; Wilkinson & Pickett, 2009); and

3. elevating the risk of developing mental illness (e.g., depression or post-traumatic stress disorder), which in addition to constituting a critical health outcome in its own right can also impair somatic health (Carney & Freedland, 2000; Rosen & Shulkin, 2004; McEwen, 2008).

Work to test these hypotheses has ranged from sharpening conceptualization and measurement of psychosocial exposures (Cohen et al., 1995; Berkman & Kawachi, 2000) to elaborating neurobiological pathways potentially linking psychosocial exposures to bodily and mental illness and also to all-cause and cause-specific mortality (National Research Council and Institute of Medicine, 2000; Shulkin, 2004a; McEwen, 2008).

Psychosocial theories of disease distribution thus stand as distinct from—even as they engage with—biomedical and sociopolitical frameworks. In their emphasis on mental interpretations of socially structured phenomena (e.g., social interactions, social hierarchy) and their biological and behavioral sequelae, psychosocial postulates explicitly challenge three core features of the biomedical model (as discussed in **Chapter 5**): its mind/body dualism, its methodological individualism, and its decontextualized framing of health behaviors as freely chosen "lifestyles." Thus, in contrast to the biomedical orientation, psychosocial analyses posit that social causes matter and that both psychosocial and material exposures can harm health (Marmot & Wilkinson, 1999; Adler, 2006).

Nevertheless, the psychosocial engagement with social phenomena is chiefly concerned with the biology of stress and individual's psychological perceptions of and behavioral responses to their social milieu and status (*see* **Textbox 6–5**). As its name implies, the psychosocial orientation not surprisingly focuses on psychological pathways and mechanisms and not political or sociological analyses of what socially patterns or precipitates their activation. The overwhelming emphasis is on how psychological phenomena (and not differences in material resources or exposures) create "social gradients in health" (*see* **Textbox 6–6**). Together, these patterns comprise, in the words of Sir Michael Marmot, the "status syndrome" (Marmot, 2004, p. 1), for which (Marmot, 2004, p. 6):

> ... Quite simply, the key lies in that most important organ, the brain. The psychological experience of inequality has profound effects on body systems. The evidence we shall examine suggests that this may be a major factor in generating the status syndrome.

Thus, compared to the social epidemiology's sociopolitical theories of disease distribution, psychosocial analyses accord less attention, theoretically and empirically, to who and what generates psychosocial insults and buffers, and also to how the social, spatial, and temporal distribution of these exposures——along with that of ubiquitous or non-ubiquitous pathogenic physical, chemical, or biological agents—is shaped by extant and changing social, political, and economic priorities and policies (Krieger, 2001a; Krieger, 2001b). Likewise receiving scant analysis is how and why diverse forms of social

Textbox 6–6. Leading Twenty-First Century Psychosocial Explanations for the "Social Gradient" in Disease: Poverty as a State of Mind—and Relative Standing in the Social Hierarchy.

Sapolsky RM. Social status and health in humans and other animals. *Annu Rev Anthropol* 2004; 33:393–418.

p. 410: "Most researchers view psychosocial factors related to stress as major media-tors of the SES/health relationship. In addition to the insufficiency of the most notable nonpsychosocial explanations, indirect support for psychosocial factors includes the following: (a) The poor have an excess of physical and psychological stressors; (b) studies report an SES gradient related to basal glucocorticoid levels; and (c) the strongest SES gradients occur for diseases with the greatest sensitivity to stress, such as heart disease, diabetes, metabolic syndrome, and psychiatric disorders.

The case for stress-related psychosocial factors has become more direct. To appreci-ate this, one must consider a truism: Given food, shelter, and safety sufficient to sustain health, if everyone is poor, then no one is. In modern societies, it is never the case that everyone is equally (non)poor. This paves the way for a key point about the gradient, namely that poor health is not so much the outcome of being poor, but of feeling poor, that is, feeling poorer than others. Therefore, poverty, rather than being an absolute measure, is a subjective assessment that is mired in invidiousness."

Marmot MG. *The Status Syndrome: How Social Standing Affects our Health and Longevity.* New York: Times Books/Henry Holt, 2004.

p. 1: "We have remarkably good health in the rich countries of the world… Except that it is better for some than others–considerably so. Where you stand in the social hierarchy is intimately related to your chances of getting ill, and your length of life…

Let me translate 'where you stand in the social hierarchy.' You are not poor. You are employed. Your children are well fed. You live in a decent house or apartment. You turn on the faucet and drink the water in the secure knowledge that it is clean. The food you buy is not similarly contaminated. Most people you come across in your daily routine also meet this description. But, among these people, none of whom is destitute or even poor, you acknowledge that some are higher in the social hierarchy: they may have more money, bigger houses, a more prestigious job, more status in the eyes of others, or simply a higher-class way of speaking. You also note that there are other people lower than you on these criteria, not just the very poor or homeless, but people whose standing is merely lower than yours, to a varying extent. The remarkable finding is that among *all* (italics in original) of these people, the higher the status in the pecking order, the healthier they are likely to be. In other words, health follows a social gradient. I call this the status syndrome."

p. 2: "… for people above a threshold of material well-being, another kind of well-being is central. Autonomy–how much control you have over your life–and the opportunities you have for full social engagement and participation are crucial for health, well-being, and longevity. It is inequality in these that plays a big part in pro-ducing the social gradient in health. Degrees of control and participation underlie the status syndrome."

p. 6: "… the causes of the social gradient are to be found in the circumstances in which we live and work… It is about the fact that control over life circumstances and full social engagement and participation in what society has to offer are distributed unequally, and as a result health is distributed unequally…

How do these experiences translate into illness? Quite simply, the key lies in that most important organ, the brain. The psychological experience of inequality has profound effects on body systems. The evidence we shall examine suggests that this may be a major factor in generating the status syndrome."

p. 11: "We then need to look at the crucial question of relative inequalities: the importance of where one stands relative to others in the hierarchy. This may be more important for health than absolute level of resources."

Wilkinson RG. *The Impact of Inequality: How to Make Sick Societies Healthier. New York: The New Press,* **2005.**

pp. 60–61: "The term psychosocial is often used in preference to psychological to emphasize the extent to which the features of emotional life that affect health are socially patterned and dependent on the social context rather than simply on individual happenstance... ."

pp. 61–62: "The normal basis on which we distinguish between material and psychosocial factors hinges on whether the health impact is dependent on some conscious or unconscious perception or cognitive processing, or whether, in contrast, it affects health regardless of what we think or feel or know. So, for instance, things such as air pollution, infectious microorganisms, poisoning, and vitamin deficiencies are all capable of harming our health even if we are totally unaware of them: they are therefore classified as material factors having a direct effect on health. But job or housing insecurity affects your health only if you are aware of it. Similarly, the practical causes of feelings of hostility, depression, or lack of sense of control may be clear enough, but if it is those feelings that are doing the health damage, they are classified as psychosocial, even if the remedies are often material. That is an important point: the remedies for psychosocial stressors often involve changes in material circumstances."

p. 63: "Concentrating on these psychosocial influences does not mean that direct effects of poorer material circumstances do not matter. Things such as poor diet, air pollution, smoking, and bad housing obviously do matter. But we should not be too simplistic about them and imagine that there are very clear connections between, for instance, exposure to the physical hazards of poor-quality housing and the causation of cancers or heart disease."

pp. 65–66: "Psychosocial influences on health are not like the health risks of eating too much fatty food—enjoyable but better avoided because of the health effects. Psychosocial factors are important because they go to the heart of our subjective experience of the quality of life. They matter not just because of their health consequences, but in themselves. If you are depressed, you want your depression to end because it is an unhappy state to be in, not merely because someone tells you that it is also a risk factor for heart disease... .

In contrast, gaining an understanding of the direct material causes of ill health could not take us to the heart of the malaise of modern society and so does not have the same potential to improve the psychosocial well-being of whole populations. The more important direct effects of material factors are already better understood, despite being less powerful, and many of them could be dealt with–provided there is the political will–simply by ensuring that the benefits of economic growth extended to all sections of society."

"hierarchies— postulated to be an evolved and innate feature of human society (Wilkinson, 2001; Sapolsky, 2004; Marmot, 2004; Wilkinson, 2005; Wilkinson & Pickett, 2009)—have dramatically differed and changed over time, whether comparing varieties of "premodern" societies (e.g., foraging, horticulturalist, pastoral, or agricultural (Smith et al., 2010) or feudalistic versus capitalistic societies, or different variants of the latter (e.g., pre vs. post-slavery, pre- vs. post-enactment of neoliberal economic policies), (Giddens and Held, 1982; Hobsbawm, 1994; Zinn, 2003; Hobsbawm, 2008). Also accorded little, if any, attention are epidemiologic data demonstrating that depending on the health outcome under consideration—and in what time and place—"social gradients" can be not only positive but also null, negative, and even change direction, as well as differ by gender and race/ethnicity (Elstad, 1998; Krieger, 2000; Lynch et al., 2000; Krieger, 2001a; Davey Smith, 2003; Hardy, 2004; Macleod et al., 2005; Macleod et al., 2006; Kunitz, 2007; Krieger, 2007).

In summary, although united in their views that societal context shapes population health and is responsible for the existence of health inequities, the sociopolitical and psychosocial frameworks offer very different—and at times clashing—sets of ideas to explain these links. Whether other approaches can be taken to parsing the relationships between what Cannon termed "the body physiologic and the body politic" (Cannon, 1941), simultaneously mindful of sociopolitical, psychosocial, and biological processes—in historical, spatiotemporal, and ecological context—is what I shall consider next.

7

Ecosocial Theory of Disease Distribution

Embodying Societal & Ecologic Context

Starting in the mid-1990s, new proposals for ecologically oriented integrative, multilevel, and dynamic epidemiologic frameworks, explicitly linking societal and biophysical determinants of disease distribution and health inequities—over the life-course and across generations in geographic and historical context—began to appear in the English-language epidemiologic literature (Krieger, 2001a). The first of these was the *ecosocial theory of disease distribution* that I initially proposed in 1994 (Krieger, 1994) and have elaborated since (*see* **Textbox 7–1**). It was joined in 1995 by Tony McMichael's urging adoption of an ecological perspective (McMichael, 1995)—that of "human ecology" (McMichael, 2002, p. 1145)—so that epidemiologists could escape being "prisoners of the proximate" (McMichael, 1999), and in 1996 by Mervyn Susser and Ezra Susser's call for "*eco-epidemiology*" (Susser & Susser, 1996).

Common to all three perspectives has been an explicit concern with: (*1*) "ecology" (albeit variously defined and conceptualized), (*2*) societal influences on health, and (*3*) their interrelationship (*see* **Textbox 7–1**). Another shared premise is overt recognition that replacing "reductionism" and "risk factor" epidemiology with an undifferentiated "holism" and indifference to specific exposures, specific diseases, specific locales, and specific time periods is unlikely to advance epidemiology: theoretically, methodologically, substantively, or practically (Krieger, 1999a). Needed instead is clear epidemiological theorizing about societal and biological processes involving phenomena within and across levels within and over different scales of time and space, in specified historical time periods and locales.

Nor has this nascent trend toward integrative theorizing been unique to epidemiology. Instead, during the late twentieth century, similar efforts have arisen within—and have been reaching across—a fast-growing array of scientific disciplines, both "natural" and "social," all sharing the aim of comprehending "complex systems" and overcoming the fragmentation and decontextualization of knowledge caused by ever more narrow disciplinary specialization; examples of such intellectual endeavors can be found in physics, biology, ecology, geography, history, sociology, psychology, and anthropology, to name but a few fields (McAdam et al., 2001; Grene & Depew, 2004; Taylor, 2005; Biersack & Greenberg, 2006; Érdi, 2008; Mitchell, 2009). Like the new ecologically-oriented epidemiologic theorizing, many of these efforts are seeking to integrate levels of analysis in relation to time and place. They are also engaged in deep debates over whether the objective

Textbox 7–1. Integrating Ecological Thinking into Epidemiologic Theories of Disease Distribution: Three Frameworks Proposed in the 1990s—Ecosocial Theory, Human Ecology, and Eco-Epidemiology

(1) Krieger's *"ecosocial theory of disease distribution"*—the most elaborated of the three, as articulated through a series of papers and discussed in more detail in this article.

This theory: (1) explicitly incorporates constructs pertaining to political economy, political ecology, ecosystems, spatiotemporal scales and levels, biological pathways of embodiment, and the social production of scientific knowledge, (2) critiques the prevalent framing of determinants as "proximal" versus "distal" (and their meta-phoric counterparts of "downstream" vs. "upstream"), and (3) proposes specific alternative theoretical constructs to guide hypotheses generation, study design, and data interpretation (Krieger, 1994; Krieger, 1999a; Krieger, 1999b; Krieger, 2000a; Krieger, 2000b; Krieger, 2001a; Krieger, 2001b; Krieger, 2001c; Krieger, 2001d; Krieger & Gruskin, 2001; Krieger, 2003a; Krieger, 2003b; Krieger, 2004a; Krieger, 2004b; Krieger & Davey Smith, 2004; Krieger, 2005a; Krieger, 2005b; Krieger, 2005c; Krieger, 2006; Krieger, 2007; Krieger, 2008a; Krieger, 2008b; Krieger, 2009; Krieger 2010a; Krieger 2010b; Krieger 2010c).

Disciplines that have used ecosocial theory to date (with the references providing only selected examples) include not only:

– epidemiology (Yen & Syme, 1999; Thacker & Buffington, 2001; Azambuja et al., 2002; Ben-Shlomo & Kuh, 2002; Goldberg et al., 2003; Wise, 2003; Sommerfeld, 2003; Stewart & Napoles-Springer, 2003; Poundstone et al., 2004; McLaren & Hawe, 2005; Velasco et al., 2006; Leslie & Lentle 2006; Yamada & Palmer 2007; Gillespie et al., 2007; Buffardi et al., 2008; Gravlee, 2009),

but also

– environmental and occupational health (Bernardi & Ebi, 2001; Northridge et al., 2003; Quinn, 2003; Parkes et al., 2003; Robert & Smith, 2004; Kegler & Miner, 2004; Parkes et al., 2004; Porto, 2005; Morello-Frosch et al., 2006);
– behavioral science and health promotion (Prothrow-Stith et al., 2003; Raphael, 2003; Barbeau et al., 2004; Maupin et al., 2004; Sorensen et al., 2004; Edwards et al., 2004; Glass & McAtee, 2006);
– nursing (Abrums, 2004; Edwards et al., 2004; MacDonald, 2004);
– psychology and substance abuse (Walters & Simoni, 2002; Burris et al., 2004; Nichter et al., 2004; Godette et al., 2006);
– sociology (Spitler, 2001);
– urban health and urban planning (Northridge et al., 2003; Northridge & Sclar, 2003; Corburn, 2004; Galea & Vlahov, 2005);
– health and human rights (Chilton, 2006; Teti et al., 2006);
– medical anthropology (Baer & Singer, 2009; Thompson et al., 2009); and
– critical analyses of population health (Levins, 1996; Levins & Lopez, 1999).

(2) McMichael's *"human ecology"* **approach** (McMichael, 2002, p. 1145), delineated in several articles and expanded into a book (McMichael, 1995; McMichael, 1999; McMichael, 2001; McMichael, 2002; McMichael, 2004).

This framework holds that "the health of populations is primarily a product of ecological circumstance: a product of the interaction of human societies with the wider environment, its various ecosystems and other life-support processes" (McMichael, 2001, pp. xiv). Theoretical work required includes: (*1*) conceptually and methodologically establishing approaches for analyzing the "complex social and environmental systems that are the context for health and disease; (*2*) thinking about population health in increasingly ecologic terms; (*3*) developing dynamic, interactive, life-course models of disease risk acquisition; and (*4*) extending their spatial-temporal frame of reference as they perceive the health risks posed by escalating human pressures on the wider environment" (McMichael, 1999, p. 887). Informed by increasing ecosystem concerns about the "overloading of the biosphere" (McMichael, 1995, p. 633), the metaphor employed is of a successive series of "footprints," referring to human evolution, culture, and humankind's "ecological footprint" on the ecosphere (McMichael, 2001, pp. xiv–xv).

(3) The Sussers' "*eco-epidemiology*," sketched in one article (Susser & Susser, 1996) and briefly re-capitulated in three editorials (Susser, 2004; March & Susser, 2006a; March & Susser, 2006b) (with two of these essays [Susser & Susser, 1996; March & Susser, 2006a] republished in Susser & Stein's 2009 book on *Eras in Epidemiology* [Susser & Stein, 2009]).

This approach advocates use of an "ecologic perspective... encompassing many levels of organization—molecular and societal as well as individual" (Susser & Susser, 1996, p. 674), with attention to "localization... and the bounds that limit generalizations about biological, human, and social systems" (Susser & Susser, 1996, p. 675); also included is attention to "trajectories of health and disease over life course" and "historical trends" (March & Susser, 2006a, p. 1379). Initially representing "levels" strictly as "nested hierarchies" via the metaphor of "Chinese boxes—a conjurer's nest of boxes, each containing a succession of smaller ones" (Susser & Susser, 1996, p. 675), eco-epidemiology subsequently has shifted to the "upstream/downstream" metaphor (March & Susser, 2006b).

is to bridge—versus reject and refute—longstanding dualisms counterposing "mind" versus "body," "nature" versus "nurture," and "biological" versus "societal" (Csordas, 1994; Cronon, 1996; Weiss & Haber, 1999; Lakoff & Johnson, 1999; Lewontin, 2000; Damasio, 2003; Haraway, 2004; Grene & Depew, 2004; Taylor, 2005; Biersack & Greenberg, 2006; Calvo & Gomila, 2008).

To date, however, much of the work in social epidemiology calling for interdisciplinary, integrated theorizing has sought to expand its conceptual groundings chiefly by turning to the social sciences—in part as a reaction to the biomedical dominance in framing biology (Cassel, 1964; Tesh, 1988; Berkman & Kawachi, 2000; Hofrichter, 2003; Graham, 2007; Hall & Lamont, 2009). It has accorded little or no attention to the biological aspects of the self-designated natural ecological sciences, despite their explicit focus on relationships between biological organisms, populations, and their environments. The emphasis instead has been on "ecology" construed as "nested social hierarchies," reflecting the influence of social science theorizing and, more specifically, the impact of the highly influential "ecological systems theory," proposed in 1979 by the renowned psychologist Urie Bronfenbrenner (1917–2005) (Bronfenbrenner, 1979; Bronfenbrenner, 2005).

Concerned with the "ecology of human development," Bronfenbrenner's model has been widely used not only in developmental psychology but also public health (including epidemiology), where it is often termed the *social ecological model* (Stokols, 1996; Earls, 2003; Bauer et al., 2003; McLaren & Hall, 2005; Glass & McAtee, 2006). In developing this theory, Bronfenbrenner was influenced (Bronfenbrenner, 2005) by the work of the Soviet development child psychologist Lev Vygotsky (1896–1934), who sought to apply the ideas of "historical dialectical materialism" to his field, so as to study children in context and reframe their development as contingent on the dynamic interplay of the child over time with her or his various biophysical and societal contexts at multiple levels (e.g., family and household, school, neighborhood, nation, political-economic system, etc.) (Vygotsky, 1978; Richards, 1996).

In Bronfenbrenner's original model, an individual's "ecology" was initially conceptualized in relation to nested "micro," "meso," "exo," and "macro" social systems (e.g, a child's family environment, the social environment connecting home and school, parents' work environment, and the larger societal context, respectively) (Bronfenbrenner, 1979, pp. 3–8). In later iterations, Bronfenbrenner added a "chrono" system, to encompass environmental events over time, and he also became more focused on biological development, such that in 2001 he renamed his framework the "bioecological theory of human development" (Bronfenbrenner, 2001; Bronfenbrenner, 2005). A feature of this theory, from the start, has been its conception of the *ecological environment* as "a set of nested structures, each inside the next, like a set of Russian dolls" (Bronfenbrenner, 1979, p. 3). Yet, as contemporary ecological theorizing in both the natural and social sciences makes clear, nested hierarchies are but one form of ecological structure; not only do non-nested hierarchies exist, but the forms of hierarchies themselves are not "fixed" and instead depend on the biological processes at issue (Villa & Ceroni, 2005; Taylor, 2008; Lidicker, 2008). A useful question to consider, then, is: What might it mean, conceptually, for epidemiology to take engage with ecologists' views of ecological theory?

The Origins of "Ecology" and Current Conceptual Debates in Ecological Thinking

For anyone interested in integrative thinking, the appeal of *ecology*, a discipline concerned with analyzing organisms in context, should not be surprising. Ever since the German physician and zoologist Ernst Haeckel (1834–1919) (Richard, 2008) first coined the term in 1866 (*see* **Textbox 7–2**), drawing on the Greek word "*oikos*," meaning "household," to refer to "the whole science of the relations of the organism to the environment" (Stauffer, 1957, p. 140), the idea and study of *ecology* has informed—and been transformed and expanded by—the thinking of and debates within diverse scientific disciplines, natural and social alike (McIntosh, 1985; Bramwell, 1989; Worster, 1994; Merchant, 2002; Taylor, 2008). Haeckel, himself inspired (Stauffer, 1957; Richard, 2008) by Charles Darwin's *Origin of Species* (Darwin, 1859), for which he was one of the most prolific popularizers (Richard, 2008), viewed his research as encompassing what he termed "the economy of nature.... in a word, ecology is the study of all those complex interrelations referred to by Darwin as the conditions of the struggle for existence" (Stauffer, 1957, p. 141). To Haeckel, this concept of *struggle for existence* was central to life, and no species was exempt—whether human or otherwise. He accordingly, like many of his contemporaries, emphasized competitive over mutualistic relationships as the norm—and he likewise embraced the Social Darwinist ideology of his era to explain and justify the conventional racial hierarchies of his era (Richards, 2008), once again underscoring how social context affects scientific theorizing. Granted, naturalists and others long before Haeckel had carefully observed and sought to explain the complex mingling of and relationships between so many creatures "in nature," but it was not until the latter part of the nineteenth century that the field developed into a

Textbox 7–2. "Ecology": Definitions (1866–2009)—Continuities and Change

Original:

1866: Original definition by Ernst Haeckel (1834–1919), appearing in *Generelle Morphologie der Organismen. Allgemeine Grundzüge der organischen Formen-Wissenschaft, mechnisch begründet durch die von Charles Darwin reformirte Descnedenz-Theorie* (Berline: Reimer, 2 vol), Vol II, pp. 286–297, and translated by Stauffer 1957 (Stauffer, 1957, pp. 140–141).

"By ecology, we mean the whole science of the relations of the organism to the environment including, in the broad sense of the term, all the 'conditions of existence.' These are partly organic, partly inorganic in nature; both, as we have shown, are of the greatest significance for the form of the organisms, for they force them to become adapted. Among the inorganic conditions of existence to which every organism must adapt itself below, first of all, the physical and chemical properties of its habitat, the climate (light, warmth, atmospheric conditions of humidity and electricity), the inorganic nutrients, nature of the water and of the soil, etc.

As organic conditions of existence we consider the entire relations of the organism to all the other organisms with which it comes into contact, and of which most contribute either to its advantage or its harm. Each organism has among the other organisms its friends and its enemies, those which favor its existence and those which harm it. The organisms which serve as organic foodstuff for others or which live upon them as parasites also belong in this category of organic conditions of existence. In our discussion of the theory of selection we have shown what enormous importance all these adaptive relations have for the entire formation of organisms, and specially how much the organic conditions of existence exert a much more profound transforming action on organisms than do the inorganic. The extraordinary significance of these relations does not correspond in the least to their scientific treatment, however. So far physiology, [the science] to which this belong, has, in the most one sided fashion, almost exclusively investigated the conserving functions of organisms (preservation of the individual and the species, nutrition, and reproduction), and among the functions of the relationship [it has investigated] merely those which are produced by the relations of single parts of the organism to each other and to the whole. On the other hand, physiology has largely neglected the relations of the organism to the environment, the place each organism takes in the household of nature, in the economy of all nature, and has abandoned the gathering of the relevant facts to an uncritical "nature history," without making an attempt to explain them mechanistically.

This great gap in physiology will now be completely filled by the theory of selection and the theory of evolution which results directly from it. It shows us how all the infinitely complicated relations in which each organism occurs in relation to the environment, how the steady reciprocal action between it and all the organic and inorganic conditions of existence are not the premeditated arrangements of a Creator fashioning nature according to a plan but are the necessary effects of existing matter with its inalienable properties and their continual motion in time and space. Thus the theory of evolution explains the housekeeping relations of organisms mechanistically as the necessary consequences of effectual causes and so forms the monistic groundwork of ecology."

1869: Refined definition by Ernst Haeckel (1834–1919), appearing in the inaugural lecture he was invited to present to the philosophical faculty of Jena, as translated by W.C. Allee (Stauffer, 1957, p. 141).

"By ecology we mean the body of knowledge concerning the economy of nature–the investigation of the total relations of the animal both to its inorganic and to its organic environment; including, above all, its friendly and inimical relations with those animals and plants with which it comes directly or indirectly into contact–in a word, ecology is the study of all those complex interrelations referred to by Darwin as the conditions of the struggle for existence."

A century later:

Odum EP. *Fundamentals of Ecology*. 3rd ed. Philadelphia: Saunders, 1971 (Odum, 1971).

p. 3: "… As a recognized distinct field of biology, the science of ecology dates from about 1900, and only the past decade has the word become part of the general vocabulary…

The word ecology is derived from the Greek *oikos*, meaning "house" or "place to live." Literally, ecology is the study of organisms "at home." Usually ecology is defined as the study of the relation of organisms or groups of organisms to their environment, or the science of the interrelations between living organisms and their environment. Because ecology is concerned especially with the biology of *groups* (italics in original) of organisms and with the *functional* (italics in original) processes on the lands, in the oceans, and in fresh waters, it is more in keeping with the modern emphasis to define ecology as the study of the structure and function of nature, it being understood that mankind (*sic*) is a part of nature. One of the definitions in Webster's Unabridged Dictionary seems especially appropriate for the closing decades of the 20th century, namely, "*the totality or pattern of relations between organisms and their environment*" (italics in original). In the long run the best definition for a broad subject field is probably the shortest and least technical one, as, for example, 'environmental biology.'"

Contemporary:

McMichael AJ. *Human Frontiers, Environments, and Disease: Past Patterns, Uncertain Futures*. Cambridge: Cambridge University Press, 2001 (McMichael, 2001).

p. 17: "Ecology refers to the interconnected relationships between populations of plants and animals and between them and their natural environment. There is an emphasis on integration, interdependency, and feedback processes, all within a systems context. Ecological systems can be studied at different levels of organization: individual, organisms, populations, biotic communities, ecosystems, biomes, the biosphere, and the ecosphere."

p. 20: "Ecology is a way of observing and thinking about the complex natural word; it is integrative, not disaggregative."

Oxford English Dictionary On-Line. Draft revision June 2009. Available at: http://dictionary.oed.com.ezp-prod1.hul.harvard.edu/ (Accessed: June 16, 2009). (OED, 2009)

1a. The branch of biology that deals with the relationships between living organisms and their environment. Also: the relationships themselves, esp. those *of* a specified organism.
1b. Chiefly *Sociol.* The study of the relationships between people, social groups, and their environment; (also) the system of such relationships in an area of human settlement. Freq. with modifying word, as *cultural ecology, social ecology, urban ecology.*
1c. In extended use: the inter-relationship between any system and its environment; the product of this.

2. The study of or concern for the effect of human activity on the environment; advocacy of restrictions on industrial and agricultural development as a political movement; (also) a political movement dedicated to this.

self-designated scientific discipline (McIntosh, 1985; Bramwell, 1989; Worster, 1994; Merchant, 2002; Richard, 2008).

Since then, scholars in myriad fields have elaborated, contested, and applied various definitions and tenets of *ecology*. Critical and creative engagement with the ideas are evident not only in a variety of self-designated ecological disciplines (e.g., plant, animal, and aquatic ecology; theoretical, ecosystem, community, population, and behavioral ecology [McIntosh, 1985; Worster, 1994; Roughgarden, 1998; Hannan, 2001; Merchant, 2002; Jax, 2008; Taylor, 2008]) and other biological sciences (e.g., evolutionary biology and developmental biology [Eldredge & Grene, 1992; Eldredge, 1999; Lewontin, 2000; Buerton et al., 2000; Gilbert, 2001]) but also in public health (Honari & Boylen, 1999; McMichael, 2001; Rayner, 2009) and a range of social sciences—especially sociology, anthropology, geography, and psychology (Bronfenbrenner, 1979; Steiner & Nauser, 1993; Lawrence, 1993; Honari, 1999; McAdam, 2001; Merchant, 2002; Turner & Boyns, 2002; Turner, 2005).

Premises shared by all these "ecological" disciplines are:

1. understanding the mutual engagement of organisms and their environments requires analysis in relation to "level," "time," and "space"—and hence consideration of processes simultaneously involving spatiotemporal scale and both geographical and historical milieu;
2. individual "organisms" (including people) necessarily belong to "populations" and both together are dynamically are shaped by and shape their "environment;" hence:
3. ecological context matters, because it arrays the particular causal mechanisms that together (in their spatiotemporal relationships) produce the specified patterns of phenomena.

Corollaries are that causal arrows between organisms, populations, and their environments flow in both directions—albeit not necessarily with the same force (Eldredge, 1999;

Turner & Boyns, 2002; Turner, 2005)—and can produce both positive and negative feed-back. Moreover, the theorizing as to what relationships and processes result in organisms constituting "populations" and "communities" (by genealogical descent and by concurrent interactions [Eldrege & Grene, 1992; Grene & Depew, 2004]) is as essential as the theorizing as to what constitutes their "environs," with such definitional issues of considerable import to epidemiology as well (Krieger, 2007).

Agreement on these basic precepts, however, co-exists with sharp debates over their use, embroiling ecologically-oriented theorists within and across myriad disciplines, with different positions holding prominence at various points in time (McIntosh, 1985; Grene, 1987; Levin, 1992; Krieger, 1994; Worster, 1994; Barbour, 1996; Ellis, 1996; Bock & Goode, 1998; Merchant, 2002; Jax, 2008; Taylor, 2008; Krieger, 2008a). Far from there being one "ecological" perspective, "the evolution of scientific ecology in twentieth century," as summarized by the historian Carolyn Merchant, has included "human ecology, organismic ecology, economic ecology, and chaotic ecology" (Merchant, 2002, p. 159). Each of these distinct theoretical trends, moreover, has held "differing assumptions about nature and the human and ethical relationship to it" (Merchant, 2002, p. 172), whereby:

> Human ecology incorporates humans into nature and adapts to nature's limits; organismic ecology views humans as separate from nature, but as followers of its balanced, homeostatic processes; economic ecology asserts humans as scientific managers of a nature that can be controlled for human benefit; finally, chaotic ecology sees nature as having unpredictable characteristics, leaving humans as only partially able to manage its systems. Nature is thus far more complex than previously considered, and is best described as a disorderly, rather than a harmonious balance.

A similar analysis of ecology's intellectual debates and shifts is offered by the ecological theorist and conservation biologist Kurt Jax [Jax 2008, pp. 5-6]:

> Until about 1950, ecological theory, like that of many other disciplines at that time, was permeated by organismic notions, which emphasized the whole in contrast to the parts and likened ecological units and their 'development' to the individual organism. This also implied an equilibrium view of these units (and nature as a whole) and thus, although ecology was never really 'static,' it emphasized those processes that seemed to account for this overall balance of nature, while changes that did not fit into this scheme, e.g., 'catastrophes' like natural forest fires or insect outbreaks, were mostly considered to be irrelevant to ecological theory... By the mid-century the way in which ecological units was perceived was also changing... The new theory emphasized the individualistic reactions of different species, gradients more than sharp boundaries, and change instead of equilibria. It thus allows for stronger connections to evolutionary theory, and the view of ecological units as historical and contingent... Recent discourses struggling for a unification of ecological theory include the role of hierarchy, scale, and heterogeneity, as well as a new emphasis on individual species within ecosystems. The last development, in particular, points to the lasting importance of natural history in ecology, which–in spite of some attempts by the 'New Ecology' to base ecology exclusively on physical and mathematical categories–will always remain an essential part of ecological science.

In other words, ecology, like any science (including epidemiology), has had its share of theoretical debate, with different frameworks leading to very different research questions and discoveries.

Among the ecologists' wide-reaching arguments, several are resonant with parallel debates in epidemiology. All concern issues of level and spatiotemporal scale and their implications for both causal processes and causal inference (McIntosh, 1985; Levin, 1992; Lidicker, 1992; Worster, 1994; Barbour, 1996; Roughgarden, 1998; Keil et al., 1998; Peterson & Parker, 1998; O'Neill & King, 1998; Hobbs, 1998; Merchant, 2002; Neumann, 2005; Paulson & Gezon, 2005; Jax, 2008; Taylor, 2008). Three examples of such ecological debates, grounded substantively in ecological problems, are provided in **Textbox 7–3**. The first concerns problems of pattern in relation to spatial scale (Levin, 1992); the second involves problems of levels and temporal scale (including a wry commentary on a period when U.S. government funding for ecology favored strictly experimental design, resulting in a wave of ecological studies whose scope effectively equaled that of a dissertation— that is, limited spatial area and with at most 5 years of observation time—despite most ecological processes involving far vaster expanses of space and time) (May, 1998); and the third pertains to problems of levels in relation to causal processes, with debates over whether the causes of ecological succession and speciation are to be found in external environmental perturbations versus the intrinsic biological properties of organisms (Eldredge, 1999).

Framed in more abstract terms that can readily be transferred to epidemiologic examples, related debates concern:

1. the nature and boundaries of "levels," including whether "levels" are ontologically "real" versus analytic abstractions (noting that for the discussion to be about ecology, at least one level must be comprised of "organisms" and another their "environment," however defined);
2. the relationships between "levels," including
   a. whether or not they necessarily form "nested" versus "non-nested" hierarchies;
   b. whether or not "emergent properties" exist, whereby "higher" levels exhibit characteristics not reducible to those of "lower" level phenomena;
   c. whether phenomena at a given level are adequately explained by processes occurring at that level versus require explanation in relation to phenomena at another level ("higher" or "lower"), and the criteria by which this can be determined; and
   d. whether observed changes in phenomena at any given level are driven chiefly by interactions of phenomena at the "same" level (i.e., endogenous) versus by perturbations at "higher" or "lower" levels;
3. the dynamics of cross-level interactions, including whether or not the systems encompassing these interactions tend toward "equilibrium" versus not, and also whether or not "non-equilibrium" at "lower levels" or smaller spatiotemporal scales can co-exist with or even contribute to stability at "higher" levels and larger scales; and
4. the importance—or not—of (natural) history and historical contingency, and hence the extent to which particular events, patterns, or processes can be generalized, regardless of time and place.

Additional debates, specific to disciplines focused on analyzing people, concern how ecological concepts or metaphors at times have been used to "naturalize" social phenomena, thereby removing political and economic causes from view (Lawrence, 1993; Krieger, 1994; Chew & Laubichler, 2003); one classic example is the use of the plant succession model by 1930's Chicago school of "social ecology" to describe and explain the changing composition of city neighborhoods (Park, 1936a; Park, 1936b), as if it were a *natural* phenomenon, independent of the workings of the real estate industry in conjunction with the

Textbox 7–3. Three Examples of Debates Within Ecological Sciences About Patterns, Level, Spatiotemporal Scale, and Causal Processes.

Example from theoretical ecology:

Levin SA. The problem of pattern and scale in ecology: the Robert H. MacArthur Award lecture. *Ecology* 1992; 73:1943–1967. (Levin, 1992)

p. 1944: "Theoretical ecology, and theoretical science more generally, relates processes that occur on different scales of space, time, and organizational complexity. Understanding patterns in terms of the processes that produce them is the essence of science, and is key to the development of principles for management. Without an understanding of mechanism, one must evaluate each new stress on each new system de novo, without any scientific basis for extrapolation; with such understanding, one has the foundation for understanding and management. A popular fascination of theorists in all disciplines, because of the potential for mechanistic understanding, has been with systems in which the dynamics at one level of organization can be understood as the collective behavior of aggregates of similar units. Statistical mechanics, interacting particle systems, synergetics, neural networks, hierarchy theory, and other subjects all have concerned themselves with this problem...

... To scale from the leaf to the ecosystem to the landscape and beyond, we must understand how information is transferred from fine scales to broad scales, and vice versa...

... The reference to 'particular scales of interest' emphasizes a fundamental point: there is no single 'correct' scale on which to describe populations or ecosystems..."

p. 1945: "When we observe the environment, we necessarily do so on only a limited range of scales; therefore, our perception of events provides us with only a low-dimensional slice through a high-dimensional cake. In some cases, the scales of observation may be chosen deliberately to elucidate key features of the natural system; more often, the scales are imposed on us by our perceptual capabilities, or by technological or logistical constraints. In particular, the observed variability of the system will be conditional on the scale of description."

Example from ecological systems ecology:

May R. Levels of organization in ecological systems. In: Bock GR, Goode JA. *The Limits of Reductionism in Biology.* **(Novartis Foundation Symposium 213). Chichester, UK: John Wiley & Sons, 1998; pp. 193–202.** (May, 1998)

pp. 193–194: "In physics, there are rules which operate largely independently of time or place, but in biology one is dealing with systems which are in a sense reactive so that the whole picture becomes hugely more complicated. In biology, one cannot assume the laws are the same all places and at all times because they are hugely context dependent and the contexts change over evolutionary time. Moving beyond biology to the social sciences, it gets even worse: there are all the problems of the life sciences plus the fact that the entities under study are aware of what is happening and are modifying things in a conscious way."

p. 196: "**Spatial and temporal** scale (bold in original). The whole idea that one can understand one level in terms of the level below it can become difficult in some areas of science because the appropriate scale–either spatial or temporal–for controlled experiment is too large or long. This is a practical question that has caused a great deal of anguish in ecology. This problem is not unique to ecology; it is also encountered in cosmology. If you want to understand the history of the Universe, there are limits to the scope for manipulative experiments.

In the USA, the National Science Foundation (NSF) went through a rather irritating hiccup from the mid 1970s to the mid 1980s when a bunch of people (who didn't understand physics but thought that ecology ought to be more like what they thought physics was) decided that the NSF ecology programme really ought to be doing reductionist things, and reductionism got confused with doing manipulative experiments. The outcome of this was an interesting phase: if you look at the manipulative experiments in ecological studies published over this time, 75% were of a spatial scale of less than 10 metres and 95% of them were on a time scale of five years or less, the time scale of a PhD thesis (May 1994). It is not at all clear that the most important questions in understanding community structure and response to disturbance necessarily happen on a scale of less than a metre or over a timescale of three years or less."

p. 197: "In conclusion, I am an antireductionist in the sense that reductionism is often confused with saying all we need is brilliantly clever manipulative experiments that describe what is going on. I believe it is important to understand not just *what* is happening, but also how it is happening, and, ultimately, *why* it is happening (italics in original)…

Sometimes real understanding may necessitate looking at lower levels, building from physiology to individual behavior to population dynamics to community structure. More commonly, phenomenological understanding of the level in question–be it individual or population or ecosystem–will be sufficient for most purposes, and too simplistic a reductionist programme will be doomed by difficulties of spatial or temporal scales, or uniqueness of history."

Example from evolutionary biology:

Eldredge N. *The Pattern of Evolution*. New York: W.H. Freeman & Co., 1999. (Eldredge, 1999)

pp. 3–4: "This is a book that asks the question: How has evolutionary theory, involving ideas on how biological evolution happens, remained so disconnected from the domain of the rest of science–the world of matter-in-motion studied by physicists, chemists, and earth scientists?

This narrative is a search for that very connection, one that asks how patterns in the history of earth and of life can reveal what the connection must look like. And, by the final chapter, I propose the answer: The connection between the evolution of life and the physical history of the earth lies through ecology. I make the very strong claim that nothing much happens in biological evolutionary history until extinction claims what has come before. And species extinction is an ecological phenomenon: the fallout of ecosystem disruption, degradation, and eventual outright destruction."

p. 4: "… (the) conviction that everything from evolutionary history to the structures of ecosystems emanates from the competitive urges of genes, if anything, isolates evolutionary biology still further from the physical realm of matter-in-motion.

Ecological succession does not happen without physical destruction of mature ecosystems. This is true whether we're talking of fires in grasslands and forests, of storm damage to coral reefs… there is no way a clearing will appear through the simple lives and deaths of individual organisms. It takes an event, a physical event, to trigger succession.

Ecological succession–where pioneer species colonize degraded habit, eventually to be replaced as other species come to be re-established–is a process that produces pattern...

Patterns in the natural world is extremely important. As we shall see, they pose both the questions and the answers that scientists formulate as they seek to describe the world: the nature and behaviors of entities such as atoms and continents, or organisms, species, and ecosystems, according to one's particular bent and expertise. Science is a search for resonance between mind and natural pattern as we try to answer these questions."

banking and business sectors and politicians and civic leaders, including their enforcement of then legal racial residential segregation laws.

Ecosocial Theory of Disease Distribution: Ecology, Biology, the Political Economy of Health, and the Social Production of Science

How might the kinds of theoretical issues raised in these ecological debates be relevant to epidemiologic theories of disease distribution? *Ecosocial theory* offers one example. Paying heed to societal and ecologic context, to lifecourse and historical generation, to levels of analysis, to interrelationships between—and accountability for—diverse forms of social inequality, including racism, class, and gender, and to epidemiologists' context and conceptual frameworks, this theory asks, **"Who and what drives current and changing patterns of social inequalities in health?"** (Krieger, 1994). Clues are to be sought in the ways of living afforded by current and changing societal arrangements of power, property, and the production and reproduction of both social and biological life, involving people, other species, and the biophysical world in which we live. Core constructs of the theory, as currently elaborated, are provided in **Figure 7–1,** along with newly summarized key propositions in **Textbox 7–4.**

My choice of the term *ecosocial*—a term not employed in the health sciences until 1994, when I introduced it (and with only a handful of one-off uses in other literature at the time)—rather than, say, *biosocial*, was deliberate. The first and foremost reason was to capture, conceptually and substantively, the more expansive ecological frame of considering the dynamic social, biotic, and abiotic context in which all organisms (including people) and populations live, interact, and die. By calling explicit attention to biological processes and principles (Scheiner, 2010), while rejecting the tenets of biomedical reductionism, the goal was build on extant analyses of the "political economy of health" and the "social production of disease" (as reviewed in **Chapter 6**), whose frameworks, although extremely useful, are, as I have noted previously, biologically opaque, affording little insight into the biophysical phenomena relevant to translating societal conditions into population patterns of health, disease and well-being (Krieger, 1994; Krieger, 2001a). The second reason was to avoid any association with the narrow biological determinist perspective that *biosocial*, with its eugenics roots, has come to represent—especially in relation to analyses regarding race/ethnicity, gender, and social class (Harrison & Peel, 1969; Harrison & Peel, 1970; Fox, 1975; Brothwell, 1977; Mascie-Taylor, 1990; Walsh, 2004; Walsh & Beaver, 2009). Indicative of this genealogy is that the present-day *Journal of Biosocial Research*

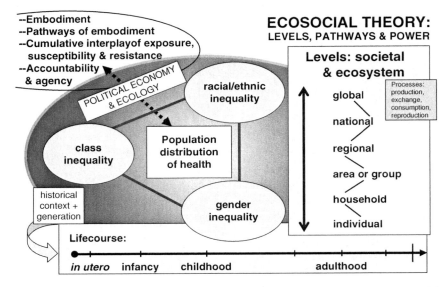

Figure 7–1. Ecosocial theory and embodying inequality: core constructs. (Krieger, 1994; Krieger, 2008a)

Core constructs, referring to processes <u>conditional upon extant political economy and political ecology</u>:

1. <u>Embodiment</u>, referring to how we literally incorporate, biologically, in societal and ecological context, the material and social world in which we live;

2. <u>Pathways of embodiment</u>, via diverse, concurrent, and interacting pathways, involving adverse exposure to social and economic deprivation; exogenous hazards (e.g., toxic substances, pathogens, and hazardous conditions); social trauma (e.g., discrimination and other forms of mental, physical, and sexual trauma); targeted marketing of harmful commodities (e.g., tobacco, alcohol, other licit and illicit drugs); Inadequate or degrading health care; and degradation of ecosystems, including as linked to alienation of indigenous populations from their lands

3. <u>Cumulative interplay of exposure, susceptibility, and resistance across the lifecourse</u>, referring to the importance of timing and accumulation of, plus responses to, embodied exposures, involving gene expression, not simply gene frequency; and

4. <u>Accountability and agency</u>, both for social disparities in health and research to explain these inequities.

(*Journal of Biosocial Science*, 2009) was, until 1968, called the *Eugenics Review* (founded in 1909) (Mazumdar, 2000).

To begin, the ecosocial question "Who and what is responsible for current and changing patterns of health inequities?" necessarily engages with the query "Who and what drives overall patterns and levels of morbidity and mortality?"—both among people and also, as warranted, among other species. It consequently is obligate, not optional, to link the theorizing to specific diseases, and their historically-specific and spatially-patterned rates and trends, both singly and in concert with other specific outcomes. Awareness of disease-specific patterns, including which are leading causes of morbidity and mortality in specified social groups at particular ages, at which historical moment, in turn is essential for comprehending the patterning of commonly used "summary" outcomes (e.g., all-cause mortality, premature mortality, and life expectancy). As ecosocial theory underscores,

Textbox 7–4. Ecosocial Theory: Core Propositions

1. People literally embody, biologically, their lived experience, in societal and eco-logic context, thereby creating population patterns of health and disease.
2. Societies' epidemiologic profile are shaped by the ways of living afforded by their current and changing societal arrangements of power, property, and the produc-tion and reproduction of both social and biological life, involving people, other species, and the biophysical world in which we live.
3. Determinants of current and changing societal patterns of disease distribution, including health inequities, are: (1) exogenous to people's bodies, and (2) manifest at different levels and involve different spatiotemporal scales, with macro-level phenomena are more likely to drive and constrain meso- and microlevel phenom-ena than vice versa; to the extent genes are relevant to societal distributions of disease, at issue is gene expression, rather than gene frequency.
4. In societies exhibiting social divisions based on property and power, and in which those with the most power and resources comprise a small percent of the popula-tion, the more prevalent the health outcome, the greater the absolute burden (and potentially the relative burden) on those with less power and fewer resources, as they comprise the majority of the population; a corollary is that for more rare or infrequent (nonendemic) diseases, it cannot be presumed, in advance, whether social inequalities in the outcome exist and, if they do, the direction of the gradi-ent.
5. Explanations of disease distribution cannot be reduced solely to explanations of disease mechanisms, as the latter do not account for why rates and patterns change, in complex ways, over time and place.
6. Practice of a reflexive epidemiology that situates in broader societal context an investigation's motivating theories, hypotheses, methods of analysis, and interpre-tation of findings will improve the likelihood of epidemiologists being better positioned to understand and convey the meanings and limitation of our study results and explanations for population patterns of health, disease and well-being.

indifference to rates of cause-specific morbidity and mortality, as evident in several of the sociopolitical theories reviewed in **Chapter 6**, precludes fully engaging with explaining—and altering—the actual burdens of ill-health experienced by real people in real time in real places.

The *first core construct of ecosocial theory* accordingly concerns **"embodiment."** The central claim is that we literally embody, biologically, our lived experience, in societal and ecologic context, thereby creating population patterns of health and disease (**Figure 7–1**). Embracing biology but not the dominant biomedical model, the idea of *embodiment* posits that determinants of current and changing societal patterns of disease distribution are exog-enous to people's bodies and cannot be reduced to allegedly "innate" characteristics, even as individual biological characteristics and variability do matter. Thus, even as ecosocial theory recognizes negative feedback can occur as a secondary phenomenon, whereby the societal context harms health, with poor health then further undermining possibilities for adequate resources for healthy living, it also emphasizes that the overwhelming weight of evidence places the primary causal arrow as leading from societal conditions to health status, as experienced from conception onward (Smith, 1999; World Health Organization Commission on the Social Determinants of Health [WHO CSDH], 2008).

Several corollaries stem from the idea of *embodiment*. The first is that understanding disease distribution requires analyzing it in dynamic context, a core ecological principle. To the extent genes are relevant to societal distributions of disease—and of course they are, because every biological process in some way involves genes (Buerton et al., 2000)—the construct of *embodiment* clarifies that when it comes to explaining population's overall and social patterning of health—and especially temporal shifts in this patterning (e.g., falling, stagnant, or rising rates of disease or of the magnitude of health inequities)—at issue is gene expression rather than gene frequency (a clarification I added after the initial formulation of ecosocial theory [Krieger, 1994], prompted by ongoing debates about causes of racial/ethnic health inequities and new research on epigenetics [Krieger, 2005a; Krieger, 2005b]).

A second corollary of *embodiment* is that observed differences in health status between population groups can causally result from group-relations, not intrinsic biology, even as the biological differences are manifested in individual bodies. Such a statement of course hinges on what (and who) defines "population" groups and choice of comparison groups (Krieger, 2007), a conceptual problem key to ecology as well. In the case of both humans and other species, one aspect of defining "population groups" involves both concurrent interactions and genealogical ancestry (Eldrege & Grene, 1992). Nevertheless, in the case of people, history matters in still another way, as reflected in the past and present social divisions that both: (*1*) create groups co-defined in relation to each other (e.g., owner/ employee, colonizer/Indigenous, free/slave, native-born/immigrant), (2) and establish the rules (*de jure* or *de facto*) determining how these groups differentially accumulate and inherit property, privileges, and other resources, concurrently and across generations. Exemplifying this point is how inequitable race relations can simultaneously socially produce, in historically specific ways, both racial/ethnic groups and their disparate health status (Krieger, 1999b; Krieger, 2000b; Krieger, 2003a; Krieger, 2005b; Gravlee, 2009; Kuzawa & Sweet, 2009; Krieger, 2010b).

Extending the idea of *embodiment* to include biological processes shaped by not only people's societal interactions but also our existence as a biological organisms who reproduce sexually, an ecosocial approach additionally encourages better contextualization of analyses, including comparisons, of the health of women and men (Krieger et al., 1993; Fee & Krieger, 1994; Krieger, 2003b). Rather than take as the starting assumption that all manifestations of reproductive health and any observed differences in the health status of women and men necessarily reflect "innate" and "natural" sexual distinctions, the construct of embodiment encourages asking both: (1) if women and men's membership in other socially-defiend groups (e.g., social classes) affects the extent of similarity (and not just difference) in their health status within and across these groups, and (2) if any on-average difference between women and men is observed, if it might arise from gender relations, not just sex-linked biology, or perhaps both, synergistically (Krieger, 2003b). Indeed, illustrating the importance of asking whether gender, sex-linked biology, both, or neither are relevant are the 12 examples provided in **Table 7–1** (Krieger, 2003b), with one such example being the association of parity with risk of both melanoma and heart disease among not only women but men, indicating that more than the potential biological effects of pregnancy are at issue (Kravdal, 1995; Lawlor et al., 2003). Together, these examples underscore why the ecosocial approach to embodiment and the interplay of biological and societal conditions matters for etiologic understanding and the modeling and interpreting of epidemiologic data.

The contextualized construct of embodiment likewise recognizes that socially-structured causal links between exposures and outcomes can vary over time and place, a proposition consonant with contemporary ecological theorizing. Nor are these shifts idiosyncratic;

Table 7–1. Selected Examples of Differential Roles of Gender Relations and Sex-Linked Biology on Health Outcomes: Only Gender, Only Sex-Linked Biology, Neither, and Both (Krieger, 2003b).

Case	Diagrammed illustration	Exposure—outcome association	Relevance of: Gender relations	Relevance of: Sex-linked biology	Explication
1	Gender relations Sex-linked biology exposure → health outcome	Greater prevalence of HIV/AIDS due to needle-stick injury among women compared to men health-care workers providing patient care (Ippolito et al., 1997)	Yes: of exposure	No	• Gender relations: determinant of risk of exposure (needle-stick injury), via gender segregation of the workforce (e.g., greater likelihood of women being nurses) • Sex-linked biology: not a determinant of risk of exposure • Risk of outcome, given exposure: risk of seroconversion same among women and men
2	Gender relations Sex-linked biology exposure → health outcome	Greater prevalence of contact lens microbial keratitis among men compared to women contact lens wearers (Liesegang, 1997)	Yes	No	• Gender relations: determinant—among those wearing contact lenses—of risk of exposure to improperly cleaned contact lenses (men less likely to properly clean them than women) • Sex-linked biology: not a determinant of exposure • Risk of outcome, given exposure: risk of contact lens microbial keratitis same among women and men, once exposed to improperly cleaned contact lenses
3	Gender relations Sex-linked biology exposure → health outcome	Greater prevalence of short stature and gonadal dysgenesis among women with Turner's syndrome compared to unaffected women (Ranke & Saenger, 2001)	No	Yes: of exposure	• Gender relations: not a determinant of exposure (X-monosomy, total or mosaic, or nonfunctional X chromosome) • Sex-linked biology: determinant of exposure • Risk of outcome, given exposure: not influenced by gender relations

Case	Diagrammed illustration	Exposure—outcome association	Relevance of:		Explication
			Gender relations	Sex-linked biology	
4	Gender relations Sex-linked biology exposure ⟶ health outcome	Both similar and different adverse health outcomes among women and men and due to ubiquitous exposure to cooking oil contaminated by polychlorinated biphenyls (PCBs) ("Yusho" disease) (Aoki, 2001)	No	Yes: of exposed	• Gender relations: not a determinant of risk of exposure (ubiquitous exposure to the contaminated cooking oil, in staple foods) • Sex-linked biology: not a determinant of risk of exposure • Risk of outcome, given exposure: partly influenced by sex-linked biology, in that although both women and men experienced chloracne and other dermal and ocular lesions, only women experienced menstrual irregularities
5	Gender relations Sex-linked biology exposure ⟶ health outcome	Higher risk of stroke among both women and men in the U.S. "stroke belt" in several Southern states, compared women and men in other regions of the United States (as distinct from differences in risk for women and men within a given region) (Pickle & Gillum, 1999)	No	No	• Gender relations: not a determinant of risk of exposure (living in the U.S. "stroke belt") • Sex-linked biology: not a determinant of risk of exposure • Risk of outcome, given exposure: neither gender relations nor sex-linked biology determine regional variation in stroke rates among men and among women (even as both may contribute to within-region higher risks among men compared to women)

6	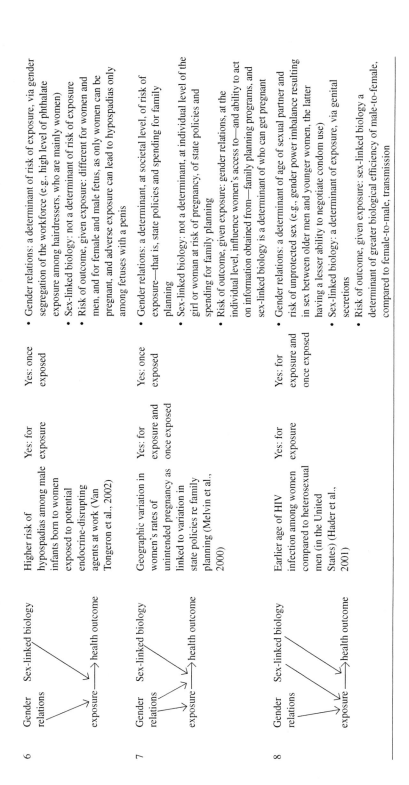Gender relations / Sex-linked biology / exposure → health outcome	Higher risk of hypospadias among male infants born to women exposed to potential endocrine-disrupting agents at work (Van Tongeron et al., 2002)	Yes: for exposure	Yes: once exposed	• Gender relations: a determinant of risk of exposure, via gender segregation of the workforce (e.g., high level of phthalate exposure among hairdressers, who are mainly women) • Sex-linked biology: not a determinant of risk of exposure • Risk of outcome, given exposure: different for women and men, and for female and male fetus, as only women can be pregnant, and adverse exposure can lead to hypospadias only among fetuses with a penis
7	Gender relations / Sex-linked biology / exposure → health outcome	Geographic variation in women's rates of unintended pregnancy as linked to variation in state policies re family planning (Melvin et al., 2000)	Yes: for exposure and once exposed	Yes: once exposed	• Gender relations: a determinant, at societal level, of risk of exposure—that is, state policies and spending for family planning • Sex-linked biology: not a determinant, at individual level of the girl or woman at risk of pregnancy, of state policies and spending for family planning • Risk of outcome, given exposure: gender relations, at the individual level, influence women's access to—and ability to act on information obtained from—family planning programs, and sex-linked biology is a determinant of who can get pregnant
8	Gender relations / Sex-linked biology / exposure → health outcome	Earlier age of HIV infection among women compared to heterosexual men (in the United States) (Hader et al., 2001)	Yes: for exposure	Yes: for exposure and once exposed	• Gender relations: a determinant of age of sexual partner and risk of unprotected sex (e.g., gender power imbalance resulting in sex between older men and younger women, the latter having a lesser ability to negotiate condom use) • Sex-linked biology: a determinant of exposure, via genital secretions • Risk of outcome, given exposure: sex-linked biology a determinant of greater biological efficiency of male-to-female, compared to female-to-male, transmission

			Relevance of:		
Case	Diagrammed illustration	Exposure—outcome association	Gender relations	Sex-linked biology	Explication
9	Sex-linked biology Gender relations exposure (a) → health outcome exposure(b)	Parity among both women and men associated with increased risk of melanoma (Kravdal, 1995)	Yes: for exposures	Yes: for exposure	• Gender relations: a determinant of parity (via expectations of who has children, at what age) • Sex-linked biology: a determinant of who can become pregnant and pregnancy-linked hormonal levels • Risk of outcome, given exposure: decreased risk of melanoma among nulliparous women and men indicates non-reproductive factors linked to parity may affect risk among both women and men, even as pregnancy-related hormonal factors may also affect women's risk
10	Sex-linked biology Gender relations exposure → health outcome	Greater referral of men compared to women for interventions for acute coronary syndromes (Feldman & Silver, 2000)	Yes: of exposure and once exposed	Yes: of exposure	• Gender relations: a determinant of how people present and physicians interpret symptoms of acute coronary syndromes • Sex-linked biology: a determinant of age at presentation (men are more likely to have acute infarction at younger ages) and possibly type of symptoms • Risk of outcome, given exposure: gender relations are a determinant of physician likelihood of referral for diagnostic and therapeutic interventions (women less likely to be referred, especially at younger ages)
11	Sex-linked biology Gender relations exposure → health outcome	Earlier age at onset of perimenopause among women experiencing greater cumulative economic deprivation over the life-course (Wise et al., 2002)	Yes: of exposure	Yes: as outcome	• Gender relations: a determinant of poverty, across the life-course, among women (via the gender gap in earnings and wealth) • Sex-linked biology: a determinant of who can experience perimenopause • Risk of outcome, given exposure: risk of earlier age at perimenopause among women subjected to greater economic deprivation across the lifecourse, including non-smokers, may reflect impact of poverty on oocyte depletion

| 12 | Gender relations Sex-linked biology 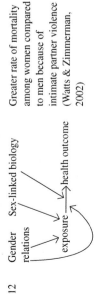 →health outcome | Greater rate of mortality among women compared to men because of intimate partner violence (Watts & Zimmerman, 2002) | Yes: of exposure | Yes: of exposure and once exposed | • Gender relations: a determinant of likelihood of men vs. women using physical violence against intimate partners, plus being encouraged to and having access to resources to increase physical strength
• Sex-linked biology: a determinant of muscle strength and stamina, at a given level of training and exertion, and also body size
• Risk of outcome, given exposure: risk of lethal assault related to on average greater physical strength and size of men and gender-related skills and training in inflicting and warding off physical attack |

Krieger, 2003

instead, as posited by ecosocial theory's fourth proposition (*see* **Textbox 7–4**), within a context of inequitable societies in which a small minority possess more power and resources than the larger majority, the more prevalent the outcome, the greater the burden—absolutely, if not also relatively—among those worse off, precisely because they comprise the bulk of society. Two ready examples are smoking and HIV/AIDS, both of which have displayed a clear reversal in their socioeconomic gradient during the twentieth century as their prevalence increased, shifting from positive (higher among the more affluent) to negative (higher among the more impoverished), a reversal that happened first in the global North followed by the global South (Graham, 1996; Brandt, 2007; Piot et al., 2007; Gillespie et al., 2007; Hargreaves et al., 2008). The implication is that explanations of disease distribution cannot be reduced solely to explanations of disease mechanisms or to static notions of "status" or "fundamental causes," as the latter do not account for why actual disease rates and patterns of health inequities change, in complex ways, over time and place.

Embodiment, for epidemiology, thus entails consideration of more than simply "phenotypes," "genotypes," and a vaguely defined "environment" eliciting "gene–environment interactions" in some vaguely defined "population" (Krieger, 2005a; Krieger, 2007). We live embodied: "genes" do not interact with the environs outside the body; only organisms do, and do so intrinsically as members of populations. These interactions have consequences, moreover, for not only gene regulation and expression (Krieger, 2005a) but also, equally if not more critical, for changing the very "environment" at issue. Embodiment is thus more than just about how social conditions "get under the skin" (Adler & Ostrove, 1999; Lupien et al., 2001; Adler & Rehkopf, 2008) or become "biologically embedded" (Hertzman, 1999; Hertzman & Siddiqi, 2009; Shonkoff et al., 2009), as phrased in some of the contemporary psychosocial and population health literature. *Embodiment* instead is far more active and reciprocal, the word itself being a verb-like noun that emphasizes our bodily engagement (soma and psyche combined), individually and collectively, with the biophysical world and each other (Krieger, 2005a).

In its use of the construct of *embodiment*, ecosocial theory not only draws on biological and ecological theories (Scheiner, 2010) but also builds on and extends sociological and anthropological scholarship. In these disciplines, *embodiment* has referred principally to the bodily implications of cultural practices and beliefs (e.g., in relation to diet and cuisine, religion, family formation, sexuality, and social identities) (Bourdieu, 1984; Csordas, 1994; O'Donovan-Anderson, 1996; Nettleton & Watson, 1998; Fox, 1999; Weiss & Haber, 1999; Kauppi, 2000; Crossley, 2005; Cregan, 2006)—albeit with analyses, until recently, tending to eschew any reference to actual biological processes. The ecosocial approach to *embodiment* likewise offers a useful bridge to novel twenty-first century research in the cognitive and neurosciences, which are providing new evidence on the centrality of bodily sensory-motor experiences and interactions (with both other organisms and the broader biophysical context) to the development and expression of both cognition and behavior (Lakoff & Johnson, 1999; Damasio, 2003; Niedenthal, 2007; Gomila & Calvo, 2008). Thus, *embodiment* conceptually stands as a deliberate corrective to dominant disembodied and decontextualized accounts of "genes," "behaviors," and mechanisms of disease causation, offering in their place an integrated approach to analyzing the multilevel processes, from societal and ecological to subcellular, that co-produce population distributions of health, disease, and well-being (Krieger, 2005a).

Building on this first construct, the **second core ecosocial construct** postulates that there typically are **multiple pathways of embodiment** contributing to disease distribution (requiring attention to specificity of exposures), with the **third core construct** calling attention to the joint **interplay of exposure, susceptibility, and resistance**, at *multiple levels,* across the *life-course*, in relation to historical generation (**Figure 7–1**). At the broadest level, this structured complexity, akin to that of ecological systems, simultaneously allows for both recognizable patterns of disease distribution *and* historical contingency in their specific societal manifestations. Any given forest, after all, is unique–while at the same time sharing, with other forests, common features that characterize what a forest is, how it functions, and how it changes over time. The existence of discernable yet distinct patterns recurrently arising out of the interplay of particular causal mechanisms—within and across levels that are brought together and entangled via the context of specific times and places— is a hallmark of ecologic, and indeed all historically emergent, phenomena.

The implications of ecosocial theory's second and third constructs are illustrated by their juxtaposition to the still influential "epidemiologic transition" theory (Omran, 1971; Omran, 1977; Omran, 1983; Mackenbach, 1994), which typically has been deterministically interpreted as holding that as societies economically "develop," their declining mortality rates universally exhibit successive temporally discrete patterns of epidemiologic profiles, shifting from predominantly infectious to non-communicable chronic disease. By contrast, ecosocial theory—like contemporary ecologic theory (Roughgarden, 1998; Eldredge, 1999; Merchant, 2002; Taylor, 2008)—would not presume orderly succession as the norm or "law." It instead would anticipate—and provides the basis for understanding— the existence of multiple co-existing epidemiologic profiles, within and across societies, over time. Such historically and geographically contingent patterns would be expected, as shaped by each society's range of societal divisions and the extent to which different societal groups have access to a functional public health infrastructure (including sanitation and potable water), are employed in safe jobs, are democratically enfranchised, and do not live in environmentally polluted and ecologically degraded regions.

Supporting this alternative conceptualization, extant evidence indicates that the extent of mortality declines and contributions of specific causes of mortality within countries display marked social inequities (especially in relation to class and race/ethnicity), with impoverished persons worldwide increasingly dying from chronic non-communicable diseases even as they continue disproportionately to bear the burden of infectious disease mortality (Frenk et al., 1989; Kunitz, 1992; Gaylin & Kates, 1997; Heuveline et al., 2002; Palazzo et al., 2003; Kunitz, 2006; Birns et al., 2009). That the non-universality of the "epidemiologic transition" is still flagged as noteworthy 20 years after articles began to detail exceptions in turn attests to the persistence of a linear "succession" model in contemporary epidemiologic thought.

Moreover, as applied to the case of health inequities, the multiple pathways delineated by ecosocial theory's second construct—potentially spanning multiple levels and playing out at different spatiotemporal scales—can involve adverse exposures to, along with differential societal and biological susceptibility and resistance to (Krieger, 1999b; Krieger, 2006; Krieger, 2008a; Krieger, 2009):

1. economic and social deprivation;
2. toxic substances, pathogens, and hazardous conditions;
3. discrimination and other forms of socially inflicted trauma (mental, physical, and sexual, directly experienced or witnessed, from verbal threats to violent acts);
4. targeted marketing of harmful commodities (e.g., "junk" food and psychoactive substances such as tobacco, alcohol, and other licit and illicit drugs);
5. inadequate or degrading health care; and
6. degradation of ecosystems, including as linked to systematic alienation of Indigenous populations from their lands and corresponding traditional economies.

Textbox 7–5. Case Example: Disease Distribution Resulting from Lead
Exposure in the Twentieth Century United States—
An Ecosocial Approach

Starting with specifying time and place, say, in the twentieth century in the United States, ecosocial theory would direct attention to the possibilities of lead exposure being shaped by societal and ecosystem phenomena at multiple levels (individual, household, area or group, regional, national, global), via processes involving production, exchange, consumption, and reproduction (Elreedy et al., 1999; Markowitz & Rosner, 2002; Krieger et al., 2003; Richardson, 2005; Rosner & Markowitz, 2007; Morello-Frosch & Lopez, 2006; Bellinger, 2008; Wigle et al., 2008; Hanchette, 2008; Vaziri, 2008).

—These processes, shaped by inequitable class, racial/ethnic, and gender relations, could involve: exposures in the neighborhood (e.g., from lead-contaminated soil, caused by past and present car exhaust from leaded fuel), exposures at work (e.g., in production processes; in recycling of old batteries), or at home (e.g., from old lead paint and lead-contaminated tap water).

—Contributing to each of these exposures is corporate-driven use of lead in gasoline, in industrial processes, and in products (e.g., house paint, plumbing fixtures), recognizing that exposures from the past can be subject to transgenerational transmission, because during pregnancy lead from pregnant woman's bones can be mobilized into her bloodstream, travel across the placenta, and enter the fetus (Markowitz & Rosner, 2002; Richardson, 2005; Maas et al., 2005; Morello-Frosch & Lopez, 2006; Rosner & Markowitz, 2007; Rastogi et al., 2007; Carter-Pokras et al., 2007; Jacobs et al., 2007; Bellinger, 2008; Hanchette, 2008; Vaziri, 2008).

—Conditions affecting susceptibility to lead exposure can thus include age at exposure (e.g., greater neurotoxicity of low doses at young ages, especially adversely affecting developing brains) as well as potentially co-exposure to neurotoxicants and cognitive deprivation caused by economic impoverishment of not only families but school districts (Richardson, 2005; Rosner & Markowitz, 2007; Bellinger, 2008; Wigle, 2008).

—Phenomena relevant to resistance include not only decades of community and consumer activism and lawsuits to: (1) ban lead from gasoline, household paint, and other commercial products, (2) pass laws requiring landlords to implement lead abatement in rental units with lead-based paints (albeit with many such programs typically underfunded and unenforced), and (3) establish state public health department lead screening programs and tap-water testing programs (likewise increasingly underfunded) (Markowitz & Rosner, 2002; Richardson, 2005; Maas et al., 2005; Jacobs et al., 2007) but also, at the individual-level, lead screening for pregnant women and provision of calcium and iron supplements to lessen release of lead from the bones (Rastogi et al., 2007).

—Considering these different pathways of embodiment, along with the cumulative interplay of exposure, susceptibility, and resistance, can help provide insight into why, despite declining levels of lead exposure, chiefly because of the removal of lead from gasoline, those most exposed and subjected to its harms continue to be U.S. children of color, born and/or residing in low-income racially segregated urban neighborhoods (Markowitz & Rosner, 2002; Krieger et al., 2003; Richardson, 2005; Morello-Frosch & Lopez, 2006; Carter-Pokras et al., 2007; Hanchette, 2008).

—Analogous racialized and economic inequities in other countries (e.g., France) provide evidence of how such disease distributions are produced and reproduced by similar societal processes (Fassin & Naudé, 2004).

Of these six pathways, I initially demarcated the first five as part of conceptualizing the ways in which racism can harm health (Krieger, 1999a). I recently added the sixth after useful engagement with social geographers regarding racism, place, and health, especially as applied to Indigenous peoples (Kearns et al., 2009; Krieger, 2009).

The point of conceptualizing these diverse pathways is not to attempt to include them all in any given study—that would be unrealistic and absurd (Krieger, 2006), a point also underscored in analyses of ecological complexity. Instead, as per Sydenstricker's 1933 recommendation discussed in **Chapter 4** (Sydenstricker, 1933, p. 206), the aim should be to guide substantive theorizing about likely exposures, potential confounders, and effect modifiers, each in relation to social groups, levels, time, and space, and also their likely impact (e.g., population attributable fraction), as some determinants are likely more responsible for the population burden of disease (i.e., rate and distribution) than others. As illustrated by the example of lead exposure and its associated ailments provided in **Textbox 7–5**, such systematic conceptualization can aid formulation of study hypotheses, study design, and statistical analyses, and also promote awareness of likely omitted variables (*in toto*, or at particular levels or time periods), thereby improving quality of causal inference. It can likewise guide public health efforts by directing attention to the causal processes with the greatest population impact (Sydenstricker, 1993, p. 206; Morris, 1957), overall and in relation to health inequities.

The *fourth core ecosocial construct* consequently pertains to **accountability and agency**, both for the actual health inequities and for ways in which they are monitored, analyzed and addressed (**Figure 7–1**). Drawing explicitly on a "political economy of health" framework (*see* **Chapter 6**) and its analyses of how political and economic systems drive population profiles of disease and patterns of health inequities (Doyal, 1979; Krieger, 2001a), this ecosocial construct directs attention to issues of power at each and every level, and hence to institutions' and individual people's capacity to act ("agency") and their responsibility ("accountability") for both actions taken and avoided. Recognition of the capacity for action at each level—action that may be directed at the same, higher, or lower levels—does not mean this capacity (and consequent accountability) is equivalent across levels. Instead, ecosocial theory posits, in line with more recent sociological, ecological, and biological theorizing (Eldrege & Grene, 1992; O'Neill & King, 1998; May, 1998; Rose, 1998; Eldredge, 1999; McAdam et al., 2001; Turner & Boyns, 2002; Grene & Depew, 2004; Turner, 2005), that macrolevel phenomena are more likely to drive and constrain meso- and microlevel phenomena than vice versa—even as, under particular circumstances, the micro can powerfully affect the macro. If that were not the case, then individuals organizing collectively to change their context despite the odds would never succeed—yet they have, as attested to by the historical facts of popular movements that have abolished slavery and legal racial discrimination, ended colonial rule and dictatorships, enfranchised women, decriminalized homosexuality, and established welfare states providing social protection, including viable public health infrastructures and policies (Hobsbawm, 1994; Porter, 1999; Zinn, 2003).

Ecosocial theory additionally recognizes, in its analysis of accountability and agency, that causal relations need not be "linear" but can skip levels (Krieger, 2008a). One example is that a national government's recognition of a right that inheres in individuals (usually occurring after the affected individuals have organized—as a social group—to demand this right) can enable individuals to exercise rights in ways that affect "intermediate" institutions (Krieger, 2008a). A case in point was the U.S. Supreme Court's 1973 ruling recognizing individuals' right to privacy, which enabled women to obtain abortions by overturning federal and state laws interfering with this right to privacy (Goldstein, 1994). This decision both: (*1*) directly affected individual women's and girls' reproductive right, and (*2*) reverberated up to other levels, by requiring changes in state laws and expanding the permitted range of services that could be provided by health professionals and health facilities (Krieger, 2008a). The positive health effects were immediate, as women were no longer forced, by law, to face the risk of unsafe illegal abortion, and they were also less likely to bear unwanted children, thereby reducing risk of adverse maternal and health outcomes (Lanham et al., 1974; Institute of Medicine, 1975; Pakter & Nelson, 1975; Lee et al., 1980). More recent U.S. Supreme Court decisions restricting the right to abortion likewise illustrate this principle of skipping levels, with contrary effects (Wright & Katz, 2006).

Ecosocial theory thus points to the danger of the socially, temporally, and spatially constrained "upstream/downstream" metaphor so common in social epidemiology (Evans et al., 1994; Marmot & Wilkinson, 1999; McKinlay & Marceau, 2000; Evans & Stoddart, 2003; Hofrichter et al., 2003; Glass & McAtee, 2006; March & Susser, 2006b; Gehlert et al., 2008; Franks & Fiscella, 2008; WHO CSDH, 2008), one premised on the "proximal/distal" logic that informs the dominant biomedical approach (Krieger, 2008a). Not only does the "upstream/downstream" metaphor make discrete and sequential societal and biological processes that, in fact, are occurring simultaneously at different spatiotemporal scales and levels, but it also obscures agency and renders it difficult to conceptualize how "downstream" factors can influence "upstream" phenomena. Yet, as the construct of "embodiment" makes clear, there is nothing distant about having reproductive rights—just as there is nothing distal about being impoverished and its impact on health.

Thus, in the case of public health, the social fact that individuals have repeatedly created organizations, and even social movements, to counter the health-harming actions of dominant institutions (Doyal, 1979; Sanders, 1985; Krieger & Bassett, 1986; Tesh, 1988; Krieger et al., 1993; Krieger & Margo, 1994; Fee & Krieger, 1994; Doyal, 1995; Krieger & Birn, 1998; Porter, 1999; McAdam et al., 2001; Navarro & Shi, 2001; Markowitz & Rosner, 2002; Hofrichter, 2003; Biersack & Greenberg, 2006; Solar & Irwin, 2006; Lefkowitz, 2007; Birn et al., 2009) underscores ecosocial theory's emphasis on considering agency and accountability at all levels. Keeping these principles in mind is likely to enhance epidemiologists' ability to generate and test hypotheses—and offer richer evidence—to public health policies, programs, and interventions increasingly attempting to adopt an "ecological" orientation to improve population health and reduce health inequities (Kickbush, 1989; McMichael, 2001; McLaren & Hawe, 2005; Rayner, 2009).

Ecosocial theory's explicit attention to spatiotemporal scale is likewise in accord with ecologists' recognition that the time-scales on which most human political and economic institutions act are considerably shorter than those of most ecosystem processes (Hobbs, 1998). Emphasizing that the same temporal concerns apply to most human life-course and transgenerational biological processes, ecosocial theory thus underscores the importance of considering appropriately long timeframes for epidemiologic analyses and interpretation (Krieger, 2005b; Kunitz, 2006; Krieger, 2007; Krieger et al., 2008). Underscoring why concern about disease specificity and spatiotemporal scale matters, were racial discrimination and poverty to be eliminated in an instant, their embodied health consequences would nevertheless persist for at least one if not several generations for many diseases, especially for chronic conditions that develop over time and for which risk of incidence may be transgenerational, such as diabetes, cancer, and cardiovascular disease—even as for some outcomes change could happen quickly (e.g., diseases preventable by access to clean water and to vaccines, or mortality preventable by effective medical interventions) (Krieger, 2005a; Krieger et al., 2008; Krieger, 2008b; Krieger, 2010b). It is not ideology, but reality, that explains why societal determinants of health are as powerful and enduring as they are.

Additionally, by calling attention to epidemiologists' active role in framing and conducting science, in context, the construct of *agency and accountability* highlights the importance of critically analyzing epidemiologic theories of disease distribution. Useful insights for guiding such critiques can be obtained from recent scholarship—including debates over—both the social production of science (Ziman, 2000; Kitcher, 2001; Keller, 2002; Jasanaoff, 2004a; Jasanoff, 2004b; Jasanoff, 2004c; Haraway, 2004; Starbuck, 2006; Wersky, 2007; Hamlin, 2007) and the framework of *critical realism* (Bhaskar, 1978; Grene, 1987; Archer et al., 1998; Ziman, 2000). The biophysical material world we inhabit and our societies and their contending ideas are not simply anything we imagine or declare them to be—but neither are our theories simply a "mirror" of "objective reality." Consider only the long history of debates over racial/ethnic health inequities, discussed in **Chapters 4** and **6** (Krieger & Bassett, 1986; Krieger, 1987; Ernst & Harris, 1999; Krieger, 2003a; Jackson & Weidman, 2004; Krieger, 2005b; Krieger, 2010b). The fact that epidemiologists in the same societies, at the same point in time, have proffered profoundly different approaches to analyzing and explaining disease distribution—with some "naturalizing" health inequities, and others contesting their inevitability—is a testament to the responsibility of epidemiologists, as scientists, for our ideas, both what we consider and what we ignore.

A final point is that as with any coherent scientific theory, none of ecosocial theory's four core constructs stands alone or should be used in isolation (Krieger, 2010c). Instead, the intellectual and empirical challenge is to integrate them to afford a richer understanding of the causal processes at play and hence better inform efforts both to improve population health and reduce health inequities.

To aid in this task of intellectual integration, ecosocial theory from the start has employed a fractal metaphor "marrying the metaphor of the continually-constructed 'scaffolding' of society that different social groups daily seek to reinforce or alter to that of the ever-growing 'bush' of evolution, together defining the potential and constraints of human life" (Krieger, 1994, p. 897). Fractals, a type of object that exhibits self-similarity at multiple scales, are but one of the many discoveries of the new sciences of "chaos" and "complexity," emerging in the late twentieth century and concerned with non-equilibrium dynamics and self-organizing systems (Mandelbrot, 1982; Prigogine, 1984; Gleik, 1987; Kelso, 2002; Erdí, 2008; Mitchell, 2009). Evident in both biological and geological structures, and involving iterative processes happening over time, examples of fractals include the simultaneously spatial and genealogical branching of trees, of alveoli in the lungs, of synapses in neural networks, of streambeds and river deltas, just as they also encompass the temporal patterns of the heart rate and the folding of DNA (Mandelbrot, 1982; Gleik, 1987; Goldberger et al., 1990; Lipsitz & Goldberger, 1992; Goldberger, 1996; Goldberger et al., 2002; Kelso, 2002; Mitchell, 2009; Ball, 2009; Lieberman-Aiden et al., 2009). Relevant especially to phenomena whose biophysical manifestation depends on both initial conditions and subsequent perturbations, fractals can thus provide a useful way of conceptualizing and generating hypotheses about the origins of complex patterned structures that exist in space and time—which, after all, is one way to conceive of disease distributions (Philippe, 1993; Krieger, 1999a; Mutch & Lefevre, 2003).

Key aspects of the ecosocial fractal metaphor (illustrated in **Figure 7–2**) are that it dynamically captures the *integral intertwining of societal and biological features at each and every level*. Well-expressing its orientation is the biologist Joseph Needham's 1936 recognition that "in the living organism there is no spatial structural with an activity as something over against it, but that the concrete organism is a spatio-temporal structure and that this spatio-temporal structure is the activity itself" (Needham, 1936, p. 6). With societal and biological history revealed through both the making of the "scaffold" and the branching of "bush," the image avoids the problematic usage of solely "organic" or "mechanical" metaphors to describe human societies and population health (Lopez, 2003). Instead, its underlying intertwined fractal form simultaneously conveys, by the "scaffold," the purposive activity by people (Lajoi, 2005) while at the same time drawing on the deep-rooted imagery of the "Tree of Life," both as it appears in diverse mythological traditions from around the globe (Cook, 1988; Tudge, 2005, p. 7) and as first proposed by Charles Darwin in 1859 to show the genealogical connection of species in evolutionary history (Darwin, 1859 [2004], pp. 140–141, 162–163; Eldredge, 2005, pp. 103–109). Elaborated since in light of expanding knowledge about species and speciation (Graves, 2003; Maddison & Schulz, 2007), Darwin's "tree" has grown to become an ever more prolific "bush," to the point where some biologists are questioning whether the "tree" or "bush" still serves to capture evolutionary relationships, given growing appreciation of "horizontal" gene transfer between many unicellular forms of life, which comprise the most common type of life on earth (Doolittle & Bapteste, 2007; Lawton, 2009). Even so, the "bush" continues to convey a dynamic sense of integral relationships involving biological organisms that occur in time and place, i.e., the very phenomena at the heart of ecological thinking. What happens in a subcellular organelle of a cell is as much a part of the interplay of the societal and biological as are population distributions of disease; the "social" and "biological" cannot neatly be cleaved (Krieger, 1994). A distinguishing feature of ecosocial theory is thus that it posits that it is mandatory, not optional, to frame epidemiologic analysis in relation to historical, societal, biological, evolutionary, and ecologic context—both that of the populations being studied and the scientists doing the research.

Political Ecology: A Useful Model

Granted, the intellectual and empirical agenda proposed by the ecosocial theory of disease distribution is ambitious. Suggesting, however, its approach is warranted and feasible is the growing stream of scholarship appearing under the rubric *political ecology* (Atkinson, 1993; Greenberg & Park, 1994; Keil et al., 1998; Low & Gleeson, 1998; Escobar, 1999; Stonich, 2001; Whiteside, 2002; Forsyth, 2003; Robbins, 2004; Neumann, 2005; Paulson & Gezon, 2005; Biersack & Greenberg, 2006; Taylor, 2008). Like ecosocial theory, this body of work explicitly emerged in the mid-1990s (Atkinson, 1993; Greenberg & Park, 1994; Forsyth, 2003; Neumann, 2005; Biersack, 2006), but because until recently its focus has not included public health, I only became conversant with its literature starting in 2007, well over a decade after starting to conceptualize ecosocial theory.

In brief, *political ecology*, like ecosocial theory, has devoted considerable theorizing to understanding how societal conditions become expressed as biophysical realities—albeit with the terrain of argument literally being that of the Earth's myriad local, regional, and global ecoscapes and with the substantive focus turned to societal—and especially political and economic—determinants of ecological processes (Greenberg & Park, 1994; Keil et al., 1998; Escobar, 1999; Stonich, 2001; Forsyth, 2003; Robbins, 2004; Neumann, 2005; Paulson & Gezon, 2005; Biersack & Greenberg, 2006). Topics analyzed have included, among others, the societal determinants and ecological impacts of economic development, agribusiness, industrial pollution, global climate change, fishery management, deforestation, water rights and water use, land tenure, land dispossession, land degradation, expropriation of Indigenous resources, bioprospecting, consumer culture, and sustainable trade (Keil et al., 1998; Robbins, 2004; Neumann, 2005; Pauslon & Geizon, 2005; Biersack & Greenberg, 2006).

The orientation, as with ecosocial theory, is to analyzing dynamic interactions, typically involving conflicts about power, property, and privilege expressed at multiple spatiotemporal scales, sites, and levels. Moreover, consonant with other ecological theorizing, the

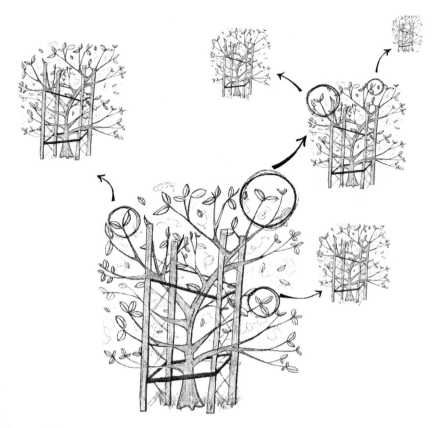

Figure 7–2. Ecosocial Theory: Illustration of Fractal Metaphor of Entwined "Scaffolding of Society" and "Bush of Life"—and Rationale for the Metaphor (Krieger, 1994)

Ecosocial metaphor pp. 896–897: "Perhaps one step toward developing an ecosocial metaphor would be augmenting the metaphor of the 'web' with two 'spiders': one social, one biologic. They would certainly reintroduce the concepts of history and agency, and would emphasize the importance of considering the origins of both social and biologic determinants of disease. Even so, the imagery of the 'spiders' may be too simplistic, and may fail to do justice to the complex origin and nature of the 'spiders' themselves. It is of little help to posit that health and disease are socially produced within evolving and socially-conditioned biologic parameters without offering insight into why and how this occurs; reducing the 'spiders' to a new form of 'black box' would only reinforce existing limitations. Nor would introducing the 'spiders' necessarily resolve the 'web's' embodiment of a biomedical and individualistic worldview. The 'web' was never intended to and does not jar epidemiologists from the long-established practice of viewing population patterns of disease as simply the sum of individual cases; it is far from obvious that adding the 'spiders' would address this fundamental problem.

As an alternative, the closest image that comes to mind stems from marrying the metaphor of the continually-constructed 'scaffolding' of society that different social groups daily seek to reinforce or alter to that of the ever-growing 'bush' of evolution, together defining the potential and constraints of human life. This intertwining ensemble must be understood to exist at every level, sub-cellular to societal, repeating indefinitely. Different epidemiologic profiles that the population-level would accordingly be seen as reflecting the interlinked and diverse patterns of exposure and susceptibility that are brought into play by the dynamic intertwining of these changing forms. It is an image that does *not* [italics in original] permit the cleavage of the social from the biologic, and the biologic from the social. It is an image that does not obscure agency. And it is an image that embraces history rather than hides it from view.

This image insists that understanding societal patterns of health and disease requires acknowledging the inextricable and ongoing intermingling–at all levels–of the social and the biologic. Through its fractal nature, it does not allow the individual to become separated from society, nor detract from people's irreducible individuality. A given branch of this intertwining structure can thus be seen as representing one set of possible epidemiologic profiles produced at a particular time by a particular combination of social structures, cultural norms, ecologic milieu, and genetic variability and similarity (among humans and among other organisms in the region). At a greater level of detail, particular groups–linked by their membership in socially-defined categories–embody these characteristics, thus acquiring, in the memorable phrase of Cristina Laurell, their distinct 'class physiognomies.'

At an even greater level of detail, the particularities of health and disease among individuals becomes apparent, reflecting yet again the interplay of these same social and biologic influences. And, moving to yet another level, these same sets of influences can be traced through their relationship to the normal functioning and disturbances of organ systems, cellular growth and differentiation, and metabolic processes. Highlighting the inherent links between levels, this image thus *requires* [italics in original] considering multiple levels when seeking to understand patterns at any given level, and likewise highlights the need to frame questions broadly, regardless of the level at which any particular investigation is conducted."

p. 899: "The field of epidemiology today suffers from the absence of not only a clearly articulated and comprehensive epidemiologic theory, but, it seems, even the awareness that it lacks such a theory. The science instead is taught and viewed as a collection of methods to be applied to particular problem involving human health and disease.

To counter this state of affairs, the image proposed in this paper is intended to spur discussion about important aspects of epidemiology's purpose and domain, as the science that seeks to explain and to generate knowledge to improve population patterns of health, disease, and well-being. Attempting to advance an ecosocial framework for the development of epidemiologic theory, this image makes clear that although the biologic may set the basis for the existence of humans and hence our social life, it is this social life that sets the path along which the biologic may flourish–or wilt. As such, it emphasizes why epidemiologists must look first and foremost to the link between social divisions and disease to understand etiology and to improve the public's health, and in doing so exposes the incomplete and biased slant of epidemiologic theories reliant upon a biomedical and individualistic world-view."

Textbox 7–6. Political Ecology: Definitions and Problems of Spatiotemporal Scale, Cross-Level Theorizing, and Historical Contingency.

Escobar A. After nature: Steps to an antiessentialist political ecology. *Current Anthropology* 1999; 40:1–16. (Escobar, 1999)

p. 3: "Political ecology can be defined as the study of the manifold articulations of history and biology and the cultural mediations through which such articulations are necessarily established. This definition does not rely on the common categories of nature, environment, or culture (as in cultural ecology, ecological anthropology, and much environmental thinking) or on the sociologically oriented nature and society (as in Marxist theories of the production of nature)."

pp. 14–15: "... can nature be theorized within an antiessentialist framework without marginalizing the biological?... A recentering of biology on the organism–marginalized by neo-Darwinianism, modern genetics, and molecular biology–and a recontextualization of the anthropology of persons within a biology of organisms are essential principles for this new synthesis... An important goal of political ecology is to understand and participate in the ensemble of forces linking social change, environment, and development."

Greenberg JB. The political ecology of fisheries in the Upper Gulf of California. In: Biersack A, Greenberg JB. *Reimagining Political Ecology.* **Durham, NC: Duke University Press, 2006; pp. 121–147. (Greenberg, 2006)**

p. 126: "... Marxist analyses of commodities, for instance, focus on how labor power transforms nature into commodities but give surprisingly little importance to the fundamental processes by which living things are reproduced or to how claims to things like land and water (which need not be products of labor) are established and legitimized.

Political ecology seems to offer a way around such problems. Unlike an earlier cultural ecology that framed the relations of human beings to nature within an adaptive evolutionary framework, political ecology seeks instead to understand how human societies use and shape nature to their own ends. Rather than attempting to explain human culture with problematic assumptions about adaptation, homeostasis, functions, and bounded ecosystems taken from natural sciences, political ecology focuses on human institutions and actions through which a "humanized" nature is constructed, transformed, and managed. Whereas political economy looks at the historical intersection of capital and the state, political ecology adds nature to the equation. In doing so, it addresses the lack of attention paid to the natural world by traditional political economy approaches and avoids making unnecessary assumptions about forms of integration or previous ecological equilibria. It simply examines how real political and economic systems interact with nature through time."

Robbins P. *Political Ecology: A Critical Introduction.* **Malden, MA: Blackwell Pub., 2004. (Robbins, 2004)**

pp. 211–212: "The ascent in scales also imposes a 'chain of command' where players at distantly removed scales (peasants, states, the World Trade Organization) have little interaction.

But using this approach, how do we understand the relationship of varying producers of nature–those on the farm, in the lab, and in the office–as they mutually create the landscape while mutually coercing one another?... The chain of explanation is a poor conceptual tool to manage such linkages and relationships. A shift away from this way of thinking towards a comparative anatomy of *networks* (italics in original) is therefore a more viable mode of explanation..."

Neumann RP. *Making Political Ecology*. London: Hodder Arnold; New York: Oxford University Press, 2005. (Neumann, 2005)

p. 65: "A final feature to emphasize in non-equilibrium ecology is the importance of spatial and temporal scale in the analysis of ecological change. First, a linear or regular relationship between the intensity of ecological impact and distance in time or space cannot be assumed. That is, impacts do not necessarily diminish with distance from an activity or event, particularly when biophysical systems are coupled with social and economic systems. Second, non-equilibrium ecology raises the question of how large a spatial scale is necessary before we can confidently identify a system in balance. Third, it further suggests that in complex natural systems, different rates of change, propelled by different abiotic and biotic processes, are occurring simultaneously at different spatial and temporal scales. Small-scale events can cascade upwards to create large-scale change."

Hvalkof S. Progress of the Victims: Political Ecology in the Peruvian Amazon. In: Biersack A, Greenberg JB. *Reimagining Political Ecology*. Durham, NC: Duke University Press, 2006; pp. 195–231. (Hvalkof, 2006)

p. 225: "The American-Brazilian anthropologist Paul E. Little uses the fractal analogy to describe such cross-scale social relationships, in which local actors link directly to a larger international system, skipping over scales to promote their specific local interests. He writes:
'These connections are rarely neatly organized and mechanically mobilized but rather are highly volatile and irregular and vary according to the historical moment, the strength and density of the cross-scale contacts, and the specific issues at hand... I call these fractal power relationships since they are, on one hand, highly irregular and unpredictable, yet on the other, they seek and partially achieve the furthering of common interests of the social groups operating at different social scales.' (Little,1998, p. 13)."

Lansing JS, Schoenfelder J, Scarborough V. Rappaport's rose: structure, agency, and historical contingency in ecological anthropology. In: Biersack A, Greenberg JB. *Reimagining Political Ecology*. Durham, NC: Duke University Press, 2006; pp. 325–357. (Lansing et al., 2006)

p. 353: "One a timescale of hours and days, human agency is apparent to an anthropologist observing the farmers of Sebatu as they carry out their daily routines in the terraces or at the water temples. Their choices seem quite constrained, since both rice and rice rituals have their own fixed schedules. But in monthly meetings of the subaks, there is a strong sense of salient agency: concerns are voiced, plans are made, decisions taken.

The constraints that limit the scope of these choices largely derives from the objective reality that the farmers inhabit, an engineered landscape of terraces, irrigation systems, and water temples. On a timescale of the everyday, this world seems fixed and permanent. But on an archaeological timescale, this reality is seen to evolve in response to human agency; indeed, there is virtually nothing present in the world of the farmers that is not the product of the labor of past generations."

analyses are cognizant that levels are not necessarily neatly nested, that interactions can skip levels, and that the level, spatiotemporal scale, and locale of analysis determines what interactions—and what patterns—can be seen (Greenberg & Park, 1994; Neumann, 2005; Hvalkof, 2006; Lansing et al., 2006; Taylor, 2008). An additional resemblance to ecosocial theory is its stance that political ecology must, by definition, be a reflexive and critical science, one in which researchers must pay heed both to how societal context informs scientific understanding and to the societal and ecological implications of their investigations (Escobar, 1999; Forsyth, 2003; Neumann, 2005; Biersack, 2006; Pálsson, 2006). Not surprisingly, given the influence of Marxist theorizing on the initial formulations of political ecology (Cockburn & Ridgeway, 1979; Greenberg & Park, 1994; Robbins, 2004; Biersack, 2006), thinking in the field has been influenced by variants of *dialectical historical materialism*, akin to what occurred during the development of the *political economy of health* and *social production of disease* frameworks discussed in **Chapter 6**.

Core to political ecology's intellectual agenda is the task of integrating theorizing that links societal and ecological phenomena—with the view that, as in the case of ecosocial theory, theorizing about only social or only biophysical processes is insufficient. As stated in the opening essay of the first issue of the *Journal of Political Ecology* (published in 1994), the two key frameworks for accomplishing this goal have been those of "political economy, with it insistence on the need to link the distribution of power with productive activity and ecological analysis, with its broader visions of bio-environmental relationships" (Greenberg & Park, 1994, p. 1). Yet, rather than simply cobble these together, the conceptual work in political ecology, as illustrated by the examples provided in **Textbox 7–6**, has involved analyzing these frameworks' complementary and at times discordant causal assumptions.

As with ecosocial theory, the conceptual work of political ecology has accordingly required engaging with: (*1*) the long reach of social, evolutionary, and geophysical history, extending well into contemporary events; (*2*) variations reflecting historical contingency; and (*3*) the complexities of cross-level theorizing and spatiotemporal scale. Such an approach, although perhaps daunting, at least clarifies when potentially misleading simplifying assumptions are introduced; commenting on the challenge, Roderick Neumann (b. 1954), a leading political ecologist, has observed (Neumann 2005, p. 10):

> The danger of such an inclusive approach is to produce a political ecology that is unmanageably complex and theoretically incoherent. This danger can be minimized, however. The position taken… is that there are fundamental philosophical and theoretical starting points that provide the field with coherence, while at the same time leaving a great deal of space for exploration, difference, and debate. First, the problem of complexity, when conducting multiscalar analyses of human-environment relations, is unavoidable. Rather than seek to reduce or repress complexity, however, the approach emphasized… is to focus on teasing out 'intersecting processes' operating at different spatial and temporal scales. With this approach, no two situations will share the same sets of processes with identical levels of importance and influence, yet there remains 'a role for some degree of social scientific generalization'. Second, the central theoretical challenge for political ecology is to integrate political and ecological dimensions, as well as material and discursive elements. As was previously suggested, critical realism provides the philosophical foundation for an approach to nature-society relations that acknowledges the ontological independence of the biophysical world while at the same time recognizing that our understanding of the natural world is partial, situational, and contingent.

The similarity of concerns to those of ecosocial theory is striking, reflecting how diverse scholars, engaged with different aspects of the complex intellectual problem of analyzing biological processes in societal, historical, and geographic context, have independently formulated a set of common conceptual approaches to help think through and test their ideas. Although these commonalities in theorizing are in no way evidence of validity of the ideas, the resemblances are informative, and illustrate how a common set of broader onto-logic and epistemologic assumptions can similarly shape research in disparate fields.

To date, however, the health of human populations and their epidemiologic profiles have understandably not been a major focus of theoretical and fieldwork conducted by self-identified political ecologists, given their concern with ecological phenomena. Even so, links between the fields of political ecology and social epidemiology can be traced back to the 1970s. One early example is Meredith Turshen's 1977 article on "The Political Ecology of Disease" (Turshen, 1977), which appeared in the same pathbreaking issue of the *Review of Radical Political Economy*, discussed in **Chapter 6**, that was instrumental to launching work on "the political economy of health" (Stark et al., 1977). In this essay, Turshen offered a Marxist critique of the paradigms of medical ecology and clinical medicine, one that she further elaborated in her 1984 book on *The Political Ecology of Disease in Tanzania* (Turshen, 1984). It was not until the mid-1990s, however, that a handful of articles began more systematically to explore theoretical links between political ecology and public health, including epidemiology (Baer, 1996; Mayer, 1996). Picking up the pace, in the past few years a number of articles, each of which has explicitly invoked ecosocial theory as an integrative framework, have begun to elaborate conceptual connections between political ecology and social epidemiology and to use them to inform empirical research (Porto & Martinez-Alier, 2007; Porto, 2007; Baer & Singer, 2009). Examples include studies on linked societal and ecological determinants of health among First Nation (Indigenous) populations in Canada (Richmond et al., 2005), air quality and health in Houston, Texas (Harper, 2004), and lead poisoning in North Carolina (Hanchette, 2008). Together, this nascent research, combined with further systematic articulation and application of the ecosocial theory of disease distribution, may well have the potential to take epidemiology to a new level—literally.

Coming Full Circle: Epidemiology and the Integral Connections Between Our Outer and Inner Worlds, in Context

As the panoply of sociopolitical, psychosocial, and ecosocial theories of disease distribu-tion make amply clear, viable and vital alternatives exist to the still dominant biomedical and lifestyle approaches to conceptualizing and conducting epidemiologic research. Biology and behavior need not—and should not—be decontextualized. Neither can they be ignored. Instead, as these alternative theories demonstrate, it is both possible and useful to analyze health-related biology and behavior in context, without being constrained by and reduced to the narrow individualistic, reductionist, and ahistorical assumptions of the pre-vailing perspectives.

Moreover, as emphasized by ecosocial theory and as echoed by its political ecology analogues, it is likewise problematic to pit "social" versus "biological" explanations for disease distribution and focus only on the former. Instead, societal, ecological, spatiotem-poral, geographic, and historical context all matter—as do specific diseases, specific expo-sures, and the myriad social and biological processes by which embodiment occurs. The advantage of epidemiologists also looking to the field of ecology—and not just to the social sciences—is, as underscored by ecosocial theory, precisely because of ecology's engage-ment with what has long been deemed the *natural* world and the lives and interactions of the organisms and populations who inhabit it. At the same time, as this chapter also makes clear, there is no singular or simple *ecological* perspective for epidemiologists to invoke.

The larger view afforded by taking embodiment and ecology seriously—substantively, not just metaphorically, and in political and economic context—is one that invites us to see, both newly and once again, the integral connections between our inner and outer worlds. As discussed in **Chapter 2**, one characteristic trait of early epidemiologic theories of disease distribution, given their historical (including technological) context, was their originators' attempt to envision the then unobservable internal workings of the body in terms of the then observable features of the environs in which they lived. In the twenty-first century, the enormously expanded possibilities and capacity to peer into both our inner and outer worlds—worlds that we inhabit simultaneously, not sequentially—renders it all the more imperative that epidemiologists engage in the intellectual and empirical work to build and test our understanding of these connections. To see current and changing population patterns of disease as the biological expression of societal and ecological conditions, as postulated by ecosocial theory (Krieger, 2005a), is to recognize that although we do not, in the first instance, create the biophysical processes enabling us to live as biological beings, we nevertheless now set the terms for their existence (Krieger, 1994). At issue is how people, acting within the constraints and possibilities of both our societies and our biology—especially in this era of global climate change—have "humanized" not only *nature* but also the epidemiologic profiles of both people and other species.

Grappling with the conceptual, substantive, and methodological challenges posed by ecosocial theory and its kindred frameworks is, I would argue, not only intellectually exciting but also vitally important. Why? Because, as I demonstrate in the next and final chapter, if we get our theories wrong, we can do great harm; if we get them right (or at least use better ones), we stand a better chance at generating valid knowledge relevant to explaining disease distribution and altering it for the good.

8

Epidemiologic Theory Counts

Harm, Knowledge, Action, and the People's Health

In this final chapter, I address in one more way the question undergirding this book: why care about epidemiologic theories of disease distribution—past, present, or future? After all, theoretical debates—including over even what constitutes "evidence" and how to think about it—are commonplace in scientific disciplines, and in fact core to the critical conduct of science (Cohen, 1985; Ziman, 2000; Mjøset, 2002; Sober, 2008). Vying for the most intellectually and empirically sound, robust, coherent, and comprehensive account of the phenomena of interest has long been standard scientific practice—and there is no reason the field of epidemiology should be any exception.

But in epidemiology, a distinction does matter. Theoretical debates about substantive explanations for disease occurrence are not simply about solving a puzzle correctly. Nor are they merely ivory-tower "academic" disputes. The difference has to do with our domain: "population distributions of disease, disability, death, and health and their determinants and deterrents, across time and space" (Krieger, 2001a; *see* **Chapter 1**). Ethically and intellectually, we are bound, in the time-honored phrase of the Hippocratic Oath, at the very least "to do no harm" (The Oath, 1983, p. 67; Nutton, 2004, pp. 66–69). Making this responsibility amply clear is the necessity of epidemiologic research to conform to the 1964 Declaration of Helsinki regarding "Ethical Principles for Medical Research Involving Human Subjects" (World Medical Association, 1964 [2008]), along with whatever are our country-specific regulations regarding human research.

However, in the case of epidemiology, I would extend the current argument to state that our accountability reaches beyond the injunction not to harm individuals who participate in epidemiologic studies. Also at issue are the ways epidemiologic theories and the research they animate contribute—potentially helpfully, potentially harmfully—to efforts to understand and address who and what is responsible for observed burdens and distributions of health, disease, and well-being.

Hence, to conclude the case that epidemiologic theory counts, in this final chapter I consider several examples in which choice of epidemiologic theory has made all the difference in whether people's health is harmed or helped.

First Do No Harm—and Second, Do Some Good: Some Examples of Why Theory Matters

Spanning a variety of disease outcomes, and involving a range of epidemiologic theories, I consider below four examples that illustrate the limitations of relying solely on either a biomedical approach stripped of societal context or a social approach focused only on social exposures—and why instead we are better served by theories attentive to society and biology, in context.

Example 1: Hormone Therapy, Cardiovascular Disease, and Breast Cancer— Biomedical Disregard for Social Determinants of Health Leads to Iatrogenic Disease. Widespread use of hormone therapy (HT) in the United States and other affluent countries took off in the 1960s (Seaman & Seaman, 1977; McCrae, 1983; Lock, 1993; Seaman, 2003; Krieger et al., 2005; Stefanick, 2005; Houck, 2006; Watkins, 2007). The promise was to alleviate menopausal symptoms and to keep women *"Feminine Forever,"* as proclaimed in 1966 by the title of one widely influential U.S. book (Wilson, 1966), whose publication and distribution was later revealed to be sponsored by Ayerst, a pharmaceutical company (Seaman & Seaman, 1977) (*see* **Textbox 8–1**). During this time, the idea that hormonal "deficiencies" led to menopause morphed into the biomedical view that menopause was itself a hormonal "deficiency disease" that could and should be treated by administration of "female" sex hormones (e.g., estrogen) (U.S. Federal Security Agency, 1950; Ayerst Labs, 1960; Rhoades, 1965; Wilson, 1966; Castallo, 1967; Seaman & Seaman, 1977; McCrea, 1983; Seaman, 2003; Krieger et al., 2005; Houck, 2006; Watkins, 2007; Foxcroft, 2009).

As background to this practice, starting in the early 1900s physicians had begun prescribing tablets made from cow ovaries to women undergoing menopause (Seaman, 2003; Stefanick, 2005; Houck, 2006; Watkins, 2007). Not surprisingly, results were mixed, given no control over the myriad substances present in cow ovaries, let alone in what quantities. By the 1930s, new laboratory techniques enabled pharmaceutical companies to start producing and marketing more carefully formulated versions of what was then termed "female sex hormone therapy" (Oudshorn, 1994; Houck, 2006; Watkins, 2007). They did so, ironically (in hindsight), at the same time laboratories were first discovering estrogen's carcinogenicity (Krieger et al., 2005; Gaudillière, 2006). Opening the door to even wider use, in 1942 the U.S. Food and Drug Administration (FDA) approved Premarin (an estrogen-only HT product) for treating menopause (Seaman, 2003; Stefanick, 2005; Watkins, 2007). Thereafter, the pace of the mass production and marketing of what became termed *hormone replacement therapy* picked up, as it became increasingly acceptable for physicians to prescribe and women to take hormonal pills to regulate their sexual and reproductive health, as also sanctioned by the FDA's approval in 1960 of the oral contraceptive pill (Gordon, 1976; Seaman & Seaman, 1977; Oudshorn, 1994; Seaman, 2003; Houck, 2006; Watkins, 2007). Although some researchers at the time did raise questions about the soundness of the science favoring HT and expressed concerns about HT-associated risks, their work had little impact (Krieger et al., 2005; Houck, 2006; Watkins, 2007).

As use of HT increased in the 1960s, so did hypotheses as to its benefits, leading to its reframing as not simply a "restorative" but actually "preventive" medicine. Fueling this thinking was recognition of differences for women versus men in the epidemiology of cardiovascular disease, an outcome whose rising mortality rates had led it to become, by the early 1960s, a—if not *the*—leading cause of death in most affluent countries (Marmot & Elliott, 2005). Specifically, age of onset was earlier among men compared to women,

Textbox 8–1. A Half-Century's Changing and Contested Perspectives and Data on—and Recurrent Questions About–Menopause, its Medicalization, and Hormone Therapy: Biomedical and Social Accounts, 1950–2005.

United States, Federal Security Agency, Public Health Service. *Menopause.* **(Health Information Series No. 15). Washington, DC: US Govt Printing Office, 1950.**

p. 1: "Menopause means the end of menstrual periods, and therefore, the end of childbearing years. It is also called the *climacteric* or *'change of life'* (italics in original). It is nature's plan for protecting women against childbearing beyond their years of greatest physical energy."

p. 2: "Many women have very few mild symptoms; some have none at all; with a few, the discomfort is very severe.

The symptoms are caused by the disappearance of the female sex hormone which the ovaries produce. The same ones occur when the ovaries are removed surgically because of disease (surgical menopause). After a period of months or a year or two, the body adjusts itself and the symptoms disappear. While this adjustment is taking place, hot flushes, etc., can appear.

Modern medical treatment is very successful in relieving symptoms of menopause. The doctor gives his patient medicine containing the ovarian hormones (or chemicals which act like it). In other words, he puts back in her body what nature is no longer producing. The treatment is continued until her body adjusts itself and hot flashes and other symptoms disappear. Treatment is necessary for a period of several months or for a year or two. *Medical care at this time also helps to correct the causes of nervousness and low spirits that often go along with the menopause* (italics in original)..."

p. 3: "Don't discuss your emotional or physical worries with relatives and neighbors during menopause; they haven't the medical knowledge to help you. Too, they might pass on some ancient 'change of life' superstition that could worry you. Rely upon your doctor or hospital clinic for information, advice, and medical treatment...

Remember that the menopause is not a complete change of life. The normal sex urges remain and women retain their usual reaction to sex long after the menopause. *There is nothing abnormal about the change of life and nothing unusual about the continuation of happy married relations afterward.*" (italics in original)

p. 3: "Each woman should see her doctor or consult a hospital clinic as soon as she notices she is starting her 'change of life'... *The modern woman relies upon her doctor for advice and goes through menopause with a minimum of physical and emotional discomfort.*" (italics in original)

Wilson RA. *Feminine Forever.* **New York: M. Evans (distributed in association with Lippincott), 1966.**

p. 18: "... menopause–far from being an act of fate or a state of mind–is in fact a deficiency disease. By way of rough analogy, you might think of menopause as a condition similar to diabetes. Both are caused by a lack of a certain substance in the body chemistry. To cure diabetes, we supply the lacking substance in the form of insulin. A similar logic can be applied to menopause–the missing hormones can be replaced."

p. 25: "In short, menopause must at last be recognized as a major medical problem in modern society. Women, after all, have the right to remain women. They should not have to live as sexual neuters for half their lives. The treatment and cure of menopause thus becomes a social and moral obligation."

pp. 43–44: "… while women during their fertile years are virtually immune to coronary disease and high blood pressure, the menopausal woman–lacking female hormones–soon loses this advantage and becomes as prone to heart trouble and strokes as a man of similar age. These are the secondary effects of her castration.

As for the primary effects, they are quite simple. Deprived of its natural fluids, the entire genital system dries up. The breasts become flabby and shrink, and the vagina becomes stiff and unyielding. The brittleness often causes chronic inflammation and skin cracks that become infected and make sexual intercourse impossible.

Additional physical consequences of castration [include]… nervousness, irritability, anxiety, apprehension, hot flushes, night sweats, joint paints, melancholia, palpitations, crying spells, weakness, dizziness, severe headache, poor concentration, loss of memory, chronic indigestion, insomnia, frequent urination, itching of the skin, dryness of eye, nose, and mouth, and a backache…

The effects of menopausal castration, as is evident from this list of symptoms, are by no means confined to the sexual organs. Because the chemical balance of the entire organism is disrupted, menopausal castration amounts to a mutilation of the whole body. I have known cases where the resulting physical and mental anguish was so unbearable that the patient committed suicide.

While not all women are affected by menopause to this extreme degree, no woman can be sure of escaping the horror of this living decay. Every woman faces the threat of extreme suffering and incapacity."

pp. 62–63: "… estrogen may be termed the hormone of feminine attraction and well-being. As it courses through the body in the bloodstream, its effects are indeed varied and manifold. Aside from keeping a woman sexually attractive and potent, it preserves the strengths of her bones, the glow of her skin, the gloss of her hair. It prevents the development of high blood pressure, heart disease, and strokes. It tends to prevent diabetes and diseases of the urinary bladder, it keeps the kidneys from wasting or losing salt in the urine—a vital matter in the regulation of tissue fluids throughout the body…

Through an ingenious mechanism by which estrogen acts on the pituitary gland at the base of the brain, it has a direct effect on a woman's emotional state. To a woman, estrogen acts as the carrier of that mysterious life force that motivates work, study, ambition, and that marvelous urge toward excellence that inspires the best of human beings.

Granted, the achievement of any woman cannot be attributed to estrogen alone— estrogen cannot command the fickle element of plain luck. Even with an abundance of estrogen, she still has to cope with the vicissitudes of existence—heredity, accident, environment, childhood training, financial status, and so forth. But at least estrogen puts her in a position where she can take advantage of whatever lucky breaks come her way. No matter what her particular sphere of activity may be—in the home, in business, in the arts or professions–a woman cannot live up to her opportunities unless she has her full quota of estrogen."

p. 158: "Estrogen therapy, far from causing cancer, tends to prevent it."

pp. 163–164: "These, then, are the facts to keep in mind when you hear estrogen discussed with suspicion: the inept and illogical mouse experiment that gave rise to the estrogen-cancer myth, and the inverse relationship of estrogen to breast and genital cancer (high estrogen in youth: low cancer incidence… low estrogen in age: high cancer incidence).

Keeping a woman rich in her ovarian hormones, especially estrogen and progesterone, lessens the incidence of malignant lesions, including breast and genital cancer."

Boston Women's Health Book Collective. *Our Bodies, Ourselves.* **Revised and expanded. New York: Simon & Schuster, 1976.**

p. 327: "Chapter 17. Menopause. Even though menopause has been a neutral or positive experience for many women, the physical and emotional changes associated with it are often misunderstood and mystifying… Even when physical symptoms are minimal or under control, menopause is often a more negative experience than it needs to be because of our society's attitude toward us during that time. The popular stereotype of the menopausal woman has been primarily negative: she is exhausted, irritable, unsexy, hard to live with, irrationally depressed, unwillingly suffering a 'change' that marks the end of her active (re)productive life."

p. 328: "In a society which equates our sexuality with our ability to have children, menopause is wrongly thought to mean the end of our sexuality–the end of our sexual pleasure, or even the total end of our sex life."

p. 330: "About one out of every five women will have no (or just a few) menopausal symptoms. Although most women do experience some bothersome symptoms, many of these will not actually require treatment. We should seek help whenever symptoms interfere with our normal activities, particularly because continuous and unrelieved distress may result in depression."

pp. 330–332: "Estrogen replacement therapy (ERT)… Those doctors who view menopause as a deficiency disease strongly argue the usefulness of widespread estrogen therapy. Others recommend a much more cautious approach.

ERT involves serious risks. Most notably, ERT has been linked with endometrial (uterine) cancer, especially among women taking estrogen for longer than one year… As with the pill, taking estrogen increases the risk of blood clots and hypertension…

Much more research is needed in the area of ERT, particularly its effect on osteoporosis, heart disease, cancer, and mental depression. Because of present uncertainties, many women are very cautious about ERT, choosing it only when symptoms are severe and when no contraindications are present."

p. 333: "Those of us looking ahead to menopause or just beginning to experience it can find little material that explains what most women go through during menopause. Most research has been done on 'clinical samples'–that is, on the minority of women who have chosen or been forced to seek medical care because of the severity of their symptoms. Consequently, we know very little about what menopause is like for all the women who never seek medical help."

Petitti DB, Perlman JA, Sidney S. Postmenopausal estrogen use and heart disease. *N Engl J Med* **1986; 315:131–132.**

p. 131: "Findings from our recently completed study of mortality and hospitalization for cardiovascular disease in postmenopausal estrogen users, based on information from the Walnut Creek Contraceptive Drug Study, may shed light on the reason for the contradictory results of other studies on the relation between cardiovascular disease and postmenopausal estrogen use.

The Walnut Creek Contraceptive Drug Study has been described in detail elsewhere. Briefly, 16,638 women between the ages of 18 and 54 were recruited to the study in the late 1960s and early 1970s and provided information on their use of oral contraceptives and other sex-steroid hormones at recruitment and approximately yearly through 1978. The current analyses uses data from follow-up for mortality through December 31, 1983…"

p. 132: "After adjustment for smoking, alcohol consumption, and history of hypertension, the [age-adjusted] relative risk of death from cardiovascular disease was 0.5 in women with postmenopausal estrogen use… The [age-adjusted] relative risk of death from accidents, homicide, and suicide was also substantially lower in postmenopausal estrogen users than in women who had never used sex-steroid hormones, and this lower risk persisted after adjustment for smoking, alcohol consumption, Quetelet index, and history of hypertension.

There is no biologically plausible reason for a protective effect of postmenopausal estrogen use on mortality from accidents, homicide, and suicide. We believe our results are best explained by the assumption that postmenopausal estrogen users in this cohort are healthier than those who had no postmenopausal estrogen use, in ways that have not been quantified and cannot be adjusted for. The selection of healthier women for estrogen use in this population is not necessarily a characteristic shared by other populations. If there are differences in the degree of selection for postmenopausal estrogen use between populations, then the disparate results of studies published to date are understandable. In the face of such selection, the question of the effect of postmenopausal estrogen use may be answerable with validity only through a randomized clinical trial."

Rosenberg L. Hormone replacement therapy: the need for reconsideration. *Am J Public Health* 1993; 83:1670–1673.

p. 1670: "Millions of menopausal women are taking hormone supplements. Observational studies suggest that unopposed estrogens reduce the risk of cardiovascular disease and fractures and increase the risk of endometrial cancer and, possibly, breast cancer. In the absence of information from randomized trials, how much of the apparent beneficial effect on heart disease is due to the tendency of healthier women to use these drugs is unknown. The effect on the cardiovascular system of estrogen taken with a progestin is unknown, and this regimen may increase the risk of breast cancer. An approach to health and illness that focuses on a single cause or preventive and on single organ systems is severely limited. Alternative ways to improve cardiovascular health and skeletal health that do not increase the risk of cancer are available. A reconsideration of the appropriate use of hormone supplements is needed."

p. 1671: One reason for the use of hormone supplements is the view held by some that menopause is a deficiency disease that requires treatment, as exemplified by the use of the term "estrogen-deficient" to characterize menopausal women. Menopausal women are indeed deficient in endogenous estrogens, relative to premenopausal women, if the focus is solely on the role of endogenous estrogens as preventives of fractures and heart disease. If the focus is shifted to the role of endogenous estrogens in the etiology of, for example, breast cancer (which occurs more frequently in women who have an early menarche or a late menopause), then premenopausal women are "hyperestrogenic" and postmenopausal women have a more desirable level. The same could be said for other diseases as well, including endometrial cancer, ovarian cancer, and uterine fibroids..."

Writing Group for the Women's Health Initiative Investigators. Risk and benefits of estrogen plus progestin in healthy postmenopausal women: principal results from the Women's Health Initiative randomized controlled trial. *JAMA* 2002; 288:321–333.

p. 321 (abstract):

CONTEXT: Despite decades of accumulated observational evidence, the balance of risks and benefits for hormone use in healthy postmenopausal women remains uncertain.

OBJECTIVE: To assess the major health benefits and risks of the most commonly used combined hormone preparation in the United States.

DESIGN: Estrogen plus progestin component of the Women's Health Initiative, a randomized controlled primary prevention trial (planned duration, 8.5 years) in which 16608 postmenopausal women aged 50–79 years with an intact uterus at baseline were recruited by 40 U.S. clinical centers in 1993–1998.

INTERVENTIONS: Participants received conjugated equine estrogens, 0.625 mg/d, plus medroxyprogesterone acetate, 2.5 mg/d, in 1 tablet (n = 8506) or placebo (n = 8102).

MAIN OUTCOMES MEASURES: The primary outcome was coronary heart disease (CHD) (nonfatal myocardial infarction and CHD death), with invasive breast cancer as the primary adverse outcome. A global index summarizing the balance of risks and benefits included the 2 primary outcomes plus stroke, pulmonary embolism (PE), endometrial cancer, colorectal cancer, hip fracture, and death due to other causes.

RESULTS: On May 31, 2002, after a mean of 5.2 years of follow-up, the data and safety monitoring board recommended stopping the trial of estrogen plus progestin vs placebo because the test statistic for invasive breast cancer exceeded the stopping boundary for this adverse effect and the global index statistic supported risks exceeding benefits. This report includes data on the major clinical outcomes through April 30, 2002. Estimated hazard ratios (HRs) (nominal 95% confidence intervals [CIs]) were as follows: CHD, 1.29 (1.02–1.63) with 286 cases; breast cancer, 1.26 (1.00–1.59) with 290 cases; stroke, 1.41 (1.07–1.85) with 212 cases; PE, 2.13 (1.39–3.25) with 101 cases; colorectal cancer, 0.63 (0.43–0.92) with 112 cases; endometrial cancer, 0.83 (0.47–1.47) with 47 cases; hip fracture, 0.66 (0.45–0.98) with 106 cases; and death due to other causes, 0.92 (0.74–1.14) with 331 cases. Corresponding HRs (nominal 95% CIs) for composite outcomes were 1.22 (1.09–1.36) for total cardiovascular disease (arterial and venous disease), 1.03 (0.90–1.17) for total cancer, 0.76 (0.69–0.85) for combined fractures, 0.98 (0.82–1.18) for total mortality, and 1.15 (1.03–1.28) for the global index. Absolute excess risks per 10,000 person-years attributable to estrogen plus progestin were 7 more CHD events, 8 more strokes, 8 more PEs, and 8 more invasive breast cancers, while absolute risk reductions per 10,000 person-years were 6 fewer colorectal cancers and 5 fewer hip fractures. The absolute excess risk of events included in the global index was 19 per 10,000 person-years.

CONCLUSIONS: Overall health risks exceeded benefits from use of combined estrogen plus progestin for an average 5.2-year follow-up among healthy postmenopausal U.S. women. All-cause mortality was not affected during the trial. The risk-benefit profile found in this trial is not consistent with the requirements for a viable intervention for primary prevention of chronic diseases, and the results indicate that this regimen should not be initiated or continued for primary prevention of CHD.

NIH State-of-the-Science Panel. National Institutes of Health State-of-the-Science Conference Statement: Management of Menopause-Related Symptoms. *Ann Int Med* 2005; 142:1005–1013.

p. 1005: "Menopause is a natural process that occurs in women's lives as part of normal aging. Many women go through the menopausal transition with few or no symptoms... The focus of this report is to identify menopausal symptoms and assess treatments for them on the basis of existing scientific evidence..."

p. 1005: "Estrogen, either by itself or with progestins, has been the therapy of choice for decades for relieving menopause-related symptoms. Epidemiologic studies in the 1980s and 1990s suggested that estrogen-containing therapy might protect women from heart disease and other serious medical problems. The Women's Health Initiative (WHI) was a large clinical trial of postmenopausal women (age rage, 50 to

79 years [mean, 63.2 years]) that was designed to see whether estrogen with or without progestin therapy could prevent chronic conditions, such as heart disease and dementia. The estrogen with progestin portion of the trial ended early because of increased incidence of breast cancer. There were increases in blood clots, stroke, and heart disease among women who received this treatment as well. These findings raised serious questions about the safety of estrogen to treat symptoms of menopause. Many women stopped hormone replacement therapy, and some searched for alternative therapies. To reflect a shift of focus from 'replacement' to use of hormones for relief of symptoms, we will use the term *menopausal hormone therapy*, which includes a range of doses and preparations of estrogens and progestins."

p. 1010: " 1. Menopause is the permanent cessation of menstrual periods that occurs naturally in women, usually in their early 50s. Many women have few or no symptoms; these women are not in need of medical treatments... 6.... much more research is needed to clearly define the natural history of menopause, associated symptoms, and effectiveness and safety of treatment for bothersome symptoms. Natural histories are important for both science and policy. Knowing how many women transit menopause with few or no symptoms, and how many manage menopause largely on their own, can lead to public health information that empowers women and increases their self-reliance... ."

pp. 1010–1011: "Menopause is 'medicalized' in contemporary U.S. society. There is great need to develop and disseminate information that emphasizes menopause as a normal, healthy phase of women's lives and promotes its demedicalization. Medical case and future clinical trials are best focused on women with the most severe and prolonged symptoms. Barriers to professional care for these women should be removed."

and their and overall rates of were mortality higher (Bush, 1990; Epstein, 2005; Stamler, 2005). Based on the biomedical view that sex hormones were chiefly responsible for myriad male/female differences, including not only for reproductive health but also for nonreproductive health outcomes and other behavioral and cognitive characteristics and capacities (Dreifus, 1977; Ruzek, 1978; Hubbard et al., 1982; Oudshorn, 1994; Fee & Krieger, 1994), this framework led to positing that "female sex hormones" were protective against cardiovascular disease.

In the mid-1960s the "Coronary Drug Project" became the first clinical trial of estrogen to prevent cardiovascular disease—and was conducted solely with men (Coronary Drug Project, 1970; Coronary Drug Project, 1973). Its results defied expectation: the estrogen arm of the study was abruptly halted in the mid-1970s because the men given Premarin had unexpectedly high cardiovascular mortality (resulting from thromboembolic events and myocardial infarction) (Coronary Drug Project, 1970; Coronary Drug Project, 1973; Petitti, 2004; Stefanick, 2005). Further crimping enthusiasm for HT, shortly thereafter, epidemiologic research implicated HT (still estrogen-only) in rising rates of endometrial cancer (Seaman & Seaman, 1977; McCrae, 1983; Seaman, 2003; Stefanick, 2005; Houck, 2006; Watkins, 2007).

The turnabout occurred in the 1980s with the introduction of estrogen-progestin HT formulations, whereby progestin was added to prevent estrogen-induced endometrial cancer (Seaman, 2003; Stefanick, 2005; Houck, 2006; Watkins, 2007). During the 1980s, a raft of observational studies reported that HT use was associated with reduced risk of osteoporosis, cardiovascular disease risk markers, and cardiovascular disease among women (Seaman, 2003; Stefanick, 2005; Houck, 2006; Watkins, 2007). By the early 1990s, major epidemiologic reviews (including meta-analyses) concluded that HT warranted use as preventive medication (Stampfer & Colditz, 1991; Grady et al., 1992). Even so, a number of articles in the epidemiologic literature warned about the dangers of causal inference based on observational data and also raised concerns about risk of breast cancer (Petitti et al., 1986; Barrett-Connor, 1992; Brinton & Schairer, 1993; Rosenberg, 1993), albeit with little impact. Consequently, in 1991 and 1992, considering the extant human observational evidence as well as animal and other laboratory studies, the FDA and American College of Physicians respectively recommended use of HT to prevent cardiovascular disease (Seaman, 2003; Stefanik, 2005). The argument was that any small risk for breast cancer was out-weighed by the larger danger of future cardiovascular disease.

In 2002, however, routine acceptance of HT was shattered by results from the Women's Health Initiative (WHI; Writing Group/WHI, 2002), the largest randomized clinical trial of HT, conducted in a population of mainly healthy U.S. women, which like the smaller 1998 Heart and Estrogen/progestin study (Hulley et al., 1998) and its 2002 follow-up (Grady et al., 2002), found that contrary to expectations, HT did not decrease—and may, in fact, have increased risk of cardiovascular disease—while also confirming that long-term use of the combined estrogen plus progestin HT increased risk of breast cancer. Publication of the results triggered a dramatic global drop in HT prescriptions and marketing, with the U.S. decline in HT use by 2004 exceeding 50% compared to just before the WHI results (Ettinger et al., 2003; Hersh et al., 2004; Buist et al., 2004; Majumdar et al., 2004; Haas et al., 2004; Stefanick, 2005; Kelly et al., 2005; Kim et al., 2005; Wei et al., 2005; Hing & Brett, 2006; Guay et al., 2007).

The findings also led to fierce debates in the epidemiologic literature over reasons for the discrepancies between the observational and clinical trial results (Humphrey et al., 2002; Grodstein et al., 2003; Stampfer, 2004; Vandenbroucke, 2004; Barret-Connor, 2004; Kuller, 2004; Petitti, 2004; Lawlor et al., 2004a; Prentice et al., 2005a; Barrett-Connor et al., 2005; Willett et al., 2006; Manson & Bassuk, 2007; Barrett-Connor, 2007; Banks & Canfell, 2009). Diametrically opposed hypotheses posited: (*1*) confounding, selection bias, and measurement error biased the observational studies, versus (*2*) the clinical trial results were misleading because the women in the WHI were typically older and more likely to have atherosclerosis (and, hence, have plaque vulnerable to HT-caused disruption) than women in the observational studies (this latter hypothesis, also known as the "timing" hypothesis, has not been supported, at the time of preparing this chapter, by the most recent re-analysis of WHI data; Prentice et al., 2009). Further spurring the debates, new legal evidence has revealed that between 1998 and 2005, 26 peer-reviewed scientific papers backing use of HT and downplaying its risks, published in 18 different medical journals (including such respectable publications as the *American Journal of Obstetrics and Gynecology*), were secretly written by medical ghostwriters paid by Wyeth, the pharmaceutical company that manufacturers Premarin; the listed academic authors, who did little or no writing, were solicited solely to provide credibility (Singer, 2009).

Where does epidemiologic theory fit into this saga? Centrally: by illuminating who and what is studied—as well as who and what is ignored. In this case, the contending perspectives pit the biomedical model against a social epidemiologic perspective (Krieger, 2005a).

Notably, starting in the latter part of the 1980s, some epidemiologists began to question whether the supposed protective effect of long-term use of HT on risk of cardiovascular disease largely reflected a combination of selection bias and confounding by social class (Petitti et al., 1986; Rosenberg, 1993). Behind this concern lay an awareness—amply confirmed by subsequent research (Humphrey et al., 2002; Nelson et al., 2002; Lawlor et al., 2004b; McPherson & Hemminki, 2004)—that women from more affluent backgrounds (childhood as well as current), with better health (including no contraindications against exogenous hormone use), were the women most likely to be prescribed (and who could afford) HT—and least likely to be stricken by cardiovascular disease (Krieger, 2003a; Petitti, 2004; Krieger et al., 2005; Barrett-Connor et al., 2005; Rossouw, 2006). This alternative hypothesis, grounded in a social epidemiologic perspective, was nevertheless discounted by biomedically-oriented researchers, in part because they believed controlling for one or two socioeconomic variables was sufficient to deal with confounding by social class (Stampfer & Colditz, 1991; Grodstein et al., 2003; Stampfer, 2004). It received serious attention only after the WHI published its results in 2002. Indeed, the rapidity of the turn-around from being controversial to argue that socioeconomic position could be an important confounder (Grodstein et al., 2003; Stampfer, 2004) to this being a "common sense" proposition (Petitti & Freedman, 2005; Barrett-Connor et al., 2005; Watkins, 2007; Banks & Canfell, 2009) is nothing short of remarkable.

Reckoned in human terms, the cost of biomedical disregard for social epidemiologic critiques of the HT hypothesis can be seen in breast cancer incidence rates. Prompted by the WHI results, new epidemiologic analyses published between 2002 and 2005, using data from the United States, Europe, and Australia, have estimated that HT might account for 10% to 25% of observed breast cancer cases (Beral et al., 2003; Bakken et al., 2004; Coombs et al., 2005a; Coombs et al., 2005b). Moreover, as per **Figure 1–2** in **Chapter 1** (Krieger, 2008a), between 2006 and 2009, 14 population-based studies—eight from the United States (Clarket et al., 2006; Ravdin et al., 2007a; Ravdin et al., 2007b; Clarket et al., 2007; Hausauer et al., 2007; Stewart et al., 2007; Jemal et al., 2007; Glass et al., 2007), five European (Bouchardy et al., 2006; Katalinic & Rawal, 2008; Kumle, 2008; Verkooijen et al., 2008; Parkin, 2009), and one Australian (Canfell et al., 2008), have documented notable and otherwise unexpected annual declines of breast cancer incidence, especially among women age 50 and older with estrogen receptor-positive (ER+) tumors. All have attributed these trends to the dramatic reduction in use of HT following the July 2002 publication of the WHI results.

Whether these declines can be causally linked to reduced HT use is now, not surprisingly, an active area of research. Suggesting the hypothesis has merit, one line of evidence indicates that observed trends are unlikely to result from declines in breast cancer detection or changes in other major risk factors (Smigal et al., 2006; Hausauer et al., 2007; Jemal et al., 2007; Glass et al., 2007; Chlebowski et al., 2009; Roberts, 2009). Specificity of the decline is also shown by new results indicating that at least with the United States, the declines in breast cancer incidence rates occurred solely among the women most likely to use HT—that is, White and living in affluent counties with ER+ tumors, and with no decline evident among the remaining women, both of color and/or living in poorer counties (Krieger et al., 2010). Further supporting the hypothesis is a second line of evidence regarding the biological plausibility of a short lag time between cessation of HT exposure and a decline in risk of developing a detectable incident breast cancer, considering how steroids, including HT, can act as breast cancer tumor promoters (Bradlow & Sepkovic, 2004; Dietel et al., 2005; Yager & Davidson, 2006; Cordera & Jordan, 2006; Ravdin et al., 2007b).

At one level, the recent disturbing findings linking HT use to iatrogenic breast cancer point to the dangers of inadequately understood pharmacologic manipulation of complex hormonal systems (Seaman, 2003; Krieger et al., 2005; Krieger, 2008)—a caution that ought be remembered (Krieger et al., 2010) when considering past and present proposals to prevent breast cancer by administering regimens of powerful hormones to healthy young women (Hendersen et al., 1993; Pike & Spicer, 2000; de Waard & Thijssen, 2005; Medina, 2005; Tsubura et al., 2008). At another level, these findings underscore how a narrow bio-medical conceptualization of menopause as a "disease" ignored alternative possibilities that, from an evolutionary standpoint, menopause could be a beneficial or neutral trait—and that its consequences for health, regardless, must be addressed in relation to many, not just single, health outcomes (Leidy, 1999, NIH, 2005).

Also exposed is the problematic longstanding reductionist framing of sex hormones (construed solely as *sex* hormones) as fundamental to explaining women's and men's behavior and biology (Oudshorn, 1994; Fee & Krieger, 1994; Doyal, 1995; Krieger et al., 2005; Payne, 2006). This theoretical perspective has been importantly challenged by social epidemiologic research attending to critical distinctions between—and the health consequences of—gender and sex-linked biology (Fee & Krieger, 1994; Doyal, 1995; Krieger, 2003b; Payne, 2006), as discussed in **Chapter 7** (*see* **Table 7–1**). Additional examples illustrating the importance of considering whether one, the other, both, or neither are germane are two figures appearing in **Chapter 1**. The first, **Figure 1–2**, also related to the breast cancer story, depicts secular changes in U.S. twentieth century age-specific breast cancer incidence rates among White women, revealing an especially steep rise—then fall—only among women age 55 years and older (Krieger, 2008a). The second, **Figure 1–3,** shows disease-specific changes in mortality rate ratios for women compared to men for mid-nineteenth to mid-twentieth century England and Wales (Morris, 1955, Morris, 1957, pp. 1–2). In both cases, the observed temporal changes in women's rates of disease and male/female risk differences cannot plausibly be explained simply by intrinsic "fixed" sex-linked traits; alterations in exogenous exposures must also be at play.

A question thus worth asking is: Had "sex hormones" been conceptualized as one par-ticular variety of hormones that affect cell proliferation, rather than as specialized molecules preoccupied with sex, might it have been possible to avoid pharmacologic change of wom-en's hormone levels being portrayed benignly as *hormone replacement therapy* and instead have this more appropriately seen as *hormone manipulation*, with attendant implications for cell proliferation, including increased risk of cancer (Krieger et al., 2005)? Also rele-vant is the role of the "invisible industrialist" in promoting use of HT (Krieger et al., 2005), a hidden factor strikingly revealed by a political economy of health perspective. The larger implication is that biomedical disregard for social epidemiologic theoretical frameworks can literally harm people's health—along with the corollary that debate over findings as framed by contending theories can lead to new insights and more valid and beneficial results.

Example 2: Peptic Ulcers, Stress, Helicobacter pylori, *and Allergies—From Psychosocial to Biomedical Extremes, Leaving Questions About Susceptibility and Unintended Consequences of Treatment Still Open.* The second example offers a con-trary case: when singular attention to social determinants can lead to neglect of relevant biophysical exposures—even as wholesale reversion to a decontextualized biomedical approach can both miss etiologic clues and promote therapeutic interventions with unan-ticipated problems. The example concerns the now well-rehearsed story of peptic ulcers, psychosocial stress, and *H. pylori* (Thagard 1999, pp. 39–97, 364–366; Atherton, 2006), albeit with a twist.

Briefly stated, during much of the twentieth century, the cause of peptic ulcers, following the tenets of psychosocial theories, was attributed to "stress." The hypothesis was that "stress" increased stomach acids, leading to perforation of the stomach wall and hence peptic ulcers (Richardson, 1985; Levenstein, 2000; Grob, 2003). With peptic ulcer conceptualized as a "disease of civilization," the early twentieth century rise and then subsequent fall of peptic ulcer mortality in industrialized countries—shown to reflect changing risks by birth cohort in pathbreaking analyses published in 1962 by Mervyn Susser (b. 1921) and Zena Stein (b. 1921) (Susser & Stein, 1962; Susser & Stein, 2002; **Figure 8–1**)—was attributed to the initial strain of and then adaptation to the quicker pace of life in the twentieth century. Treatments included not only surgery and modified diets but also stress-reduction therapies (Grob, 2003).

Starting in 1984, however, when Barry Marshall (b. 1951) and Robin Warren (b. 1937) discovered an unidentified bacteria (later identified as *H. pylori*) in the stomach of patients with gastritis and peptic ulceration (Marshall & Warren, 1984), the etiologic orientation began to shift, such that by 1994, an NIH consensus document deemed *H. pylori* to be the leading cause of peptic ulcer (NIH, 1994). "Civilization" became re-interpreted as improved hygiene, with better sanitation reducing risk of early life fecal–oral transmission while simultaneously increasing age at infection in childhood (as prevalence was waning); later age at infection, moreover, was posited to increase risk of developing peptic ulcer, leading to its rise in early twentieth century birth cohorts in industrialized countries (Sonnenberg et al., 2002; Leung, 2006; Atherton, 2006). The successful treatment of peptic ulcers by antibiotics vindicated the biomedical approach to both etiology and intervention and discredited the psychosocial accounts, whose etiologic understandings had promoted psychological and dietary treatments incapable of eradicating the harmful infection (NIH, 1994; Thagard, 1999; Danesh, 1999; Marshall, 2002; Leung, 2006; Kandulski et al., 2008).

Yet, suggesting that the story may not be quite so simple as "biomedical = correct" and "psychosocial = wrong" are two sets of considerations—one involving etiology, the other medical interventions (both curative and preventive). Starting with etiology, one relevant finding is that only 15% to 20% of persons with *H. pylori* infection develop ulcers (Levenstein, 2000; Atherton, 2006; Choung & Talley, 2008; Kandulski et al., 2008). Moreover, some countries, such as India, have very high infection rates but show marked regional variation in rates of peptic ulcer (Akhter et al., 2007; Leong, 2009). These well-known phenomena, whereby not everyone infected by a microorganism becomes ill, and population variation in disease rates exists despite virtually ubiquitous infection, in turn raises the equally well-known question: What additional conditions are required for infection to become disease?

One hypothesis proposed in the *H. pylori* literature focuses on genetic susceptibility, whereby a "match" is needed between host polymorphisms and whichever strain of *H. pylori* (a bacteria with very high genetic variability [Dykhuizen & Kalia, 2008]) has colonized the stomach (Leung, 2006; Atherton, 2006; Kandulski et al., 2008; Snaith et al., 2008). Still other evidence, however, has led to a re-emergence and refinement of the "stress" hypothesis (Levenstein, 2000; Levenstein, 2002; Choung & Talley, 2008). In contrast to the prior version, where "stress" was thought to induce ulcer formation directly, the two updated "stress"-related pathways posit that adverse stress can alter behavior and physiology in a way that increases susceptibility to infection by *H. pylori*, resulting in disease. One route is by stress increasing alcohol and aspirin consumption, both of which have been shown to increase risk of developing an ulcer; the other is by stress impairing immune responses relevant to wound healing (Levenstein, 2000; Levenstein, 2002; Choung & Talley, 2008). Thus, although adverse psychosocial exposures clearly are not obligate for development of peptic ulcers arising from *H. pylori* infection, and by themselves cannot explain the changing incidence rates over time, that does not mean they are completely irrelevant to explaining disease occurrence. Both the genetic "match" *and* the psychosocial

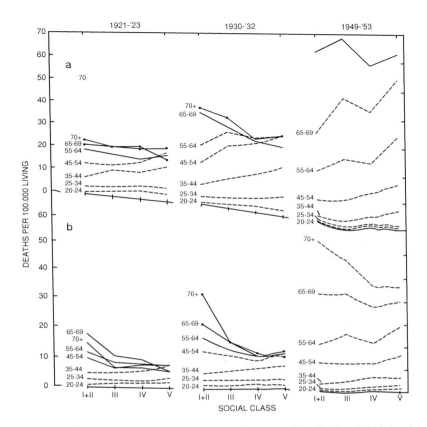

Figure 8–1. Changing class gradients in mortality because of peptic ulcer by birth cohort: analysis of 1921–1923 through 1949–1953 mortality data from the United Kingdom by Susser and Stein. (Susser & Stein, 1962, p. 118). (©1962 Elsevier, Inc. Reprinted with permission.)

Classes: Class I + II = "Professional, Managerial, and Technical Occupations"; Class III = "Skilled Occupations"; Class IV = "Partly-Skilled Occupations"; Class V = "Unskilled Occupations"

Description and interpretation of the changing class gradients (in effect arguing against a monotonic gradient invariant to time, in this case, historical generation):

p. 116: *Social Class.*

Analysis of changes in mortality by social class over the last three censuses again shows upward age-shifts, which suggest that each generation is carrying forward its own particular risk. At each successive census, a more or less regular pattern of mortality recurred in age-groups, which were older by the interval, which had elapsed between the censuses.

Statistics relate only to males, and are first available for the period of the 1921 census (Morris and Titmuss, 1944). From 1921 to 1923 death-rates from gastric ulcer showed a social class gradient increasing from the higher to the lower classes up to the age of 55; this gradient flattened between 55 and 70, and was reversed over the age of 70. A decade later, in the period 1930–32, the gradient increasing from higher to lower classes was apparent up to age 65 and then reversed—i.e., ten years older than at the previous census. In the period 1949–52 the gradient increasing from higher to lower classes persisted up to the age of 70 before it flattened… Although death rates in old age must be interpreted with caution, the trend fits the expectation.

248

hypotheses can be correct (i.e., be complementary, not antagonistic, each explaining a different part of the pattern).

Second, raising questions about appropriate medical interventions to cure or prevent *H. pylori* infection, several new investigations (albeit not all) have reported an increased risk of asthma among persons lacking childhood infection by *H. pylori* (Jarvis et al., 2004; Chen & Blaser, 2007; Blaser et al., 2008; Kandulski et al., 2008). A new interpretation, based on long-term historical and evolutionary thinking, including recognition that *H. pylori* has ubiquitously colonized the human gut since Paleolithic times (Atherton, 2006; Blaser et al., 2008; Dykhuizen & Kalia, 2008) is that early life exposure to relevant microbes—in this case, possibly *H. pylori* or else another microbe that tracks with *H. pylori* exposure—may be important for healthy immune system development and function (a.k.a. the "hygiene hypothesis") (Jarvis et al., 2004; Atherton, 2006; Chen & Blaser, 2007; Blaser et al., 2008). Additionally, some—but not all—studies have suggested that adults treated by antibiotics for *H. pylori* infection may be at increased risk of gastro-esophageal reflux disease, Barrett's esophagus, and adenocarcinoma of the esophagus, a consequence of *H. pylori* eradication affecting stomach acidity (Ahmed & Sechi, 2005; Atherton, 2006; Kandulski et al., 2008). Consequently, a biomedical emphasis on eradicating *H. pylori* infection by antibiotics, necessary for treating adults with ulcers, and also on preventing infection in children via vaccines could have consequences other than averting *H. pylori*-related illness (Chen & Blaser, 2007; Blaser et al., 2008). As with HT, biomedical "magic bullets" can well hit targets others than those anticipated by reductionist analysis, a possibility more readily considered by non-reductionist frameworks.

Thus, in this second example, as with the first, critical social, biological, evolutionary, and historical thinking are necessary for robust hypotheses and apt interventions. The omission of any one can lead to incomplete understanding and potentially harmful consequences.

Example 3: Diabetes and Indigenous Health—From "Thrifty Genes," Fictional History, and Racialized Disease to Reckoning With the Transgenerational Biological Embodiment of Social and Ecological Injustice. Epidemiologic analysis of the mid-twentieth century sudden emergence of high and rising rates of diabetes among some—but not all—Indigenous peoples, especially those living in countries of the global North (Joe & Young, 1993; Young, 1994; Kunitz, 1994; Young, 2000; Gohdes & Action, 2000; Ferriera & Lang, 2006; Gracey & King, 2009; King et al., 2009; Cunningham, 2009), constitutes the third example of why epidemiologic theory matters for etiologic analysis. At issue is the harm caused by problematic causal inferences of epidemiologic theories of disease distribution that selectively—or erroneously—invoke history and neglect addressing jointly the societal and biophysical (including ecological) determinants of current and changing population patterns of health and health inequities.

In 1962, the geneticist James V. Neel (1915–2000) (Lindee, 2001), attempting to unravel the puzzle of rising rates of diabetes among people who, in his words "have come to enjoy the blessings of civilization" (Neel, 1962, p. 357), proposed his then novel hypothesis of the "thrifty genotype," a vivid phrase he coined precisely because it was "a somewhat colloquial but expressive term" (Neel, 1962, p. 354). Neel's thesis, foreshadowing present-day biomedical/lifestyle versions of "evolutionary medicine" and "gene–environment interaction" frameworks (as discussed in **Chapter 5**), was premised on the assumption (asserted without any supporting references) that humanity, for most of its existence as hunter-gatherers, experienced cycles of "feast-and famine" (*see* **Textbox 8–2**).

Positing a survival advantage for individuals predisposed to metabolize energy frugally (because "during a period of starvation" they would have "an extra pound of adipose reserve" (Neel, 1962, p. 355)), Neel theorized that this trait would become harmful as food

Textbox 8–2. "Thrifty Gene" Hypothesis: Fictional Pasts Versus Historical Realities, 1962–2009.

"Thrifty Gene" hypothesis: Neel's initial (1962) and modified (1999) propositions

1962: original statement of hypothesis by James V. Neel (1915–2000), in: Neel JV. Diabetes mellitus: a "thrifty" genotype rendered detrimental by "progress"? *Am J Human Genet* 1962; 14:353–362.

p. 353: "For the population geneticist, diabetes mellitus has long presented an enigma. Here is a relatively frequent disease, often interfering with reproduction by virtue of an onset during the reproductive or even pre-reproductive years, with a well-defined genetic basis, perhaps as simple in many families as a single recessive or incompletely recessive gene. If the considerable frequency of the disease is of relatively long duration in the history of our species, how can this be accounted for in the face of the obvious and strong genetic selection against the condition? If, on the other hand, the frequency is a relatively recent phenomenon, what changes in the environment are responsible for the increase?"

p. 354: "... in the early years of life the diabetic genotype is, to employ a colloquial but expressive term, a 'thrifty' genotype, in the sense of being exceptionally efficient in the intake and/or utilization of food... The precise physiologic basis for this 'thriftiness' remains unclear. There are obvious possibilities. Thus, if after stimulation of the islets of Langerhans they continued to function longer in the predisposed than the normal, this could depress the blood sugar level unduly, resulting in hunger and increased food intake..."

p. 355: "A second possible mechanism to be considered involves a pancreas more rapidly responsive to increases in the level of blood glucose. In this connection it must be remembered that during the first 99 per cent or more of man's life on earth, while he existed as a hunter and gatherer, it was often feast or famine. Periods of gorging alternated with periods of greatly reduced food intake. The individual whose pancreatic responses minimized post-prandial glycosuria might have, during a period of starvation, an extra pound of adipose reserve..."

p. 357: "We now come to the problem posed by the relatively high frequency of the disease diabetes... three lines of thought suggest there has been a true increase in the frequency of the disease as more and more people have come to enjoy the blessings of civilization. Firstly, obesity appears to be, on the whole, a rarer phenomenon in primitive cultures than our own. There is less opportunity to indulge a hypertrophied appetite, and/or the lower mean caloric intake and greater physical activity of these primitive groups provide less of a stimulus to insulin production; this in turn means less stimulation of the antagonist-producing mechanism. Secondly, the action of the adrenal steroids in bringing to light the subclinical diabetic, in addition to the well-recognized effect of these compounds on gluconeogensis, may also be through stimulation of antagonist production. Since the response of the adrenal cortex to alarm situations is now less often followed by motor activity than in the past, one may postulate a disturbance in the physiologic balance established in the course of human evolution. Thirdly, the well-known glucose-mobilizing effects of adrenalin release are now not followed to the same extent by physical activity as seems to have been the case for primitive societies; since this calls for a greater insulin production than would otherwise be the case, here again it is an opportunity for increased stimulation of the insulin antagonist mechanism. These latter two thoughts would tend to place diabetes in the poorly defined areas of the 'stress diseases'–and indeed, the physiologic evidence to this effect is right now at least as convincing as it is for regarding peptic ulcer and coronary hypertension as stress disease."

pp. 359–360: "Should the foregoing thoughts prove correct, then diabetes underlines one of the ethical dilemmas of modern medicine. If the dietary and cultural conditions which elicit the relatively high frequency of diabetes in the Western World are destined to spread and persist over the entire globe, then, to the extent that modern medicine makes it possible for diabetics to propagate, it interferes with genetic evolution. But if, on the other hand, the mounting pressure of population numbers means an eventual decline in the standard of living with, in many parts of the world, a persistence or return to seasonal fluctuations in the availability of food, then efforts to preserve the diabetic genotype through this transient period of plenty are in the interests of mankind. Here is a striking illustration of the need for caution in approaching what at first glance seem to be 'obvious' eugenic considerations!"
NB: (a) Neel provided no evidence or documentation that hunter-gatherers routinely experienced "feast or famine" nor did the article ever discuss diabetes among Indigenous populations, yet (b) most of the application of the "thrifty gene" hypothesis has been in relation to selection effects of "feast vs famine" as translated to presumed differences in genotype of Indigenous vs non-Indigenous populations, even though two of Neel's three lines of evidence focused on diabetes as a "modern" "stress disease." (See also example 2, above, on peptic ulcer as a "stress" disease).

1998–1999: Neel's qualification—yet upholding—of the hypothesis, in:

a) **Neel JV. The "thrifty genotype" in 1998. *Nutr Rev* 1999; 57:S2–S9.**

p. S3: "A more telling observation concerning the role of lifestyle in the emergence of NIDDM [non-insulin dependent diabetes mellitus, i.e., Type 2 diabetes] in Amerindians involves the Pima Indians of southern

Arizon and a closely related group, the Pima Indians of the Sierra Madre Mountains of northern Mexico, two groups estimated to have separated some 700–1000 years ago. The results of studies done in those groups give no support to the notion that the high frequency of NIDDM in reservation Amerindians might be due simply to an ethnic predisposition—rather, it must predominantly reflect lifestyle changes."

p. S4: "Despite all these advances in our understanding of NIDDM, the nature of the environmentally precipitated genetic maladjustments that result in the disease remain obscure. Given the intensity of the current effort to localize and characterize the genes, the functioning of which seems to be compromised in NIDDM, speculation at this time concerning their nature seems of little value. However, the concept of a 'thrifty genotype' remains as viable as when first advanced..."

b) Neel JV, Weder AB, Julius S. Type II diabetes, essential hypertension, and obesity as "syndromes of impaired genetic homeostasis": the "thrifty genotype" hypothesis enters the 21st century. *Perspect Biol Med* 1998; 42:44–74.

pp. 45–46: "The Arizona Pima are the textbook material for the emergence of NIDDM and obesity among Amerindians following acculturation. Forced on a government dole by the rapacious diversion by the early settlers of the West of the water essential to their irrigation-style agriculture, the Pima of necessity adapted a high-fat, highly refined, government dispensed diet at the same time that they were forced to abandon any pretense of the agricultural work ethic. Currently among adults, the BMI (kg wt/ht in m2) averages 33.4 ± 7.5 and 37 percent of men and 54 percent of women meet the criteria for NIDDM. The Mexican Pima, by contrast, still pursue a much more traditional lifestyle. The average BMI was 24.9 ± 4.0, and only 2 of 19 women (36 ± 13 years of age) and 1 of 16 men (48 ± 14 years of age) were diabetic. The diet of the Mexican Pima was largely beans, corn, and potatoes, grown by traditional and physically very demanding techniques."

p. 49: "... it is now clear that the original thrifty genotype hypothesis, with its emphasis on feast or famine, presented a grossly overly simplistic view of the physiological adjustments involved in the transition from the lifestyle of our ancestors to life in the high-tech fast lane."

pp. 60–61: "The various recent developments regarding NIDDM, essential hypertension and obesity suggest both a modification and a broadening of the original concept of a thrifty genotype. It now seems preferable to conceptualize these diseases as resulting from previously adaptive multifactorial genotypes, the integrated functioning of whose the complexly altered environment in which these genotypes now find themselves. Some terminological problems must be dealt with. The term 'thrifty genotype' has served its purpose, overtaken by the growing complexity of modern genetic medicine... The ultimate genetic complexity of each of these diseases qualifies it for the term *syndrome* [italics in original]. Perhaps collectively we can speak of 'syndromes of impaired genetic homeostasis' or, more colloquially, the 'civilization syndromes,' or the 'altered life style syndromes,' to which other diseases may be added.

This viewpoint creates some terminological issues. As the genes associated with these three diseases are identified, let us not repeat the mistakes in genetic terminology that have and still are occurring in the field of cancer genetics. Although it is convenient as genes associated with the various malignancies are identified to speak of proto-oncogenes and, following the demonstration of the appropriate mutations, of oncogenes, these genes are for the most part cell cycle or housekeeping genes, playing important roles in normal cell activities; the sooner these roles are elucidated, the better for clear thinking. The same considerations will apply as the nature of the genes associated with the failed homeostatic syndromes are elucidated. They are not "NIDDM genes" or "hypertension genes," and in the end, developing the appropriate perspective will be facilitated by avoiding this shortcut terminology and developing a nomenclature more appropriate to the function of the gene."

Rebuttals of the premises of and evidence for the "thrifty gene" hypothesis

Benyshek DC, Watson JT. Exploring the thrifty genotype's food-shortage assumptions: a cross-cultural comparison of ethnographic accounts of food security among foraging and agricultural societies. *Am J Physical Anthropol* 2006; 131:120–126.

p. 120: "The 'thrifty genotype hypothesis' has become firmly entrenched as one of the orienting concepts in biomedical anthropology, since first being proposed by Neel ([1962] Am. J. Hum. Genet. *14*:353–362) over 40 years ago. Its influence on inquiries into the evolutionary origins of diabetes, lactose intolerance, and other metabolic disorders can hardly be underestimated, as evidenced by its continued citation in many top scientific and medical journals. However, its fundamental assumption, that foragers are more likely to experience regular and severe food shortages than sedentary agriculturalists, remains largely untested. The present report tests this assumption by making a cross-cultural statistical comparison of the quantity of available food and the frequency and extent of food shortages among 94 foraging and agricultural societies as reported in the ethnographic record. Our results indicate that there is no statistical difference ($P < 0.05$) in the quantity of available food, or the frequency or extent of food shortages in these reports between preindustrial foragers, recent foragers, and agriculturalists. The findings presented here add to a growing literature that calls into question assumptions about forager food insecurity and nutritional status in general, and ultimately, the very foundation of the thrifty genotype hypothesis: the presumed food shortages that selected for a 'thrifty' metabolism in past foraging populations."

Paradies YC, Montoya MJ, Fullerton SM. Racialized genetics and the study of complex diseases: the thrifty genotype revisited. *Perspectives Biol Med* **2007; 50: 203–227.**

pp. 212–213: "Although it has been argued that famines are incapable of producing the differential mortality required to select for a thrifty genotype, it is, nonetheless, plausible that metabolic efficiency, as well as energy balance and storage, would have been a selective advantage in most human populations during the last few million years. Hence, under the racialized THG [thrifty genome hypothesis], there is a need for an intense environmental impetus to reverse this selection pressure for Europeans first (or only), in order to explain why this ethnoracial group does not suffer from T2DM [Type 2 diabetes mellitus] at the same rate as other ethnoracial groups. It has been suggested that agriculture, which became a dominant mode of subsistence 10,000 years ago for some human societies, could be this impetus.

Underlying the proposal of agriculture as this environmental impetus is the assumption that its advent was associated with an abundant food supply. There is little evidence, however, that agricultural societies were free of feast-and-famine cycles.... Furthermore, some hunter-gather societies were free of feast-and-famine cycles altogether. For instance, Nauruans and other Pacific populations, who now suffer from a very high prevalence of T2DM, formerly lived in thinly populated tropical islands that boasted a generous food supply all year round.

To complicate this simple evolutionary story further, a number of disadvantaged ethnoracial groups, who are thought to now have the putative thrifty genotype, have been using agriculture for many thousands of years. For example, the Pima Indians, the leitmotif of the TGH, have been farming intensively for over 2,000 years."

Ferriera ML, Sanchez T, Nix B. **Touch the heart of the people: cultural rebuilding and the Potawot Health Village in California. In: Ferriera ML, Lang CG (eds).** *Indigenous Peoples and Diabetes: Community Empowerment and Wellness.* **Durham, NC: Carolina Academic Press, 2006; pp. 459–492.**

pp. 467–469: "As a Yurok outreach worker at United Indian Health Services recently put it, 'to say I am an American Indian means I am or will be diabetic.' A recent statistical analysis of the Yurok database, however, reveals that there is a weak, negative correlation between diabetes and quantum of Indian blood... The Pearson correlation between diabetes and blood quantum is -0.218 ($p < 0.001$), which indicates that as quantum increases towards full bloods, the frequency of diabetes decreases...

In fact, few medical studies actually correlate individual genetic admixture with the occurrence of diabetes, when stating that Indian blood quantum structures risk for diabetes. Most studies take 'Indian heritage' for granted, and use it as a major variable to establish genetic causative links for the diabetes epidemic. The problem here is, of course, one of social identity, because it is closely related to the question 'Who is an Indian'?—which appears as the most frequently asked question in the Bureau of Indian Affairs' website. While there are nations, such as the Pima of the Gila River Indian Community, which require a minimum of ¼ 'Indian blood' for tribal membership, in other groups who have 'open enrollment,' such as the Cherokee Tribe of Oklahoma, there are members today who are 1/2048 Cherokee (the fractions are always multiples of 2). Genetically speaking, 'Indian heritage' obviously has different meanings for enrolled members of the Pima and Cherokee nations."

But the hypothesis lives on...

National Institute of Diabetes and Digestive and Kidney Diseases. The Pima Indians: obesity and diabetes. Available at: http://diabetes.niddk.nih.gov/DM/pubs/ pima/obesity/obesity.htm (Accessed: July 22, 2009).

NIDDK research conducted on the Pima Indians for the past 30 years has helped scientists prove that obesity is a major risk factor in the development of diabetes. One-half of adult Pima Indians have diabetes and 95% of those with diabetes are overweight.

These studies, carried out with the help of the Pima Indians, have shown that before gaining weight, overweight people have a slower metabolic rate compared to people of the same weight. This slower metabolic rate, combined with a high fat diet and a genetic tendency to retain fat may cause the epidemic overweight seen in the Pima Indians, scientists believe.

Along with genetic make-up, diet is a key factor to healthy lifestyle. The influence of traditional desert crops on the metabolism of the Pima Indians is being studied to determine how to prevent the onset of diabetes and obesity.

Scientists use the "thrifty gene" theory proposed in 1962 by geneticist James Neel to help explain why many Pima Indians are overweight. Neel's theory is based on the fact that for thousands of years populations who relied on farming, hunting, and fishing for food, such as the Pima Indians, experienced alternating periods of feast and famine. Neel said that to adapt to these extreme changes in caloric needs, these people developed a thrifty gene that allowed them to store fat during times of plenty so that they would not starve during times of famine.

Dr. Eric Ravussin, a visiting scientist at the Phoenix Epidemiology and Clinical Research Branch at NIDDK, has studied obesity in the Pima Indians since 1984. He believes the thrifty gene theory applies to the Pimas.

The Pima Indians maintained much of their traditional way of life and economy until the late 19th century, when their water supply was diverted by American farmers settling upstream, according to Ravussin. At that time, their 2,000-year-old tradition of irrigation and agriculture was disrupted, causing poverty, malnutrition and even starvation. The Pima community had to fall back on the lard, sugar and white flour the U.S. government gave them to survive, says Ravussin.

However, World War II brought great social and economic change for American Indians. Those who entered military service joined Caucasian units. Many other American Indians migrated from reservations to cities for factory employment and their estimated cash income more than doubled from 1940 to 1944.

When the war and the economic boom ended, most Native Americans returned to the reservations, but contact with the larger society had profoundly affected the Pimas' way of life. Ravussin says it is no surprise that the increase in unhealthy weight among the Pima Indians occurred in those born post-World War II.

During this century people world-wide experienced more prosperity and leisure time, and less physical work. Since the 1920s, all Americans have consumed more fat and sugar and less starch and fiber. The greatest changes have occurred in consumption of fat. In the 1890s, the traditional Pima Indian diet consisted of only about 15 percent fat and was high in starch and fiber, but currently almost 40 percent of the calories in the Pima diet is derived from fat. As the typical American diet became more available on the reservation after the war, people became more overweight.

"The only way to correct obesity is to eat less fat and exercise regularly," Ravussin says.

Recently, Ravussin visited a Pima community living as their ancestors did in a remote area of the Sierra Madre mountains of Mexico. These Mexican Pimas are genetically the same as the Pima Indians of Arizona. Out of

35 Mexican Pimas studied, only three had diabetes and the population as a whole was not overweight, according to Ravussin.

"We've learned from this study of the Mexican Pimas that if the Pima Indians of Arizona could return to some of their traditions, including a high degree of physical activity and a diet with less fat and more starch, we might be able to reduce the rate, and surely the severity, of unhealthy weight in most of the population," Ravussin says.

"However, this is not as easy as it sounds because of factors such as genetic influences that are difficult to change. Our research focuses on determining the most effective way to bring about permanent weight loss in light of these factors," Ravussin adds.

Candib LM. Obesity and diabetes in vulnerable populations: reflections on proximal and distal causes. *Ann Fam Med* **2007; 5:547–556.**

p. 550: "**Thrifty genotype.** This hypothesis proposes that the ability to conserve calories by laying down abdominal fat offers a genetic advantage for selection of this genotype during periods of food scarcity in human history. All humans are likely to have genetically determined mechanisms to survive caloric restriction, but some people may have thriftier genotypes than others, resulting in a higher likelihood of obesity when they are faced with higher caloric loads. With increases in caloric intake and decreases in physical activity brought about by economic and social changes, the genetically driven tendency toward central fat deposition becomes a health hazard. Such visceral fat is directly related to the development of insulin resistance and eventually diabetes. This hypothesis has been criticized for its potential to confuse genes with race and its application of biological determinism in the explanation of diabetes without addressing the social determinants of health, however, unique ethnic patterns of abdominal fat deposition resulting from a variety of genetic mutations are demonstrable. Compared with white Europeans, ethnic groups from developing countries–as well as native Americans, native Canadians, Maori, Asian Pacific islanders, and many other native populations–are more vulnerable to the development of diabetes, possibly because of genetic selection for those who could withstand starvation. Why the rate of diabetes among Europeans is lower despite famines in European history is subject to speculation, perhaps because of the differing patterns of famine, differing ways regions addressed food scarcity, or out-migration of those most at risk for diabetes."

> Vogel F, Motulsky AG. **Human and medical genetics.**
> In: Detels R, McEwen J, Beaglehole R, Tanaka H (eds).
> *Oxford Textbook of Public Health.* Oxford: Oxford University Press, 2004. Available at: http://www.r2library.com (Accessed: July 25, 2009).
> "Some decades ago Neel (1962) proposed the hypothesis that type 2 diabetes might be caused by a 'thrifty genotype.' He suggested that the gene or genes underlying diabetes might be an adaptation to long-lasting conditions of food shortage and starvation. Genes that increased mobilization of carbohydrate may have enabled their carriers to survive and reproduce. There is circumstantial evidence in favor of this hypothesis. India is a country in which the majority of the population have suffered for a long time from food shortages. Indians who have emigrated and are living under affluent conditions have a higher frequency of type 2 diabetes. Among some Amerindian tribes, diabetes and obesity have also become very common under the conditions of the current Western American diet. Type 2 diabetes, despite its genetic determination, can often be prevented by avoiding overnutrition."

availability increased—a hypothesis aptly captured by his article's title: "Diabetes mellitus: a 'thrifty' genotype rendered detrimental by 'progress'?" (Neel, 1962, p. 353). Aggravating this tendency toward increased obesity and hence elevated diabetes risk, Neel argued, would be the physiological consequences of civilization's "new types of stresses" (Neel, 1962, p. 359) and increased propensity for sedentary living, with people in modern as compared to what he termed *primitive* societies less likely to respond with physical activity (whether "fight" or "flight") to "alarm situations" that "increased stimulation of the insulin antagonist mechanism" (Neel, 1962, p. 357) (*see* **Textbox 8–2**).

Comparing selection for the putative "thrifty genotype" to selection for sickle cell trait in populations living in regions "hyperendemic for falciparum malaria" (another genetic condition he had studied [Lindee, 2001]), Neel ended his article with a section titled "some eugenic considerations" (Neel, 1962, p. 359). Speculating that "the mounting pressure of population numbers" would lead to global food shortages, he argued—contrary to what he termed "'obvious' eugenic considerations!"—that under such conditions, "modern medicine" would be justified in its efforts to "preserve" (as opposed to eliminate) the "diabetic phenotype" because the "thrifty gene" would once again confer a survival advantage (Neel, 1962, pp. 369–360; *see* **Textbox 8–2**).

In his original 1962 article, Neel made no mention of any Indigenous populations; he would do so later, in a highly influential article published in 1982 (Neel, 1982). Instead, Neel's initial intent was to explain rising rates of diabetes in the "Western World" (Neel, 1962, p. 359). Nevertheless, the "thrifty gene" hypothesis was swiftly deployed (starting in the mid-1960s) to account for fast rising rates of diabetes in the twentieth century among American Indians and Aboriginal Australians, populations in which diabetes had been previously extremely rare or non-existent (Knowler et al., 1983; Knowler et al., 1990; Knowler et al., 1993; Ravussin et al., 1994; Young, 1994; Swinburn, 1996; McDermott, 1998; Bennett, 1999; Paradies et al., 2007). It soon became "one of the orienting concepts in biomedical anthropology" (Benyshek & Watson, 2006, p. 120) (*see* **Textbox 8–2**) and has achieved "textbook" status both for explaining diabetes epidemiology among Indigenous peoples worldwide *and* as an exemplar of "gene–environment interaction," as elaborated in numerous contemporary reference texts (see, for example: Williams, 2003; Vogel & Motulsky, 2004; Hetzel et al., 2004; Inzucchi & Sherwin, 2007; Leonard, 2008) (*see* **Textbox 8–2**). As such, the hypothesis features prominently in the website for the longest-running joint NIH and Indian Health Service studies on diabetes among American Indians, established in 1965 among the Pima Indians (NIDDK, 2009) (*see* **Textbox 8–2**).

Yet, despite the "thrifty genotype" hypothesis' popularity, substantial evidence contradicts its core assumptions, overall and as applied to Indigenous peoples (*see* **Textbox 8–2**), as Neel himself came to recognize (Neel et al., 1998; Neel, 1999). Three major flaws may be summarized as follows:

—*Faulty assumption 1: Risk for diabetes is determined by specific "diabetes genes," and these genes are more prevalent in Indigenous populations.* First, Neel's initial presumption that diabetes has "a well-defined genetic basis, perhaps as simple in many families as a single recessive or incompletely recessive gene" (Neel, 1962, p. 353) has been refuted by contemporary research. Findings instead implicate myriad candidate genes expressed in diverse biological pathways involving energy intake and expenditure (Vogel & Motulsky, 2004; Hetzel et al., 2004; Prentice et al., 2005b; Paradies et al., 2007; Inzucchi & Sherwin, 2007; Prentice et al., 2008). The argument is not that genes are irrelevant but that it is erroneous to posit there exists a specific "thrifty genotype." Second, despite 40-plus years of intensive investigation, to date no unique set of "Indigenous genes" has been identified that singularly predict diabetes occurrence among diverse Indigenous populations (McDermott, 1998; Ferriera & Lang, 2006; Paradies et al., 2007), even as claims have been made for entirely different candidate genes in disparate groups (e.g., in Canada [Hegele et al., 2003] and Australia [Busfield et al., 2002]). Although a lack of evidence is not equivalent to negative evidence, nevertheless the implication (as with other types of health inequities) is that gene expression, not gene frequency, is what matters (Krieger, 2005a).

—*Faulty assumption 2: Risk of famine is greatest in "primitive" societies.* Neel's unreferenced—and oft-repeated—assertion that the "primitive" hunter-gatherer societies accounting for "the first 99 percent or more of man's [*sic*] life on earth" endemically experienced cycles of "feast-and-famine" (Neel, 1962, p. 355), whereas subsequent agriculturalist societies did not, is belied by both historical and contemporary evidence. The evidence refuting his claim was clearly available at the time Neel proposed his hypothesis and has been mounting since (Sigerist, 1951 [1979]; Crosby, 1986; Swinburn, 1996; Ströhle & Wolters, 2004; Prentice et al., 2005; Speakman, 2006; Benyshek & Watson, 2006; Paradies et al., 2007; Ó Gráda, 2009). Empirical research, for example, has found no difference exists "in the quantity of available food, or the frequency or extent of food shortages… between preindustrial foragers, recent foragers, and agriculturalists" (Benyshek & Watson, 2006, p. 120). Moreover, not only were ancient agricultural civilizations, such as Egypt, Mesopotamia, and China, plagued by famines (Sigerist, 1951 [1979]; Prentice et al., 2005b; Ó Gráda, 2009), but as summarized by Mark Nathan Cohen, an anthropologist with expertise in population and agriculture (Cohen, 1989, p. 97):

"The recent histories of India, Russia, China, France, and most of the rest of Europe at least until the nineteenth century display a record of frequent and severe famine that is not exceeded or even matched in simpler societies, much of the famine being attributed not to climate but to the failure of—and even burden imposed by—central administrative mechanisms".

Although debates continue over the importance of recent famine regarding its potential selective effects on fertility and metabolism versus mortality (Speakman, 2006; Prentice et al., 2008; Speakman, 2008), Neel's initial supposition about "primitive" societies and cycles of "feast-and-famine" stands as refuted—even as it is still repeated uncritically in contemporary literature (see, for example: Lindsay & Bennett, 2001; Zimmet & Thomas, 2003; Chakravarthy & Booth, 2004; Candib, 2007; Kuzawa et al., 2008; Leonard, 2008; Servio et al., 2009).

—*Faulty assumption 3: Incorporation of Indigenous peoples into modern states reduced their risk of famine and increased their caloric intake.* The assumptions that Indigenous peoples prior to colonization were solely hunter-gatherers and/or experienced famine only before—but not after—colonization are likewise demonstrably false (Crosby, 1986; Weatherford, 1988; Viola & Margolis, 1991; Nabokov, 1991; Kunitz, 1994; Jackson, 1993; Mann, 2005; Carson et al., 2007). Within the United States, for example, the Pima Indians of southern Arizona, who since the 1970s have been repeatedly stated to have the highest rates of diabetes among U.S. Indian nations, if not the world (Bennett et al., 1971; Knowler et al., 1983; Knowler et al., 1990; Smith et al., 1993; Bennett, 1999), were, along with the Hohokam, their likely predecessors, agriculturalists for centuries before the Spaniards arrived in 1535 (Castetter & Underhill, 1935; Smith et al., 1993; Sheridan, 2006). Instead, their experiences of famine, like those of other American Indian nations, date chiefly to the late nineteenth and early twentieth centuries, a consequence of U.S. policies involving forced relocation into reservations, followed by forced reliance on U.S. government-supplied "ration" and "commodity" foods that, like the diets of children forced to attend Indian boarding schools, were inadequate both in quantity and quality (i.e., primarily starch and meat, with few or no vegetables, fresh fruit, eggs, or milk) (Nabokov, 1991; Smith et al., 1993; Jackson, 1993; Sheridan, 2006; Omura, 2006; Lang, 2006; Martinez et al., 2009).

The subsequent post-World War II reliance on cheap energy-dense nutrition-poor food and lack of access to affordable high-quality food by predominantly impoverished American Indians—both on and off reservation (Joe & Young, 1993; Snip, 2000; Ferriera & Lang, 2006; Candib, 2007), moreover, is not unique to Indigenous peoples but instead common to impoverished populations in many wealthy and middle-income countries, with attendant increased risks of obesity and diabetes (Tanumihardjo et al., 2007; Larson et al., 2009; Gracey & King, 2009). What differs is the intensity and compressed generational timeframe of these events: from traditional foods to famine to the poverty version of the so-called "Western diet," and from a traditional to cash economy. Similarly, Indigenous peoples in the Pacific whose rates of diabetes (especially among impoverished urban populations) have suddenly risen in the twentieth century (Hales & Barker, 1992; Kunitz, 1994; Gracey & King, 2009; Cunningham, 2009) were unlikely to have experienced famine prior to colonization. Illustrating this point is the example of the Naurans, who, given their low population density and the availability of tropical vegetation and fish throughout the year (Baschetti, 1998; Paradies et al., 2007), had sufficient food pre-contact—but under Japanese rule during World War II, experienced "forced labour, exile, and starvation," followed by "post-war prosperity from phosphate exports… accompanied by sedentariness, obesity, and diabetes" (McDermott, 1998).

Thus, although the diversity of experiences of Indigenous peoples and their contingent health profiles, both before and after their forced incorporation into modern states, defies simple generalizations (Young, 1994; Kunitz, 1994; Ferriera & Lang, 2006; Carson et al., 2007; Gracey & King, 2009; King et al., 2009; Cunningham, 2009), the assumption of a long period of "feast-and-famine" sufficient to select for a "thrifty genotype" uniquely or uniformly among Indigenous populations is untenable. So, too, is the assumption that their experiences of famine occurred only pre-colonization and was followed simply by "plenty."

Recognizing threats to the tenets of the "thrifty gene" hypothesis, in 1998 and 1999, shortly before his death, Neel published a set of articles—one lengthy (Neel et al., 1998) and one abridged (Neel, 1999)—in which he both tempered and defended his hypothesis (*see* **Textbox 8–2**). Together, these articles superseded Neel's initial 1982 updating of his hypothesis, in which he included "alternative physiological mechanisms, not understood 20 years ago" (Neel, 1982, p. 284) and also tellingly admitted that "although I have talked rather glibly about a 'thrifty genotype,' I have been quite discrete as to the precise genetic basis of the genotype" (Neel, 1982, p. 290). Accepting, 16 years later, that both the terminology of *thrifty genotype* and the emphasis on "feast-and famine" was "overly simplistic" (Neel et al., 1998, p. 49), Neel further concluded that there was "no evidence for a strong ethnic predisposition" (Neel et al., 1998, p. 45) to Type 2 diabetes in "Amerindians." He instead attributed the rapid emergence of diabetes among the Pima to forced "acculturation," including the destruction of their farming culture through settlers' diversion of their water (Neel et al., 1998, p. 46) (*see* **Textbox 8–2**).

Arguing that "NIDDM [non-insulin dependent diabetes, i.e., Type 2 diabetes] is an etiologically (genetically) heterogeneous entity" (Neel et al., 1998, p. 46) with "complex genetics," Neel accordingly cautioned against referring simplistically to "NIDDM genes." Going further, he stated it was important to avoid the errors made in "cancer genetics," whereby "clear thinking" was hindered by labeling particular genes "proto-oncogenes" and "oncogenes," as if they were exclusively relevant to cancer, when instead such "genes are for the most part cell cycle or housekeeping genes, playing important roles in normal cell activities" (Neel et al., 1998, p. 61). Nevertheless, despite discussing the etiologic importance of the "environment," specifically in relation to diet and physical activity, Neel continued to argue that diabetes and such kindred conditions as obesity and hypertension should be conceptualized as "'syndromes of impaired genetic homeostasis,' or, more colloquially, the 'civilization syndromes,' or the 'altered life styles syndromes,' to which other diseases may be added" (Neal et al., 1998, p. 61; *see* **Textbox 8–2**).

One current alternative to the *thrifty genotype* hypothesis is now the *thrifty phenotype* hypothesis, first proposed in 1992 by C. Nicholas Hales (1935–2005) and David JP Barker (b. 1938) (Hales & Barker, 1992) and elaborated and debated since (Swinburn, 1996; Hales et al., 1997; Bennett, 1999; Hales & Barker, 2001; Lindsay & Bennett, 2001; Prentice et al., 2005b). Premised on a life-course framework (*see* **Chapter 6**), this alternative hypothesis posits that poor nutrition in early life (pre- and post-natal) produces "permanent changes in glucose-insulin metabolism… which, combined with the effects of obesity, ageing and physical inactivity, are the most important factors in determining type 2 diabetes" (Hales & Barker, 2001, p. 5). A corollary is that there can be nongenetically determined familial transgenerational transmission of risk (e.g., because of shared poor nutrition across generations or the physiologic consequences of being a fetus born to an overweight, obese, or diabetic mother) (Hillier et al., 2007; Smith et al., 2009).

Thus, in contrast to the *thrifty genotype* hypothesis, which holds that malnutrition acted as "a selection pressure over many generations to alter the genetic make up of the population" (Lindsay & Bennett, 2001, p. 24), the *thrifty phenotype* hypothesis focuses on present-day early life exposures and proposes physiological mechanisms involving expression of common genes. In effect "de-racializing" both the genotype and disease, the hypothesis has no need to maintain the claim, unsupported by contemporary data (McDermott, 1998; Ferriera & Lang, 2006; Paradies et al., 2007), that there exists a specific genotype predisposed to diabetes that is uniquely shared by the highly heterogeneous populations comprising Indigenous peoples. Instead calling into question the continued use of resources to search for unique Indigenous *thrifty genes*, the *thrifty phenotype* hypothesis has instead shifted attention to health-damaging effects of recent (i.e., late nineteenth to twenty-first centuries) adverse conditions (Hales & Barker, 1992; McDermott, 1998; Speakman, 2006; Paradies et al., 2007).

What has been the harm caused by a nearly half-century prioritizing of "thrifty genes," premised on inaccurate history, to explain twentieth and twenty-first century spatiotemporal patterns of varying degrees of excess and rising rates of diabetes among diverse Indigenous peoples? First and foremost, the entrenched focus by scientists and health professionals on an assumed genetically-determined Indigenous vulnerability to common (a.k.a. "normal") "Western" foods effectively relegated primary prevention to a secondary consideration (McDermott, 1998; Ferriera & Lang, 2006). Efforts instead prioritized clinical care and diabetes self-management—albeit within the funding constraints typically undercutting provision of appropriate health services to Indigenous populations (Knowler et al., 1990; Knowler et al., 1993; Gohdes & Acton, 2000; Roubideaux et al., 2000; Wilson et al., 2005; Warner, 2006; Pavkov et al., 2008). Although providing medical care to those in need is, of course, imperative, the point is that the racialized *thrifty genotype* perspective deemed this was all that could be done, ignoring possibilities for primary prevention.

Second and related, a prevalent corollary of the *thrifty gene* hypothesis is the fatalistic view that "'being Indian means to be diabetic'" (Ferriera & Lang, 2006, p. 15; see also McDermott, 1998; Unnatural Causes, 2009). As stated in one of the handful of books on diabetes and Indigenous Peoples providing Indigenous perspectives, "[p]atients and their families reason that if diabetes is genetic or in their blood, 'there is nothing that can be done about it'" (Ferriera et al., 2006, p. 470). Commenting in 1994 on a three-decade long federally funded study of diabetes among the U.S. Pima Indians, James W. Justice, who did similar research among the nearby related Tohono O'odham Indians, sadly observed (Justice 1993, p. 73):

> "It is sometimes disheartening to consider that with all of our abilities to detect diabetes and begin early intervention, we (i.e., IHS (Indian Health Services) and NIH (National Institutes of Health)) failed to prevent the disaster that has overtaken the Tohono O'odham people and other American Indian Tribes in the United States."

The neglect of context is further underscored by the existence, to date, of only *one* age-period-cohort analysis of diabetes mortality among American Indians. Based on New Mexican mortality records, its limited findings suggest the existence of a birth cohort effect beginning in 1912 (not explained) and a strong period effect starting in 1960 (attributed to not only rising prevalence but also to the increase in health centers and improved accuracy of death certificates) (Gilliand et al., 1997).

Etiologic analyses and interventions premised on the alternative assumptions of sociopolitical, psychosocial, and ecologically and historically oriented epidemiologic theories of disease distribution offer a different vantage (Joe & Young, 1993; McDermott, 1998; Ferriera & Lang, 2006; Carson et al., 2007; Bartlett et al., 2007; King et al., 2009; Cunningham, 2009; Martinez et al., 2009). Reinterpreting diabetes as not only a bodily disease but also "representative and symptomatic of the disruption in the physiology *and* cultures of Indigenous Peoples around the world" (italics in original) (Raymer, 2006, p. 313), these alternatives detail how actual—including recent—histories and contemporary realities of political, economic, territorial, cultural, and ecological expropriation, combined with global changes in the political economy and ecology of food (production, commerce, consumption, and ultimately food sovereignty [La Via Campesina, 2003; IPC, 2009; Rosset, 2009; McMichael, 2009]), have, since the mid-twentieth century, jointly increased of risk diabetes. At issue are their impact on: (*1*) local economies of food, work, and land ownership; (*2*) resources for and participation in Indigenous traditions; and (*3*) access to and resources for appropriate health services (Joe &Young, 1993; McDermott, 1998; Warner, 2006; Ferriera & Lang, 2006; Carson et al., 2007; Bartlett et al., 2007; King et al., 2009; Cunningham, 2009; Martinez et al., 2009).

Together, these sociopolitical phenomena have become embodied, affecting both birth outcomes and birth cohorts, via both transgenerational and concurrent influences on social and biophysical conditions across the life-course (Joe &Young, 1993; McDermott, 1998; Ferriera & Lang, 2006; Carson et al., 2007; Bartlett et al., 2007; King et al., 2009). Particularly salient is the research noted earlier showing the long reach of past damage, whereby children born to mothers affected by obesity, diabetes, and even just high (although not clinically abnormal) insulin levels are themselves at greater risk for these outcomes because of metabolic alterations, independent of heredity *per se* (Hillier et al., 2007; Smith et al., 2009).

Rejecting ill-founded genetic determinism, new Indigenous-led initiatives, many informed by what are referred to as "decolonizing methodologies" (Smith, 1999; Bartlett et al., 2007), are thus developing innovative approaches to prevent diabetes and improve its prognosis. They are doing so by reclaiming history, reclaiming traditional practices and foods, reorienting health interventions to address societal determinants of health, redesigning health systems to be culturally safe and inclusive, and, in the case of the Tohono O'odham, Pima, and Maricopa Indians, literally reclaiming the waters of the Gila River to enable them to farm once again, having finally won an 80-plus year battle contesting the diversion of the river's waters to non-reservation non-Indigenous farmlands, suburbs, and cities, including Phoenix (Castetter & Underhill, 1935 (1978); Kraker, 2004; Applied Research Center, 2005; Sheridan, 2006; Archibold, 2008; TOCA, 2009; Unnatural Causes, 2009; Martinez et al., 2009) (*see* **Textbox 8–3**). Because these initiatives are new, it is too soon to tell whether they will succeed where prior efforts have not. Nevertheless, what stands out is the stark contrast between the analytic approaches—and practical public health implications—of epidemiologic theories of disease distribution that do versus do not engage with actual societal, historical, geographic, and ecologic contexts and relevant spatiotemporal scales and levels.

Example 4: Short-Sighted Analyses—The Impact of Curtailing and Depoliticizing Relevant Time-Frames on Analyses of Temporal Trends in Health Inequities. The fourth and final case concerns a different sort of harm—at the population and policy level, with implications for individuals but without harm directed at individuals *per se*. The example is a recent debate involving different theoretical trends within social epidemiology, with the empirical dispute focused on the question: As population health improves, do relative and absolute social inequalities in health widen or shrink? (Shaw et al., 1999; Phelan & Link, 2005; Mechanic, 2005; Kunitz & Pesis-Katz, 2005; Cutler et al., 2006; Kunitz, 2006; Siddiqi & Hertzman, 2007; Krieger et al., 2008a; Beckfield & Krieger, 2009).

An increasingly common view, typically drawing on recent data from the United States, is that relative, if not also absolute, health disparities are bound to increase as mortality rates decline, largely because groups with the most education and most resources are most

Textbox 8–3. Contemporary Alternative Analysis of Diabetes Epidemiology by Tohono O'odham Indians (Arizona, United States) and Corresponding Prevention Strategies

Diabetes prevalence: from nonexistent prior to 1950 to among the world's highest

Pre-to-mid-1950s:

"Earlier government reports do not mention diabetes as a health problem among the Tohono O'odham nor is diabetes mentioned by the Tohono O'odham tribal economic plans for 1949, although infant mortality, malnutrition and other problems were listed... The first extensive health status survey of the Tohono O'odham was conducted by Kraus and Jones during 1952-1953... They reported a diabetes prevalence rate of 5 per 1,00 population for Tohono O'odham and 9 per 1000 for the Pimas." (Justice 1994, p. 74)

1960s–1980s

Estimated diabetes prevalence rates among persons > 25 years old (per 1000 population) (Justice, 1994, pp. 77, 79):

	1965	1985
Men	153.9	257.8
Women	144.7	373.0

21st century:

'... the Tohono O'odham Nation has the highest diabetes rate in the world; over 50 percent of adults have adult-onset diabetes. (Applied Research Center 2005; p. 41)

Ecological and economic context

Before encounter with Europeans in late 1600s:

"When Jesuit missionary Eusebio Francisco Kino criss-crossed the Pimería Alta in the early 1690s, he and his frequent traveling companion, Juan Mateo Manje, distinguished among different groups of O'odham, including the Sobas along the Río de la Concepcíon and the Papabotas (Papagos [Tohono O'odham])..." (Sheridan, 2006, p 26)

"Before Kino and his companions rode down the Santa Cruz, O'odham... living along the few rivers and streams of the Sonoran Desert pursued three complementary subsistence strategies, all of which depended upon an intricate knowledge of plants, animals, and climate. During the spring and summer, they farmed floodplain fields or arroyo deltas. Throughout the year, they harvested wild plants and hunted wild game. When rains were abundant, washes ran and rivers flowed, watering their desert cultigens. When heat and drought withered crops, the O'odham relied entirely upon the seeds, fruits, roots, and caudices produced by the desert itself. Their agriculture was based upon three thousand years of accumulated knowledge about plant physiology and microclimates in the Sonoran Desert. O'odham in the Santa Cruz, San Pedro, and Magdalena-Altar-Concepción watersheds practiced irrigation agriculture, constructing brush weirs that diverted water into earthen canals that led to their fields. O'odham along the Gila River... may not have needed to expend the energy to build weirs and canals. instead, they simply may have planted their seeds in swales and islands after the Gila's seasonal floodwaters receded." (Sheridan, 2006, p. 34)

"*Historical Tohono O'odham Food System.* The traditional food system supported a local economy, maintained the people's physical well-being, and provided the material foundation for Tohono O'odham culture. For many centuries, the Tohono O'odham and their ancestors combined a series of well-adapted strategies of producing food in the arid lands of the Sonoron Desert. The three parts of this traditional Tohono O'odham food system were:

Ak Chin Farming—Using the flood waters that accompany the summer monsoons, thousands of acres were planted with crops that are nutritious and well-adapted to the short, hot growing season. Many of these foods were eaten fresh and preserved for use throughout the rest of the year.

Harvesting Wild Foods—Throughout the year, the desert provides a wide variety of wild foods that were collected and eaten. These wild foods included cholla buds, the fruit of different cacti, mesquite bean pods and acorns. Many of these foods were preserved for use throughout the year.

Hunting—The animals of the desert also provided an important source of nutrition. The hunting of rabbits, deer, havalina and other desert dwellers was a significant supplement to the foods grown in O'odham fields and collected in the desert. The combination of flood-based farming during the summer rains, collection of wild foods, and hunting provided the O'odham with a rich and varied diet.

In addition to providing healthy foods, all of these activities (and their cultural supports such as traditional dancing) promoted high levels of physical activity and fitness." (TOCA, 2009)

20th century CE:

"Tohono O'odham Community Action (TOCA) is based in Sells, Arizona, on the 4,600-square-mile Tohono O'odham Reservation, in the heart of the Sonora Desert. The tribe now has around 24,000 members. Until the mid 1900s, the O'odham used traditional agricultural practices they had developed over a thousand years. But a series of government policies seriously undermined their ability to continue these practices. Federal food programs introduced processed foods, displacing traditional nutrition. O'odham we re encouraged to take jobs as field laborers for large irrigated cotton farms that surrounded O'odham land, resulting in many families leaving for six to eight months a year and being unable to maintain their own fields. Nearby development lowered the flood table and, as a result of governmental flood control projects, water became scarce, and flood waters were eliminated from important lands. On top of these devastating changes, large numbers of children were forcibly sent to boarding schools, where they were severely punished for speaking their language and participating in their culture. All of these factors resulted in a break in the transfer of knowledge and traditions.

These changes wreaked havoc on O'odham agriculture. In the 1920s, over 20,000 acres of flood plain were cultivated using flash-flood irrigation conducive to the area's pattern of frequent summer monsoons. But by 1949 only 2,500 acres were cultivated, and by 2000 only a few acres were cultivated. There are other major challenges as well. The reservation is extremely rural and has the lowest per capita income of all U.S. reservations. The Tohono O'odham Nation has the highest diabetes rate in the world; over 50 percent of adults have adult-onset diabetes. The major changes in diet and community have certainly played a role in the diabetes epidemic." (Applied Research Center, 2005; p. 41)

"The steady change from a farming, hunting, and gathering society to one in which most individuals became wage earners occurred very slowly until the1930s. During the 1930s, cotton farming off reservation needed manual labor, and by 1939, one third of all dollars earned by reservation residents came from this work... By 1960, most of the dollars earned by reservation Papagos [Tohono O'odham] came from off reservation work or from allotments paid by outside agencies, including the Bureau of Indian Affairs Welfare Program... Once wage earning because the primary source for food purchasing, the six trading posts on or near the reservation change their inventories. As late as 1949, most stores carried only beans, syrup, sugar, flour, coffee, lard, and powdered or canned milk. By the early 1960s, these same on-reservation stores started to carry high caloric pre-packed sweets, such as carbonated beverages (i.e., 'soda pop'), candy, potato chips, and cakes. None of these foods were mentioned by Ross in her 1941 survey of dietary habits nor by Van Cleft, who in 1954 calculated an in-depth survey of the buying habits of 16 families at 'the trading posts'... Finally in 1959, large quantities of refined flour, sugar, and canned fruits high in sugar became available from the U.S. Department of Agriculture surplus commodity food program, and by 1965 were being distributed widely." (Justice, 1994, pp. 115–117)

"More than a hundred years ago, the Gila River, siphoned off by famers upstream, all but dried up here in the parched flats south of Phoenix, plunging an Indian community that had depended on it for centuries of farming into starvation and poverty... Most of the water was diverted in the late 19th century, slowing the Gila River to a trickle. It was a startling turn of events for a tribe whose ancestors had thrived on the river for generations through an elaborate system of ditches and laterals, some of them still visible today. The construction of the Coolidge Dam, completed in 1928, by the federal government was intended to restore some of the lost water, but the reservation never received enough to bring back farming in any big way. Later diversions also depleted the Salt River, which runs north of the reservation and helped support farming as well. As the water disappeared and the Pima switched to government rations as their staple, obesity, alcoholism and diabetes exploded…" (Archibold, 2008)

21st century CE:
"Per capita income on the Tohono O'odham Nation is $6998 (compared with $21,994 nationally), the lowest of all U.S. reservations. Median family income is $21,223 (compared with $50,046 nationally). 41.7% of all households and 50.6% of households with children are below the poverty level (compared to the U.S. averages of 9.2% and 13.6%, respectively). Only 31.3% of the adult population is currently employed." (TOCA, 2009)
"Fewer than half of the Tohono O'odham community's adults have completed high school, the lowest rate of all U.S. Native American tribes." (TOCA, 2009)

Etiologic analysis

"The primary cause of diabetes within the community is the change from a diet consisting primarily of traditional food and the destruction of a sustainable Tohono O'odham food system." (TOCA, 2009)

Interventions

TOCA programs:
"TOCA's goal is to develop a food system and then encourage people to make healthy choices. TOCA's food system project focuses on three incentives: health, culture, and economy. In addition to their health benefits, traditional foods and crops are closely related to O'odham cultural identity. Many of TOCA's programs work to encourage the continuity of these linked traditions. TOCA is also working to encourage production and supply of traditional foods." (Applied Research Center, 2005, p. 44)
"TOCA's Tohono O'odham Food System and wellness initiatives combat the highest rates of diabetes in the world while simultaneously creating economic opportunity. By reintroducing traditional food production to the community, TOCA is stimulating improved community health, cultural revitalization and economic opportunity… This program has established a working farm to grow food once part of the daily O'odham diet, is actively documenting song, stories, harvesting, cultivation and processing methods, and is providing traditional foods for sale in the community and to hospitals, schools, and elderly lunch programs." (TOCA, 2009)

Reclamation of river waters for farming:

"... the long lush fields of the Pimas and Maricopas began to wither in the late 1800s, when Mormon farmers upstream began diverting huge amounts of water from the Gila...

The Gila River Indian Community first went to court in 1925, and has spent millions of dollars in an effort to quantify its water rights. Originally, the tribes made a claim on the Gila and Salt rivers, which form the boundaries of the reservation. In 1974, they sued for nearly the entire annual flow of the Gila, almost 2 million acre-feet. If the tribes had pursued that claim, it would have posed a major threat to the water supply of fast-growing Phoenix, according to City Water Manager Tom Buschatzke. Phoenix took the threat so seriously that, in 1988, it created an adjudication section within its law department, staffed by an attorney, a paralegal, a historian and a hydrologist, to try to work out a settlement with the Gila River Community and other tribes...

It took eight years, but the city, working with the Arizona Department of Water Resources, the Central Arizona Water Conservation District, the Bureau of Indian Affairs, the Bureau of Reclamation, irrigation districts and other metropolitan cities, finally came to an agreement with the Gila River Community..." (Kraker, 2004)

"...[the settlement] provides the reservation 653,500 acre-feet of water a year (an acre-foot is equivalent to about one family's water use annually) coming from a mix of sources, with the Central Arizona Project tapping the Colorado River providing the biggest share. It also includes the $680 million to rebuilt the irrigation system and to provide drainage, water monitoring, and other benefits... The reservation has discussed farming some 150,000 acres, 40 percent of its 372,000 acres... And it will take much effort to reverse the legacy of poor health, though programs abound, intended for the young and old, to combat diabetes... 'When we lost that water, we lost generations of farming,' said Janet Haskie, a community gardener. 'Then people had the attitude like, "They owe us. I'm going to take these rations." So now we have to start over again, a little at a time.'" (Archibold, 2008)

able to take advantage of new knowledge and technology (Phelan & Link, 2005; Mechanic, 2005; Cutler et al., 2006). By contrast, others, reviewing contemporary data from other countries (such as Canada), have posited that as mortality rates drop, health inequities tend to "flatten up" (Siddiqi & Hertzman, 2007), largely because improvements in population health are driven by "'pulling up' the health of the lower groups" (Siddiqi & Hertzman, 2007, p. 592). Still others, examining both the North American and European data over longer spans of time, hold that no one general pattern can be expected; instead, the circumstances leading to improvements in population health and affecting the magnitude of health inequities are historically contingent and depend on the societal context and its public health, political, and economic priorities (Shaw et al., 1999; Kunitz & Pesis-Katz, 2005; Kunitz, 2006; Krieger et al., 2008a; Beckfield & Krieger, 2009). At a theoretical level, the contrast is between hypotheses premised on a depoliticized and ahistorical population health perspective versus those that are explicit about political and historical context, as discussed in **Chapters 6** and **7**.

Such a debate has profound policy implications. If, for example, increased health inequities inevitably accompany improvements in population health, it would suggest that the focus on health inequities be secondary to concerns about overall secular trends (Cutler et al., 2006)—in effect, a "trickle-down" approach to rectifying health inequities. Conversely, if improvements in overall population rates chiefly result from larger gains among those faring worst, then it would suggest that as long as population rates improve, health inequities should decline (Siddiqi & Hertzman, 2007)—that is, these trends necessarily move together. If, however, the relationship between population health and the magnitude of health inequities is more variable, it would imply resources are needed to tackle both concerns (Krieger et al., 2008a; Beckfield & Krieger, 2009).

Providing insight into this debate are **Figures 1–1a** and **1–1b** in **Chapter 1**, showing the past half-century of trends in U.S. premature mortality (death before age 65 years) and infant death rates by county income level and race/ethnicity (Krieger et al., 2008a). These figures address the partial picture provided by most prior U.S. analysis, which, in part because of data limitations, typically have focused on post-1980 trends, mainly regarding racial/ethnic disparities in mortality, but with a few also including socioeconomic data and with a handful also extending back to 1968 and two using data from 1960 in conjunction with post-1969 data (Pappas et al., 1993; Singh & Yu, 1995; Singh & Yu, 1996a; Singh & Yu, 1996b; Schalick et al., 2000; Levine et al., 2001; Hillemeier et al., 2001; Kington & Nickens, 2001; Williams, 2001; Singh & Siapush, 2002; Singh, 2003; Ronzio, 2003; Satcher et al., 2005; Murray et al., 2006; Singh & Kogan, 2007; Ezzati et al., 2008). Together, this prior work on racial/ethnic and socioeconomic inequities in U.S. mortality has tended to support the hypothesis that as overall deaths rates have declined, social inequities in mortality have increased.

The yearly mortality data presented in the figures in **Chapter 1**, by contrast, span from 1960 to 2002, an interval that precedes as well as encompasses the period of the mid-1960s, a time when new U.S. federal policies were enacted with the intent of reducing socioeconomic and racial/ethnic inequalities, overall and also in relation to medical care (Davis & Schoen, 1978; O'Connor, 2001; Fairclough, 2001; Conley & Springer, 2001; Turncock & Atchison, 2002; Quadagno & McDonald, 2003; Navarro & Muntaner, 2004; Duncan & Chase-Lansdale, 2004; Kunitz & Pesis-Katz, 2005; Krieger et al., 2008a). Examples include the various federal policies constituting the "War on Poverty," the 1964 U.S. Civil Rights Act, and the establishment of Medicare, Medicaid, and community health centers (Davis & Schoen, 1978; Cooper et al., 1981; O'Connor, 2001; Fairclough, 2001; Turncock & Atchison, 2002; Quadagno & McDonald, 2003; Duncan & Chase-Landsdale, 2004; Almond et al., 2006; Navarro & Muntaner, 2004; Smith, 2005; Lefkowitz, 2007). The selected timeframe likewise encompasses subsequent periods of active debate and change regarding government policies and spending on anti-poverty and civil rights initiatives, including post-1980 policies to "roll back" the welfare state (O'Connor, 2001; Fairclough, 2001; Turncock & Atchison, 2002; Henwood, 2003; Duncan & Chase-Landsdale, 2004; Navarro & Muntaner, 2004; Auerbach et al., 2006; Beckfield & Krieger, 2009).

The study's *a priori* prediction, borne out by the results shown in **Figures 1–1a** and **1–1b,** was that the societal changes during the study time period (1960–2002) would be embodied and manifested in reductions in socioeconomic and racial/ethnic health inequities that preceded the documented post-1980 widening of health disparities noted above.

As revealed by more detailed analyses (Krieger et al., 2008a) between 1966 and 1980, the relative and absolute socioeconomic disparities in premature mortality shrank, overall and especially among U.S. populations of color; and thereafter, starting in 1981, the relative and absolute socioeconomic gaps for premature mortality widened; similar trends occurred for infant deaths. These patterns, unlikely to be explained simply by changes in health behaviors or medical treatment (Krieger et al., 2008a), refute the view that improvements in population health by default entail growing or shrinking health disparities, whether absolute or relative.

The net implication is that the societal patterning of socioeconomic inequities in mortality within and across racial/ethnic groups is historically contingent: context matters (Shaw et al., 1999; Kunitz & Pesis-Katz, 2005; Kunitz, 2006; Krieger et al., 2008a; Beckfield & Krieger, 2009). Comparing the results for 1966 to 1980 versus 1981 to 2002, the early trends give grounds for hope; the latter augur poorly for the *Healthy People 2010* objective of eliminating U.S. socioeconomic and racial/ethnic health disparities (U.S. DHHS, 2000)—a target clearly not met. Enabling these patterns to be seen is research motivated by epidemiologic theories of disease distribution attuned to history and sociopolitical context. The harmful consequences, including for policy formulation, of overlooking relevant historical time periods is apparent. Getting it right matters: Death is inevitable. Premature mortality—and widening inequities in premature mortality—are not.

Summary of Selected Cases: Illustrative, Not Isolated—Hence, Error, Harm, and the Vital Importance of Epidemiologic Theory. If the above four examples were isolated problems, their impact would be "restricted" to the specific harm done to the diverse populations affected. But they are not.

Instead, and as the previous chapters recount, epidemiologists since the inception of the field have long reckoned with the knowledge that erroneous and inadequate explanations can cause damage—either literally harming particular individuals or else not averting preventable suffering, illness, and death. At one level, the awareness of the potential of epidemiologic research to do harm, not just good, is well-recognized in the obligate discussion of "Type I" and "Type II" errors that routinely appears in epidemiologic textbooks (*see*, for example, those reviewed in **Chapter 1**). Conceptualized in relation to the empirical statistical testing of hypotheses, these two types of error are defined as (Porta 2008, p.85):

- **Error, Type I** (Syn: alpha error). The error of wrongly rejecting a null hypothesis—that is, declaring that a difference exists when it does not.
- **Error, Type II** (Syn: beta error). The error of failing to reject a false null hypothesis—that is, declaring that a difference does not exist when, in fact, it does.

Commonly considered causes of these types of errors include various types of systematic error, different kinds of confounding, and inadequate sample size.

Bringing the discussion of error to literally another level, however, since the late 1990s, a third type of error has been added to the epidemiologic roster, defined as (Porta 2008, p. 85):

- **Error, Type III** Wrongly assessing the causes of interindividual variation within a population when the research question requires an analysis of causes of differences between population or time periods... Risk differences between individuals within a particular population may not have the same causes as differences in the average risk between two different populations.

This definition, introduced in 1999 by Sharon Schwartz and Kenneth Carpenter (Schwartz & Carpenter, 1999), recognizes that Type I and Type II errors do not exhaust the number of ways it is possible to get a right or wrong answer. Precursors to this definition of Type III error include the 1948 proposal, by the eminent biostatistician Frederick Mosteller (1916–2006), of "a third kind of error"—that of "correctly rejecting the null hypothesis for the wrong reason" (as "it is possible for the null hypothesis to be false") (Mosteller, 1948, p. 61). More akin to the Schwartz and Carpenter approach is the 1957 definition provided by Allyn W. Kimbal: "the error committed by giving the right answer to the wrong problem" (Kimball, 1957, p. 134). Indeed, as the epidemiologist Major Greenwood (1880–1949) cogently observed in 1935: nature "always answers truthfully the question you ask her, not the question you *meant* to ask her but the one you *did* ask" (italics in original) (Greenwood, 1935, p. 67).

In offering their expanded definition of Type III error, Schwartz and Carpenter built on Geoffrey Rose's social epidemiologic insight, discussed in **Chapter 6**, that causes of incidence are not necessarily the same as causes of cases (Rose, 1985). Also germane was the parallel recognition that "the sort of evidence gathered on the benefits of interventions aimed at individuals may not help in guiding policies directed towards reducing health inequalities" (Davey Smith et al., 2001). Motivated by then ongoing debates about individual-level versus societal determinants of population rates of homeless, obesity, and infant mortality, Schwartz and Carpenter's concern was that studies designed to analyze individual-level differences in risk within a specified population were often wrongly interpreted as being causally informative about why rates change over time or differ between populations (Schwartz & Carpenter, 1999). For example, although inter-individual genetic variability could potentially contribute to explaining inter-individual variation in body mass index in a given population at a given point in time, such individual-level genetic variability could not by itself account for why obesity rates within a population were quickly rising, as "genetic variation does not change that rapidly"; instead, to explain the rising rates, data are needed on "whatever other changes have occurred between time periods (e.g., an increase in the pervasiveness of advertisements enticing people to eat, the number of fast food restaurants per square mile, or exposure to sedentary leisure activities)" (Schwartz & Carpenter, 1999, p. 1178). Schwartz and Carpenter consequently argued that valid epidemiologic research "requires consideration of the full range of risk factors at all levels organization" and that "to examine such exposures requires their overt consideration and different sampling, measurement, and conceptual frameworks" (Schwartz & Carpenter, 1999, p. 1179).

Stated another way, avoiding the kind of Type III error described by Schwartz and Carpenter requires explicitly engaging with epidemiologic theory. At issue is the role of theory in guiding the hypotheses that are tested in the first place, before even attempting to ascertain whether any particular study provides a valid test of the hypothesis under consideration. Methodological precision alone cannot suffice because choice of methods follows choice of question (Morris, 1957, p. 14; Krieger, 2007). Paying heed to epidemiologic theory, and theorizing deeply across a diverse array of determinants of distributions of disease in real societies at real points in time, is thus not a matter of "politically correct" science, as some conservative commentators have charged (Satel, 2000). It is, instead, a matter of doing *correct* science (Krieger, 2005a) and answering well the questions that epidemiology is best suited to answer.

Hence, as should by now be clear, epidemiologic theory counts—for good and for bad. It matters not just because of the potential to cause harm but also because it can lead to valuable knowledge that spurs possibilities for beneficial change. Otherwise, to paraphrase Morris, what's the use of epidemiology? (Morris, 1957)

Looking Ahead: Epidemiologic Theory, the People's Health, and the Stories that Bodies Tell

In the half-century since publication of Morris' *Uses of Epidemiology* (Morris, 1957) and MacMahon et al.'s *Epidemiologic Methods* (MacMahon et al., 1960), the field of epidemiology has grown enormously (Boslaugh, 2008; Susser & Stein, 2009). Epidemiologists have, in keeping with the "seven uses" of epidemiology that Morris outlined in 1957 (*see* **Chapter 6, Textbox 6–2**) (Morris, 1957, p.96), constructively contributed to the public's health. The roster of accomplishments includes: producing valuable knowledge about current and changing population distributions of health and disease at the community, national, and global levels; conducting etiologic research to elucidate the underlying causes of these patterns; quantifying the need for health services and evaluating the effectiveness of services provided; and helping identify both healthy "ways of living" and obstacles preventing individuals and communities from living healthy lives.

Like any other academic discipline, epidemiology has also been embroiled in myriad debates about the substance of its scholarship. Potentially calling the credibility of the field into question, the past decade alone has witnessed major disputes over why, in a number of high profile cases, discordant results about likely benefits versus harm have been produced by observational studies versus randomized clinical trials, including the case of HT, discussed above, and also use of vitamin supplements and other micronutrients (Davey Smith & Ebrahim, 2001; Lawlor et al., 2004a; Lawlor et al., 2004b; Lawlor et al., 2004c; von Elm & Egger, 2004; Ebrahim & Clarke, 2007). Added to this list of concerns is, most recently, why results of so many genetic association studies are, like the observational studies, often inconsistent, if not nonreproducible (Mayes et al., 1989; Davey Smith & Ebrahim, 2001; von Elm & Egger, 2004; Pocock et al., 2004; Ebrahim & Davey Smith, 2008; Little et al., 2009a; STROBE, 2009; STREGA, 2009). Typically, in the case of the observational studies, blame for discrepancies has been attributed to their inability to control adequately for confounding, above and beyond problems of reverse causation, measurement error, and selection bias (Davey Smith & Ebrahim, 2002; Ebrahim & Clarke, 2007; STROBE, 2009); the genetic studies, in turn, are postulated to suffer from problems of small sample size, inadequate characterization of study populations, biased analyses (STREGA, 2009), and perhaps even faulty hypotheses (Dickson et al., 2010). Reacting to the controversies and mixed evidence, some high-profile external critics, such as Gary Taubes, have gone so far as to argue that only epidemiologic evidence from randomized trials be given credence (Taubes, 1995; Taubes, 2007).

Within the field, however, more realistic and nuanced arguments have recognized the need for diverse study designs, each with their own limitations and strengths and each attuned to answering some types of questions but not others (Davey Smith et al., 2001; Barreto, 2004; Vandenbroucke, 2008). For example, just as randomized trials are ill-suited to investigate causes of disease and are incapable of addressing such critical epidemiologic questions as to whether (and, if so, why) age-period-cohort effects exist or rates of disease are changing over time, observational studies are poorly suited to evaluate whether intended therapies have their intended effects. Both types of studies, moreover, face the challenge of delineating the likely causal relationships between the phenomena of interest, so as to guide which variables should be included as exposures, outcomes, confounders, mediators, or effect modifiers and also how they should be measured. Both also must reckon with the profound problem of selection bias (Porta, 2008, pp. 225–226), which, by affecting who is and is not part of the study population, can skew the range of observed exposures and outcomes and hence the magnitude of observed exposure–outcome associations. Such bias can profoundly compromise not only the extent to which results "may apply, be relevant, or be generalized to populations or groups that did not participate in the study" (Porta, 2008, p. 252), but also, the internal validity of the results themselves. Stated more bluntly, the argument that internal validity is paramount and comes before concerns about generalizability only makes sense if the study populations included provide a valid test of the hypothesis in question—and theory is vital to making this determination.

Taking stock of the field, recent articles have tallied up both epidemiology's successes and failures (for examples, *see* **Textbox 8–4**) (Davey Smith & Ebrahim, 2001; Ness, 2009), with virtually all calling attention to the importance of the multiplicity of study populations, study designs, measures (including of relevant covariates), and modeling approaches needed to test hypotheses well and get the answers right. Representing one constructive step toward addressing recent criticisms of epidemiology are several new initiatives, including the STROBE ("STrengthening the Reporting of Observational Studies in Epidemiology") and STREGA ("STrengthening the REporting of Genetic Association Studies") guidelines, both of which have been published in major epidemiology and biomedical journals (Egger et al., 2007; von Elm et al., 2007a–2007g; Vandenbroucke et al., 2007a–2007c; von Elm et al., 2008; STROBE, 2009; Little et al., 2009a–2009g; STREGA, 2009). Intended to improve the rigor and transparency of how epidemiologic findings are presented, their recommendations set high standards for how studies are done.

Tellingly, however, none of these contemporary discussions about the strengths and limitations of epidemiologic research, nor the new STROBE and STREGA guidelines, include any explicit discussion about the relevance of epidemiologic theories of disease distribution for study hypotheses, methods, or interpretation of findings. Similarly, new efforts to improve causal analysis and inference—such as those using directed acyclic graphs (DAGs), which graphically encode relationships between variables (Greenland et al., 1999; Robins, 2001; Hérnan, 2002; Glymour, 2006; Fleisher & Diez Roux, 2008; Richiardi et al., 2008)—likewise remains mum about what determines which variables are even considered, let alone why and how they may be causally linked or contingently entangled, even as they do acknowledge that background knowledge is needed to understand the causal processes at play. Nor do contemporary epidemiologic textbooks offer much guidance, as discussed in **Chapter 1**.

Instead, epidemiologists are once again left to their own devices, free to populate more carefully structured causal webs with undertheorized assorted "variables," as if hypotheses were independent of theoretical frameworks, and as if approaches to causal theorizing about determinants of population distributions and risk of disease are either self-evident, requiring no analysis, or else simply a matter of idiosyncratic inspiration (or ideological proclivities). If, however, transparency of assumptions is vital for valid scientific research, then explicit attention to epidemiologic theories of disease distributions is essential for the field—and as the above examples make clear, the cost of ignoring these theories can be high, whether measured in wasted effort or, more profoundly, in people's lives.

But there is room for hope—at multiple levels. Within the past two decades, a renewed interest in epidemiologic theories of disease distribution has become apparent (*see* **Chapters 6** and **7**), largely prompted by the revitalization of social epidemiology and its focus on developing frameworks, concepts, models, and methods to explain—and inform efforts to alter—current and changing societal patterning of health, disease, and health inequities (Krieger, 1994; Krieger, 2001b). Although some of these approaches have been dismissive of research focusing on specific "risk factors" (including health behaviors) and biological aspects of pathogenesis, others have decidedly engaged with the biophysical and behavioral processes involved in disease etiology, albeit rejecting the decontextualized analytic mode of the biomedical and lifestyle perspectives. Conceptualizing disease processes and rates in relation to multiple levels of societally-shaped exposures, susceptibility,

Textbox 8-4. Twenty-First Century Appraisals of Epidemiology's Triumphs and Failures Since 1950

Triumphs	Failures
Davey Smith G, Ebrahim S. Epidemiology—is it time to call it a day? *Int J Epidemiol* 2001; 30:1–11	Davey Smith G, Ebrahim S. Epidemiology—is it time to call it a day? *Int J Epidemiol* 2001; 30:1–11

Triumphs	Failures
- cigarette smoking as a cause of lung cancer (and other diseases as well) (p. 2) - evidence on the fetal origins of adult disease and the "rebirth of social physiology" (pp. 2–3) - applied epidemiology in "poorer parts of the world": eradication of smallpox; expanded programs of immunization; sanitary improvements (e.g., "slit latrines and deep tube wells") (p. 3) **Topics included in 2009 special issue of Annals of Epidemiology on the "triumphs of epidemiology" (Ness 2009):** 1. folic-acid fortification to reduce risk of folic-acid preventable spina bifida and anencephaly (Oakley, 2009) 2. use of hepatitis B vaccine to prevent hepatocellular carcinoma (Palmer-Beasley, 2009); health impact of low-level lead exposure (Needleman, 2009); 3. elucidation of which types of human papilloma virus (HPV) cause which types of cancer, relevant to development of the new HPV vaccine (Koutsky, 2009); 4. prone sleeping position as a preventable cause of sudden infant death syndrome (Dwyer & Ponsoby, 2009); 5. identification of individuals uninfected by HIV despite high exposure and possible immunologic and genetic traits conferring "natural" protection (Detels, 2009); 6. health benefits of physical activity, including for cardiovascular and other chronic diseases (Blair & Morris, 2009); 7. health effects of particulate air pollution, including elevated risk of mortality (Dockery, 2009).	i. despite extensive epidemiologic research on peptic ulcer in relation to temporal trends, birth cohort effects, and possible risk factors, these investigations played no role in identification of *H. pylori* as a key causal agent (pp. 4–5) ii. refutations by intervention studies (e.g., randomized clinical trials (RCTs)) of posited protective effects based on observational epidemiologic evidence for: (pp. 5–6) a. hormone replacement therapy and risk of cardiovascular disease: observational = protective; RCTs = increased risk b. beta-carotene and risk of cardiovascular disease: observational = protective; RCTs = increased risk c. vitamin E and risk of cardiovascular disease: observational = protective; RCTs = increased risk d. vitamin C and risk of cardiovascular disease: observational = protective; RCTs = no protection e. fiber intake and risk of colon cancer: observational = protective; RCTs = no protection

and resistance across the life-course and transgenerationally, these latter frameworks essentially posit there is more to biology than biomedicine and more to behavior than lifestyle. Offering fresh approaches to analyzing disease distribution as the embodiment of societal, ecologic, and historical context, this new work additionally makes clear that alternatives to current inequities are possible—and that it is theory that enables us to see this, in eminently practical terms.

After all, as Raymond Williams (1921–1988) observed in his historical etymologic explication of the many meanings of "theory" (*see* **Chapter 1, Textbox 1–1**), the act of theorizing is "always in active relation to *practice* [italics in original]: an interaction between things done, things observed and (systematic) explanation of these" (Williams, 1983a, p. 317). To Williams, theory's power to be transformative occurs when it when it makes "hope practical, rather than despair convincing" (Williams, 1983b, p. 240). It can do so by providing new means to think about and address unsolved problems (whether conceptual, methodological, or practical), by revealing connections between previously unlinked ideas or phenomena, and by sparking awareness that, to use the language of the day, "another world is possible" (World Social Forum, 2001). Williams' conclusion that "if there are no easy answers there are still available and discoverable hard answers, and it is these that we can now learn to make and share" (Williams, 1983b, pp. 268–269), far from being disheartening, is one that encourages creative and cooperative efforts to develop theory, apply it, and learn from the experience—advice as apt for the work of epidemiologists and other scientists as it is for those who seek to translate the knowledge gained from scientific research into practical improvements in people's ability to live meaningful, healthy, and dignified lives.

I accordingly offer three final examples of the difference, conceptually and empirically, that explicit attention to epidemiologic theory can make—for description, for etiologic analysis, and for action. The examples are:

Textbox 8–5: Data on social class, race/ethnicity and gender in public health surveillance systems

Textbox 8–6: Discrimination as a determinant of health inequities (*see also* **Figure 8–2**)

Textbox 8–7: New national policies and global recommendations for health equity, in ecologic context

In each case, I show how application of diverse social epidemiologic frameworks has revealed serious gaps in knowledge and expanded the range of questions, data, understanding, and evidence available for improving population health and promoting health equity.

In closing, epidemiology is complex science, one with a profound capacity to illuminate—or obscure—the stories that our bodies tell. Deeply engaged with so many facets of human existence and life on this planet, epidemiology as a discipline is a remarkable intellectual project, one constantly grappling with how lived experience translates into society's epidemiologic profiles. As its past history and present state readily reveal, what knowledge the field offers depends on theories of disease distribution deployed, not just the methods used. Created by real people, in real historical, political, and ecologic contexts, epidemiologic theories of disease distribution necessarily draw on metaphors and mechanisms that reflect the contending worldviews and technological level of the societies in which these theories are developed, employed, and contested. Recognition of the critical role of theory in shaping epidemiologic inquiry in turn raises issues of accountability and agency, in relation to not only who and what is responsible for observed disease distributions but also how they are monitored, analyzed, and addressed.

Textbox 8–5. The Difference Epidemiologic Theory Can Make: Description—"Painting a Truer Picture" of the People's Health Using Social Epidemiologic Frameworks to Conceptualize Public Health Surveillance Data, Identify Gaps, and Fill Them, Using the Four Cases Examples of Class, Race/Ethnicity, Gender, and Global Health Inequities.

Public health surveillance: objective

Public health surveillance systems (vital statistics, disease registries, health surveys) should, as Edgar Sydenstricker (1881–1936) observed when he was designing the first U.S. population-based morbidity studies in the 1920s (Sydenstricker, 1930), **"give glimpses of what the sanitarian has long wanted to see—a picture of the public-health situation as a whole, drawn in proper perspective and painted in true colors"** (bold added) (Sydenstricker, 1952, p. 280)

Conceptual statement of problem

"The making of public health data: paradigms, politics, and policy" (Krieger, 1992)

p. 412: "If you don't ask, you don't know, and if you don't know, you can't act. These basic precepts lie at the core of current and long-standing controversies about the nature and politics of public health data within the United States. At issue is the routine omission of social class data from most data sources, such as national vital statistics, disease registries, hospital records, and even individual studies, along with the persistent treatment of 'race' and 'sex' as essentially biological variables, their consistent conflation with ethnicity and gender, and the pervasive silence about the social realities of class inequalities, racism, and sexism.

Although concerns about measures used in public health data may seem removed from the tumult of everyday life and everyday struggles for dignity and health, the ways these data are collected and reported can profoundly affect how public health professionals and the public at large perceive public health problems and their support for or opposition to diverse public health problems. Label infant mortality a problem of 'minorities' and present data only on racial/ethnic differences in rates, and the white poor disappear from view; label it a 'poverty' issue and proffer data stratified only by income, and the impact of racism on people of color at each income level is hidden from sight; define the 'race' or socioeconomic position of the infant solely in terms of the mother's characteristics, and the contribution of the father's traits and household class position to patterns of infant mortality will likewise be observed. Any particular approach necessarily affects our ability to understand and alter social inequalities in health.

Despite being fraught with political considerations, the making of public health data–that is, the processes whereby health professionals and institutions decide whether to obtain and present data in particular forms–usually is cast in apolitical terms. On rare occasions, the politics are patently transparent, as exemplified by the recent federal cancellation of two national sex surveys. Usually, however, conscious and unconscious decisions about what types of data to include and exclude are based on prevailing theories of disease causation, and the links between these theories and concurrent political concerns are often obscured by the claim that scientific knowledge is 'objective' and 'neutral.'"

p. 422: "Science is at once objective and partisan. There is no escaping this fact. It is critical to recognize that the allegedly neutral stance of leaving out class and focusing on race, and treating race and sex as chiefly biological characteristics without reference to ethnicity and gender, is as thoroughly political as overt efforts to augment public health data bases without variables pertaining to social class and the everyday realities of both racism and sexism. The seemingly 'apolitical' stance is also fundamentally invalid, for by failing to address the full range of variation in population patterns of disease, it blocks our scientific efforts and professional duties to understand and improve the public's health."

WHO Commission on Social Determinants of Health. *Closing the gap in a generation: health equity through action on the social determinants of health. Final report of the Commission on Social Determinants of Health.* **(WHO CSDH, 2008)**
p. 20: "No data often means no recognition of the problem. Good evidence on levels of health and its distribution, and on the social determinants of health, is essential for understanding the scale of the problem, assessing the affects of action, and monitoring progress."
p. 181: "A minimum health equity surveillance system provides basic data on mortality and morbidity by socioeconomic and regional groups within countries… In addition to population averages, data on health outcomes should be provided in a stratified manner including stratification by: sex; at least two social markers (e.g., education, income/wealth, occupational class, ethnicity/race); at least one regional marker (e.g., rural/urban, province); include at least one summary measure of absolute health inequities between social groups, and one summary measure of relative health inequities between social groups. Good-quality data on the health of Indigenous Peoples should be available, where applicable."

Case 1. U.S. Public Health Surveillance Systems: Limitations Imposed by a Biomedical Approach—the Problem of Missing Socioeconomic Data and an Ecosocial Solution

Empirical evidence of problem	**"Can we monitor socioeconomic inequalities in health? A survey of U.S. Health Departments' data collection and reporting practices"** (Krieger et al., 1997); study abstract (p. 481)

"Objective. To evaluate the potential for and obstacles to routine monitoring of socioeconomic inequalities in health using U.S. vital statistics and disease registry data, the authors surveyed current data collection and reporting practices for specific socioeconomic variables.
Methods. In 1996 the authors mailed a self-administered survey to all of the 55 health department vital statistics offices reporting to the National Center for Health Statistics (NCHS) to determine what kinds of socioeconomic data they collected on birth and death certificates and in cancer, AIDS, and tuberculosis (TB) registries and what kinds of socioeconomic data were routinely reported in health department publications.

Results. Health departments routinely obtained data on occupation on death certificates in most cancer registries. they collected data on educational level for both birth and death certificates. None of the databases collected information on income, and few obtained data on employment status, health insurance carrier, or receipt of public assistance. When socioeconomic data were collected, they were usually not included in published reports (except for mother's educational level in birth certificate data). Obstacles cited to collecting and reporting socioeconomic data included lack of resources and concerns about the confidentiality and accuracy of the data. All databases, however, included residential address, suggesting records could be geocoded and linked to Census-based socioeconomic data.

Conclusions. U.S. state and Federal vital statistics and disease registries should routinely collect and publish socioeconomic data to improve efforts to monitor trends in and reduce social inequalities in health."

Project designed to address the problem, informed by ecosocial theory

Executive summary: *The US Public Health Disparities Geocoding Project* (Krieger et al., 2004)

The problem	A lack of socioeconomic data in most U.S. public health surveillance systems.
Why is this a problem?	Absent these data, we cannot: *(a)* monitor socioeconomic inequalities in US health; *(b)* ascertain their contribution to racial/ethnic and gender inequalities in health; and *(c)* galvanize public concern, debate, and action concerning how we, as a nation, can achieve the vital goal of eliminating social disparities in health (Healthy People 2010 overarching objective #2)
Possible solution	Geocoding public health surveillance data and using census-derived area-based socioeconomic measures (ABSMs) to characterize both the cases and population in the catchment area, thereby enabling computation of rates stratified by the area-based measure of socioeconomic position.
Knowledge gaps	Unknown which ABSMs, at which level of geography, would be most apt for monitoring U.S. socioeconomic inequalities in health, overall, and within diverse racial/ethnic-gender groups.
Methodologic study: The Public Health Disparities Geocoding Project	We accordingly launched the Public Health Disparities Geocoding Project to ascertain which ABSMs, at which geographic level (census block group [BG], census tract [CT], or ZIP Code [ZC]), would be suitable for monitoring U.S. socioeconomic inequalities

in the health. Drawing on 1990 census data and public health surveillance systems of 2 New England states, Massachusetts and Rhode Island, we analyzed data for: *(a)* 7 types of outcomes: mortality (all cause and cause-specific), cancer incidence (all-sites and site-specific), low birth weight, childhood lead poisoning, sexually transmitted infections, tuberculosis, and nonfatal weapons-related injuries, and *(b)* 18 different ABSMs. We conducted these analyses for both the total population and diverse racial/ethnic-gender groups, at all 3 geographic levels.

Key findings

Our key methodologic finding was that the ABSM most apt for monitoring socioeconomic inequalities in health was the census tract (CT) poverty level, since it: (a) consistently detected expected socioeconomic gradients in health across a wide range of health outcomes, among both the total population and diverse racial/ethnic-gender groups, (b) yielded maximal geocoding and linkage to area-based socioeconomic data (compared to BG and ZC data), and (c) was readily interpretable to and could feasibly be used by state health department staff. Using this measure, we were able to provide evidence of powerful socioeconomic gradients for virtually all the outcomes studied, using a common metric, and further demonstrated that: (a) adjusting solely for this measure substantially reduced excess risk observed in the Black and Hispanic compared to the White population, and (b) for half the outcomes, over 50% of cases overall would have been averted if everyone's risk equaled that of persons in the least impoverished CT, the only group that consistently achieved Healthy People 2000 goals a decade ahead of time.

Recommendation

U.S. public health surveillance data should be geocoded and routinely analyzed using the CT-level measure "percent of persons below poverty," thereby enhancing efforts to track—and improve accountability for addressing—social disparities in health.

State Health Departments that have issued reports using the methodology of the Public Health Disparities Geocoding Project	"The Health of Washington State Supplement: a statewide assessment addressing health disparities by race, ethnic group, poverty and education." September 2004. http://www.doh.wa.gov/HWS

The Virginia Department of Health Epidemiology Profile 2007. http://www.vdh.virginia.gov/epidemiology/DiseasePrevention/Profile2007.htm

The 2008 Virginia Health Equity Report. http://www.vdh.state.va.us/healthpolicy/2008report.htm

Massachusetts Deaths 2008 (in press) http://www.mass.gov/dph/repi |
| **Public Health Disparities Geocoding Project Publications** | Krieger et al., 2001; Krieger et al., 2002a; Krieger et al., 2002b; Krieger et al., 2003a; Krieger et al., 2003b; Krieger et al., 2003c; Krieger et al., 2003d; Krieger et al., 2005b; Subramanian et al., 2005; Krieger, 2006; Subramanian et al., 2006a; Subramanian et al., 2006b; Rehkopf et al., 2006; Chen et al., 2006; Krieger et al., 2007; Krieger, 2009 |

Case 2. Racial/Ethnic Data in Public Health Surveillance Systems—Unmasking the Politics of Data by Using Social Epidemiologic Approaches: PAHO, Brazil, and the United States (Krieger, 2000; Nobels, 2000; PAHO, 2002; Krieger, 2004b; Paixão, 2004; Travassos & Williams, 2004; Romera & da Cunha, 2006)

PAHO: rationale for collecting and reporting ethnic origin data–and problem with missing data	**Division of Health and Human Development, Program on Public Policy and Health. Final Report Experts Workshop: Cultural diversity and disaggregation of statistical health information. Quito, Ecuador, 4-June 5, 2002. Washington, DC: Pan American Health Organization, 2002. (PAHO, 2002)**

p. 2: "The collection and dissemination of data by ethnic origin are essential in order to identify, monitor, and progressively eliminate inequities in health status and access to health services. This information is critical to the effort to ensure that prevention, promotion, and treatment programs are effective and to establish binding norms that will make it possible to achieve equity.

The lack of high-quality, congruent data and analysis based on ethnic origin is a problem in the majority of the countries. The existence of information systems is vital for evidence-based decision-making, to achieve the proper allocation of limited resources, and to evaluate the effectiveness of interventions."

p. 3: "The goals of this project are to: 1) improve data collection and analytic capacity; 2) generate new information that expands our collective knowledge of the health situation of indigenous populations and populations of African descent." |

Brazil: problem of inadequate or missing racial data—and also economic data

Conceptual statement of problem:
Paixão M. Waiting for the Sun: An Account of the (Precarious) Social Situation of the African Descendant Population in Contemporary Brazil. J Black Studies 2004; 34:743–765. (Paixão, 2004)

"Analysis of the statistical data on the economic and social situation of African descendants in Brazil demonstrates severe racial inequalities, which traditionally have been denied according to the conventional wisdom of the myth of "racial democracy." The absence of reliable statistical data has fueled the force of this myth; statistics produced recently are the result of pressure by the black movement. The demographic presence of African descendants in the Brazilian population is examined and social indices are broken down by color/race, income levels, educational standards, and health conditions. Specific Human Development Index analysis, disaggregating data for African descendants and whites in Brazil, demonstrates the severity of racial inequality in comparison with other countries of the world and Africa. The black population in Brazil is still characterized by the absence of collective social rights and by the wide gap separating its living standards from those of the Brazilian European descendant population."

Empirical manifestation:
Romera DE, da Cunha CB. Quality of socioeconomic and demographic data in relation to infant mortality in the Brazilian Mortality Information System (1996/2001). Cad Saúde Pública 2006; 22:673–681. (Romera & da Cunha, 2006)

"This study aimed to evaluate the quality of socioeconomic and demographic data in the Brazilian Mortality Information System (SIM), in relation to infant mortality. The article assesses the system's potential for monitoring inequalities in infant mortality in various States in the country. Accessibility, timeliness, methodological clarity, incompleteness, and consistency were explored as quality indicators. Selected variables were: race, birth weight, gestational age, medical care, parity, and maternal schooling, age, and occupation. The study also reviewed the system's working documentation and the scientific literature on infant mortality. Proportions of data incompleteness were calculated by region and State, identifying factors that might influence (in)completeness using logistic regression. Despite the database's accessibility and the relevance of most of its variables, the system has serious quality problems: confusing instructions in the information manual concerning missing data, misclassification of maternal occupation, lack of data on the informant's race/ethnicity, and high proportions of incomplete information. The system does not appear to be a reliable source for monitoring, evaluating, and planning measures to minimize infant health inequalities."

United States: argument against excluding racial/ethnic data and the necessity of analyzing it critically

Krieger N. Data, "race," and politics: a commentary on the epidemiologic significance of California's Proposition 54. *J Epidemiol Community Health* 2004; 58: 632–633. (Krieger, 2004b)

"Data for social justice and public health is akin to the proverbial two-edged sword. To the extent we base any of our claims about social injustice in evidence, we must use data–whether of the quantitative or qualitative sort. But data do not simply exist. Contrary to the literal definition of 'data' as 'that which is given,' data instead are duly conceived and collected, via the ideas and labor of those who would obtain the requisite evidence. In the case of epidemiology, moreover, we must often use population data appearing in categories that are far from ideal–precisely because the assumptions of those with the power to shape and accrue the data often differ from those who seek to use these data to illuminate and oppose social inequalities in health.

Instructively highlighting these tensions are issues that recently arose in relation to the California ballot initiative Proposition 54. Officially designated as the 'Classification by Race, Ethnicity, Color, or National Origin Initiative'–but called the "Racial Privacy Initiative" by its supporters (who previously sponsored the successful anti-affirmative action Proposition 209)–Proposition 54 sought to ban collection or use of racial/ethnic data by government agencies. Under the slogan "Think outside the box," the initiative's proponents claimed Proposition 54 would "end government's preferential treatment based on race, and junk a 17th-century racial classification system that has no place in 21st-century America."

Despite its seemingly "progressive" approach to discounting outdated modes of classifying "race," Proposition 54 nevertheless was soundly defeated (64% opposed) by a coalition lead in large part by public health advocates and researchers, who exposed how the absence of these data would translate to public harm, especially in relation to public health.

… Tellingly, both proponents and opponents of Proposition 54 condemned racism and unscientific beliefs about "race" as an "innate" characteristic. But, whereas proponents argued that racial/ethnic data should not be collected because "race" is not "real" (i.e., not "biological"), opponents countered that this stance patently ignored the social realities of "race," i.e., as a socially constructed category reflecting societal and individual histories of racial discrimination and dispossession.

The contradiction is therefore sharp–and unavoidable–and affects all research employing categories that bear the mark of social inequality. Data on social disparities in health has long been disparately interpreted as evidence of: (a) "innate" inferiority, (b) "cultural" inferiority, or (c) embodied consequences of social inequity. There is no "thinking outside of the box" devoid of context. In the case of racial/ethnic inequalities in health, when "color" is no longer a signal for denial of human dignity and human rights, we will live in–and the data will show–a multi-hued society with equality for all. Only by bringing into the open the issues of power and injustice that lie behind the "that which is given" of public health data can we work honestly with the data to promote social justice and human rights, which together comprise the foundation of public health."

Case 3. Engendering Global Health Statistics: Enormous Gaps in Data Continue to Exist (Hedman et al., 1996; DESA, 2006; Lin et al., 2007; Jara, 2007).

Why gender statistics matter, including for health	**Hedman B, Perucci F, Sundström P.** *Engendering Statistics: A Tool for Change.* **Stockholm, Sweden: Statistics Sweden, 1996. (Hedman et al., 1996)** p. 9: *"Statistics and indicators on the situation of women and men in all spheres of society are an important tool in promoting equality. Gender statistics have an essential role in the elimination of stereotypes, in the formulation of policies and in monitoring progress towards full equality. The production of adequate gender statistics concerns the entire official statistical system as well as different statistical sources and fields. It also implies the development and improvement of concepts, definitions, classifications and methods."* (italics in original)

Smith MK. Enhancing gender equity in health programmes: monitoring and evaluation. Gender Development 2001; 9:95–105. (Smith, 2001)

p. 95: "Over the past ten years there has been increasing international recognition of the vital role to be played by investment in health care in the poverty-reduction strategies supported by governments and international donors. Parallel to this, there has been a growing debate at national level on the need for gender analysis in mainstream health programming and policy. Previously, concern for women's and gender issues was confined to a narrow focus on women's reproductive role, and hence on mother-and-child services, rather than taking account of women's needs, caring roles, and access and utilisation of health services. Gender-sensitive monitoring and evaluation is an essential component of this new agenda. It is a key principle in gender work to question any assumptions that a particular project or programme reaches all members of a community and has a similar impact on all of them."

Extent of missing data: 1996 and 2006...	**Hedman B, Perucci F, Sundström P.** *Engendering Statistics: A Tool for Change.* **Stockholm, Sweden: Statistics Sweden, 1996. (Hedman et al., 1996)** p. 77: "The following is a list of topics where data [stratified by gender] are particularly scarce." (NB: health outcomes are put in **bold**; the rest are all social determinants of health.)

- **Male fertility**
- **Household** composition and structure
- **Diseases and causes of death**
- Internal and international migration

- School dropout rates
- Educational achievement
- Fields of higher education
- Access to credit
- Access to land
- Informal sector

- Subsistence agriculture
- Unpaid work
- Time use
- Individual and household income
- Income control
- Poverty

- **Violence against women/ domestic violence**
- Economic decision making
- Decision making at the local level
- Decision making in the household
- Resources allocation within the household

and still missing data 10 years later...

Department of Economic and Social Affairs, Statistics Division.
The World's Women 2005: Progress in Statistics. **New York: United Nations, 2006. (DESA, 2006)**

pp. 21–22: 'In the period 1995–2003, even basic statistical data such as the number of deaths of women and men and girls and boys are not being reported for many countries or areas. More than a third of the 204 countries or areas examined did not report the number of deaths by sex even once for the period 1995 to 2003. About half did not report deaths by cause, sex and age at least once in the same period... The region with the lowest proportion of countries or areas reporting deaths by sex is Africa. Only 18 out of 55 countries or areas, comprising 35 per cent of the region's population, reported national data on deaths by sex at least once in the period 1995–2003. In Asia, 33 countries or areas, representing 55 per cent of the region's population, and in Oceania 7 countries or areas, representing 76 per cent of the region's population, reported deaths by sex Deaths by sex and age are reported by most countries or areas in North America, South America and Europe..'

pp. 22–23: 'According to the Beijing Platform for Action, son preference is one factor that contributes to differential mortality by sex. As a result, in some countries it is estimated that men outnumber women by 5 in every 100. A preference for sons remains deeply rooted in many societies and girls may have less access to nutrition, preventive care (such as immunization) and health care. Data on infant deaths by sex are needed to see where excess mortality among girls exists so that it can be addressed and eliminated. While total infant deaths were reported by 143 countries or areas in the period 1995–2003, fewer—114, representing 40 per cent of the world population—reported infant deaths by sex. The pattern of low reporting in Africa and Asia and high reporting in the other geographic regions, as seen with reporting deaths by sex, also prevails for infant deaths.'

p. 27: 'In general, countries fall into one of two groups: either they have a strong statistical capacity and have been able to report mortality data almost every year by sex, age and cause; or their reporting capacity is very limited and has not improved since 1975. Moreover, there is a clear association between the national reporting of mortality data by sex and age and the level of development. This is, at least partially, a consequence of the lack of well-functioning civil registration systems that record births and deaths in the less developed regions. However, there have been some notable improvements. There has been better reporting of deaths caused by HIV/AIDS. In addition, the implementation of international programmes such as Multiple Indicator Cluster Surveys and Demographic and Health Surveys have contributed to a wider availability of national data on some aspects of mortality, morbidity and disability.'

Lin V, Gruszin S, Ellickson C, Glover J, Silburn K, Wilson G, Poljski C. Comparative evaluation of indicators for gender equity and health. *Int J Public Health* **2007; 52:S19–S26. (Lin et al., 2007)**

p. S19: 'Methods: A comprehensive health information framework
was developed on a generic framework by the ISO (2001) to use for
the analysis of gender equity within mainstream health systems.
A sample of 1 095 indicators used by key international organizations
were mapped to this framework and assessed for technical quality
and gender sensitivity.'

p. S21–22: '—most routine indicators, including basic health indicators such as infant mortality, were not reported disaggregated by sex
or age, nor with a comparator or over time; although sex disaggre-
gations were reported in indicators on life expectancy, education,
workforce, and democracy;

— there were few age-disaggregated indicators and none that were
disaggregated for ethnicity or socioeconomic groups;

— most sex-specific indicators described women, and were age-lim-
ited to women of reproductive age, or described reproductive
outcomes (e. g. deliveries, births), while indicators on the health
problems of females out of reproductive age (e. g., older women,
girls) or pertaining to non-reproductive states (e. g., mental health)
were largely missing.

— indicators with comparators compared females to males (i.e. used
the male as the norm), and most were found in only six topics
(including literacy, education, employment); and

— few indicators included a time element that would allow the
assessment of change over time.

Case
examples:
burn statistics

Smith MK. Enhancing gender equity in health programmes:
monitoring and evaluation. Gender Development 2001; 9:
95–105. (Smith, 2001)

pp. 98–99: "A gender-sensitive monitoring exercise focusing on the
Assuit Burns Centre, a health project in Upper Egypt, provided an in-
depth understanding of the gender dimensions of burns in a poor rural
area of Upper Egypt, revealing women's particular vulnerability to
burns, and their lack of access to health services... A gender analysis of
burns in Upper Egypt tells us that it is usually women who are affected
by burns, while they are performing their domestic tasks of cooking
and baking... Although the physical complications of burns, such as
disfigurement and disability, are the same for women and men, the
social complications are different. Disfigured women have to face many
prejudices which affect their social lives. For example, unmarried
women who are burned may never get married, and may live almost
as outcasts from society, which demands conformity to gendered
expectations of female beauty and capacity for physical work."

Case 4. New Approaches for Visualizing Between and Within Country Health
Inequities and Their Social Determinants (Worldmapper, 2008; Gapminder,
2008)

Maps:

Chapter 1, Figures 1–4a through 1–4h: Maps from the "World-
mapper" project (Worldmapper, 2008).

Using available sociodemographic and health data in a novel way,
whereby each territory is sized in relation to the variable depicted,
these maps from the "Worldmapper" project, premised on a social
determinants of health analysis, are intended to give new insights

into–and spur action to address–global inequalities in health. Although these maps cannot, by themselves, answer the question "why" the observed inequities exist, the point here is the theoretical perspective used to create and juxtapose these maps in the first place–precisely so as to galvanize this very question of "why." As stated by Danny Dorling (b. 1967), one of the team members who produced these maps (Dorling, 2007):

> "Drawing maps is one way to engage more of our imagination to help understand the extent and arrangement of world inequalities in health... what I think matters most are the new ways of thinking that we foster as we redraw the images of the human anatomy of our planet in these ways. What do we need to be able to see–so that we can act?"

Graphs: **Figures 1–5 through 1–6 in Chapter 1: Graphs from the "Gapminder" project (Gapminder, 2008)**

Likewise animated by a social epidemiologic orientation, these graphs from the "Gapminder" project, developed by Hans Rosling (b. 1948), offer still another new way to present data on global health inequities. Intended to promote **"sustainable global development and achievement of the United Nations Millennium Development Goals"** (Gapminder, 2008), the figures' stark depictions of the variable magnitudes of health inequities, within and between countries, at similar and different per capita income levels, and also over time, underscores both the variability in the magnitude of health inequities–and nothing inevitable about their size. The "why" questions prompted by data display reflect a theoretical orientation engaged with the social determinants of health and attuned to both historical and geographical contingency. Or, as stated by Rosling (Barone, 2007):

> "Most people know only two types of countries, Western and third world, whereas I know 200 types of countries. I know each country's gross national product, educational level, child mortality, main export products, and so on. We have a continuum of life conditions in the world... We want to know: How can we better measure and communicate the conditions of the poorest 1 to 2 billion people in the world?... There is a tsunami every month that could be cured by penicillin, for which there are no images and no reporting..."

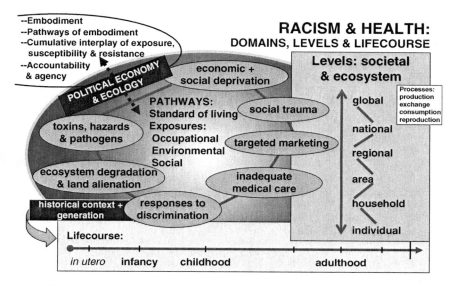

Figure 8–2. Pathways by which racial discrimination can harm health: an ecosocial perspective. (Krieger, 1999/2000; Krieger, 2010a)

Textbox 8–6. The Difference Epidemiologic Theory Can Make: Etiology—Racial Discrimination as a Societal Determinant of Health Inequities, Identified Using Social Epidemiologic Theories but Ignored by Biomedical and Lifestyle Approaches

A Personal Reflection on the Rapid Growth of Epidemiologic Research on Discrimination and Health Since the 1980s—and the Work that Lies Ahead:

When I first began conducting epidemiologic research in the latter part of the 1980s and early 1990s on discrimination as a determinant of health inequities (Krieger, 1990; Krieger et al., 1993; Krieger & Sidney, 1996: Krieger, 2003) there were virtually no epidemiologic studies on this topic; what little research existed chiefly was in the psychology literature and usually not population-based. Enabling me to identify and start to address this important gap in the epidemiologic literature was the social production of disease framework (*see* **Chapter 6**); I soon found, however, that it gave insufficient guidance for thinking through how social inequalities become biologically expressed needed, a realization that spurred my work on developing ecosocial theory (Krieger, 1994)(*see* **Chapter 7**).

In 1999, I published the first major epidemiologic review article on discrimination and health (Krieger, 1999), in which I used ecosocial theory to delineate five major pathways by which discrimination could harm health: (*1*) economic and social deprivation; (*2*) toxic substances and hazardous conditions; (3) socially inflicted trauma; (*4*) targeted marketing of harmful products; and (*5*) inadequate or degrading medical care—to which I have now added: *(6)* degradation of ecosystems, including as linked to systematic alienation of Indigenous populations from their lands and corresponding traditional economies *(see* below, and also as discussed in **Chapter 7**) (Krieger, 1999; Krieger, 2003c; Krieger, 2009; Krieger, 2010a). For this review, I was able to identify 21 population-based studies that explicitly tested hypotheses about associations between self-reported experiences of discrimination and health. Among these 21 investigations (3 of which addressed multiple types of discrimination), 15 focused on racial discrimination (the first published in 1984), 3 on gender discrimination (the first published in 1990), 4 on discrimination based on sexual orientation (the first published in 1994), and 1 on discrimination based on disability status (published in 1998); the range of health outcomes investigated spanned from somatic health to mental health to health behaviors.

Reflecting, in part, the growing influence of social epidemiologic frameworks in the field since the early 1990s, the pace of epidemiologic research on the health impacts of discrimination has quickened enormously. To date, much of the work has remained focused on racial discrimination and health, with the number of articles quickly rising, as evidenced by three recently published epidemiologic review articles: one published in 2003 included 53 studies, of which more than half (24) were published during or after 2000 (Williams et al., 2003), one published in 2006 included 138 studies published up through 2004 (Paradies, 2006), and a third published in 2009 included 115 articles that were indexed in PubMed between 2005 and 2007 alone (Williams & Mohammed, 2009). Initially, studies examining links between racial/ethnic discrimination and health were conducted almost exclusively in the United States; the research now, however, is starting to become global in scope, with studies now also conducted in Latin American and European countries, and also South Africa, New Zealand, and Australia (Krieger, 1999; Williams et al., 2003; Paradies, 2006; Williams & Mohammed, 2009).

Increasing interest in epidemiologic research on racial discrimination and health has also led to the development and refinement of methods to study racial discrimination at multiple levels (e.g., self-reported by individuals, in relation to residential racial segregation, in relation to health-care system factors, and at the government policy level), both across the life-course and transgenerationally. As discussed in the above four review articles (Krieger, 1999; Williams et al., 2003; Paradies, 2006; Williams & Mohammed, 2009), a 2004 National Research Council report focused on methods for measuring racial discrimination (National Research Council, 2004) and other recent review articles (Kressin et al., 2008; Pager & Sheperd, 2008; Pachter & Garcia, 2009), researchers currently employ a variety of methods and instruments (some validated, many not) to measure diverse aspects and levels of racial discrimination. Addressing current controversies about how epidemiologic research can best measure discrimination—at the individual, institutional, and societal levels—will require creative and critical empirical research; investigations tackling these challenges is clearly underway (Williams & Mohammed, 2009; Kressin et al., 2008; Carney et al., 2010, Sharrif-Marco et al., 2009; Krieger et al., 2010).

Overall, epidemiologic research on discrimination and health, although perhaps no longer in its infancy (Krieger, 1999; Krieger, 2003c), is still very young, both conceptually and methodologically. The extant literature is thus not surprisingly full of inconsistent results and only just beginning to yield some robust findings that hold for specified outcomes across different studies. A safe prediction is that there will continue to be rapid and increasingly global growth in epidemiologic research engaged with the conceptual, methodologic, and substantive challenges of investigating the health consequences of diverse types of discrimination, singly and combined (Krieger, 2010a).

Textbox 8–7. The Difference Epidemiologic Theory Can Make: Action—
Contrasts Between Priorities Based on Research Guided by
Individually Oriented Biomedical and Lifestyle Approaches
Versus Social Epidemiologic Frameworks

(a) "10 Tips for Better Health"—a Satirical Contrast Between Recommendations Based on a Biomedical and Lifestyle Approach Versus a Social
Determinants of Health Approach

Chief Medical Officer's Top Ten Tips for Health—United Kingdom (1999) (Donaldson, 1999)	Alternative Tips—Townsend Center for International Poverty Research (1999) (Gordon, 1999)
1) Don't smoke. If you can, stop. If you can't, cut down.	1) Don't be poor. If you are poor, try not to be poor for too long.
2) Follow a balanced diet with plenty of fruit and vegetables.	2) Don't live in a deprived area. If you do, move.
3) Keep physically active.	3) Don't be disabled or have a disabled child.
4) Manage stress by, for example, talking things through and making time to relax.	4) Don't work in a stressful low-paid manual job.
5) If you drink alcohol, do so in moderation.	5) Don't live in damp, low quality housing or be homeless.
6) Cover up in the sun, and protect children from sunburn.	6) Be able to afford to pay for social activities and annual holidays.
7) Practise safer sex.	7) Don't be a lone parent.
8) Take up cancer screening opportunities.	8) Claim all benefits to which you are entitled.
9) Be safe on the roads: follow the Highway Code.	9) Be able to afford to own a car.
10) Learn the First Aid ABC–air- ways, breathing and circulation.	10) Use education as an opportunity to improve your socio-economic position.

(b) Experts "10 Steps to Health Inequalities" Developed for the United Kingdom's 1998 *Independent Inquiry into Inequalities in Health* (the "Acheson
Report") (Independent Inquiry, 1998), Reflecting the Dominance of Individual-Level Biomedical and Lifestyle Studies)—and a Social Epidemiologic
Critique

Laurance J. Experts' 10 steps to health equality. *The Independent*, November 12, 1998. (Laurance, 1998)	Davey Smith G, Ebrahim S, Frankel S. How policy informs the evidence: "evidence based" thinking can lead to debased policy making. *BMJ* 2001; 322:184–185. (Davey Smith et al., 2001)
"The 10 best ways of closing the health gap between the rich and the poor, highlighted as a priority by ministers, have been drawn up by an expert committee… The expert group that drew up the list included the editors of Britain's two leading medical journals, the Lancet and the British Medical Journal, who assessed a range	Who would not want health policy to be based on evidence? "Evidence based medicine" and "evidence based policy" have such reassuring and self-evidently desirable qualities that it may seem contrary to question their legitimacy in relation to reducing health inequalities. However, these terms are now so familiar that it is easy to forget the important

of studies on health inequalities and ranked the measures they recommended according to their chances of success... Dr Smith [editor of BMJ] said the group's recommendations could be criticized for concentrating on relatively small, medical interventions–rather than macro changes, such as adjustments to the tax and benefit system—but that was where the evidence was strongest."

1 Nicotine gum and patches free on the NHS. They double the chances of stopping smoking.
2 Pre-school education and child care. Strong evidence that it improves long-term prospects for children.
3 Fluoridation of drinking water. Cuts tooth decay.
4 Accident prevention—e.g., fit cars with soft bumpers. Accidents are the principal cause of deaths among young people.
5 Drugs education in schools. Prevents pupils becoming hooked.
6 Support around childbirth to promote breastfeeding and mental health. Good evidence of long-term benefits.
7 Improved access to NHS for ethnic minorities—e.g., by appointing link workers.
8 Adding folate to flour. Prevents spina bifida in babies; early evidence suggests it may prevent heart disease and Alzheimer's.
9 Free school milk.
10 Free smoke alarms. Good evidence they save lives.

question about what sort of data provide appropriate evidence for particular types of decisions. The sort of evidence gathered on the benefits of interventions aimed at individuals may not help in guiding policies directed towards reducing health inequalities... .

The task of the Acheson inquiry was to make recommendations that would reduce inequalities in health, not merely have a positive overall health benefit. For most of the evaluation group's suggested interventions there are no high quality controlled studies showing that they would reduce health inequalities...

... Despite occasional rhetorical interest in wider determinants of health, evidence based assessments are largely restricted to individualized interventions. The *Cochrane Library* is unlikely ever to contain systematic reviews or trials of the effects of redistributive national fiscal policies, or of economic investment leading to reductions in unemployment, on health.

The insidious nature of this mismatch between evidence and policy is highlighted by the fact that the evaluation group is, as one would expect of such informed commentators, aware of the problem, while implicitly ignoring it. One of the evaluation group stated when launching the '10 steps to health equity,' 'Our recommendations are quite medical because are the sort that tend to have evidence behind them.'"

(c) **New Twenty-First Century Examples of National Policies and Global Recommendations for Improving Population Health and Promoting Health Equity: Moving Beyond a Biomedical and Lifestyle Approach to One Informed by Social Epidemiologic Frameworks**

Sweden's new Public Health Policy (2003)

Conceptual approach:
Swedish National Institute of Public Health. *Sweden's New Public Health Policy: National Public Health Objectives for Sweden.* Revised edition: 2003. (Swedish NIPH, 2003)

WHO Commission on the Social Determinants of Health (2008)

Conceptual statement:
WHO Commission on Social Determinants of Health. *Closing the Gap in a Generation: Health Equity Through Action on the Social Determinants of Health. Final report of the Commission on Social Determinants of Health.* (WHO CSDH, 2008)

pp. 5–6: "During the post-Second World War decades, the nature of health issues became increasingly more medical and professional. The discovery of new drugs and other irrefutable medical progress laid the foundations for a strong belief in the ability of doctors and the health service to solve all the major health problems. Health policy became increasingly synonymous with medical care policy, with the debates centering on how we should finance and recruit personnel to an ever-swelling hospital sector. Preventive health care tended increasingly to take a back seat.

Public health work began to regain a stronger position during the 1980s. The spread of AIDS dealt a deathblow to the belief in the health service's ability to overcome major health problems and instead, many people began to question whether growing medical costs really did lead to an improvement in public health. The realization that there were large and growing class differences even in Swedish society also helped bring about a rethink in health policy...

... Whereas objectives had previously been based on diseases or health problems, health determinants were now chosen instead. Health determinants are factors in society or in our living conditions that contribute to good or bad health... .

The benefit of using determinants as a basis is that the objectives will then be accessible for political decisions and can be influenced by certain types of societal measures. If we set objectives in terms of disease, e.g., to reduce the number of heart attacks, they do not provide any guidance as to what measures may be effective for achieving them... Using health determinants as the basis means the vast majority of public health work must take place outside the medical care service. Most of the factors that impact health are to be found outside the spheres of medical competence and knowledge.

p. viii: "...The poorest of the poor have high levels of illness and premature mortality. But poor health is not confined to those worst off. In countries at all levels of income, health and illness follow a social gradient: the lower the socioeconomic position, the worse the health.

It does not have to be this way and it is not right that it should be like this. Where systematic differences in health are judged to be avoidable by reasonable action they are, quite simply, unfair. It is this that we label health inequity. Putting right these inequities–the huge and remediable differences in health between and within countries–is a matter of social justice. Reducing health inequities is, for the Commission on Social Determinants of Health (hereafter, the Commission), an ethical imperative. Social injustice is killing people on a grand scale."

p. 1: "The Commission takes a holistic view of social determinants of health. The poor health of the poor, the social gradient in health within countries, and the marked health inequities between countries are caused by the unequal distribution of power, income, goods, and services, globally and nationally, the consequent unfairness in the immediate, visible circumstances of peoples lives– their access to health care, schools, and education, their conditions of work and leisure, their homes, communities, towns, or cities–and their chance of leading a flourishing life. This unequal distribution of health-damaging experiences is not in any sense a 'natural' phenomenon but is the result of a toxic combination of poor social policies, and programmes, unfair economic arrangements, and bad politics. Together, the structural determinants and conditions of daily life constitute the social determinants of health and are responsible for a major part of health inequities between and within countries...

... Our core concerns with health equity must be part of the global community balancing the needs of social and economic development of the whole global population, health equity, and the urgency of dealing with climate change."

When it comes to influencing unemployment figures, social security, housing segregation and alcohol habits, decisions taken in municipal assemblies and other democratic bodies play a much more important role than efforts made in the medical care sector...

... The overarching aim is to create the conditions for good health on equal terms for the entire population."

Policy

p. 6: *"Eleven general objectives for public health work"*
1. Participation and influence in society
2. Economic and social security
3. Secure and favorable conditions during childhood and adolescence
4. Healthier working life
5. Healthy and safe environments and products
6. Health and medical care that more actively promotes good health
7. Effective protection against communicable diseases
8. Safe sexuality and good reproductive health
9. Increased physical activity
10. Good eating habits and safe food
11. Reduced use of tobacco and alcohol, a society free from illicit drugs and doping and a reduction in the harmful effects of excessive gambling

p. 7: "The first six objectives relate to what are normally considered to be structural factors, i.e., conditions in society and our surroundings that can be influenced primarily by moulding public opinion and by taking political decisions on different levels. The last five objectives concern lifestyles which an individual can influence him/herself, but where the social environment normally plays a very important part."

Recommendations

p. 2: *"The Commission's overarching recommendations"*
1. Improve Daily Living Conditions.
2. Tackle the Inequitable Distribution of Power, Money, and Resources.
3. Measure and Understand the Problem and Assess the Impact of Action

Components:

pp. 3–9: Improve Daily Living Conditions
- "Equity from the start"
- "Healthy places healthy people"
- "Fair employment and decent work"
- "Social protection across the lifecourse"
- "Universal health care"

pp. 10–19: Tackle the Inequitable Distribution of Power, Money, and Resources
- "Health equity in all policies, systems, and programmes"
- "Fair financing"
- "Market responsibility"
- "Gender equity"
- "Political empowerment—inclusion and voice"
- "Good global governance"

pp. 20–21: "Measure and Understand the Problem and Assess the Impact of Action"
- "The social determinants of health: monitoring, research, and training"

Perspectives that need to be incorporated:
pp. 20–21: "a gender perspective on public health"
pp. 21–22: "a lifetime perspective on public health"
pp. 22–23: "Swedish public health in international perspective"

p. 22: Actors—"The role of governments through public sector action is fundamental to health equity. But the role is not government's alone. Rather it is through the democratic processes of civil society participation and public policy-making, supported at the regional and global levels, backed by the research on what works for health equity, and with the collaboration of private actors, that real action for health equity is possible."

Implications for the epidemiologic research agenda:
p. 6: "It is important to clarify how a determinant impacts health. There is a relationship between greater economic inequality and poorer public health, but the mechanisms behind this relationship have not been particularly well clarified. This means in turn that the public health argument does not carry quite so much weight in the public debate as for example economic arguments do. Formulating public health objectives in terms of health determinants requires public health work to be very much knowledge-based."

p. 20: "The majority of the research carried out in the health sector is basic medical research or research into disease, disease processes and their treatment. A vast amount of this research is financed by the pharmaceutical industry or by other economic interests associated with the medical care sector.
Research into preventive measures is performed to a substantially less extent and there is hardly any research at all into the social mechanisms of ill health. The latter constitutes just a small percentage of the total research performed.
Research policy reflects both an overconfidence in the medical care services' ability to solve fundamental health problems and the strong economic interests that exist in the field of medical treatment. An individual

Implications for the epidemiologic research agenda:
pp. 178–179: "The underlying causes of health inequity need to be understood, and evidence is needed on what types of interventions work best to reduce the problem. The evidence base needs strengthening in several respects. First, most health research (funding) remains overwhelming biomedically focused, whereas the largest health improvements arguably come from improvements in the social determinants of health. More interdisciplinary and multidisciplinary research on the social determinants of health is needed... Moreover, evidence on the social determinants of health
can be context dependent. Responses to inequities will reflect a wide range of factors, including the culture and history of a society. Understanding the impact that context has on health inequities and the effectiveness of interventions requires a rich evidence base that includes both qualitative and quantitative data. Evidence needs to be judged on fitness for purpose—that is, does it convincingly answer the question asked–rather than on the basis of strict traditional hierarchies of evidence."
p. 196: "Some of the overarching research needs that have emerged from the work of the Commission are:

1. The determinants of health in addition to the determinants of average population health:
- understanding reasons for the relationship between social stratification and health outcomes;

and often deep-rooted biological approach dominates within the field of medicine, resulting in socially determined health discrepancies being studied relatively seldom or in many cases being ignored completely.

There is a substantial need for long-term competence building and research into the social causes of health and ill-health. Concerning basically all the social determinants of health, there is a need for research into the modes of action and the efficacy of various health policy strategies. Effective knowledge-based preventive measures need to be systematically developed.

In partnership with the Swedish Council for Working Life and Social Research, the Institute of Public Health has been instructed to analyse the Swedish public health research and propose improvements."

For updates on the policy and additional background on its context, see:
(a) Swedish National Institute of Public Health. Public health policy–11 objectives. Updated March 12, 2009. (Swedish NHIP, 2009)
(b) Sundin J, Willner W. Social Change and Health in Sweden: 250 Years of Politics and Practice. (2007) (Swedish NHIP, 2007)
(c) Wall S, Persson G, Weinehall L. Public health in Sweden: facts, visions and lessons. (2003) (Wall et al., 2003)

- understanding the interaction between aspects of stratification (for example, gender, ethnicity, and income) and health inequities;
- quantifying the impact of supra-national political, economic and social systems on health and health inequities within and between countries.
2. Interventions, global to local, to address the social determinants of health and health equity…
3. Policy analysis…
4. Monitoring and measurement:
- developing new methodologies for measuring and monitoring health inequities, and for assessing the impact of population-level interventions."

For updates and commentaries on the WHO CSDH final report, see:
(a) World Health Organization Executive Board Resolution: "Reducing health inequities through action on the social determinants of health" (EB124.46) (WHO, 2009)
(b) The Wellcome Trust Centre for the History of Medicine at UCL: "The World Health Organization and the social determinants of health: assessing theory, policy and practice" (Wellcome Trust, 2008)

For epidemiologists—and others—to know the history of our field and its theories of disease distribution is vital. Such knowledge can help us avoid errors, spark new ideas, and enable us to be as critical conceptually as we are methodologically of the studies that comprise the substantive contributions of our field. At issue are not only the questions asked and interpretations offered but also those ignored. By making conscious use of epidemiologic theory and having informed debates over the different theoretical perspectives at play, we stand a better of chance of producing epidemiologic knowledge truly useful for preventing disease, promoting health equity and improving the public's health. If epidemics are that which befall the people, it is our professional obligation to do the best work we can, with the clearest thinking possible, to identify what will allow the people to stand once again. Our commitment to the people's health—and to explaining the people's health—demands no less. Embracing, extending, debating, and improving epidemiologic theory is one very good place to start.

References

Chapter 1

Abramson JH. Re: "Definitions of epidemiology." *Am J Epidemiol* 1979; 109:99–101.

Allen GE. Eugenics. In: *Encyclopedia of Life Sciences*. Chichester: John Wiley & Sons, Ltd, 2001. http://www.els.net/ (doi:10.1038/npgels.0003485). (Accessed: July 9, 2008)

Altbach PG et al. (eds). *Textbooks in American Society: Politics, Policy, and Pedagogy*. Albany, NY: State University of New York Press, 1991.

American College of Epidemiology. Ethics Guidelines. January 2000. Available at: http://www.acepidemiology.org/policystmts/EthicsGuide.htm. (Accessed: July 16, 2008).

Anderson RN, Rosenberg HM. *Age Standardization of Death Rates: Implementation of the Year 2000 Standard*. National Vital Statistics Reports: Vol 47, no. 3. Hyattsville, MD: National Center for Health Statistics, 1998.

Apple MW, Christian-Smith LK. *The Politics of The Textbook*. New York: Routledge, 1991.

Archer A, Bhaskar R, Collier R, Lawson T, Norrie A. *Critical Realism: Essential Readings*. London: Routledge, 1998.

Banton MP. *Racial theories*. 2nd ed. Cambridge: Cambridge University Press, 1998.

Barbeau E, Krieger N, Soobader M-J. Working class matters: Socioeconomic deprivation, race/ethnicity, gender and smoking in the National Health Interview Survey, 2000. *Am J Public Health* 2004; 94:269–278.

Bennett T, Grossberg L, Morris M (eds). *New Keywords: A Revised Vocabulary of Culture and Society*. Malden, MA: Blackwell Publishing, 2005.

Ben-Shlomo Y, Kuh DH. A lifecourse approach to chronic disease epidemiology: conceptual models, empirical challenges, and interdisciplinary perspectives. *Int J Epidemiol* 2002; 31: 285–293.

Berkman L, Kawachi I (eds). *Social Epidemiology*. Oxford, UK: Oxford University Press, 2000; pp. 3–12.

Blake W. Auguries of innocence. (1800-1803); In: Ostriker A (ed). *The Complete Poems of William Black*. Harmondsworth: Penguin, 1977; pp. 506–510.

Brandt A. *The Cigarette Century: The Rise, Fall, and Deadly Persistence of the Product that Defined America*. New York: Basic Books, 2007, pp. 360, 393.

Braun L, Fausto-Sterling A, Fullwiley D, Hammonds EM, Nelson A, Quivers W, Reverby SM, Shields AE. Racial categories in medical practice: how useful are they? *PLoS Med* 2007; 4:3271. doi:10.1371/journal.pmed.0040271

Brenner S. Autobiography: Sydney Brenner, The Nobel Prize in Physiology or Medicine 2002. Available at: http://nobelprize.org/nobel_prizes/medicine/laureates/2002/brenner-autobio.html (Accessed: July 12, 2008).

Burchard EG, Ziv E, Coyle N, et al. The importance of race and ethnic background in biomedical research and clinical practice. *New Engl J Med* 2003; 348:1170–1175.

Byrne MM. Uncovering racial bias in nursing fundamentals textbooks. *Nurs Health Care Perspect* 2001; 22:299–303.

Carpiano RM, Daley DM. A guide and glossary on postpositivist theory building for population health. *J Epidemiol Community Health* 2006; 60:564–570.

Carrington D. Reading the book of life. BBC News Online, May 30, 2000. Available at: http://news.bbc.co.uk/1/hi/in_depth/sci_tech/2000/human_genome/760893.stm (Accessed: July 12, 2008).

Chase A. *The Legacy of Malthus: The Social Costs of the New Scientific Racism*. New York: Knopf, 1977.

Chia KS, Reilly M, Tan CS, et al. Profound changes in breast cancer incidence may reflect changes into a Westernized lifestyle: a comparative population-based study in Singapore and Sweden. *Int J Cancer* 2005; 113:302–306.

Clemmesen J. Carcinoma of the breast symposium: 1. Results from statistical research. *Br J Radiology* 1948; 11:583–590.

Cohen IB. *Revolution in Science*. Cambridge, MA: Harvard University Press, 1985.

Collins HM. Scientific knowledge, sociology of. In: Smesler NJ, Baltes PB (eds). *International Encyclopedia of the Social & Behavioral Sciences*. Elsevier, 2001; pp. 13,741–13,746. doi:10.1016/B0-08-043076-7/03156-9 (Accessed: August 23, 2008).

Daintith J (ed). *A Dictionary of Science*. Oxford: Oxford University Press, 2005.

Daston L, Gallison P. *Objectivity*. New York: Zone Books, 2007.

Daston L. How probabilities came to be objective and subjective. *Historia Mathematica* 1994; 21: 330–344.

Daston L. On scientific observation. *Isis* 2008; 99:97–110.

Davey Smith G, Egger M. Commentary: understanding it all—health, meta-theories, and mortality trends. *Br Med J* 1996; 313:1584–1585.

Davis RM, Wakefield M, Amos A, Gupta PC. The hitchhiker's guide to tobacco control: a global assessment of harms, remedies, and controversies. *Annu Rev Public Health* 2007; 28:171–194. doi:10.1145/annurev.publhealth.28.021406.144033

Desrosières A. *The Politics of Large Number: A History of Statistical Reasoning*. (transl. Camille Naish). Cambridge, MA: Harvard University Press, 1998.

Dunn JR. Speaking theoretically about population health. *J Epidemiol Community Health* 2006; 60:572–573.

Duster T. Lessons from history: why race and ethnicity have played a major role in biomedical research. *J Law Med Ethics* 2006; 34:487–496, 479.

Eldredge N. *Darwin: Discovering the Tree of Life*. New York: WW Norton & Co, 2005.

Eldredge N. *The Pattern of Evolution*. New York: W.H. Freeman & Co, 1999.

Evans AS. Re: "Definitions of epidemiology." *Am J Epidemiol* 1979; 109:379–382.

Fleck L. *Genesis and Development of a Scientific Fact*. Chicago: University of Chicago Press, 1979 (1935).

Fleck L. On the crisis of "reality" (1929). In: Cohen RS, Schnelle T (eds). *Cognition and Fact—Materials on Ludwig Fleck*. Boston: D. Reidel Pub Co., 1986; pp. 47–57.

Frerichs RR, Neutra R. Re: "Definitions of epidemiology." *Am J Epidemiol* 1978; 108:74–75.

Frow J. Theory. In: Bennett T, Grossberg L, Morris M (eds). *New Keywords: A Revised Vocabulary of Culture and Society*. Malden, MA: Blackwell Publishing, 2005; pp. 347–349.

Gadenne V. Causation (theories and models): conceptions in the social sciences. In: Smesler NJ, Baltes PB (eds). *International Encyclopedia of the Social & Behavioral Sciences*. Elsevier, 2002; pp. 1561–1567. doi:10.1016/B0-08-043076-7/00697-5 (Accessed: July 9, 2008).

Gannett L. What's in a cause? The pragmatic dimensions of genetic explanations. *Biology Philosophy* 1999; 14:349–374.

Gapminder. Available at: http://www.gapminder.org/; (Accessed: July 5, 2008).

Gibson JJ. *The Ecological Approach to Visual Perception*. Boston: Houghton Mifflin, 1979.

Gilbert SF. *Developmental Biology*. 6th ed. Sunderland, MA: Sinauer Associates, 2000.

Gilbert W. A vision of the grail. In: Kevles DJ, Hood L (eds). *The Code of Codes: Scientific and Social Issues in The Human Genome Project*. Cambridge, MA: Harvard University Press, 1992; pp. 83–97.

Gilbert W. Autobiography: Walter Gilbert, The Nobel Prize in Chemistry 1980. Available at: http://nobelprize.org/nobel_prizes/chemistry/laureates/1980/gilbert-autobio.html (Accessed: July 12, 2008).

Gould S. *The Hedgehog, The Fox, and The Magister's Pox: Mending the Gap between Science and the Humanities*. New York: Harmony Books, 2003.

Gould SJ. *The Mismeasure of Man*. Rev. and expanded. New York: Norton, 1996.

Gould SJ. *The Structure of Evolutionary Theory*. Cambridge, MA: The Belknap Press of Harvard University Press, 2002.

Gould SJ. *Time's Arrow, Time's Cycle: Myth and Metaphor in the Discovery of Geological Time*. Cambridge, MA: Harvard University Press, 1987.

Graham H. *Unequal Lives: Health and Socio-economic Inequalities*. Berkshire, England: Open University Press, 2007.

Greenland S. Induction versus Popper: substance versus semantics. *Int J Epidemiol* 1998; 27: 543–548.

Grene M, Depew D. *The Philosophy of Biology*. Cambridge, UK: Cambridge University Press, 2004.

Groff R (ed). *Revitalizing Causality: Realism about Causality in Philosophy and Social Science*. London: Routledge, 2008.

Hacking I. *An Introduction to Probability and Inductive Logic*. Cambridge: Cambridge University Press, 2001.

Hacking I. *The Taming of Chance*. Cambridge: Cambridge University Press, 1990.

Hanson NR. *Patterns of Discovery: An Inquiry into the Conceptual Foundations of Science*. Cambridge: Cambridge University Press, 1958.

Haraway D. *Primate Visions: Gender, Race, and Nature in the World of Modern Science*. New York: Routledge, 1989.

Haraway DJ. *The Haraway Reader*. New York: Routledge, 2004.

Harding S (ed). *The "Racial" Economy of Science: Towards a Democratic Future*. Bloomington, IN: Indiana University Press, 1993.

Harris B, Ernst W (eds). *Race, Science, and Medicine, 1700–1960*. London: Routledge, 1999.

Holton G, Brush SG. *Physics, the Human Adventure: From Copernicus to Einstein and Beyond*. 3rd ed. New Brunswick, NJ: Rutgers University Press, 2001.

Holton GJ. *Thematic Origins of Scientific Thought: Kepler to Einstein*. Rev ed. Cambridge, MA: 1988. Harvard University Press.

Hubbard R. *The Politics of Women's Biology*. New Brunswick, NJ: Rutgers University Press, 1990.

Jackson JP, Weidman NM. *Race, Racism, and Science: Social Impact and Interaction*. Santa Barbara, CA: ABC-CLIO, 2004.

Keith B, Ender MG. The sociological core: conceptual patterns and idiosyncrasies in the structure and content of introductory sociology textbooks, 1940–2000. *Teaching Sociology* 2004; 32:19–36.

Keller EF. *Making Sense of Life: Explaining Biological Development with Models, Metaphors, and Machines*. Cambridge, MA: Harvard University Press, 2002.

Keller EF. *Refiguring Life: Metaphors of Twentieth-Century Biology*. New York: Columbia University Press, 1995.

Keller ER. Nature, nurture, and the Human Genome Project. In: Kevles DJ, Hood L (eds). *The Code of Codes: Scientific and Social Issues in The Human Genome Project*. Cambridge, MA: Harvard University Press, 1992; pp. 281–299.

Kevles DJ. *In The Name of Eugenics: Genetics and the Uses of Human Heredity*. Cambridge, MA: Harvard University Press, 1995.

Krieger N, Rehkopf DH, Chen JT, Waterman PD, Marcelli E, Kennedy M. The fall and rise of US inequities in premature mortality: 1960–2002. *PLoS Med* 2008 5(2): e46. doi:10.1371/journal.pmed.0050046.

Krieger N, Strong EF, Makosky C, Weuve J. Breast cancer, birth cohorts, & Epstein-Barr virus: methodological issues in exploring the "hygiene hypothesis" in relation to breast cancer, Hodgkin's disease, and stomach cancer. *Cancer Epidemiol Biomarkers Prevention* 2003; 12:405–411.

Krieger N, Williams DR. Changing to the 2000 Standard Million: are declining racial/ethnic and socioeconomic inequalities in health real progress or statistical illusion? *Am J Public Health* 2001; 91:1209–1213.

Krieger N. A glossary for social epidemiology. *J Epidemiol Community Health* 2001; 55:693–700. (2001c)

Krieger N. Commentary: society, biology, and the logic of social epidemiology. *Int J Epidemiol* 2001; 30:44–46. (2001b).

Krieger N. Epidemiology and social sciences: towards a critical reengagement in the 21st century. *Epidemiologic Reviews* 2000; 11:155–163.

Krieger N. Epidemiology and the web of causation: has anyone seen the spider? *Soc Sci Med* 1994; 39:887–903.

Krieger N. Hormone therapy and the rise and perhaps fall of US breast cancer incidence rates: critical reflections. *Int J Epidemiol* 2008; 37:1–11.

Krieger N. Shades of difference: theoretical underpinnings of the medical controversy on black-white differences, 1830-1870. *Int J Health Services* 1987; 17:258–279.

Krieger N. Stormy weather: 'race,' gene expression, and the science of health disparities. *Am J Public Health* 2005; 95:2155–2160.

Krieger N. The making of public health data: paradigms, politics, and policy. *J Public Health Policy* 1992; 13:412–427.

Krieger N. Theories for social epidemiology in the 21st century: an ecosocial perspective. *Int J Epidemiol* 2001; 30:668–677. (2001a)

Krieger N. Ways of asking and ways of living: reflections on the 50th anniversary of Morris' ever-useful *Uses of Epidemiology*. *Int J Epidemiol* 2007; 36:1173–1180. (2007a)

Krieger N. Why epidemiologists cannot afford to ignore poverty: a commentary for the "Global Theme Issue on Poverty and Human Development." *Epidemiology* 2007; 18:658–663. (2007b)

Lakoff G., Johnson M. *Metaphors We Live By*. Chicago: Chicago University Press, 1980.

Lavery JV et al. (eds). *Ethical Issues in International Biomedical Research: A Casebook*. Oxford: Oxford University Press, 2007.

Lawrence SC, Bendixen K. His and hers: male and female anatomy texts for U.S. medical students, 1890–1989. *Soc Sci Med* 1992; 35:925–934.

Lewontin R. *The Triple Helix: Gene, Organism and Environment*. Cambridge, MA: Harvard University Press, 2000.

Lewontin RC, Rose S, Kamin LJ. *Not In Our Genes: Biology, Ideology, and Human Nature*. New York: Pantheon Books, 1984.

Lieberson S. Einstein, Renoir, and Greeley: some thoughts about evidence in sociology. *Am Social Review* 1992; 57:1–15.

Lilienfeld AM, Lilienfeld DE. Epidemiology and the public health movement: A historical perspective. *J Public Health Policy* 1982; 3:140–149.

Lilienfeld DE. Definitions of epidemiology. *Am J Epidemiol* 1978; 107:87–90.

Link BG, Phelan J. Social conditions as fundamental causes of disease. *J Health Social Behav* 1995; 35:80–94.

Lock M., Gordon D. (eds). *Biomedicine Examined.* Dordrecht: Kluwer Academic Pub., 1988.

Longino HE. The social dimensions of scientific knowledge. In: *Stanford Encyclopedia of Philosophy* (2006), Zalta EN (ed). URL = http://plato.stanford.edu/entries/scientific-knowledge-social/ (Accessed: July 9, 2008).

Maasen S, Mendelsohn E, Weingart P (eds). *Biology as Society, Society as Biology: Metaphors.* Dordrecht: Kluwer Academic Publishers, 1995.

MacCormac E.R. *A Cognitive Theory of Metaphor.* Cambridge, MA: MIT Press, 1985.

Macgillivray IK, Jennings T. A content analysis of exploring lesbian, gay, bisexual, and transgender topics in foundations of education textbooks. *J Teacher Education* 2008; 59:170–188.

Machamer P, Wolters G (eds). *Thinking about Causes: From Greek Philosophy to Modern Physics.* Pittsburgh, PA: University of Pittsburgh Press, 2007.

Maclure M. Karl Popper and his unending quest: an epidemiologic interpretation. *Epidemiology* 1995; 6:331–334.

MacMahon B. Breast cancer at menopausal ages: an explanation of observed incidence changes. *Cancer* 1957; 10:1037–1044.

Martin J, Harré R. Metaphor in science. In: Miall DS (ed). *Metaphor: Problems and Perspectives.* Sussex, NJ: The Harvester Press, 1982; pp. 89–105.

Mawson AR. On not taking the world as you find it–epidemiology in its place. *J Clin Epidemiol* 2002; 55:1–4.

Mayr E. *The Growth of Biological Thought: Diversity, Evolution, and Inheritance.* Cambridge, MA: The Belknap Press of Harvard University Press, 1982.

McMichael AJ. People, populations, and planets: epidemiology comes full circle. *Epidemiology* 1995; 6:633–636.

Melnechuck T. Notes of a conversation with Dr. Sydney Brenner, December 17, 1968. Available at: http://profiles.nlm.nih.gov/JJ/B/B/L/N/_/jjbbln.ocr (Accessed: July 11, 2008).

Mendelsohn E, Weingart P, Whitley R (eds). *The Social Production of Scientific Knowledge.* Dordrecht, Holland: D. Reidel Pub., 1977.

Mendelsohn KD, Nieman LZ, Isaacs K, Lee S, Levison SP. Sex and gender bias in anatomy and physical diagnosis text illustrations. *JAMA* 1994; 272:1267–1270.

Mjøset L. Theory: conceptions in the social sciences. In: Smesler NJ, Baltes PB (eds). *International Encyclopedia of the Social & Behavioral Sciences.* Elsevier, 2002; pp. 15641–15647. doi:10.1016/ B0-08-043076-7/00702-6 (Accessed: July 9, 2008).

Monod J. *Chance and Necessity: An Essay on the Natural Philosophy of Modern Biology.* (translated from the French by Austryn Wainhouse). New York: Vintage Books, 1972.

Mooney C. *The Republican War on Science.* New York: Basic Books, 2005.

Morabia A (ed). *A History of Epidemiologic Methods and Concepts.* Basel: Birkhäuser Verlag, 2004.

Morning A. Reconstructing race in science and society: biology textbooks, 1952–2002. *Am J Sociol* 2008; 114(S1):S106–S137.

Morris JN. Uses of epidemiology. *Br Med J* 1955; 2:395–401.

Morris JN. *Uses of Epidemiology.* Edinburgh: E. & S. Livingston Ltd., 1957.

Moyal JE. Causality, determinism and probability. *Philosophy* 1949; 24:310–317.

Muntaner C, Nieto FJ, O'Campo P. The Bell Curve: on race, social class, and epidemiologic research. *Am J Epidemiol* 1996; 144:531–536.

Najman J. Theories of disease causation and the concept of general susceptibility: a review. *Soc Sci Med* 1980; 14:231–237.

Osherson S., Amarasingham L. The machine metaphor in medicine. In: Mishler EG, Amarasingham L, Hauser ST, et al. (eds). *Social Contexts of Health, Illness, and Patient Care.* Cambridge: Cambridge University Press, 1981; pp. 218–249.

Oxford English Dictionary (OED). *OED online.* Available at: http://dictionary.oed.com.ezp1.harvard. edu/ (Accessed: July 9, 2008).

Pearce N, Crawford-Brown D. Critical discussion in epidemiology: problems with the Popperian approach. *J Clin Epidemiol* 1989; 42:177–184.

Pearce N. Traditional epidemiology, modern epidemiology, and public health. *Am J Public Health* 1996; 86:678–683.

Popay J. Whose theory is it anyway? *J Epidemiol Community Health* 2006; 60:571–572.

Popper K. *Popper Selections* (edited by David Miller). Princeton, NJ: Princeton University Press, 1985.

Popper K. *The Logic of Scientific Discovery*. New York: Basic Books, 1959.

Proctor R. *Racial Hygiene: Medicine Under the Nazis*. Cambridge, MA: Harvard University Press, 2003.

Rabinoff M, Caskey N, Rissling A, Park C. Pharmacologic and chemical effects of cigarette additives. *Am J Public Health* 2007; 97:1981–1991.

Rabow MW, Hardie GE, Fair JM, McPhee SJ. End-of-life care content in 50 textbooks from multiple specialties. *JAMA* 2000; 283:771–778.

Rose H, Rose S, eds. *Ideology of/in the Natural Sciences*, with an introductory essay by Ruth Hubbard. Cambridge, MA: Schenkman. 1980.

Rosenberg CE, Golden J (eds). *Framing Disease: Studies in Cultural History*. New Brunswick, NJ: Rutgers University Press, 1992.

Rothman K (ed). *Causal Inference*. Chestnut Hill, MA: Epidemiology Resources Inc., 1988.

Rothman KJ, Adami H-O, Trichopolous D. Should the mission of epidemiology include the eradication of poverty? *Lancet* 1998; 352:810–813.

Rothman KJ. *Modern Epidemiology*. Boston, MA: Little, Brown and Company, 1986.

Roughgarden J. *Evolution's Rainbow: Diversity, Gender, and Sexuality in Nature and People*. Berkeley, CA: University of California Press, 2004.

Russo F, Williamson J (eds). *Causality and Probability in the Sciences*. London: College Publications, 2007.

Scott J, Marshall G (eds). *Oxford Dictionary of Sociology*. Oxford: Oxford University Press, 2005.

Shapin S. Science. In: Bennett T, Grossberg L, Morris M (eds). *New Keywords: A Revised Vocabulary of Culture and Society*. Malden, MA: Blackwell Publishing, 2005; pp. 314–317.

Shulman S. *Undermining Science: Suppression and Distortion in the Bush Administration*. Berkeley, CA: University of California Press, 2006.

Sober E. *Evidence and Evolution: The Logic Behind the Science*. Cambridge: Cambridge University Press, 2008.

Stallones RA. To Advance Epidemiology. *Ann Rev Public Health* 1980; 1:69–82.

Stern A. *Eugenic Nation: Faults and Frontiers of Better Breeding in Modern America*. Berkeley, CA: University of California Press, 2005. (2005a)

Stern AM. Sterilized in the name of public health: race, immigration, and reproductive control in modern California. *Am J Public Health* 2005; 95:1128–1138. (2005b)

Stigler SM. *The History of Statistics: The Measurement of Uncertainty Before 1900*. Cambridge, MA: Belknap Press of Harvard University Press, 1986.

Susser M. Choosing a future for epidemiology: II. From black boxes to Chinese boxes and eco-epidemiology. *Am J Public Health* 1996; 86:674–677.

Susser M. Epidemiology in the United States after World War II: the evolution of technique. *Epidemiol Rev* 1985; 7:147–177.

Susser M. Epidemiology Today: "A Thought-Tormented World." *Int J Epidemiol* 1989; 18:481–488.

Susser M. The logic of Sir Karl Popper and the practice of epidemiology. *Am J Epidemiol* 1986; 124:711–718.

Terris M. The epidemiologic tradition: The Wade Hampton Frost Lecture. *Public Health Reports* 1979; 94:203–209.

Tompkins CJ, Rosen AL, Larkin H. An analysis of social work textbooks for aging content: how well do social work foundation texts prepare students for our aging society? *J Social Work Educ* 2006; 42:3–23.

Topham J. A textbook revolution. In: Frasca-Spada M, Jardine N (eds). *Books and The Sciences in History*. Cambridge: Cambridge University Press, 2000; pp. 317–337.

US Census. *Geographic Areas Reference Manual*. Available at: http://www.census.gov/geo/www/garm.html (Accessed: July 4, 2008).

Vågerö D. Where does new theory come from? *J Epidemiol Community Health* 2006; 60:573–574.

Van Speybroeck L, Ven de Vijver G, De Waele D. *From Epigenesis to Epigenetics: The Genome in Context*. New York: the New York Academy of Sciences, 2002.

Victora CG, Huttly SR, Fuchs SC, Olinto MTA. The role of conceptual frameworks in epidemiological analysis: a hierarchical approach. *Int J Epidemiol* 1997; 26:224–227.

Watson JD. A personal view of the project. In: Kevles DJ, Hood L (eds). *The Code of Codes: Scientific and Social Issues in The Human Genome Project*. Cambridge, MA: Harvard University Press, 1992; pp. 164–173.

Watson JD. *The Double Helix: A Personal Account of the Discovery of the Structure of DNA*. New York: Atheneum, 1968.

Weber M. Determinism, realism, and probability in evolutionary theory. *Phil Sci* 2001; 68: S213–S224.

Williams R. *Keywords: A Vocabulary of Culture and Society*. Rev. ed. New York: Oxford University Press, 1983.

Worldmapper: The World As You've Never Seen it Before. Available at: http://www.worldmapper.org/index.html (Accessed: July 5, 2008).

Young R. *Darwin's Metaphor*. Cambridge: Cambridge University Press, 1985.

Ziman J. *Real Science: What it is, and What it Means*. Cambridge, UK: Cambridge University Press, 2000.

Chapter 2

Ackerknecht E. Natural diseases and rational treatment in primitive medicine. *Bull Hist Med* 1946; 19: 467–497.

Akerejola GB (Eminefo III, Ologori of Ogori). *The History of Ogori* (Occasional Publication No. 22). Ibadan, Nigeria: University of Ibadan, Institute of African Studies, 1973.

Austin MM, Vidal-Naquet P. *Economic and Social History of Ancient Greece: An Introduction*. Berkeley, CA: University Of California Press, 1977.

Baer HA, Singer S, Susser I. *Medical Anthropology and the World System: A Critical Perspective*. Westport, CT: Bergin & Garvey, 1997.

Bannerman RH, Burton J, Wen-Chieh C (eds). *Traditional Medicine and Health Care Coverage: A Reader for Health Administrators and Practitioners*. Geneva, Switzerland: World Health Organization, 1983.

Bastien JW. Differences between Kallawaya-Andean and Greek-European humoral theory. *Soc Sci Med* 1989; 28:45–51.

Bastien JW. *Drum and Stethoscope: Integrating Ethnomedicine and Biomedicine in Bolivia*. Salt Lake City, UT: University of Utah Press, 1992.

Bastien JW. *Mountain of the Condor: Metaphor and Ritual in an Andean Ayllu*. Prospect Heights, IL: Waveland Press, 1985.

Beckfield J, Krieger N. Epi + demos + cracy: a critical review of empirical research linking political systems and priorities to the magnitude of health inequities. *Epidemiol Review* 2009; 31:152–177.

Bodde D. *Chinese Thought, Society, and Science: The Intellectual and Social Background of Science and Technology in Pre-Modern China*. Honolulu: University of Hawaii Press, 1991.

Buck C, Llopis A, Najera E, Terris M (eds). *The Challenge of Epidemiology: Issues and Selected Readings*. Washington, DC: Pan American Health Organization, 1988.

Bynum W. *The History of Medicine: A Very Short Introduction*. Oxford: Oxford University Press, 2008.

Canguilhem G. *The Normal and the Pathological*. Translated by Carolyn R. Fawcett in collaboration with Robert S. Cohen; with an introduction by Michel Foucault. New York: Zone Books, 1991.

Crandon-Malamud L. *From the Fat of Our Souls: Social Change, Political Process, and Medical Pluralism in Bolivia*. Berkeley, CA: University of California Press, 1991.

Curtin P, Feierman S, Thompson L, Vansina J. *African History: From Earliest Times to Independence*. London: Longman, 1995.

Cusicanqui SR. *"Oppressed but not Defeated": Peasant Struggles among the Aymara and Qhechwa in Bolivia, 1900-1980*. Geneva: United Nations Research Institute for Social Development, 1987.

Davidson B. *West Africa Before the Colonial Era: A History to 1850*. London: Longman, 1998.

de Tichaer RW. Medical beliefs and practices of the Aymara Indians. *JAMWA* 1973; 28:133–139.

Edelstein L. Greek medicine in its relation to religion and magic. *In*: Temkin O, Temkin CL (eds). *Ancient Medicine: Selected Papers of Ludwig Edelstein*. Baltimore, MD: Johns Hopkins University Press, 1967; pp. 205–246. (1967d)

Edelstein L. The dietetics of antiquity. *In*: Temkin O, Temkin CL (eds). *Ancient Medicine: Selected Papers of Ludwig Edelstein*. Baltimore, MD: Johns Hopkins University Press, 1967; pp. 303–316. (1967a)

Edelstein L. The Hippocratic physician. *In*: Temkin O, Temkin CL (eds). *Ancient Medicine: Selected Papers of Ludwig Edelstein*. Baltimore, MD: Johns Hopkins University Press, 1967; pp. 87–110. (1967c)

Edelstein L. The relation of ancient philosophy to medicine. *In*: Temkin O, Temkin CL (eds). *Ancient Medicine: Selected Papers of Ludwig Edelstein*. Baltimore, MD: Johns Hopkins University Press, 1967; pp. 349–366. (1967b)

Evans-Pritchard EE. *Witchcraft, Oracles and Magic among the Azande*. Abridged with an introduction by Eva Gillies. Oxford, UK: Clarendon Press, 1976.

Evans-Pritchard EE. *Witchcraft, Oracles, and Magic among the Azande*. Oxford, UK: Clarendon Press, 1937 (1965).

Eyler JM. *Victorian Social Medicine: The Ideas and Methods of William Farr*. Baltimore, MD: The Johns Hopkins University Press, 1979.

Fairbank JK. *China: A New History*. Cambridge, MA: The Belknap Press of Harvard University Press, 1992.

Falola T, Heaton MM. *A History of Nigeria*. Cambridge: Cambridge University Press, 2008.

Farr W. Lecture on the history of hygiene. *Lancet* 1835–1836; 1:773–780.

Feierman S, Janzen M. *The Social Basis of Health and Healing in Africa*. Berkeley, CA: University of California Press, 1992.

Fernández Juárez G. *Los Kallawayas: Medicina Indígena en Los Andes Bolivianos*. Cuenca: Ediciones de la Universidad de Castilla-La Mancha, 1998.

Galeano E. *Open Veins of Latin America: Five Centuries of the Pillage of a Continent*. (transl. by Cedric Belfrage). New York: Monthly Review Press, 1973.

Gillies E. Causal criteria in African classifications of disease. In: Loudon JB (ed). *Social Anthropology and Medicine*. London: Academic Press, 1976; pp. 358–395.

Green EC. *Indigenous Theories of Contagious Disease*. Walnut Creek, CA: Altamira Press, 1999.

Greenwood M. *Epidemiology: Historical and Experimental*. The Herter Lectures for 1931. Baltimore, MD: The Johns Hopkins Press, 1932.

Grmek MD (ed). *Western Medical Thought from Antiquity to the Middle Ages*. Cambridge, MA: Harvard University Press, 1998.

Grmek MD. *Diseases in the Ancient Greek World*. Baltimore, MD: Johns Hopkins University Press, 1983 (1989).

Gwei-Djen L, Needham J. *Celestial Lancets*. Cambridge: Cambridge University Press, 1980.

Hodgson MGS. *Rethinking World History: Essays on Europe, Islam, and World History*. Cambridge: Cambridge University Press, 1993.

Hoizey D, Hoizey MJ (transl. P. Bailey). *A History of Chinese Medicine*. Vancouver: University of British Columbia, 1993.

Hsu E (ed). *Innovation in Chinese Medicine*. Cambridge: Cambridge University Press, 2001.

Hughes CC. Public health in non-literate societies. In: Galdston I (ed). *Man's Image in Medicine and Anthropology*. New York: New York Academy of Medicine International Universities Press, 1963; pp. 157–233.

Isichei E. *A History of Nigeria*. London: Longman, 1983.

Iwu MM. *African Ethnomedicine*. Enugu, Nigeria: CECTA Ltd, 1986.

Jouanna J. *Hippocrates* (transl. M.B. DeBevoise). Baltimore, Md.: John Hopkins University Press, 1999.

King H (ed). *Health in Antiquity*. London: Routledge, 2005.

King H. *Hippocrates' Woman: Reading the Female Body in Ancient Greece*. London: Routledge, 1998.

King H. Women's Health and Recovery in The Hippocratic Corpus. In: King H (ed). *Health in Antiquity*. London: Routledge, 2005; pp. 150–161.

Klein HS. *A Concise History of Bolivia*. Cambridge: Cambridge University Press, 2003.

Kolata AL. *Valley of the Spirits: A Journey into the Lost Realm of the Aymara*. New York, NY: John Wiley & Sons, 1995.

Krieger N. Epidemiology and social sciences: towards a critical reengagement in the 21st century. *Epidemiologic Reviews* 2000; 11:155–163.

Kuriyama S. *The Expressiveness of the Body and the Divergence of Greek and Chinese Medicine*. New York: Zone Books, 1999.

Lehman D (ed). *Ecology and Exchange in the Andes*. Cambridge, UK: Cambridge University Press, 1982.

Llanque D, Irrázabal D, Mendoza S. *Medicina Aymara*. La Paz, Bolivia: Hisbol, 1994.

Lloyd GER (ed). *Hippocratic Writings*. London: Penguin Books, 1983. (1983a)

Lloyd GER. *Demystifying Mentalities*. Cambridge: Cambridge University Press, 1990.

Lloyd GER. *Magic, Reason and Experience: Studies in the Origin and Development of Greek Science*. Cambridge: Cambridge University Press, 1979.

Lloyd GER. The female sex: medical treatment and biological theories in the fifth and fourth centuries B.C. *In*: Lloyd GER. *Science, Folklore, and Ideology: Studies in the Life Sciences of Ancient Greece*. Cambridge: Cambridge University Press, 1983; pp. 58–111. (1983b)

Lloyd GER. *The Revolutions of Wisdom: Studies in the Claims and Practice of Ancient Greek Science*. Berkeley, CA: University of California Press, 1987.

Lloyd GER, Sivin N. *The Way and The Word: Science and Medicine in Early China and Greece*. New Haven: Yale University Press, 2002.

Longrigg J. *Greek Rational Medicine: Philosophy and Medicine from Alcmaeon to the Alexandrians*. London: Routledge, 1993.

Loudon JB (ed). *Social Anthropology and Medicine*. London: Academic Press, 1976.

Loza CB. *Kallawaya: Reconocimiento Mundial a Una Ciencia de Los Andes*. La Paz, Bolivia: FCBCB (Fundación Cultural, Banco Central de Bolivia): Viceministerio de Cultura, Bolivia: UNESCO, [2004?]

Machle EJ. *Nature and Heaven in Xunzi: A Study of the Tian Lun*. Albany: State University of New York, 1993.

Masood E. *Science & Islam: A History*. London: Icon Books, 2009.

Murray O. *Early Greece*. Cambridge, MA: Harvard University Press, 1978 (1993).

Needham J. *Science and Civilization in China, Volume 1: Introductory Orientations*. Cambridge: Cambridge University Press, 1954.

Needham J. *Science and Civilization in China, Volume 2: History of Scientific Thought*. Cambridge: Cambridge University Press, 1969.

Nutton V. *Ancient Medicine*. London: Routledge, 2004.

Nutton V. Healers in the medical market place: towards a social history of Graeco-Roman medicine. *In*: Wear A. (ed). *Medicine in Society: Historical Essays*. Cambridge: Cambridge University Press, 1992; pp. 15–58.

Oxford English Dictionary (OED). Available At: Http://Dictionary.Oed.Com.Ezp1.Harvard.Edu; Accessed: September 4, 2008.

Osheidu AB. *Historical Facts on Ogori. 2nd Ed. With Additions*. Ilorin: A. Baba Osheidu, 1980.

Pei W. Traditional Chinese Medicine. *In*: Bannerman RH, Burton J, Wen-Chieh C (eds). *Traditional Medicine and Health Care Coverage: A Reader for Health Administrators and Practitioners*. Geneva: World Health Organization, 1983; pp. 68–75.

Pomeroy SB. *Goddesses, Whores, Wives, and Slaves: Women in Classical Antiquity*. New York: Schocken Books, 1975.

Porkert M. *The Theoretical Foundations of Chinese Medicine*. Cambridge, MA: Harvard University Press, 1974.

Pormann P, Savage-Smith E. *Medieval Islamic Medicine*. Edinburgh: Edinburgh University Press, 2007.

Porter D. *Health, Civilization and the State: A History of Public Health from Ancient to Modern Times*. London: Routledge, 1999.

Porter R. *The Greatest Benefit to Mankind: A Medical History of Humanity*. New York: W.W. Norton, 1997.

Powell A. *Athens and Sparta: Constructing Greek Political and Social History from 478 BC*. London: Routledge, 1988.

Ranger T. The influenza pandemic in Southern Rhodesia: a crisis of comprehension. In: Arnold D (ed). *Imperial Medicine and Indigenous Societies*. Manchester: Manchester University Press, 1988; pp. 172–188.

Rosen G. *A History of Public Health*. (1958) Expanded edition (Introduction by Elizabeth Fee; Biographical essay and new bibliography by Edward T. Morman). Baltimore, MD: The Johns Hopkins University Press, 1993.

Saliba G. *Islamic Science and the Making of the European Renaissance*. Cambridge, MA: The MIT Press, 2007.

Schneider D, Lilienfeld DE, Winklestein WR Jr (eds). *Public Health: The Development of a Discipline*. New Brunswick, NJ: Rutgers University Press, 2008.

Schull WJ, Rothhammer F (eds). *The Aymara: Strategies in Human Adaptation to a Rigorous Environment*. Dordrecht, The Netherlands: Kluwer Academic Publishers, 1990.

Sealey R. *Women and Law in Classical Greece*. Chapel Hill, NC: The University of North Carolina Press, 1990; pp. 1–11.

Sigerist HE. *A History of Medicine, Volume I: Primitive and Archaic Medicine*. New York: Oxford University Press, 1951.

Sigerist HE. *A History of Medicine, Volume II: Early Greek, Hindu, and Persian Medicine*. New York: Oxford University Press, 1961.

Sivin N. *Traditional Medicine in Contemporary China: A Partial Translation of Revised Outline of Chinese Medicine (1972) with an Introductory Study on Change in Present-day and Early Medicine*. Ann Arbor: University of Michigan, 1987.

Susser M, Stein Z. *Eras in Epidemiology: The Evolution of Ideas*. New York: Oxford University Press, 2009.

Taussig M. *The Devil and Commodity Fetishism*. Chapel Hill, NC: University of North Carolina Press, 1980.

Temkin O. *Galenism: Rise and Decline of a Medical Philosophy*. Ithaca, NY: Cornell University Press, 1973.

UNESCO. *Proclamation 2003: "The Andean Cosmovision of the Kallaway."* Available at: http://www.unesco.org/culture/ich/index.php?topic=mp&cp=BOTOC2; Accessed: November 7, 2008.

Unschuld P. *Chinese Life Sciences: Introductory Readings in Classical Chinese Medicine: Sixty Texts with Vocabulary and Translation, A Guide to Research Aids, and a General Glossary*. Taos, NM: Paradigm Publications: Distributed by Redwing Book Co., 2005.

Unschuld P. *Huang Di Nei Jing Su Wen: Nature, Knowledge, Imagery in an Ancient Chinese Medical Text, with an Appendix, The Doctrine of The Five Periods and Six Qi in The Huang Di Nei Jing Su Wen*. Berkeley: University of California Press, 2003.

Unschuld PU. *Medicine in China: A History of Ideas*. Berkeley, CA: University of California Press, 1985.

van den Berg H, Schiffers N (eds). *La Cosmovision Aymara*. La Paz, Bolivia: Hisbol, 1992.

van der Eijk PJ (ed). *Hippocrates in Context: Papers Read at the Xith International Hippocrates Colloquium, University Of Newcastle Upon Tyne, 27-August 31, 2002*. Leiden: Brill, 2005.

van Lindert P, Verkoren O. *Bolivia: A Guide to the People, Politics, and Culture*. London: Latin American Bureau, 1994.

Vaughan M. *Curing Their Ills: Colonial Power and African Illness*. Cambridge, UK: Cambridge University Press, 1991.

Vaughan M. Healing and curing: issues in the social history and anthropology of medicine in Africa. *Social History Medicine* 1994; 7:283–295.

Veith I (transl). *Huang Ti Ne Ching Su Wên: The Yellow Emperor's Classic of Internal Medicine*. Berkeley: University of California Press, 1966.

Webster TBL. *Athenian Culture and Society*. Berkeley, CA: University of California Press, 1973.

Wilbur CM. *Slavery in China during the Former Han Dynasty 206 B.C.-A.D. 25*. Chicago: Natural History Museum, Anthropological Series V. 24–25, 1943.

Wilkins J. The social and intellectual context of *Regimen II*. In: van der Eijk PJ (ed). *Hippocrates in Context: Papers Read at the Xith International Hippocrates Colloquium, University Of Newcastle Upon Tyne, 27-August 31, 2002*. Leiden: Brill, 2005; pp. 121–133.

Wong KC, Lien-Teh W. *History of Chinese Medicine*. Tientsin, China: The Tientsin Press, 1932.

Zmiewski P, Cheng-Yü L (eds). *Fundamentals of Chinese Medicine*. Brookline, MA: Paradigm Publications, 1985.

Chapter 3

AAA statement on race. *American Anthropologist* 1999; 100:712–713.

AAPA statement on biological aspects of race. *American Anthropologist* 1999; 100:714–715.

Academie de Médicine. *Rapport lu a l'Académie Royale de Médecine, dans les seances des 15 mai et 19 juin 1827, au nom de la Commission chargée d'examiner des documents de M. Chervin concernant la fièvre jaune. Publié Textuellement d'apres l'édition de l'Académie, et accompagné de remarques par le Docteur Chervin*. Paris: F. Didot, 1828.

Ackerknecht EH. Anticontagionism between 1821 and 1867. *Bull Hist Med* 1948; 22:562–593. (1948b)

Ackerknecht EH. Hygiene in France, 1815–1848. *Bull Hist Med* 1948; 22:117–155. (1948a)

Ackerknecht EH. *Rudolf Virchow, Doctor, Statesman, Anthropologist*. Madison, WI: University of Wisconsin Press, 1953.

Agassiz L. The diversity of the origin of the human races. *Christian Examiner* 1850; 49:110–145.

Aisenberg AR. *Contagion: Disease, Government, and the "Social Question" in Nineteenth-Century France*. Stanford, CA: Stanford University Press, 1999.

Alison SS. *An Inquiry into the Propagation of Contagious Poisons, by the Atmosphere: As also into the Nature and Effects of Vitiated air, its Forms and Sources, and other Causes of Pestilence…* Edinburgh, Scotland: S. Maclachlan, 1839.

Alison SS. *Report on the Sanitary Condition and General Economy of the Town of Tranent, and the Neighbouring District in Haddingtonshire*. London, 1840. (1840a)

Alison WP. *Observations on the Epidemic Fever of MDCCCXLIII in Scotland, and its Connection with the Destitute Condition of the Poor*. Edinburgh, Scotland: W. Blackwood, 1844.

Alison WP. Observations on the Generation of Fever. Remarks on… by Neill Arnott. London, UK: His Majesty's Stationery Office. 1840. (1840b)

Allen P. Etiological theory in America prior to the civil war. *J Hist Med Allied Sciences* 1947; 2: 489–520.

Anderson MJ. *The American Census: A Social History*. New Haven, CT: Yale University Press, 1988.

Anon. Cartwright on the Diseases, etc., of the Negro Race. *Charleston Med J* 1851; 6:829–843, continued in 1852;7:89–98.

Arnold D (ed). *Imperial Medicine and Indigenous Societies*. Manchester, UK: Manchester University Press, 1988.

Augstein HF (ed). *Race: The Origins of an Idea, 1760–1850*. Bristol, UK: Thoemmes Press, 1996.

Augstein HF. From the land of the Bible to the Caucasus and beyond: the shifting ideas of the geographical origin of humankind. In: Ernst W, Harris B (eds). *Race, Science and Medicine, 1700-1960*. London: Routledge, 1999; pp. 58–79.

Baecque A. *The Body Politic: Corporeal Metaphor in Revolutionary France, 1770–1800*. (transl. Charlotte Mandel). Stanford, CA: Stanford University Press, 1997.

Baer HA, Singer S, Susser I. *Medical Anthropology and the World System: A Critical Perspective*. Westport, CT: Bergin & Garvey, 1997.

Baker KM. *Condorcet: From Natural Philosophy to Social Mathematics*. Chicago, IL: University of Chicago Press, 1975.

Baker KM. The early use of the term "social science." *Annals of Science* 1969; 20:211–226.

Baker LD. *From Savage to Negro: Anthropology and the Construction of Race, 1860–1954*. Berkeley, CA: University of California Press, 1998.

Baldwin P. *Contagion and the State in Europe, 1830–1930.* Cambridge, UK: Cambridge University Press, 1999.

Banton MP. *Racial Theories.* 2nd ed. Cambridge, UK: Cambridge University Press, 1998.

Beik D, Beik P. *Flora Tristan: Utopian Feminist: Her Travel Diaries and Personal Crusade. Selected, Translated, and with an Introduction to her Life.* Bloomington, IN: Indiana University Press, 1993.

Bendsyhe T. Preface. In: Blumenbach JF. *The Anthropological Treatises of Johann Friedrich Blumenbach, Late professor at Göttingen and court physician to the King of Great Britain, with Memoires of him by Marx and Flourens, and an account of his anthropological museum by Professor R. Wagner, and the inaugural dissertation of John Hunter, MD, on the Varieties of Man. Translated and edited from the Latin, German, and French originals, by Thomas Bendyshe, M.A., V.P.A.S.L., fellow of King's College, Cambridge.* London: Published for the Anthropological Society, by Longman, Green, Longman, Roberts & Green, 1865; pp. vii–xiv.

Blane G. *Elements of Medical Logick, Illustrated by Practical Proofs and Examples; Including a Statement of the Evidence Respecting the Contagious Nature of the Yellow-Fever.* London: Thomas & George Underwood, 1819.

Blumenbach JF. *On the Natural Variety of Mankind* (1st ed, 1775). In: Blumenbach JF. *The Anthropological Treatises of Johann Friedrich Blumenbach, Late professor at Göttingen and court physician to the King of Great Britain, with Memoires of him by Marx and Flourens, and an account of his anthropological museum by Professor R. Wagner, and the inaugural dissertation of John Hunter, MD, on the Varieties of Man. Translated and edited from the Latin, German, and French originals, by Thomas Bendyshe, M.A., V.P.A.S.L., fellow of King's College, Cambridge.* London: Published for the Anthropological Society, by Longman, Green, Longman, Roberts & Green, 1865; pp. 65–145.

Boulay de La Meurthe H. *Histoire du cholera-morbus dans le quartier du Luxembourg, ou precis des travaux de la commission sanitaire et du bureau de secours de ce quartier, suivi de documens statistiques sur les ravages que la cholera y a exerces.* Paris, France: Renouard, 1832.

Bousfield MO. An account of physicians of color in the United States. *Bull Hist Med* 1945; 17:61–85.

Boyd R. *The Coming of the Spirit of Pestilence: Introduced Infectious Disease and Population Decline among Northwest Coast Indians, 1774–1874.* Vancouver, Canada: University of British Columbia Press; Seattle, WA: University of Washington Press, 1999.

Brock H. North America, a western outpost of European medicine. In: Cunningham A, French R (eds). *The Medical Enlightenment of the Eighteenth Century.* Cambridge, UK: Cambridge University Press, 1990; pp. 194–217.

Buck P. People who counted: political arithmetic in the eighteenth century. *Isis* 1982; 73:28–45.

Burton DM. *The History of Mathematics: An Introduction.* 4th ed. Boston: McGraw-Hill, 1999.

Bynum W. *The History of Medicine: A Very Short Introduction.* Oxford: Oxford University Press, 2008.

Byrne BB. *An Essay to Prove the Contagious Character of Malignant Cholera; with Brief Instructions for its Prevention and Cure.* Baltimore, MD: Carey, Hart & Co., 1833.

Cartwright SA. Alcohol and the Ethiopian; of the moral and physical effects of ardent spirits on the Negro race, and some account of the peculiarity of that people. *New Orleans Med Surg J* 1853;10:150–165. (1853b)

Cartwright SA. Ethnology of the Negro or prognathous race—A lecture delivered November 30, 1857, before the New Orleans Academy of Science. *New Orleans Med Surg J* 1858; 15:149–163.

Cartwright SA. Remarks on dysentery among Negroes. *New Orleans Med Surg J* 1855; 11:145–163.

Cartwright SA. Report on the diseases and physical peculiarities of the Negro race. *New Orleans Med Surg J* 1850; 7:691–715.

Cartwright SA. Slavery in the light of ethnology. In: Elliott EN (ed). *Cotton is King and Pro-Slavery Arguments (1860).* New York: Negro Universities Press, 1969 (reprinted); pp. 691–728.

Cartwright SA. The diseases and physical peculiarities of the Negro race (continued). *New Orleans Med Surg J* 1851; 8 (part 1):187–194.

Cartwright SA. Philosophy of the Negro constitution. Elicited through questions propounded by Dr. C.R. Hall of Torquay, England, through Professor Jackson, of Massachusetts Medical College, Boston, to Saml. A Cartwright, M.D., New Orleans. *New Orleans Med Surg J* 1853; 9:195–208. (1853a)

Cavalli-Sforza LL, Menozzi P, Piazza A. *The History and Geography of Human Genes*. Princeton, NJ: Princeton University Press, 1996.

Cavalli-Sforza LL. *Genes, Peoples, and Languages* (transl. Mark Seielstad). New York: North Point Press, 2000.

Chervin N. *Examen critique des prétendues preuves de contagion de la fièvre jaune observée en Espagne, or Réponse aux alllégations de M. Pariset contre le rapport fait a l'Académie Royale de Médecine, le 15 Mai 1827*. Paris: Chez J.-B. Baillière, 1828.

Chervin N. *Reponse au discours de M. le Dr. Audouard : contre le rapport fait a l'Académie Royale de Médecine de Paris, le 15 Mai 1827, sur mes documents concernant la fièvre jaune*. Paris: Crapelet, 1827

Cohen IB. A note on "social science" and on "'natural science." In: Cohen IB (ed). *The Natural Sciences and the Social Sciences: Some Critical and Historical Perspectives*. Dordrecht, the Netherlands: Kluwer Academic Pub, 1994; pp. xxv–xxxvi. (1994a)

Cohen IB. *Revolution in Science*. Cambridge, MA: Belknap Press of Harvard University Press, 1985.

Cohen IB. The scientific revolution in the social sciences. In: Cohen IB (ed). *The Natural Sciences and the Social Sciences: Some Critical and Historical Perspectives*. Dordrecht, the Netherlands: Kluwer Academic Pub, 1994; pp. 152–203. (1994b)

Cohen PC. *A Calculating People: The Spread of Numeracy in Early America*. Chicago, IL: University of Chicago Press, 1982.

Cole J. *The Power of Large Numbers: Population, Politics, and Gender in Nineteenth-Century France*. Ithaca, NY: Cornell University Press, 2000.

Coleman W. *Death is a Social Disease: Public Health and Political Economy in Early Industrial France*. Madison, WI: Univ of Wisconsin Press, 1982.

Coleman W. *Yellow Fever in the North: The Methods of Early Epidemiology*. Madison, WI: University of Wisconsin Press, 1987.

Cook ND. Disease and the depopulation of Hispaniola, 1492–1518. In: Kiple KF, Beck SV (eds). *Biological Consequences of the European Expansion, 1450-1800*. Aldershot, Hampshire, Great Britain: Ashgate/Variorum, 1997; pp. 37–69 (originally published in: Colonial Latin American Review II, nos. 1–2 (San Diego, CA, 1993); pp. 213–245). (1997a)

Cook SF. The significance of disease in the extinction of the New England Indians. In: Kiple KF, Beck SV (eds). *Biological Consequences of the European Expansion, 1450–1800*. Aldershot, Hampshire, Great Britain: Ashgate/Variorum, 1997; pp. 251–274 (originally published in: Human Biology XLV, no. 3 (Detroit, MI, 1973); pp. 485–508. (Cook 1997b)

Crosby AW Jr. *Ecological Imperialism: The Biological Expansion of Europe, 900-1900*. Cambridge, UK: Cambridge University Press, 1986.

Crumpler R. *A Book of Medical Discourses*. Boston: Cashman, Keating & Co, 1883. Available at: http://pds.lib.harvard.edu/pds/view/2573819?n=2&s=4 (Accessed: November 26, 2008).

Cunningham A, French R (eds). *The Medical Enlightenment of the Eighteenth Century*. Cambridge, UK: Cambridge University Press, 1990.

Cunningham A. Thomas Sydenham: epidemics, experiment and the 'Good Old Cause.' In: French R, Wear A (eds). *The Medical Revolution of the Seventeenth Century*. Cambridge, UK: Cambridge University Press, 1989; pp. 165–190.

Currie W. Report of the College of Physicians, in answer to the Governor's enquiries, respecting the origin of the late epidemic; and their directions for extinguishing latent infection. In: Currie W. *A Treatise on the Synochus Icteroides, or Yellow Fever: As it Lately Appeared in the City of Philadelphia: Exhibiting a Concise View of its Rise, Progress and Symptoms, Together with the Method of Treatment Found Most Successful; Also Remarks on the Nature of its Contagion, and Directions for Preventing the Introduction of the Same Malady, in Future*. Philadelphia, PA: Thomas Dobson, 1794; pp. 83–85.

Curtin PD. *Death by Migration: Europe's Encounter with the Tropical World in the Nineteenth Century*. Cambridge, UK: Cambridge University Press, 1989.

Curtin PD. *Disease and Empire: The Health of European Troops in the Conquest of Africa*. Cambridge, UK: Cambridge University Press, 1998.

Cuvier G. *The Animal Kingdom: Arranged After its Organization; Forming a Natural History of Animals, and an Introduction to Comparative Anatomy (1817), by the late Baron Cuvier;*

translated and adapted to the present state of science. New ed., with considerable additions by W.B. Carpenter and J.O. Westwood. London: H.G. Bohn, 1863; New York: Kraus Reprint, 1969.

D'Aulaire I, Daulaire I. *D'Aulaires' Book of Greek Myths*. Garden City, NY: Doubleday & Co. 1962.

Darwin C. *The Origin of Species* (1859). Edison, NJ: Castle Books, 2004.

Daston LJ. Rational individuals versus laws of society: from probability to statistics. In: Krüger L, Daston LJ, Heidelberger M. *The Probabilistic Revolution. Vol. 1. Ideas in History*. Cambridge, MA: Cambridge University Press, 1987; pp. 295–304.

Delaporte F. *Disease and Civilization: The Cholera in Paris, 1832*. (transl. Arthur Goldammer; foreword by Paul Rabinow). Cambridge, MA: MIT Press, 1986.

Desmond A, Moore J. *Darwin's Sacred Cause: How a Hatred of Slavery Shaped Darwin's Views on Human Evolution*. London: Penguin Books, 2009.

Desrosières A. *The Politics of Large Numbers: A History of Statistical Reasoning*. (transl. Camille Naish). Cambridge, MA: Harvard University Press, 1998.

Deutsch A. The first U.S. census of the insane (1840) and its use as pro-slavery propaganda. *Bull Hist Med* 1944; 15:469–482.

Dewhurst K. *Dr. Thomas Sydenham (1624–1689). His Life and Original Writings*. Berkeley, CA: University of California Press, 1966.

Donnelly M. From political arithmetic to social statistics: how some nineteenth-century roots of the social sciences were implanted, in Heilbron J, Magnusson L, Wittrock B (eds). *The Rise of the Social Sciences and the Formation of Modernity: Conceptual Change in Context, 1750–1850*. Dordrecht, the Netherlands: Kluwer Acad Pub, 1998; pp. 224–239.

Duffy J. Smallpox and the Indians in the American colonies. In: Kiple KF, Beck SV (eds). Biological Consequences of the European Expansion, 1450-1800. Aldershot, Hampshire, Great Britain: Ashgate/Variorum, 1997; pp. 233–250 (originally published in: Bulletin of the History of Medicine XXV, no. 4 (Baltimore, MD, 1951); pp. 324–341).

Eknoyan G. Adolphe Quetelet (1764–1874)–the average man and indices of obesity. *Nephrol Dial Transplant* 2008; 23:47–51.

Engels F. *The Condition of the Working Class in England*. (1845) Translated by W.O. Henderson and W.H. Chaloner. Stanford, CA: Stanford University Press, 1958.

Englander D. *Poverty and Poor Law Reform in Britain: From Chadwick to Booth, 1834–1914*. London: Addison Wesley Longman, 1998.

Ernst W, Harris B (eds). *Race, Science and Medicine, 1700–1960*. London: Routledge, 1999.

Eyler JM. *Victorian Social Medicine: The Ideas and Methods of William Farr*. Baltimore, MD: The Johns Hopkins University Press, 1979.

Falk LA. Black abolitionist doctors and healers, 1810–1885. *Bull Hist Med* 1980; 54:258–272.

Farr W. Vital statistics. *British Annals of Medicine* 1837; 1:353–360.

Farr W. *Vital Statistics: A Memorial Volume of Selections from the Reports and Writings of William Farr (London: Offices of the Sanitary Institute, 1885). With an introduction by Mervyn Susser and Abraham Adelstein. Published under the auspices of the Library of the New York Academy of Medicine*. Metuchen, NJ: Scarecrow Press, 1975.

Fenner ED. Acclimation; and the liability of Negroes to endemic fevers of the south. *Southern Med Surg J* 1858; 14:452–461.

Finlay CJ. The mosquito hypothetically considered as the agent of transmission of yellow fever. Read before the Royal Academy of Medical, Physical and Natural Sciences, sessions of August 15th, 1881. Reprinted. in: Buck C, Llopis A, Nájera E, Terris M (eds). *The Challenge of Epidemiology: Issues and Selected Readings*, Washington, DC: Pan American Health Organization, World Health Organization, 1988; pp. 60–66.

Flinn MW (ed). *Report on the Sanitary Condition of the Laboring Population of Great Britain - by Edwin Chadwick* (1842). Edinburgh: Edinburgh University Press, 1965.

Floures M. Memoir of Blumenbach. In: Blumenbach JF. *The Anthropological Treatises of Johann Friedrich Blumenbach, Late professor at Göttingen and court physician to the King of Great Britain, with Memoires of him by Marx and Flourens, and an account of his anthropological museum by Professor R. Wagner, and the inaugural dissertation of John Hunter, MD, on the Varieties of Man. Translated and edited from the Latin, German, and French originals, by Thomas Bendyshe, M.A., V.P.A.S.L., fellow of King's College, Cambridge.* London: Published for the Anthropological Society, by Longman, Green, Longman, Roberts & Green, 1865; pp. 49–63.

Forry S. On the relative proportion of centenarians, of deaf and dumb, of blind, and of insane, in the races of European and African origin, as shown by the census of the United States. *New York J Med* 1844; 2:310–320.

Forry S. Vital statistics furnished by the sixth census of the United States, bearing upon the question of the unity of the human race. *New York J Med* 1843; 1:151–167.

Frank JP. The people's misery: the mother of diseases. An Address, delivered in 1790. *Bull Hist Med* 1941; 9:88–100.

French R, Wear A (eds). *The Medical Revolution of the Seventeenth-Century.* Cambridge, UK: Cambridge University Press, 1989.

Frost WH (ed). *Snow on Cholera, being a Reprint of Two Papers by John Snow, M.D., together with a Biographical Memoir by B.W. Richardson, M.D., and an Introduction by Wade Hampton Frost, M.D.* New York: The Commonwealth Fund, 1936.

Gaunt P. *Oliver Cromwell.* Oxford, UK: Blackwell Publishers with the Historical Association, 1996.

Gilmore J. *The Poetics of Empire: A Study of James Grainger's The Sugar Cane (1764).* London: Athlone Press, 2000.

Glass DV. *Numbering the People: The Eighteenth-Century Population Controversy and the Development of Census and Vital Statistics in Britain.* Farnborough, Hants, UK: Saxon House, 1973.

Goodman P. *Of One Blood: Abolitionism and the Origins of Racial Equality.* Berkeley, CA: University of California Press, 1998.

Gould SJ. *The Mismeasure of Man, Rev. and expanded.* New York: Norton, 1996.

Grainger J. *An Essay on the More Common West-India Diseases and the Remedies which that Country itself Produces. To which are Added, Some Hints on the Management, &c., of Negroes. By a Physician in the West-Indies.* London: Printed for T. Becket and P.A. De Hondt, in the strand. MDCCLXIV (1764).

Graunt J. *Natural and Political Observations Made Upon the Bills of Mortality,* by John Graunt (1662), edited with an introduction by Walter F. Willcox. Baltimore, MD: The Johns Hopkins Press, 1939.

Greenwood M. *Some British Pioneers of Social Medicine.* London: Oxford University Press, 1948.

Grob G. Edward Jarvis and the Federal Census: a chapter in the history of nineteenth-century American medicine. *Bull Hist Med* 1976; 50:4–27.

Guerrini A. Isaac Newton, George Cheyne and the 'Principia Medicinae.' In: French R, Wear A (eds). *The Medical Revolution of the Seventeenth Century.* Cambridge, UK: Cambridge University Press, 1989; pp. 222–245.

Guy WA. On the health of nightmen, scavengers, and dustmen. *J Statistical Society London* 1848; 11:72–81.

Guy WA. On the original and acquired meaning of the term "statistics," and on the proper functions of a Statistical Society: also on the question whether there be a science of statistics; and if so, what are its nature and objects, and what is its relation to political economy and "social science." *J Statistical Society* 1865; 28:478–493.

Guy WA. On the value of the numerical method as applied to science, but especially to physiology and medicine. *J Statistical Society* 1839; 2:25–47.

Hacking I. How should we do the history of statistics? *Ideology and Consciousness* 1981; 8:15–26.

Hacking I. *The Emergence of Probability.* Cambridge, UK: Cambridge University Press, 1975.

Hacking I. *The Taming of Chance.* Cambridge, UK: Cambridge University Press, 1990.

Haller JS Jr. *Outcasts from Evolution: Scientific Attitudes of Racial Inferiority, 1859–1900.* Urbana, IL: University of Illinois Press, 1971.

Halley E. An estimate of the degrees of mortality of mankind, drawn from curious tables of the births and funerals at the City of Breslaw; with an attempt to ascertain the price of annuities on lives. *Philosoph Transactions* 1693; XVII:483–492.

Hamilton E. *Mythology.* Boston: Little, Brown & Co. 1942 (reissued as: Hamilton E. *Mythology: Timeless Tales of Gods and Heroes.* New York: 1999).

Hamlin C. Finding a function for public health: disease theory or political philosophy. *J Health Politics Policy Law* 1995; 20:1025–1230.

Hamlin C. *Public Health and Social Justice in the Age of Chadwick. Britain: 1800–1854.* Cambridge, UK: Cambridge University Press, 1998.

Hankins FH. *Adolphe Quetelet as Statistician.* (1908) New York: Ams Press, 1968.

Harding S (ed). *The "Racial" Economy of Science: Toward a Democratic Future.* Bloomington, IN: University of Indiana Press, 1993.

Harrison M. 'The tender frame of man': Disease, climate, and racial difference in India and the West Indies, 1760–1860. *Bull Hist Med* 1996; 70:68–93.

Harrison M. *Climates & Constitutions: Health, Race, Environment, and British Imperialism in India, 1600–1850.* New York: Oxford University Press, 2002.

Haskell TL. *The Emergence of Professional Social Science: The American Social Science Association and the Nineteenth-Century Crisis of Authority.* Urbana, IL: University of Illinois Press, 1977.

Hays JN. *The Burdens of Disease: Epidemics and Human Response in Western History.* New Brunswick, NJ: Rutgers University Press, 1998.

Heilbron J, Magnusson L, Wittrock B (eds). *The Rise of the Social Sciences and the Formation of Modernity: Conceptual Change in Context, 1750–1850.* Dordrecht, the Netherlands: Kluwer Acad Pub, 1998.

Hill C. *God's Englishman; Oliver Cromwell and the English Revolution.* New York: Harper & Row, 1972.

Hirsch A. *Handbook of Geographic and Historical Pathology, Vol I, Acute Infective Disease* (transl. from the second German edition by Charles Creighton). London: The New Sydenham Society, 1883.

Hobsbawm E. *The Age of Capital, 1848–1875.* New York: Vintage Books, 1996 (1975). (1996b).

Hobsbawm E. *The Age of Revolution, 1789–1848.* New York: Vintage Books 1996 (1962). (1996a)

Hobsbawm EJ. *Nations and Nationalism since 1780: Programme, Myth, Reality.* 2nd ed. Cambridge: Cambridge University Press, 1992.

Hopkins DR. *Princes and Peasants: Smallpox in History;* with a foreword by George I. Lythcott. Chicago: University of Chicago Press, 1983.

Hosack D. *Observations on Febrile Contagion and on the Means of Improving the Medical Police of the City of New York. Delivered as an Introductory Discourse, in the Hall of the College of Physicians and Surgeons, on the Sixth of November, 1820.* New York: Elam Bliss, 1820.

Hull CH (ed). *The Economic Writings of Sir William Petty, together with the Observations upon the Bills of Mortality more probably by Captain John Graunt. Vol 1.* Reprints of Economic Classics. New York: August M. Kelley, 1963.

Humphreys M. *Yellow Fever and the South.* New Brunswick, NJ: Rutgers University Press, 1992.

James CLR. *The Black Jacobins: Toussaint L'Ouverture and the San Domingo Revolution,* 2nd ed., rev., New York: Vintage Books, 1989 (1938; 1963).

Jarvis E. Insanity among the colored population of the free states. *Am J Insanity* 1852; 8:268–282.

Jarvis E. Insanity among the coloured population of the free states. *Am J Medical Sciences* 1844; 7:71–83.

Jarvis E. Statistics of insanity in the United States. *Boston Med Surg J* 1842; 27:116–121.

Kaplan JB, Bennett T. Use of race and ethnicity in biomedical publication. *JAMA* 2003; 289:2709–2716.

Koren J (ed). *The History of Statistics: Their Development and Progress in Many Countries. In Memoirs to Commemorate the Seventy-Fifth Anniversary of the American Statistical Association.* New York: Burt Franklin, 1918.

Krieger N, Birn AE. A vision of social justice as the foundation of public health: commemorating 150 years of the spirit of 1848. *Am J Public Health* 1998; 88:1603–1606.

Krieger N, Davey Smith G. Bodies count & body counts: social epidemiology & embodying inequality. *Epidemiol Review* 2004; 26:92–103.

Krieger N. Epidemiology and social sciences: towards a critical reengagement in the 21st century. *Epidemiologic Reviews* 2000; 11:155–163.

Krieger N. Historical roots of social epidemiology: socioeconomic gradients in health and contextual analysis. (letter) *Int J Epidemiol* 2001; 30:899–900. (2001a)

Krieger N. Shades of difference: theoretical underpinnings of the medical controversy on black/white differences in the United States, 1830–1870. *Int J Health Services* 1987; 17:259–278.

Krieger N. Stormy weather: "race," gene expression, and the science of health disparities. *Am J Public Health* 2005; 95:2155–2160.

Krieger N. Theories for social epidemiology in the 21st century: an ecosocial perspective. *Int J Epidemiol* 2001; 30:668–677. (2001b)

Kunitz SJ. *Disease and Social Diversity: The European Impact on the Health of Non-Europeans.* New York: Oxford University Press, 1994.

La Berge AF. *Mission and Method: the Early Nineteenth-Century French Public Health Movement.* Cambridge, UK: Cambridge University Press, 1992.

Lesky E. Introduction. In: Lesky E (ed). *A System of Complete Medical Police: Selections from Johann Peter Frank.* Baltimore, MD: Johns Hopkins University Press, 1976; ix–xxiii.

Levesque GA. Boston's Black Brahmin: Dr. John S. Rock. *Civil War History* 1980; 54:326–346.

Lewis RA. *Edwin Chadwick and the Public Health Movement, 1832–1854.* London: Longmans, Green and Co., 1952.

Lilienfeld AM (ed). *Times, Places, and Persons: Aspects of the History of Epidemiology.* Baltimore, MD: Johns Hopkins University Press, 1980.

Lilienfeld AM, Lilienfeld DE. Epidemiology and the public health movement: A historical perspective. *J Public Health Policy* 1982; 3:140–149.

Lilienfeld DE, Lilienfeld AM. Epidemiology: a retrospective study. *Am J Epidemiol* 1977; 106:445–459.

Lilienfeld DE. John Snow: the first hired gun? *Am J Epidemiol* 2000; 152:4–9.

Link EP. The civil rights activities of three great Negro physicians (1840–1940). *J Negro History* 1967; 52:169–184.

Lurie E. Louis Agassiz and the Races of Man. *Isis* 1954; 45:227–242.

Maclean C. *Evils of Quarantine Laws, and Non-Existence of Pestilential Contagion; Deduced from the Phaenomena of the Plague of the Levant, the Yellow Fever of Spain, and the Cholera Morbus of Asia.* London: T. & G. Underwood; Philadelphia, Carey & Lea, 1824.

Magnusson L. The language of mercantilism: the English economic discussion during the seventeenth century. In: Heilbron J, Magnusson L, Wittrock B (eds). *The Rise of the Social Sciences and the Formation of Modernity: Conceptual Change in Context, 1750–1850.* Dordrecht, the Netherlands: Kluwer Acad Pub, 1998; pp. 163–188.

Mann CC. *1491: New Revelations of the Americas before Columbus.* New York: Knopf, 2005.

Marcus S. *Engels, Manchester & the Working Class.* New York: Vintage Books, 1974.

Martin J. Sauvage's nosology: medical enlightenment in Montpellier. In: Cunningham A, French R (ed). *The Medical Enlightenment of the Eighteenth Century.* Cambridge, UK: Cambridge University Press, 1990; pp. 111–137.

Mayr E. *Toward a New Philosophy of Biology: Observations of an Evolutionist.* Cambridge, MA: Belknap Press of Harvard University Press, 1988.

McDonald JC. The History of Quarantine in Britain during the 19th century. *Bull Hist Med* 1951; 25:22–44.

Mitchell JK. On the cryptogamous origin of malarious and epidemic fevers. Philadelphia: Lea and Blanchard, 1849. In: *Animacular and Cryptogamic Theories on the Origins of Fevers.* New York: Arno Press, 1977.

Morais HM. *The History of the Afro-American in Medicine.* Cornwells Heights, PA: The Publishers Agency, Inc., under the auspices of The Association for the Study of Afro-American Life and History, 1978.

Morton SG. *Crania Americana; or, A Comparative View of the Skulls of Various Aboriginal Nations of North and South America: To which is Prefixed An Essay on the Varieties of the Human Species.* Philadelphia: J. Dobson, 1839.

Nardinelli C. *Child labor and the Industrial Revolution.* Bloomington, IN: Indiana University Press, 1990.

National Library of Medicine. Dr. Rebecca Lee Crumpler. Available at: http://www.nlm.nih.gov/changingthefaceofmedicine/physicians/biography_73.html (Accessed: November 26, 2008).

Nott JC, Gliddon GR. *Types of Mankind; or, Ethnological Researches, Based upon the Ancient Monuments, Paintings, Sculptures, and Crania of Races, and upon their Natural, Geographical, Philological, and Biblical History, Illustrated by Selections from the Inedited Papers of Samuel George Morton, and by Additional Contributions from L. Agassiz, W. Usher, and H. S. Patterson.* Philadelphia, Lippincott, Grambo, 1854. Reprinted: Miami, FL: Mnemosyne Pub. Co., 1969.

Nott JC. The mulatto a hybrid-probable extermination of the two races if the whites and blacks are allowed to intermarry. *Boston Med Surg J* 1843; 26:29–32.

Nott JC. Thoughts on acclimation and adaptation of races to climates. *Am J Med Sciences* 1856; 32:320–334.

Olson R. *The Emergence of the Social Sciences 1642–1792*. New York, NY: Twayne Publishers, 1993.

Oxford English Dictionary (OED). Available At: Http://Dictionary.Oed.Com.Ezp1.Harvard.Edu (Accessed: September 4, 2008).

Painter NI. *The History of White People*. New York: W.W. Norton & Co., 2010.

Pelling M. *Cholera, Fever and English medicine, 1825–1865*. Oxford, UK: Oxford University Press, 1978.

Pendleton EM. Statistics of diseases of Hancock County. *Southern Medical Surgical Journal* 1849; n.s. 5:647–654.

Petty W. *Political Arithmetick* (1676; published 1690), in: Hull CH (ed). *The Economic Writings of Sir William Petty, together with the Observations upon the Bills of Mortality more probably by Captain John Graunt. Vol 1. Reprints of Economic Classics*. New York: August M. Kelley, 1963; pp. 233–313.

Petty W. *The Political Anatomy of Ireland* (1672; published 1690), in: Hull CH (ed). *The Economic Writings of Sir William Petty, together with the Observations upon the Bills of Mortality more probably by Captain John Graunt. Vol 1. Reprints of Economic Classics*. New York: August M. Kelley, 1963; pp. 121–231.

Pier GB. Chapter 114. Molecular Mechanisms of Microbial Pathogenesis. In: Fauci AS, Braunwald E, Kasper DL, Hauser SL, Longo DL, Jameson JL, Loscalzo J (eds). *Harrison's Principles of Internal Medicine*, 17th Edition, 2008. Available at: http://www.accessmedicine.com.ezp-prod1. hul.harvard.edu/content.aspx?aID=2860470 (Accessed: November 16, 2008).

Pinckard G. *Notes on the West Indies, Written During the Expedition under the Command of the Late General Sir Ralph Abercromby: Including Observations on the Island of Barbadoes, and the Settlements Captured by the British Troops, upon the Coast of Guiana; Likewise Remarks Relating to the Creoles and Slaves of the Western Colonies and the Indians of South America: with Occasional Hints, Regarding The Seasoning, or Yellow Fever, of Hot Climates. In Three Volumes*. London: Printed for Longman, Hurst, Rees, and Orme, Paternoster-row, 1806.

Poovey M. *A History of the Modern Fact: Problems of Knowledge in the Sciences of Wealth and Society*. Chicago, IL: University of Chicago Press, 1998.

Porter D. *Health, Civilization and the State: A History of Public Health from Ancient to Modern Times*. London: Routledge, 1999.

Porter R. *The Greatest Benefit to Mankind: A Medical History of Humanity*. New York: W.W. Norton, 1997.

Porter TM. *Trust in Numbers: The Pursuit of Objectivity in Science and Public Life*. Princeton, NJ: Princeton University Press, 1995.

Powell JH. *Bring Out Your Dead : The Great Plague of Yellow Fever in Philadelphia In 1793*; reprinted with a new introduction by Kenneth R. Foster, Mary F. Jenkins, and Anna Coxe Toogood. Philadelphia: University of Pennsylvania Press, 1993 (1949).

Quetelet A. *Sur l'homme et le développement de ses facultés, ou Essai de physique sociale*. Paris: Bachelier, 1835; for translation, see: Quetelet A. *A Treatise on Man and the Development of his Faculties* (1835). (transl. R. Knox). Edinburgh, 1842 (Reprinted: New York: Burt Franklin, 1968).

Rather LJ (ed). *Rudolf Virchow: Collected Essays on Public Health and Epidemiology*. Vol 1. Canton, MA: Science History Publications, 1985.

Richmond PA. American attitudes toward the germ theory of disease, 1860–1880. *J Hist Med Allied Sci* 1954; 9:58–84.

Rock JS. I will sink or swim with my race. Speech delivered on March 5, 1858 in Boston as part of the annual Crispus Attucks Day observance ceremony and published in The Liberator on March 12, 1858. Available at: http://www.blackpast.org/?q=1858-john-s-rock-i-will-sink-or-swim-my-race (Accessed: November 26, 2008).

Roncaglia A. *Petty: The Origins of Political Economy*. Armonk, NY: ME Sharpe, Inc, 1985.

Rosen G. *A History of Public Health*. (1958) Expanded edition (Introduction by Elizabeth Fee; Biographical essay and new bibliography by Edward T. Morman). Baltimore, MD: The Johns Hopkins University Press, 1993.

Rosen G. *From Medical Police to Social Medicine*. New York: Science History Publications, 1974.

Rosenberg CE. Epidemiology in context. *Int J Epidemiol* 2009; 38:28–30.

Rosenberg CE. Pathologies of progress: the idea of civilization as risk. *Bull Hist Med* 1998; 72: 714–730.

Rosenberg CE. *The Cholera Years: The United States in 1832, 1849, and 1866*. Chicago: University Press, 1962. Reprint, with a new afterword by author. Chicago: University of Chicago Press, 1987.

Rosenkrantz BG. *Public Health and the State. Changing Views in Massachusetts, 1842–1936*. Cambridge, MA: Harvard University Press, 1972.

Ross D. *The Origins of American Social Science*. Cambridge, UK: Cambridge University Press, 1991.

Rossignol H. Statistics of the mortality in Augusta, Georgia, from 1839 to 1848. *Southern Medical Surgical Journal* 1848; n.s. 4:658–663.

Rothman K. *Modern Epidemiology*. Boston: Little Brown & Co, 1986.

Rousseau JJ. *Discourse on the Origin of Inequality* (1755). (Discours sur l'origine et les fondements de l'inégalité parmi les homes), translated by Donald A. Cress, introduced by James Miller. Indianapolis, IN: Hackett Pub Co., 1992.

Rueschemery D, Skocpol T (eds). *States, Social Knowledge, and the Origins of Modern Social Policies*. Princeton, NJ: Princeton University Press, 1996.

Runes DD (ed). *The Selected Writings of Benjamin Rush*. New York: Philosophical Society, 1947.

Rush B. *An Address on the Slavery of the Negroes in America*. Philadelphia: John Dunlap, 1773. Reprinted by the Arno Press and New York Times, 1969.

Rush B. *Medical Inquiries and Observations (Vol 3): Containing an Account of the Bilious and Remitting and Intermitting Yellow Fever, as it Appeared in Philadelphia in the Year 1794: Together with an Inquiry into the Proximate Cause of Fever; and a Defence of Blood-Letting as a Remedy for Certain Diseases*. 3rd edition. Philadelphia, PA: Johnson & Warner, 1809. (1st ed: Philadelphia, PA: Thomas Dobson, 1796).

Saakwa-Mante N. Western medicine and racial constitutions: surgeon John Atkins' theory of polygenism and sleepy distemper in the 1730s. In: Ernst W, Harris B (eds). *Race, Science, and Medicine, 1700–1960*. London: Routledge, 1999; pp. 29–57.

Schiebinger L. *Nature's Body: Gender in the Making of Modern Science*. Boston: Beacon Press, 1993.

Shattuck L. *Report of a General Plan for the Promotion of Public and Personal Health… Relating to a Sanitary Survey of the State; The Shattuck Report*. Boston: Massachusetts Sanitary Commission, 1850 (reprinted by Harvard University Press, Cambridge, MA, 1948).

Shaw M, Miles I. The social roots of statistical knowledge. In: Irvine J, Miles I, Evans J. *Demystifying Social Statistics*. London: Pluto Press, 1981; pp. 27–38.

Sheridan RB. *Doctors and Slaves: A Medical and Demographic History of Slavery in the British West Indies, 1680–1834*. Cambridge, UK: Cambridge University Press, 1985.

Sherwood RE. *Oliver Cromwell: King in All but Name, 1653–1658*. New York : St. Martin's Press, 1997.

Sigerist HE. Introduction to: The People's Misery: Mother of Diseases. An Address, Delivered in 1790 by Johann Peter Frank. *Bull Hist Med* 1941; 9:81–87.

Silverberg H. Introduction: toward a gendered social science history. In: Silverberg H (ed). *Gender and American Social Science: The Formative Years*. Princeton, NJ: Princeton University Press, 1998; pp. 3–32.

Sinclair J. *The Statistical Account of Scotland*. Edinburgh, Scotland: W. Creech, 1791–1799.

Smillie WG. *Public Health: Its Promise for the Future—A Chronicle of the Development of Public Health in the United States, 1607-1914*. New York: Macmillan Co., 1955.

Smillie WG. The period of great epidemics in the United States (1800–1875). In: Top FH (ed). *The History of American Epidemiology*. St. Louis, MN: CV Mosby, 1952; pp. 52–73.

Smith JM. On the fourteenth query of Thomas Jefferson's Notes on Virginia. *The Anglo-African Magazine* 1859; 1:225–238.

Smith JT. Review of Dr. Cartwright's report on the diseases and physical peculiarities of the negro race. *New Orleans Med Surg J* 1851; 8:219–237.

Snow J. *On continuous molecular changes, more particularly in their relation to epidemic diseases: being the Oration delivered at the 80th anniversary of the Medical Society of London.* London: John Churchill, 1853.

Spector B. Noah Webster: his contribution to American thought and progress (introductory essay). In: Noah *Webster: Letters on Yellow Fever Addressed to Dr. William Currie, with an introductory essay by Benjamin Spector.* Supplement to the Bulletin of the History of Medicine. Baltimore, MD: Johns Hopkins Press, 1947; pp. 1–17.

Stanton W. *The Leopard's Spots: Scientific Attitudes Toward Race in America 1815–59.* Chicago, IL: University of Chicago Press, 1960.

Steckel RH, Floud R (eds). *Health and Welfare During Industrialization.* Chicago: University of Chicago Press, 1997.

Stepan N. *The Idea of Race in Science: Great Britain, 1800–1960.* London: Macmillan, 1982.

Stephen L, Lee S (eds). *The Dictionary of National Biography,* Vol I. London: Oxford University Press, 1921–1922; pp. 290–292.

Sterling D (ed). *We are Your Sisters: Black Women in the Nineteenth Century.* New York: W.W. Norton, 1994.

Stigler SM. *The History of Statistics: The Measurement of Uncertainty before 1900.* Cambridge, MA: Belknap Press of Harvard University Press, 1986.

Sydenham T. *Selected Works of Thomas Sydenham, M.D., with a short biography and explanatory notes by John D. Comrie.* New York: William Wood & Co., 1922.

Szreter S. Economic growth, disruption, deprivation, disease, and death: on the importance of the politics of public health for development. *Population Development Review* 1997; 23:693–728.

Takaki RT. *A Different Mirror: A History of Multicultural America.* Boston: Little, Brown & Co., 1993.

Terris M. Epidemiology and the public health movement. *J Public Health Policy* 1987; 8:315–329.

Thornton R. *American Indian Holocaust and Survival: A Population History Since 1492.* Norman: University of Oklahoma Press, 1987.

Tidyman P. A sketch of the most remarkable Diseases of the Negroes of the Southern States, with an account of the method of treating them, accompanied by physiological observations. *Philadelphia J Medical Physical Sci* 1826; 12:306–339.

Tomes N. American attitudes towards the germ theory: Phyllis Richmond Allen revisited. *J Hist Med Allied Sci* 1997; 52:17–50.

Tristan F. *Flora Tristan's London Journal: A survey of London Life in the 1830s*; a translation of *Promenades dan Londres* (1840) by Dennis Palmer and Giselle Pincetl. London: George Prior Publishers, 1980.

Villalba J de. *Epidemiologia Española, o historia cronologica de las pestes, contagios, epidemias y epizootias que han acaecido en Espana desde la venida de los Cartagineses hasta el ano 1801. Con noticia de algunas otras enfermedades de esta especie que han sufrido los Espanoles en otros reynos, y do los autores nacionales que han escrito sobre esta materia, asi en la peninsula como fuero de ella.* Por el licenciado Don Joaquin de Villalba... Madrid, En la imprenta de D. Fermin Villapando, 1803.

Villermé LR. Des épidémies sous les rapports de l'hygiene publique, de la statistique medicale et de l'économie politique. *Annales d'hygiéne publique et de médecine légale* 1833; 9:5–58.

Villermé LR. Mémoire sur la taille de l'homme en France. *Annales d'hygiène publique et de médecine légale* 1829; 1:351–399.

Villermé LR. Mémoire sure la mortalité en France dans la classe aisée et dans la class indigente. *Mémoires de l'Académie royale de médecine* 1828; 1:51–98.

Villermé LR. Rapport fait par M. Villermé, et lu à l'Académie royale de Médecine, au nom de la Commission de statistique, sur une série de tableaux relatifs au movement de la population dans les doúze arrondisements municipaux de la ville de Paris, pendant les cinq années 1817, 1818, 1819, 1820 et 1821. *Archives Générales de Médecine* 1826; 10:216–247.

Villermé LR. *Tableau de l'état physique et moral des ouvriers employés dans les manufactures de coton, de laine et de soie.* Tome Premier et Second. Paris: Jules Renouard, 1840.

Virchow L. Report on the Typhus Epidemic in Upper Silesia. (1848), In: Rather LJ (ed). *Rudolf Virchow: Collected Essays on Public Health and Epidemiology, Vol. 1.* Canton, MA: Science History Publications, 1985; pp. 205–319. (1848 a)

Virchow R. Public Health Service. Medical Reform, No. 8, 25 Aug 1848. In: Rather LJ (ed). *Rudolf Virchow: Collected Essays on Public Health and Epidemiology, Vol. 1.* Canton, MA: Science History Publications, 1985; pp. 21–24. (1848c)

Virchow R. The Charity Physician. Medical Reform No. 18, 3 Nov 1848. In: Rather LJ (ed). *Rudolf Virchow: Collected Essays on Public Health and Epidemiology, Vol. 1.* Canton, MA: Science History Publications, 1985; pp. 33–36. (1848b)

Waitzkin H. The social origins of illness: a neglected history. *Int J Health Services* 1981; 11:77–103.

Waldram JB, Herring DA, Young TK. *Aboriginal Health in Canada: Historical, Cultural, and Epidemiological Perspectives.* Toronto: University of Toronto Press, 1995.

Walker R. The Enlightenment and the French revolutionary birthpangs of modernity, in Heilbron J, Magnusson L, Wittrock B (eds). *The Rise of the Social Sciences and the Formation of Modernity: Conceptual Change in Context, 1750–1850.* Dordrecht, the Netherlands: Kluwer Acad Pub, 1998; pp. 35–76.

Wear A, French R, Lonie I (eds). *The Medical Renaissance of the Sixteenth Century.* Cambridge, UK: Cambridge University Press, 1985.

Webster N. *A Brief History of Epidemic and Pestilential Diseases; with the Principal Phenomena of the Physical World, which Precede and Accompany Them, and Observations Deduced from the Facts Stated: In Two Volumes.*/By Noah Webster, author of Dissertations on the English language and several other works—member of the Connecticut Academy of Arts and Sciences—of the Society for the Promotion of Agriculture, Arts and Manufactures, in the state of New-York—of the American Academy of Arts and Sciences, and corresponding member of the Historical Society in Massachusetts.; Vol. I(-II). Hartford, CT: Hudson & Goodwin., 1799. (Published according to act of Congress.).

Weir DR. Economic welfare and physical well-being in France, 1750-1990. In: Steckel RH, Floud R (eds). *Health and Welfare During Industrialization.* Chicago, IL: University of Chicago Press, 1997; pp. 161–200.

Weissbach LS. *Child Labor Reform in Nineteenth-Century France: Assuring the Future's Harvest.* Baton Rouge, NO: Louisiana State University Press, 1989.

Wheen F. *Karl Marx.* London: Fourth Estate, 1999.

Williams R. *Keywords: a Vocabulary of Culture and Society.* Rev Ed. New York: Oxford University Press, 1985 (1976).

Wilson DA. *The King and the Gentleman: Charles Stuart and Oliver Cromwell, 1599–1649.* New York: St. Martin's Press, 1999.

Winslow C-EA. The colonial era and the first years of the Republic (1607-1799) the pestilence that walketh in darkness. In: Top FH (ed). *The History of American Epidemiology.* St. Louis, MN: CV Mosby, 1952; pp. 11–51.

World Health Organization. *History of the development of the ICD.* Available at: http://www.who.int/classifications/icd/en/HistoryOfICD.pdf (Accessed: November 25, 2009).

Young TK. *The Health of Native Americans: Towards a Biocultural Epidemiology.* New York: Oxford, 1994.

Zinn H. *A People's History of the United States 1492-Present.* New York: HarperPerennial, 2003.

Chapter 4

A.B.H, Butler W. Obituary: Major Greenwood. *J Royal Stat Soc* 1949; Series A (General), 112: 487–489.

Acheson RM. The epidemiology of Charles-Edward Amory Winslow. *Am J Epidemiol* 1970; 91:1–18.

Allen LC. The Negro health problem. *Am J Public Health* 1915; 5:194–203.

American Association of Public Health. Charles-Edward Amory Winslow (February 4, 1877–January 8, 1957): A Memorial. *Am J Public Health* 1957; 47:153–167.

Brunner WF. The Negro health problem in southern cities. *Am J Public Health* 1915; 5:183–190.

Bynum W. *The History of Medicine: A Very Short Introduction.* Oxford: Oxford University Press, 2008.

Carlson EA. *The Unfit: A History of a Bad Idea.* Cold Spring Harbor, NY: Cold Spring Harbor Press, 2001.

Chapin CV. *The Present State of the Germ-Theory of Disease.* Providence, RI: Kellogg Printing Co., 1885.

Chapin CV. The Principles of Epidemiology (1928). In: Gorham FP (ed). *Papers of Charles V. Chapin, M.D. A Review of Public Health Realities.* New York: The Commonwealth Fund, 1934; pp. 172–216. (originally published as: Chapin CV. The science of epidemic diseases. *The Scientific Monthly* 1928; 26:481–493)

Chapin CV. The science of epidemic diseases. *The Scientific Monthly* 1928; 26:481–493.

Chapin CV. *The Sources and Modes of Infection.* New York: J. Wiley, 1910.

Chase A. *The Legacy of Malthus: The Social Costs of the New Scientific Racism.* New York: Knopf, 1977.

Cold Spring Harbor Laboratory (CSHL). About CSHL. Available at: http://www.cshl.edu/about/index. html (Accessed: December 6, 2009).

Daniel TM. *Wade Hampton Frost: Pioneer Epidemiologist 1880–1938.* Rochester, NY: University of Rochester Press, 2004.

Davenport CB. *Heredity in Relation to Eugenics.* New York: Henry Holt & Co, 1911.

Desrosières A. *The Politics of Large Numbers: A History of Statistical Reasoning.* (translated by Camille Naish). Cambridge, MA: Harvard University Press, 1998.

Doull JA. The bacteriological era (1876–1920). In: Winslow C-EA, Smillie WG, Doull JA, Gordon JE (edited by Top FH). *The History of American Epidemiology.* (Sponsored by the Epidemiology Section, American Public Health Association). St. Louis, MO: The C.V. Mosby Company, 1952; pp. 74–113.

Du Bois WEB. *The Philadelphia Negro.* New York: Lippincott, 1899.

Duster T. Lessons from history: why race and ethnicity have played a major role in biomedical research. *J Law Med Ethics* 2006; 34:487–496.

Ernst W, Harris B (eds). *Race, Science and Medicine, 1700–1960.* London: Routledge, 1999.

Etheridge B. *The Butterfly Caste: A Social History of Pellagra in the South.* Westport, CT: Greenwood, 1972.

Evans AS. Discussion of "The Germ Theory of Disease" by P.A. Richmond. In: Lilienfeld A (ed). *Times, Places and Persons: Aspects of the History of Epidemiology.* Baltimore, MD: Johns Hopkins University Press, 1980; pp. 94–98.

Fee E. *Disease and Discovery: A History of the Johns Hopkins School of Hygiene and Public Health, 1916-1939.* Baltimore, MD: The Johns Hopkins University Press, 1987.

Fort AG. The Negro health problem in rural communities. *Am J Public Health* 1915; 5:191–193.

Frost WH. Epidemiology (1927). In: Maxcy KF (ed). *Papers of Wade Hampton Frost, MD.* New York: Commonwealth Fund, 1941; pp. 493–542.

Frost WH. *Snow on Cholera.* New York: The Commonwealth Fund, 1936.

Galton F. *Hereditary Genius: An Inquiry into its Laws and Consequences.* London: MacMillan & Co, 1869.

Gamble VN. *Germs Have No Color Line: Blacks and American Medicine, 1900–1940.* New York: Garland Pub., 1989.

Goldberger J, Wheeler GA, Sydenstricker E. A study of the relation of family income and other economic factors to pellagra incidence in seven cotton-mill villages of South Carolina in 1916. *Public Health Reports* 1920; 35:2673–2714.

Gould SJ. *The Mismeasure of Man.* (Revised and expanded). New York: Norton, 1996.

Gould SJ. *The Structure of Evolutionary Theory.* Cambridge, MA: The Belknap Press of Harvard University Press, 2002.

Gradle H. *Bacteria and the Germ Theory of Disease: Eight Lectures Delivered at the Chicago Medical College.* Chicago, IL: W.T. Keener, 1883.

Gradman C. Invisible enemies: bacteriology and the language of politics in Imperial Germany. *Science in Context* 2000; 13:9–30.

Graves ML. Practical remedial measures for the improvement of hygienic conditions of the Negroes in the South. *Am J Public Health* 1915; 5:212–217.

Greenwood M. *Epidemics and Crowd Diseases: An Introduction to the Study of Epidemiology.* London: Williams & Norgate, Ltd, 1935.

Hamilton A. *Exploring the Dangerous Trades.* Boston: Little, Brown, 1943.

Hamilton A. *Industrial Poisons in the United States.* New York: The Macmillan Co., 1925.

Hamilton A. Investigations of the lead troubles in Illinois, from a hygienic standpoint. In: *Report of Commission on Occupational Diseases; To His Excellency Governor Charles S. Deneen.* Chicago: Warner Printing Co., 1911. Available at: http://www.idaillinois.org/cdm4/document. php?CISOROOT=/isl&CISOPTR=12187 (Accessed: January 7, 2009).

Hansen NE, Janz HL, Sobsey DJ. 21st century eugenics? In: Godsland J, Osmond R, Pini P. Darwin's Gifts. *Lancet* 2008; December special supplement: S104–S107.

Hindman SS. Syphilis among insane Negroes. *Am J Public Health* 1915; 5:218–224.

Holland DF, Perrott GSJ. Health of the Negro. Part I. Disabling illness among Negroes and low-income white families in New York City–A report of a sickness survey in the spring of 1933. *Milbank Mem Fund Q* 1938; 16:5–15. (1938a)

Holland DF, Perrott GSJ. Health of the Negro. Part II. A preliminary report on a study of disabling illness in a representative sample of the Negro and white population of four cities canvassed in the National Health Survey, 1935–1936. *Milbank Mem Fund Q* 1938; 16:16–38. (1938b)

Kasius RV (ed). *The Challenge of Facts: Selected Public Health Papers of Edgar Sydenstricker.* New York: Prodist, 1974.

Keller EF. *The Century of the Gene.* Cambridge, MA: Harvard University Press, 2000.

Kevels D. *In the Name of Eugenics: Genetics and the Uses of Human Heredity.* New York: Knopf, 1985.

Krieger N, Fee E. Measuring social inequalities in health in the United States: an historical review, 1900-1950. *Int J Health Services* 1996; 26:391–418.

Krieger N. Epidemiology and social sciences: towards a critical reengagement in the 21st century. *Epidemiologic Reviews* 2000; 11:155–163.

Krieger N. Epidemiology and the web of causation: has anyone seen the spider? *Soc Sci Med* 1994; 39:887–903.

Krieger N. Theories for social epidemiology in the 21st century: an ecosocial perspective. *Int J Epidemiol* 2001; 30:668–677. (2001a)

Kunitz S. *The Health of Populations: General Theories and Particular Realities.* Oxford: Oxford University Press, 2007.

Ladd-Taylor M. Saving Babies and Sterilizing Mothers: Eugenics and Welfare Politics in the Interwar United States. *Social Politics* 1997; 4:136–153.

Lee L. The Negro as a problem in public health charity. *Am J Public Health* 1915; 5:207–211.

MacKenzie DA. Eugenics and the rise of mathematical statistics in Britain. In: Irvine J, Miles J, Evans J (eds). *Demystifying Social Statistics.* London: Pluto Press, 1979; pp. 39–50.

MacKenzie DA. *Statistics in Britain 1865–1930: The Social Construction of Scientific Knowledge.* Edinburgh: Edinburgh University Press, 1981.

Maclagan TJ. *The Germ Theory: Applied to the Explanation of the Phenomena of Disease: The Specific Fevers.* London: Macmillan, 1876.

Marable M. *W. E. B. Du Bois: Black Radical Democrat.* New updated edition. Boulder: Paradigm Publishers, 2005.

Markowitz G. C.-E.A. Winslow: scientist, activist, and theoretician of the American public health movement throughout the first half of the twentieth century–Commentary. *J Public Health Policy* 1998; 19:154–159.

Mayr E. *The Growth of Biological Thought: Diversity, Evolution, and Inheritance.* Cambridge, MA: The Belknap Press of Harvard University Press, 1982.

Mendelsohn JA. From eradication to equilibrium: how epidemics became complex after World War I. In: Lawrence C, Weisz G (eds). *Greater than the Parts: Holism in Biomedicine, 1920–1950.* New York: Oxford University Press, 1998; pp. 303–331.

Nelson HV. The Philadelphia Negro. In: Asante KF, Mazama A. *Encyclopedia of Black Studies.* Thousand Oaks, CA: Sage Publications, 2004; pp. 397–398.

Oxford English Dictionary (OED). Available At: Http://Dictionary.Oed.Com.Ezp1.Harvard.Edu (Accessed: December 3, 2009).

Painter NI. *The History of White People.* New York: W.W. Norton & Co., 2010.

Pernick MS. Eugenics and public health in American history. *Am J Public Health* 1997; 87: 1767–1772.

Perrott GSJ, Collins SD. Relation of sickness to income and income change in ten surveyed communities. Health and Depression Studies No. 1: Method of study and general results for each locally. *Public Health Reports* 1934; 49:1101–1111.

Perrott GSJ, Sydenstricker E. Causal and selective factors in illness. *Am J Sociol* 1935; 40:804–812.

Porter D. *Health, Civilization and the State: A History of Public Health from Ancient to Modern Times.* London: Routledge, 1999.

Porter R. *The Greatest Benefit to Mankind: A Medical History of Humanity.* New York: W.W. Norton, 1997.

Porter TM. *The Rise of Statistical Thinking, 1820–1900.* Princeton, NJ: Princeton University Press, 1986.

Proctor R. *Racial Hygiene: Medicine under the Nazis.* Cambridge, MA: Harvard University Press, 1988.

Richmond PA. American attitudes towards the germ theory of disease (1860-1880). *J Hist Med Allied Sci* 1954; 9:58–84.

Rosen G. *A History of Public Health.* (1958) Expanded edition (Introduction by Elizabeth Fee; Biographical essay and new bibliography by Edward T. Morman). Baltimore, MD: The Johns Hopkins University Press, 1993.

Rosenberg CE. *The Cholera Years: The United States in 1832, 1849, and 1866.* Chicago: University Press, 1962. Reprint, with a new afterword by author. Chicago: University of Chicago Press, 1987.

Rosner D. C.-E.A. Winslow: scientist, activist, and theoretician of the American public health movement throughout the first half of the twentieth century–Commentary. *J Public Health Policy* 1998; 19:147–153.

Sicherman B. *Alice Hamilton: A Life in Letters. Cambridge,* MA: Harvard University Press, 1984.

Stern AM. *Eugenic Nation: Faults and Frontiers of Better Breeding in Modern America.* Berkeley, CA: University of California Press, 2005. (2005b)

Stern AM. Sterilized in the name of public health: race, immigration, and reproductive control in modern California. *Am J Public Health* 2005; 95:1128–1138. (2005a)

Sydenstricker E, King WIA. A method for classifying families according to incomes in studies of disease prevalence. *Public Health Reports* 1920; 35:2828–2846.

Sydenstricker E. *Health and Environment.* New York: McGraw-Hill, 1933.

Sydenstricker E. Health and the Depression. *Milbank Mem Fund Q* 1934; 12:273–280.

Sydenstricker E. The incidence of illness in a general population group: General results of a morbidity study from December 1, 1921 through March 31, 1924 in Hagerstown, Md. *Public Health Reports* 1925; 40:279–291.

Terris M (ed). *Goldberger on Pellagra.* Baton Rouge, LA: Louisiana State University Press, 1964.

Terris M. C.-E.A. Winslow: scientist, activist, and theoretician of the American public health movement throughout the first half of the twentieth century. *J Public Health Policy* 1998; 19:135–146.

Tesh S. *Hidden Arguments: Political Ideology and Disease Prevention Policy.* New Brunswick, NJ: Rutgers University Press, 1988.

Tibbitts C. The socio-economic background of Negro health status. *J Negro Educ* 1937; 6:413–428.

Tomes NJ. American attitudes toward the germ theory of disease: Phyllis Allen Richmond revisited. *J History Med Allied Science* 1997; 52:17–50.

Viseltear AJ. Winslow, C.E.A. And the early years of public health at Yale, 1915–1925. *Yale J Biology Medicine* 1982; 55:137–151. (1982a)

Viseltear AJ. Winslow, C.E.A. And the later years of public health at Yale, 1940–1945. *Yale J Biology Medicine* 1982; 60:447–470. (1982b)

Wahlsten D. Leilani Muir versus the philosopher king: eugenics on trial in Alberta. *Genetica* 1997; 99:185–198.

Warren BS, Sydenstricker E. Health of garment workers in relation to their economic status. *Public Health Reports* 1916; 31:1298–1305.

Weindling P (ed). *The Social History of Occupational Health.* London: Croom Helm, 1985.

Weingart P. Eugenics–medicine or social science? *Science in Context* 1995; 8:197–207.

Wiehl DG. Edgar Sydenstricker: a memoir. In: Kasius RV (ed). *The Challenge of Facts: Selected Public Health Papers of Edgar Sydenstricker.* New York: Prodist, for Milbank Memorial Fund, 1974; pp. 1–17.

Winslow C-EA, Smillie WG, Doull JA, Gordon JE (edited by Top FH). *The History of American Epidemiology.* (Sponsored by the Epidemiology Section, American Public Health Association). St. Louis, MO: The C.V. Mosby Company, 1952.

Winslow CEA. *The Evolution and Significance of the Modern Public Health Campaign.* New Haven: Yale University Press, 1923.

Wolff MJ. The myth of the actuary: life insurance and Frederick L. Hoffman's Race Traits and Tendencies of the American Negro. *Public Health Rep* 2006; 121:84–91.

Zylberman P. Scandianvian eugenics: Nordic historians provide new approaches. *Med Sci* (Paris) 2004; 20:916–925.

Chapter 5

Abel T, Cockerham W. Life Style or Lebensführung? Critical remarks on the mistranslation of Weber's "Class, Status, Party." *Sociological Q* 1993; 34:551–556.

Adler A. *What Life Should Mean to You.* (edited by Alan Porter). London: Allen and Unwin, 1962 (1931).

Agency for Toxic Substances & Disease Registry (ATSDR). *Toxicological Profile for Lead.* August 2007. Atlanta, GA: US Department of Health and Human Services, Public Health Service, 2007. Available at: http://www.atsdr.cdc.gov/toxprofiles/tp13.htmlbookmark07 (Accessed: February 19, 2009).

Aldana SG. *The Culprit & The Cure: Why Lifestyle is the Culprit Behind America's Poor Health and How Transforming That Lifestyle Can Be the Cure.* Mapleton, Utah: Maple Mountain Press, 2005.

Anderson C. *Eyes Off the Prize: The United Nations and The African American Struggle for Human Rights, 1944–1955.* Cambridge: Cambridge University Press, 2003.

Anderson MJ. *The American Census: A Social History.* New Haven, CT: Yale University Press, 1988.

Badash L. Science and McCarthyism. *Minerva* 2000; 38:53–80.

Bannister RC. Sociology. In: Porter T, Ross D (eds). *The Modern Social Sciences, in The Cambridge History of Science Series,* vol 7 (general editors: David C. Lindberg & Ronald L. Numbers). Cambridge: Cambridge University Press, 2003; pp. 329–353.

Barfield CE, Smith BLR (eds). *The Future of Biomedical Research.* Washington, DC: American Enterprise Institute and The Brookings Institute, 1997.

Barker DJ, Osmond C, Law CM. The intrauterine and early postnatal origins of cardiovascular disease and chronic bronchitis. *J Epidemiol Community Health* 1989; 43:237–240.

Barker DJ. The developmental origins of well-being. *Philos Trans R Soc Lond B Biol Sci* 2004; 359:1359–1366.

Barker DJ. The origins of the developmental origins theory. *J Intern Med* 2007; 261:412–417.

Barker JD, Osmond C. Infant mortality, childhood nutrition, and ischaemic heart disease in England and Wales. *Lancet* 1986; 1(8489):1077–1081.

Bennett T, Grossberg L, Morris M (eds). *New Keywords: A Revised Vocabulary of Culture and Society.* Malden, MA: Blackwell, 2005.

Berman DM. *Death on the Job: Occupational Health and Safety Struggles in the United States.* New York: Monthly Review Press, 1978.

Bogenhold D. Social inequality and the sociology of lifestyle: material and cultural aspects of social stratification–focus on economic sociology. *Am J Econ Sociol* 2001; 60:829–847.

Brandt A. *The Cigarette Century: The Rise, Fall, and Deadly Persistence of the Product that Defined America.* New York: Basic Books, 2007.

Breilh J, Granda E. Epidemiology and heterogeny. *Soc Sci Med* 1989; 28:1121–1127.

Breilh J. *Epidemiología: Economía, Medicina y Política.* 4e ed., Mexico City, Mexico: Fontamara, 1988 (1979).

Breilh J. Epidemiology's role in the creation of a humane world: convergences and divergences among the schools. *Soc Sci Med* 1995; 41:911–914.

Brickman JP. "Medical McCarthyism": The Physicians Forum and the Cold War. *J History Medicine Allied Sciences* 1994; 49:380–418.

Buck C, Llopis A, Nájera E, Terris M. Discussions. In: Buck C, Llopis A, Nájera E, Terris. *The Challenge of Epidemiology: Issues and Selected Readings.* Washington, DC: Pan American Health Organization, 1988; pp. 967–985.

Bunton R, Nettleton S, Burrows R (eds). *The Sociology of Health Promotion: Critical Analyses of Consumption, Lifestyle, and Risk.* London: Routledge, 1995.

Burri R, Dumit J (eds). *Biomedicine as Culture: Instrumental Practices, Technoscientific Knowledge, and New modes of Life.* New York: Routledge, 2007.

Bynum W. *The History of Medicine: A Very Short Introduction.* Oxford: Oxford University Press, 2008.

Cambrosio A, Keating P. Biomedical sciences and technology: history and sociology. In: *International Encyclopedia of the Social and Behavioral Sciences.* Amsterdam: Elsevier, Ltd, 2001. DOI: 10.1016/B0-08-04307607/03143-0.

Campbell H. Gene environment interaction. *J Epidemiol Community Health* 1996; 50:397–400.

Cassel J. Social science theory as a source of hypotheses in epidemiological research. *Am J Public Health* 1964; 54:1482–1488.

Cockerham W, Rütten A, Abel T. Conceptualizing contemporary health lifestyles: moving beyond Weber. *Sociological Q* 1997; 38:321–342.

Committee on Models for Biomedical Research, Board on Basic Biology, Commission on Life Sciences, National Research Council. *Models for Biomedical Research: A New Perspective.* Washington, DC: National Academy Press, 1985. (Included as Appendix C in: Committee on New and Emerging Models in Biomedical and Behavioral Research, Institute for Laboratory Animal Research, Commission on Life Sciences, National Research Council. *Biomedical Models and Resources: Current Needs and Future Opportunities.* Washington, DC: National Academy of Sciences, 1998.)

Conrad P., Kern R. (eds). *The Sociology of Health and Illness: Critical Perspectives.* 4th ed. New York: St. Martin's Press, 1994.

Coreil J, Levins JS, Jaco EG. Life Style: an emergent concept in the sociomedical sciences. *Culture, Medicine, and Psychiatry* 1985; 9:423–437.

Corella D, Ordovas JM. Integration of environment and disease into "omics" analysis. *Curr Opin Mol Ther* 2005; 7:569–576.

Costa LG, Eaton DL (eds). *Gene-Environment Interactions: Fundamentals of Ecogenetics.* Hoboken, NJ: John Wiley & Sons, 2006.

Crawford R. You are dangerous to your health: the ideology and politics of victim blaming. *Int J Health Services* 1977; 7:663–680.

Daintith J, Martin E (eds). *Oxford Dictionary of Science.* 5th ed. Oxford: Oxford University Press, 2005.

Davison C, Davey Smith G. The baby and the bath water: examining socio-cultural and free-market critiques of health promotion. In: Bunton R, Nettleton S, Burrows R (eds). *The Sociology of Health Promotion: Critical Analyses of Consumption, Lifestyle, and Risk.* London: Routledge, 1995; pp. 91–99.

Dawber TR, Kannel WB, Revotksie N, Stokes J 3rd, Kagan A, Gordon T. Some factors associated with the development of coronary heart disease: six years' follow-up experience in the Framingham study. *Am J Public Health Nations Health* 1959; 49:1349–1356.

Dawber TR, Meadors GR, Moore FE Jr. Epidemiological approaches to heart disease: the Framingham Study. *Am J Public Health Nations Health* 1951; 41:279–281.

de Almeida Filho N. *Epidemiología sin Números [Epidemiology without Numbers]* Washington, DC: Organización Panamericana de la Salud, 1992.

de Almeida-Filho N. *La Ciencia Tímida: Ensayos de Deconstrucción de la Epidemiología.* Buenos Aires: Lugar Editorial, 2000.

Derickson A. The house of Falk: the paranoid style in American health politics. *Am J Public Health* 1997; 87:1836–1843.

Doyal L. *The Political Economy of Health.* London: Pluto Press, 1979.

Dubos R, Dubos J. *The White Plague: Tuberculosis, Man, and Society.* Boston: Little, Brown, 1952.

Dubos RJ. *Mirage of Health: Utopias, Progress, and Biological Change.* New York: Harper, 1959.

Eaton S, Konner M, Shotak M. Stone Agers in the fast lane: chronic degenerative diseases in evolutionary perspective. *Am J Med* 1988; 84:739–749.

Engel GL. The need for a new medical model: a challenge for biomedicine. *Science* 1977; 196: 129–136.

Fee E, Krieger N. Understanding AIDS–historical interpretations and the limits of biomedical individualism. *Am J Public Health* 1993; 83:1477–1486.

Foley DL, Craig JM, Morley R, Olsson CJ, Dwyer T, Smith K, Saffery R. Prospects for epigenetic epidemiology. *Am J Epidemiol* 2009; 169:389–400.

Forman MR, Hursting SD, Umar A, Barrett JC. Nutrition and cancer prevention: a multidisciplinary perspective on human trials. *Annu Rev Nutr* 2004; 24:223–254.

Framingham Heart Study. Epidemiological background and design: The Framingham Study. Available at: http://www.framinghamheartstudy.org/about/background.html (Accessed: December 13, 2009).

Fraumeni JF Jr. Genes and the environment in cancer etiology. In: Wilson SH, Institute of Medicine (US) Roundtable on Environmental Health Sciences, Research, and Medicine, Institute of Medicine (US), Board on Health Sciences Policy. *Cancer and the Environment: Gene-Environment Interaction.* Washington, DC: National Academy of Science Press, 2002; pp. 14–24.

Fried A. *McCarthyism: The Great American Red Scare–A Documentary History.* New York: Oxford, 1997.

Friedman GD. *Primer of Epidemiology.* 5th ed. New York: McGraw-Hill, 2004.

Galdston I (ed). *Beyond the Germ Theory: The Roles of Deprivation and Stress in Health and Disease.* New York: Health Education Council, New York Academy of Medicine, 1954.

Garrety K. Dietary policy, controversy and proof: doing something versus waiting for definitive evidence. In: Ward JW, Warren C (eds). *Silent Victories: The History and Practice of Public Health in Twentieth-Century America.* Oxford: Oxford University Press, 2007; pp. 401–422.

Gilbert SF. The genome in its ecological context: philosophical perspectives on interspecies epigenesist. *Ann NY Acad Sci* 2002; 981:202–218.

Gluckman P, Hanson M (eds). *Developmental Origins of Health and Disease.* Cambridge: Cambridge University Press, 2006.

Gluckman PD, Hanson M. *Mismatch: The Lifestyle Diseases Timebomb.* Oxford: Oxford University Press, 2008.

Gluckman PD, Hanson MA, Beedle AS. Early life events and their consequences for later disease: a life history and evolutionary perspective. *Am J Hum Biol* 2007; 19:1–19.

Goldberg AD, Allis CD, Bernstein E. Epigenetics: a landscape takes shape. *Cell* 2007; 128:635–638.

Gordon DH. Tenacious assumptions in Western medicine. In: Lock M, Gordon D (eds). *Biomedicine Examined.* Dordrecht: Kluwer Academic Publishers, 1988; pp. 19–56.

Gordon J.E. Epidemiology - old and new. *J Michigan State Medical Society* 1950; 49: 194–199.

Gordon JE. The twentieth century–yesterday, today, and tomorrow (1920—). In: Winslow C-EA, Smillie WG, Doull JA, Gordon JE (edited by Top FH). *The History of American Epidemiology.* (Sponsored by the Epidemiology Section, American Public Health Association). St. Louis, MO: The C.V. Mosby Company, 1952; pp. 114–167.

Gordon JE. The world, the flesh and the devil as environment, host, and agent of disease. In: Galdston I (ed). *The Epidemiology of Health.* New York: Health Education Council, 1953; pp. 60–73.

Gould SJ. *The Structure of Evolutionary Theory.* Cambridge, MA: The Belknap Press of Harvard University Press, 2002.

Graham S. Toward a dietary prevention of cancer. *Epidemiol Rev* 1983; 5:38–50.

Green LW, Kreuter MW. Health promotion as a public health strategy for the 1990s. *Annu Rev Public Health* 1990; 11:319–334.

Green LW, Potvin L. Education, health promotion, and social and lifestyle determinants of health and disease. Chapter 2.3 in: Detels R, McEwen J, Beaglehole R, Tanaka H. *Oxford Textbook of Public Health*. 4th Ed. Oxford: Oxford University Press, 2004. Available at: http://www.R2Library.com/marc_frame.aspx?ResourceID=112 (Accessed: February 2, 2009).

Greenhouse SW. The growth and future of biostatistics: (A view from the 1980s). *Stat Med* 2003; 22:3323–3335.

Greenlund KJ, Giles WH, Keenan NL, Malarcher AM, Zheng ZJ, Caspar ML, Heath GW, Croft JB. Heart disease and stroke mortality in the twentieth century. In: Ward JW, Warren C (eds). *Silent Victories: The History and Practice of Public Health in Twentieth-Century America*. Oxford: Oxford University Press, 2007; pp. 381–400.

Greenwald P, Sondik E, Lynch BS. Diet and chemoprevention in NCI's research strategy to achieve national cancer control objectives. *Annu Rev Public Health* 1986; 7:267–291.

Grene M, Depew D. *The Philosophy of Biology*. Cambridge, UK: Cambridge University Press, 2004.

Hansen EC, Easthope G. *Lifestyle in Medicine*. London: Routledge, 2007.

Harden VA, Hannaway C. National Institutes of Health (NIH). In: *Encyclopedia of Life Sciences*. New York: John Wiley & Sons, 2001. DOI: 10.1038/npg.els.0003407.

Harden VA. A short history of the National Institutes of Health: WWI and the Randsdell Act of 1930. Available at: http://history.nih.gov/exhibits/history/docs/page_04.html (Accessed: December 10, 2009). (Harden 2009a)

Harden VA. A short history of the National Institutes of Health: Biomedical Research. Available at: http://history.nih.gov/exhibits/history/docs/page_11.html (Accessed: December 10, 2009). (Harden 2009b)

Harden VA. A short history of the National Institutes of Health: NIH Successes. Available at: http://history.nih.gov/exhibits/history/docs/page_12.html (Accessed: December 12, 2009). (Harden 2009c)

Harden VA. *Inventing the NIH: Federal Biomedical Research Policy, 1887-1937*. Baltimore, MD: Johns Hopkins University Press, 1986.

Hernandez LM, Blazer DG (eds). *Genes, Behavior, and the Social Environment: Moving Beyond the Nature/Nurture Debate*. Committee on Assessing Interactions Among Social, Behavioral, and Genetic Factors in Health, Institute of Medicine. Washington, DC: National Academy Press, 2006.

Institute for Systems Biology. Systems biology: the 21st century science. Available at: http://www.systemsbiology.org/Intro_to_ISB_and_Systems_Biology/Systems_Biology_—_the_21st_Century_Science (Accessed: January 30, 2009).

Institute of Biomedical Science. Available at: http://www.ibms.org/index.cfm?method=ibms.about (Accessed: January 12, 2009).

Irvine J, Miles J, Evans J (eds). *Demystifying Social Statistics*. London: Pluto Press, 1979.

Isaac J. The human sciences in Cold War America. *The Historical Journal* 2007; 50:725–746.

Jablonka E. Epigenetic epidemiology. *Int J Epidemiol* 2004; 33:929–935.

Kannel WB, Dawber TF, Friedman GD, Glennon WE, McNamara PM. Risk factors in coronary heart disease: an evaluation of several serum lipids as predictors of coronary heart disease: the Framingham study. *Ann Intern Med* 1964; 61:888–899.

Kannel WB, Dawber TF, Kagan A, Revotskie N, Stokes J 3rd. Factors of risk in development of coronary heart disease–six year follow-up experience: the Framingham Study. *Ann Int Med* 1961; 55:33–50.

Keller EF. *Making Sense of Life: Explaining Biological Development with Models, Metaphors, and Machines*. Cambridge, MA: Harvard University Press, 2002.

Keller EF. *The Century of the Gene*. Cambridge, MA: Harvard University Press, 2000.

Kitano H. Systems Biology: a brief overview. *Science* 2002; 295:1662–1664.

Kornberg A. Support for basic biomedical research: how scientific breakthroughs occur. In: Barfield CE, Smith BLR (eds). *The Future of Biomedical Research*. Washington, DC: American Enterprise Institute and The Brookings Institute, 1997; pp. 35–41.

Krieger N. Epidemiology and social sciences: towards a critical reengagement in the 21st century. *Epidemiologic Reviews* 2000; 11:155–163.

Krieger N. Epidemiology and the web of causation: has anyone seen the spider? *Soc Sci Med* 1994; 39:887–903.

Krieger N. Proximal, distal, and the politics of causation: what's level got to do with it? *Am J Public Health* 2008; 98:221–230.

Krieger N. Theories for social epidemiology in the 21st century: an ecosocial perspective. *Int J Epidemiol* 2001; 30:668–677.

Krieger N. Ways of asking and ways of living: reflections on the 50th anniversary of Morris' ever-useful *Uses of Epidemiology*. *Int J Epidemiol* 2007; 36:1173–1180.

Kumanyika SK. Epidemiology of what to eat in the 21st century. *Epidemiol Rev* 2000; 22:87–94.

Labarthe D. Chapter 2: Causation and prevention of cardiovascular disease: an overview of contributions of 20th-century epidemiology. In: Labarthe D. *Epidemiology and Prevention of Cardiovascular Diseases: A Global Challenge*. Boston: Jones & Bartlett, 1998; pp. 17–26.

Lansdown R, Yule W. *Lead Toxicity: History and Environmental Impact*. Baltimore, MD: Johns Hopkins University Press, 1986.

Lappé M. *Evolutionary Medicine: Rethinking the Origins of Disease*. San Francisco, CA: Sierra Club Books, 1994.

Laurell AC. La salud-enfermedad como proceso social. *Rev Latinoam Salud* 1982; 2:7–25.

Lawrence C, Weisz G (eds.). *Greater than the Parts: Holism in Biomedicine, 1920–1950*. New York: Oxford University Press, 1998.

Leonard WR. Lifestyle, diet, and disease: comparative perspectives on the determinants of chronic health risks. In: Stearns SC, Koella JC (eds). *Evolution in Health and Disease*. 2nd ed. Oxford: Oxford University Press, 2008; pp. 265–276.

Lewontin R. *The Triple Helix: Gene, Organism and Environment*. Cambridge, MA: Harvard University Press, 2000.

Lewontin RC, Rose S, Kamin LJ. *Not In Our Genes: Biology, Ideology, and Human Nature*. New York: Pantheon Books, 1984.

Lock M, Gordon D (eds). *Biomedicine Examined*. Dordrecht, The Netherlands: Kluwer Academic Publishers, 1988.

Lock M. The future is now: locating biomarkers for dementia. In: Burri R, Dumit J (eds). *Biomedicine as Culture: Instrumental Practices, Technoscientific Knowledge, and New modes of Life*. New York: Routledge, 2007; pp. 61–85.

Maclure KM, MacMahon B. An epidemiologic perspective on environmental carcinogenesis. *Epidemiol Rev* 1980; 2:19–48.

MacMahon B, Pugh TF, Ipsen J. *Epidemiologic Methods*. Boston: Little, Brown and Company, 1960.

Magee JH. *A Review of The Field of Epidemiology: Current Activities and Training of Practitioners*. Washington, DC: Association of Schools of Public Health, 1983.

Maniolo TA, Bailey-Wilson JE, Collins FS. Genes, environment and the value of prospective cohort studies. *Nat Rev Genet* 2006; 7:812–820.

Markowitz G, Rosner D. *Deceit and Denial: The Deadly Politics of Industrial Pollution*. Berkeley, CA: University of California Press, 2002.

Marmot M, Elliott P (eds). *Coronary Heart Disease Epidemiology: From Aetiology to Public Health*. 2nd ed. Oxford: Oxford University Press, 2005.

Mayr E. *The Growth of Biological Thought: Diversity, Evolution, and Inheritance*. Cambridge, MA: The Belknap Press of Harvard University Press, 1982.

McJones P. History of FORTRAN and FORTRAN II. Computer History Museum Software Preservation Group. Last modified: July 22, 2008. Available at: http://www.softwarepreservation.org/projects/FORTRAN/ (Accessed: January 12, 2009).

McMichael AJ. People, populations, and planets: epidemiology comes full circle. *Epidemiology* 1995; 6:633–636.

McMichael AJ. Prisoners of the proximate: loosening the constraints on epidemiology in an age of change. *Am J Epidemiol* 1999; 149:887–897.

Medline Plus. Biomedicine. Available at: http://www2.merriam-webster.com/cgi-bin/mwmednlm?book=Medical&va=biomedicine (Accessed: January 12, 2009).

Mishler EG. Viewpoint: critical perspectives on the biomedical model. In: Mishler EG, Amarasingham LR, Hauser ST, Osherson S, Wexler NE, Liem R. *Social Context of Health, Illness and Patient Care*. Cambridge: Cambridge University Press, 1981; pp. 1–23.

Morgan MS. Economics. In: Porter T, Ross D (eds). *The Modern Social Sciences* in, *The Cambridge History of Science Series*, vol 7 (general editors: David C. Lindberg & Ronald L. Numbers). Cambridge: Cambridge University Press, 2003; pp. 275–305

Morris JN. *Uses of Epidemiology*. Edinburgh: E & S Livingston, Ltd, 1957.

National Institutes of Health (NIH) Study Committee. *Biomedical Science and its Administration: A Study of the National Institutes of Health. Report to the President.* Washington, DC: The White House, 1965.

National Institutes of Health. *The Genes and Environment Initiative (GEI)*. Available at: http://genesandenvironment.nih.gov/index.asp (Accessed: February 19, 2009).

National Institutes of Health. The NIH Almanac–Appropriations. Available at: http://www.nih.gov/about/almanac/appropriations/part2.htm (Accessed: January 23, 2009).

National Research Council. *Biomedical Models and Resources: Current Needs and Future Opportunities*. Committee on New and Emerging Models in Biomedical and Behavioral Research, Institute for Laboratory Animal Research, Commission on Life Sciences, National Research Council. Washington, DC: National Research Council, 1998.

Navarro V (ed). *Health and Medical Care in the US: A Critical Analysis*. Amityvile, NY: Baywood Publishing, 1977.

Navarro V. *Crisis, Health, and Medicine: A Social Critique*. New York: Tavistock, 1986.

Nesse RM, Williams GC. *Why We Get Sick: The New Science of Darwinian Medicine*. New York: Vintage Books, 1994.

Nesse RM. Evolution: medicine's most basic science. In: Godsland J, Osmond R, Pini P. Darwin's Gifts. *Lancet* 2008; December special supplement: S104–S107.

Nestle M, Dixon LB (eds). *Taking Sides: Clashing Views on Controversial Issues in Food and Nutrition*. Guilford, CT: McGraw-Hill/Dushkin, 2004.

Nestle M. *Food Politics: How the Food Industry Influences Nutrition and Health*. Berkeley, CA: University of California Press, 2007.

Noble D. *The Music of Life: Biology Beyond the Genome*. Oxford: Oxford University Press, 2006.

O'Brien M. Health and lifestyle: a critical mess? Notes on the dedifferentiation of health. In: Bunton R, Nettleton S, Burrows R (eds). *The Sociology of Health Promotion: Critical Analyses of Consumption, Lifestyle, and Risk*. London: Routledge, 1995; pp. 191–205.

Omenn GS. Chemoprevention of lung cancer: the rise and demise of beta-carotene. *Annu Rev Public Health* 1998; 19:73–99.

On-Line Medical Dictionary. Available at: http://cancerweb.ncl.ac.uk/omd/index.html (Accessed: January 14, 2009).

Osherson S., Amarasingham L. The machine metaphor in medicine. In: Mishler EG, Amarasingham L, Hauser ST, et al (eds). *Social Contexts of Health, Illness, and Patient Care*. Cambridge: Cambridge University Press, 1981; pp. 218–249.

Oxford English Dictionary (OED). Available At: Http://Dictionary.Oed.Com.Ezp1.Harvard.Edu; (Accessed: December 3, 2009).

Oxford Textbook of Public Health. 4th Ed. Oxford: Oxford University Press, 2004. Available at: http://www.R2Library.com/marc_frame.aspx?ResourceID=112 (Accessed: February 2, 2009).

Parekh B. Individual. In: Bennett T, Grossberg L, Morris M (eds). *New Keywords: A Revised Vocabulary of Culture and Society*. Malden, MA: Blackwell, 2005; pp. 183–184.

Peto R, Doll R, Buckley JD, Sporn MB. Can dietary beta-carotene materially reduce human cancer rates? *Nature* 1981; 290:201–208.

Picavet E. Methodological Individualism in Sociology. In: Smelser NJ, Baltes PB (eds). *International Encyclopedia of the Social Sciences*. New York: Elsevier, 2001; pp. 9751–9755.

Pollan M. *In Defense of Food*. New York: Penguin Books, 2008.

Poovey M. *A History of the Modern Fact: Problems of Knowledge in the Sciences of Wealth and Society*. Chicago, IL: University of Chicago Press, 1998.

Porta M (ed). *A Dictionary of Epidemiology*. 5th edition. New York: Oxford University Press, 2008.

PubMed, U.S. National Library of Medicine and the National Institutes of Health. Available at: http://www.ncbi.nlm.nih.gov/sites/entrez (Accessed: February 16, 2009, for 1960–2008 literature search on "epidemiology" and "lifestyle".)

Robbins A, Landrigan PJ. Safer, healthier workers: advances in occupational disease and injury prevention. In: Ward JW, Warren C (eds). *Silent Victories: The History and Practice of Public Health in Twentieth-Century America.* Oxford: Oxford University Press, 2007; pp. 209–229.

Rose G. Sick individuals and sick populations. *Int J Epidemiol* 1985; 14:32–38.

Rose G. *The Strategy of Preventive Medicine.* Oxford: Oxford University Press, 1992.

Rose H, Rose S (eds). *Ideology of/in the Natural Sciences,* with an introductory essay by Ruth Hubbard. Cambridge, MA: Schenkman. 1980.

Ross D. Changing contours of the social science disciplines. In: Porter T, Ross D (eds). *The Modern Social Sciences,* in *The Cambridge History of Science Series,* vol 7 (general editors: David C. Lindberg & Ronald L. Numbers). Cambridge: Cambridge University Press, 2003; pp. 205–237.

Rothstein W. *Public Health and the Risk Factor: A History of an Uneven Medical Revolution.* Rochester, NY: University of Rochester Press, 2008.

Russo F, Williamson J. Interpreting probability in causal models for cancer. In: Russo F, Williamson J (eds). *Causality and Probability in the Sciences.* College Publications, King's College: London, 2007; pp. 217–242.

Sargent MG. *Biomedicine and the Human Condition: Challenges, Risks, and Rewards.* Cambridge: Cambridge University Press, 2005.

Sayer A. *Method in Social Science: A Realist Approach.* London: Hutchinson, 1984.

Schnall P (ed). *The Social Etiology of Disease.* HMO Packet 2. New York: HealthPac, 1977.

Schrecker E. *Many are the Crimes: McCarthyism in America.* Boston: Little Brown & Co, 1998.

Scott J, Marshall G (eds). *Oxford Dictionary of Sociology.* New York: Oxford University Press, 2005.

Shostak S. Locating gene-environment interactions: at the intersections of genetics and public health. *Soc Sci Med* 2003; 56:2327–2342.

Sinclair KD, Lea RG, Rees WD, Young LE. The developmental origins of health and disease: current theories and epigenetic mechanisms. *Soc Reprod Fertil Suppl* 2007; 64:425–443.

Skeet RG. The impact of the computer on the cancer registry. *Gann Monograph on Cancer Research* 1987; 33:89–95.

Slater D. The sociology of consumption and lifestyle. In: Calhoun C, Rojek C, Turner B (eds). *The Sage Handbook of Sociology.* Thousand Oaks, CA: Sage Publications, 2005; pp. 174–187.

Smelser NJ, Baltes PB (eds). *International Encyclopedia of the Social Sciences.* New York: Elsevier, 2001.

Sobel ME. *Lifestyle and Social Structure: Concepts, Definitions, Analyses.* New York: Academic Press, 1981.

Stallones R.A. To advance epidemiology. *Annu. Rev. Public Health* 1980; 1:69–82.

Stearns SC (ed). *Evolution in Health and Disease.* Oxford: Oxford University Press, 1999.

Stearns SC, Koella JC (eds). *Evolution in Health and Disease.* 2nd ed. Oxford: Oxford University Press, 2008.

Strickland SP. *Politics, Science, and Dread Disease; A Short History of United States Medical Research Policy.* Cambridge, MA: Harvard University Press, 1972.

Subramanian SV, Jones K, Kaddour A, Krieger N. Revisiting Robinson: the perils and pitfalls of individualistic and ecologic fallacy. *Int J Epidemiol* 2009; 38:342–360; doi:10.1093/ije/dyn359.

Susser M, Stein Z. *Eras in Epidemiology: The Evolution of Ideas.* Oxford: Oxford University Press, 2009.

Susser M, Susser E. Choosing a future for epidemiology: II. From black box to Chinese boxes and eco-epidemiology. *Am J Public Health* 1996; 86:674–677. [Erratum in: *Am J Public Health* 1996; 86:1093].

Susser M. *Causal Thinking in the Health Sciences: Concepts and Strategies of Epidemiology.* New York: Oxford University Press, 1973.

Susser M. Epidemiology in the United States after World War II: the evolution of technique. *Epidemiol. Rev* 1985; 7:147–177.

Swain DC. The rise of a research empire: NIH, 1930 to 1950. *Science* 1962; 138:1233–1237.

Swedberg R. *The Max Weber Dictionary: Key Words and Central Concepts.* Stanford, CA: Stanford University Press, 2005. ("Lifestyle": pp. 150–151).

Sydenstricker E. *Health and Environment.* New York: McGraw-Hill, 1933.

Systems Biology Institute. Available at: http://www.systems-biology.org/000/ (Accessed: January 30, 2009).

Taylor I, Knowelden J. *Principles of Epidemiology.* London: J & A Churchill, Ltd, 1957.

Terris M. The lifestyle approach to prevention: editorial. *J Public Health Policy* 1980; 1:6–9.

Tesh S. *Hidden Arguments: Political Ideology and Disease Prevention Policy.* New Brunswick, NJ: Rutgers University Press, 1988.

Thagard P. *How Scientists Explain Disease.* Princeton, NJ: Princeton University Press, 1999.

Thomas L. The future impact of science and technology on medicine. *BioScience* 1974; 24:99–105.

Trevathan WR, McKenna JJ, Smith EO (eds). *Evolution in Health and Disease.* 2nd ed. Oxford: Oxford University Press, 2007.

Trevathan WR, Smith EO, McKenna JJ. *Evolutionary Medicine.* New York: Oxford University Press, 1999.

Trevathan WR. Evolutionary medicine. *Annu Rev Anthropol* 2007; 36:139–154.

Turner JH. A new approach for theoretically integrating micro and macro analyses. In: Calhoun C, Rojek C, Turner B (eds). *The Sage Handbook of Sociology.* Thousand Oaks, CA: Sage Publications, 2005; pp. 405–422.

Udehn L. The changing face of methodological individualism. *Annu Rev Sociol* 2000; 28:479–507.

United States Department of Health and Human Services (DHHS). *Surgeon General's Reports on Smoking and Tobacco Use* (1964–2006). Available at: http://www.cdc.gov/tobacco/data_statistics/sgr/index.htm (Accessed: February 19, 2009).

US Public Health Service. *Annual Report of the Surgeon General of the Public Health Service of the United States. Washington,* DC: US Government Printing Office, 1933.

Van Speybroeck L, Van De Vijver G, De Waele D (eds). *From Epigenesis to Epigenetics: The Genome in Context.* New York: The New York Academy of Sciences, 2002.

Varmus HE. The view from the National Institutes of Health. In: Barfield CE, Smith BLR (eds). *The Future of Biomedical Research.* Washington, DC: American Enterprise Institute and The Brookings Institute, 1997; pp. 9–15.

Vineis P, Kriebel D. Causal models in epidemiology: past inheritance and genetic future. *Environ Health* 2006; 5:21. doi:10.1186/1476-069X-5-21

Vineis P. A self-fulfilling prophecy: are we underestimating the role of the environment in gene-environment interaction research? *Int J Epidemiol* 2004; 33:945–946.

Waddington CH. *Organisers & Genes.* Cambridge: Cambridge University Press, 1940.

Waddington CH. *The Evolution of an Evolutionist.* Ithaca, NY: Cornell University Press, 1975.

Waddington, C. H. *The Strategy of the Genes: A Discussion of Some Aspects of Theoretical Biology.* With an appendix by H. Kacser. New York: Macmillan, 1957.

Waitzkin H. The social origins of illness: a neglected history. *Int J Health Services* 1981; 11:77–103.

Ward JW, Warren C (eds). *Silent Victories: The History and Practice of Public Health in Twentieth-Century America.* Oxford: Oxford University Press, 2007.

Waterland RA, Michels KB. Epigenetic epidemiology of the developmental origins hypothesis. *Annu Rev Nutr* 2007; 27:363–388.

Webster's Third New International Dictionary, Unabridged. Available at: http://collections.chadwyck.com.ezp-prod1.hul.harvard.edu/home/home_mwd.jsp (Accessed: January 12, 2009).

Wersky G. *The Visible College: A Collective Biography of British Scientists and Socialists of the 1930s.* London: Free Association Books, 1988.

Whitaker Foundation. A history of biomedical engineering. Available at: http://www.bmes.org/WhitakerArchives/glance/history.html (Accessed: January 14, 2009).

Willett WC. Nutritional epidemiology issues in chronic disease at the turn of the century. *Epidemiol Rev* 2000; 22:82–86.

Williams R. *Keywords: A Vocabulary of Culture and Society.* Rev. ed. New York: Oxford University Press, 1983.

Wilson SH, Institute of Medicine (US) Roundtable on Environmental Health Sciences, Research, and Medicine, Institute of Medicine (US), Board on Health Sciences Policy. *Cancer and the*

Environment: Gene-Environment Interaction. Washington, DC: National Academy of Science Press, 2002.

Wintour EM, Owens JA (eds). *Early Life Origins of Health and Disease.* New York: Springer Science, 2006.

WordNet. Available at: http://wordnet.princeton.edu/ (Accessed: January 12, 2009).

Zablocki BD, Kanter RM. The differentiation of life-styles. *Annu Rev Sociol* 1976; 2:269–298.

Ziman J. *Real Science: What it is, and What it Means.* Cambridge, UK: Cambridge University Press, 2000.

Chapter 6

Adler N. When one's main effect is another's error: Material vs psychosocial explanations of health disparities. A commentary on Macleod et al. *Soc Sci Med* 2006; 63:846–850.

Adler NE (ed). *Socioeconomic Status and Health in Industrial Nations: Social, Psychological, and Biological Pathways.* New York: NY Academy of Science, 1999.

Adler NE, Epel ES, Castellazzo G, Ickovics JR. Relationship of subjective and objective social status with psychological and physiological functioning: preliminary data in healthy white women. *Health Psychol* 2000; 19:586–592.

Adler NE, Rehkopf DH. U.S. disparities in health: descriptions, causes, and mechanisms. *Annu Rev Public Health* 2008; 29:235–252.

Ahmed P, Coelho G (eds). *Towards a New Definition of Health: Psychosocial Dimensions.* New York: Plenum Books, 1979.

Almeida-Filho N, Kawachi I, Filho AP, Dachs NW. Research on health inequities in Latin America and the Caribbean: bibliometric analysis (1971–2000) and descriptive content analysis (1971–1995). *Am J Public Health* 2003; 93:2037–2043.

Almeida-Filho N. *La ciencia tímida: Ensayos de Deconstrucción de la Epidemiología.* Buenos Aires, Argentina: Lugar Editorial S.A., 2000.

Alvarado CH, Martínez ME, Vivas-Martínez S, Gutiérrez NJ, Metzger W. Social change and health policy in Venezuela. *Social Medicine* 2008; 3:95–109.

Amick B III, Levine S, Tarlov AR, Walsh D (eds). *Society & Health.* New York: Oxford University Press, 1995.

Anderson C. Eyes *Off the Prize: the United Nations and the African American Struggle for Human Rights, 1944–1955.* Cambridge, UK: Cambridge University Press, 2003.

Arditti R, Brenna P, Cavrak S (eds). *Science and Liberation.* Boston, MA: South End Press, 1980.

Armada F, Muntaner C, Chung H, Williams-Brennan L, Benach J. Barrio Adentro and the reduction of health inequalities in Venezuela: an appraisal of the first years. *Int J Health Services* 2009; 39:161–187.

Badash L. Science and McCarthyism. *Minerva* 2000; 38:53–80.

Bambra C, Fox D, Scott-Samuel A. A politics of health glossary. *J Epidemiol Community Health* 2007; 61:571–574.

Barrett PS, Chavez D, Rodriguez-Garavito C. *The New Latin American Left: Utopia Reborn.* London: Pluto Press, 2009.

Beaglehole R (ed). *Global Public Health: A New Era.* Oxford: Oxford University Press, 2003.

Beckfield J, Krieger N. Epi + demos + cracy: linking political systems and priorities to the magnitude of health inequities——evidence, gaps, and a research agenda. *Epidemiol Review* 2009; 31: 152–177.

Ben-Shlomo Y, Kuh DH. A lifecourse approach to chronic disease epidemiology: conceptual models, empirical challenges, and interdisciplinary perspectives. *Int J Epidemiol* 2002; 31:285–293.

Berkman LF, Kawachi I (eds). *Social Epidemiology.* Oxford: Oxford University Press, 2000.

Berliner H. Notes on historical precursors of materialist epidemiology. In: *Health Movement Organization. Health Marxist Organization (HMO) Packet 1.* New York: Health/PAC, 1976; ME 1–3.

Berridge V, Blume S (eds). *Poor Health: Social Inequality Before and After The Black Report*. London: Routledge/Frank Cass, 2002.

Beyrer C, Pizer HF (eds). *Public Health & Human Rights: Evidence-Based Approaches*. Baltimore, MD: The Johns Hopkins University Press, 2007.

Bijlmakers LA, Bassett MT, Sanders DM. *Health and Structural Adjustment in Rural and Urban Zimbabwe*. Upsalla, Sweden: Nordiska Afrikainstitutet, 1996.

BIREME/PAHO/WHO. Virtual health library. Available at: http://www.bireme.br/php/index.php?lang=en (Accessed: April 9, 2009).

Birn AE, Pillay Y, Holtz TH. *Textbook of International Health: Global Health in a Dynamic World*. Oxford: Oxford University Press, 2009.

Birn A-E. Making it politic(al): *Closing the Gap in A Generation: Health Equity through Action on the Social Determinants of Health. Social Medicine* 2009; 5:166–182.

Black D, Morris JN, Smith C, Townsend P. *Inequalities in Health: A Report of a Research Working Group*. London: Department of Health and Social Security, 1980. (*The Black Report*; original available at: http://www.sochealth.co.uk/history/black.htm (Accessed: March 7, 2009; see also: Black D, Morris JN, Smith C, Townsend P. *The Black Report*) (Report of the Working Group on Inequalities in Health). London: Penguin, 1982.)

Blakely T, Tobias M, Atkinson J. Inequalities in mortality during and after restructuring of the New Zealand economy: Repeated cohort studies. *Br Med J* 2008; 336:371–375.

Blane D, Netuveli G, Stone J. The development of lifecourse epidemiology. *Rev Epidemiol Sante Publique* 2007; 55:31–38.

Borgia F. Health in Uruguay: progress and challenges in the right to health care three years after the first progressive government. *Social Medicine* 2008; 3:110–125.

Braveman P. Health disparities and health equity: concepts and measurement. *Annu Rev Public Health* 2006; 27:167–194.

Breilh J, Granda E. Epidemiologia y contrahegemonia. *Soc Sci Med* 1989; 28:1121–1128.

Breilh J. *Epidemiología: Economía, Medicina y Política*. 4e ed. Mexico City, Mexico: Fontamara, 1988 (1979).

Briggs CL, Mantini-Briggs C. Confronting health disparities: Latin American social medicine in Venezuela. *Am J Public Health* 2009; 99:549–555.

Brownlea A. From public health to political epidemiology. *Soc Sci Med* 1981; 15D:57–67.

Brunner E, Marmot M. Social organization, stress, and health. In: Marmot M, Wilkinson RG (eds). *Social Determinants of Health*. Oxford: Oxford University Press, 1999; pp. 17–43.

Brunner E. Stress and the biology of inequality. *Br Med J* 1997; 314:1472–1476.

Brunner EJ. Toward a new social biology. In: Berkman LF, Kawachi I (eds). *Social Epidemiology*. New York: Oxford University Press, 2000; pp. 306–331.

Burns EB, Charlip JA. *Latin America: An Interpretative History*. Upper Saddle River, NJ: Pearson/Prentice Hall, 2007.

Campbell JC, Webster D, Koziol-McLain J, et al. Risk factors for femicide in abusive relationships: results from a multisite case control study. *Am J Public Health* 2003; 93:1089–1097.

Cannon W. The Body Physiologic and the Body Politic. *Science* 1941; 93:1–10.

Cannon WB. *Bodily Changes in Pain, Hunger, Fear and Rage: An Account of Recent Researches into the Function of Emotional Excitement*. New York: Appleton, 1915.

Cannon WB. Stresses and strains of homeostasis. *Am J Medical Sciences* 1935; 189:1–14.

Carney RM, Freedland KE. Depression and mental illness. In: Berkman LF, Kawachi I (eds). *Social Epidemiology*. New York: Oxford University Press, 2000; pp. 191–212.

Carson B, Dunbar T, Chenhall RD, Bailie R. *Social Determinants of Indigenous Health*. Crows Nest, NSW: Allen & Unwin, 2007.

Cassel J. Psychosocial processes and "stress": theoretical formulation. *Int J Health Services* 1974; 4:471–482.

Cassel J. The contribution of the social environment to host resistance. *Am J Epidemiol* 1976; 104:107–123.

Castellanos PL. On the concept of health and disease: description and explanation of the health situation. *Epidemiological Bulletin* 1990; 10:1–8.

Catalano R. Health, medical care, and economic crisis. *New Engl J Med* 2009; 360:749–751.

Chae DH, Krieger N, Bennett GG, Lindsey JC, Stoddard AM, Barbeau EM. Implications of discrimination based on sexuality, gender, and race for psychological distress among working class sexual minorities: the United for Health Study, 2003–2004. *Int J Health Services*, 2010; 40:589–608.

Chope HD. Epidemiology in the social sciences. *Calif Med* 1959; 91:189–192.

Clarke A, McCarthy M, Alvarez-Dardet C, Sogoric S, Groenewegen P, Groot W, Delnoij D. New directions in European public health research: report of a workshop. *J Epidemiol Community Health* 2007; 61:194–197.

Clegg SR. Power in society. In: *International Encyclopedia of the Social & Behavioral Sciences* (online). Elsevier, 2004: pp. 11932–11936. Available at: http://www.sciencedirect.com.ezp1.harvard.edu/science (Accessed: March 28, 2009).

Coburn D, Denny K, Mykhalovskiy E, McDonough P, Robertson A, Love R. Population health in Canada: a brief critique. *Am J Public Health* 2003; 93:392–396.

Cohen A. The Brasilian health reform: a victory over the neoliberal model. *Social Medicine* 2008; 3:71–81.

Cohen S, Kessler RC, Gordon LU. *Measuring Stress: A Guide for Health and Social Scientists.* New York: Oxford University Press, 1995.

Committee on Environmental Justice, Health Sciences Policy Program, Health Sciences Section, Institute of Medicine. *Toward Environmental Justice: Research, Education, and Health Policy Needs.* Washington, DC: National Academy Press, 1999.

Conrad P, Kern R. The social production of disease and illness. In: Conrad P, Kern R (eds). *The Sociology of Health and Illness: Critical Perspectives.* New York: St. Martin's Press, 1981; pp. 9–11.

Costa AM, Merchán-Hamann E, Tajer D. *Saúde, Eqüidade e Gênero: Um Desafia Para as Políticas Públicas.* Brasília: Editora Universidade de Brasília, 2000.

Cunningham M. Health. In: United Nations, Department of Economic and Social Affairs. *The State of the World's Indigenous Peoples.* New York: United Nations, 2009; pp. 156–187.

Dahlgren G, Whitehead M. *Levelling Up (part 2): A Discussion Paper on European Strategies for Tackling Social Inequities in Health.* Denmark: WHO Regional Office for Europe, 2006.

Dahlgren G, Whitehead M. *Tackling inequalities in health: what can we learn from what has been tried?* Working paper prepared for the King's Fund International Seminar on Tackling Inequalities in Health, Ditchley Park, Oxfordshire, London, King's fund (mimeo), 1993.

Davey Smith G (ed). *Health Inequalities: Lifecourse Approaches.* Bristol, UK: Policy Press, 2003.

Davey Smith G. The end of the beginning for chronic disease epidemiology. *Int J Epidemiol* 2010; 39:1–3.

Davey Smith G. The uses of "Uses of Epidemiology." *Int J Epidemiol* 2001; 30:1146–1155.

Declaration of Alma-Ata. International Conference on Primary Health Care, Alma-Ata, USSR, 6-September 12, 1978. Available at: http://www.who.int/hpr/NPH/docs/declaration_almaata.pdf (Accessed: December 26, 2009).

Diaz RM, Ayala G, Bein E, Henne J, Marin BV. The impact of homophobia, poverty, and racism on the mental health of gay and bisexual Latino men: findings from 3 US cities. *Am J Public Health* 2001; 91:927–932.

Doyal L. *The Political Economy of Health.* London: Pluto Press, 1979.

Doyal L. *What Makes Women Sick? Gender and The Political Economy of Health.* New Brunswick, NJ: Rutgers University Press, 1995.

Duran B, Walters KL. HIV/AIDS prevention in "Indian country": current practice, indigenist etiology models, and postcolonial approaches to change. *AIDS Educ Prev* 2004; 16:187–201.

Eikemo TA, Bambra C. The welfare state: a glossary for public health. *J Epidemiol Community Health* 2008; 62:3–6.

Eisenberg L. Rudolf Ludwig Karl Virchow, where are you now that we need you? *Am J Med* 1984; 77:524–532.

Eldredge JD, Waitzkin H, Buchana HS, Teal J, Iriart C, Wiley K, Tregear J. The Latin American Social Medicine database. *BMC Public Health* 2004; 4:69.

Elliott GR, Eisdorfer C (eds). *Stress and Human Health: Analysis and Implications of research. A study by the Institute of Medicine/National Academy of Sciences.* New York: Springer, 1982.

Ellsberg M, Jansen HAFM, Heise L, Watts CH, Garcia-Moreno C. Intimate partner violence and women's physical and mental health in the WHO multi-country study on women's health and domestic violence: an observational study. *Lancet* 2008; 371:1165–1172.

Elstad JI. The psycho-social perspective on social inequalities in health. In: Bartley M, Blane D, Davey Smith G, eds. *The Sociology of Health Inequalities*. Oxford: Blackwell, 1998; pp. 39–58.

Emmons KM. Health behaviors in social context. In: Berkman LF, Kawachi I (eds). *Social Epidemiology*. New York: Oxford University Press, 2000; pp. 242–266.

Engel GL. The need for a new medical model: a challenge for biomedicine. *Science* 1977; 196: 129–136.

Epidemiologic Reviews. Theme issue: "Epidemiologic approaches to health disparities." *Epidemiol Rev* 2009; 31:1–194.

Esplet A, Borrell C, Rofríguez-Sanz M, Muntaner C, Pasarín MI, Benach J, Schaap M, Kunst AE, Navarro V. Inequalities in health by social class dimensions in European countries of different political traditions. *Int J Epidemiol* 2008; 37:1095–1105.

Etches V, Frank J, Di Ruggiero E, Manuel D. Measuring population health: a review of indicators. *Annu Rev Public Health* 2006; 27: 29–55.

Evans RG, Barer ML, Marmot TR (eds). *Why Are Some People Healthy and Others Not? The Determinants of Health of Populations*. New York: Aldine de Gruyter, 1994.

Evans RG, Stoddart GL. Consuming research, producing policy? *Am J Public Health* 2003; 93: 371–379.

Evans RG, Stoddart GL. Producing health, consuming health care. *Soc Sci Med* 1990; 31:1347–1363.

Evans-Cambell T. Historical trauma in American Indian/Native Alaska communities: a multilevel framework for exploring impacts on individuals, families, and communities. *J Interpers Violence* 2008; 23:316–338.

Eyer J, Sterling P. Stress-related mortality and social organization. *Rev Radical Political Economy* 1977; 9:1–44.

Fee E, Krieger N. *Women's Health, Politics, and Power: Essays on Sex/Gender, medicine, and Public Policy*. Amityville, NY: Baywood Publishers, 1994.

Fee E. Public health and the state: the United States. In: Porter D (ed). *The History of Public Health and the Modern States*. Amsterdam: Editions Rodopi B.V., 1994; pp. 224–275.

Ferriera ML, Lang CG (eds). *Indigenous Peoples and Diabetes: Community Empowerment and Wellness*. Durham, NC: Carolina Academic Press, 2006.

Flaherty D, Kelman S, Lazonick W, Price L, Rodberg L, Stark E (eds). Special issue on The Political Economy of Health. *The Review of Radical Political Economics* 1977; 9:1–140.

Franco S, Nunes E, Breilh J, Laurell C. *Debates en Medicina Social*. Organización Panamericana de la Salud-Alames. Quito, Ecuador: Non Plus Ultra, 1991.

Franco S. A social-medical approach to violence in Colombia. *Am J Public Health* 2003; 93: 2032–2036.

Franco-Giraldo A, Palma M, Alvarez-Dardet C. The effect of structural adjustment on health conditions in Latin America and the Caribbean, 1980–2000. *Revista Panamericana De Salud Publica-Pan American Journal of Public Health* 2006; 19:291–299.

Frank JW. Why "population health"? *Canadian J Public Health* 1995; 86:162–164.

Frankel RM, Quill TE, McDaniel S. *The Biopsychosocial Approach: Past, Present, Future*. Rochester, NY: University of Rochester Press, 2003.

Frolich KL, Mykhalovskiy E, Miller F, Daniel M. Advancing the population health agenda: encouraging the integration of social theory into population health research and practice. *Canadian J Public Health* 2004; 95:392–395.

Furumoto-Dawson A, Gehlert S, Sohmer D, Olopade O, Sacks T. Early-life conditions and mechanisms of population health vulnerabilities. *Health Aff (Millwood)* 2007; 26:1238–1248.

Galdston I (ed). *Beyond the Germ Theory: The Roles of Deprivation and Stress in Health and Disease*. New York: Health Education Council, New York Academy of Medicine, 1954. (1954a)

Galdston I (ed). *Social Medicine: Its Derivations and Objectives*. New York: Commonwealth Fund, 1949.

Galdston I. Beyond the germ theory: the roles of deprivation and stress in health and disease. In: Galdston I (ed). *Beyond the Germ Theory: The Roles of Deprivation and Stress in Health and*

Disease. New York: Health Education Council, New York Academy of Medicine, 1954; pp. 3–16. (1954b)

Garcia-Moreno C. Violence against women: international perspectives. *Am J Prev Med* 2000; 19: 330–333.

Gaynor D, Eyer J. Materialist epidemiology. In: In: Health Movement Organization. *Health Marxist Organization (HMO) Packet 1.* New York: Health/PAC, 1976; ME 4–7.

Ghaed SG, Gallo LC. Subjective social status, objective socioeconomic status, and cardiovascular risk in women. *Health Psychol* 2007; 26:668–674.

Giddens A, Held D (eds). *Classes, Power, and Conflict: Classical and Contemporary Debates.* Berkeley, CA: University of California Press, 1982.

Gil-González D, Palma Solís M, Ruiz Cantero MT, Ortiz Moncada MR, Franco Girdaldo A, Stein A, Alvarez-Dardet Díaz C. The challenge to public health of the Millennium Development Goals: an approach from political epidemiology. *Gac Sanit* 2006; 20(Suppl 3):61–65.

Gil-González D, Ruiz-Cantero MT, Alvarez-Dardet C. How political epidemiology research can address why the millennium development goals have not been achieved: developing a research agenda. *J Epidemiol Community Health* 2009; 63:278–280.

Glendon MA. *A World Made New: Eleanor Roosevelt and the Universal Declaration of Human Rights.* New York: Random House, 2001.

Goodman E, Adler NE, Kawachi I, Frazier AL, Huang B, Colditz GA. Adolescents' perceptions of social status: development and evaluation of a new indicator. *Pediatrics* 2001; 108:e31; DOI:10.1542/peds.108.2.e31

Gordon JE. The world, the flesh and the devil as environment, host, and agent of Disease. In: Galdston I (ed). *The Epidemiology of Health.* New York: Health Education Council, 1953; pp. 60–73.

Graham H. *Unequal Lives: Health and Socio-economic Inequalities.* Berkshire, England: Open University Press, 2007.

Graham S, Schneiderman M. Social epidemiology and the prevention of cancer. *Prev Med* 1972; 1:371–380.

Granda E. ALAMES turns 24. *Social Medicine* 2008; 3:165–172.

Greeley K, Tafler S. History of *Science for the People*: a ten year perspective. In: Arditti R, Brenna P, Cavrak S (eds). *Science and Liberation.* Boston, MA: South End Press, 1980; 369–382.

Greenwood M. *Some British Pioneers of Social Medicine.* London: Oxford University Press, 1948.

Gruskin S, Ferguson L. Using indicators to determining the contribution of human rights to public health efforts: why? what? and how? *Bull World Health Org* 2009; 87:714–719.

Gruskin S, Grodin MA, Annas GJ, Marks SP (eds). *Perspectives on Health and Human Rights.* New York: Routledge, 2005.

Gruskin S, Mills EJ, Tarantola D. Health and human rights 1: history, principles, and practice of health and human rights. *Lancet* 2007; 370:449–455.

Gruskin S, Tarantola D. Health and human rights. In: Detels R, McEwen J, Beaglehole R, Tanaka K, eds. *The Oxford Textbook of Public Health,* 4th ed. New York: Oxford University Press, 2001; pp. 311–335.

Grusky DB (ed). *Social Stratification: Class, Race, and Gender in Sociological Perspective.* Boulder, CO: Westview Press, 2001.

Halliday JL. Epidemiology and the psychosomatic afflictions: a study in social medicine. *Lancet* 1946; 248:185–220.

Hardy A. Macroscopic epidemiology and the lessons of history. *Rev Epidemiol Sante Publique* 2004; 52:353–356.

Heller RF. *Evidence for Population Health.* Oxford: Oxford University Press, 2005.

Henry HP, Cassel JC. Psychosocial factors in essential hypertension: recent epidemiologic and animal experimental evidence. *Am J Epidemiol* 1969; 90:171–200.

Hertzman C. The biological embedding of early experience and its effects on health in adulthood. *Ann NY Acad Sci* 1999; 896:85–95.

Hobsbawm E. *On Empire: America, War, and Global Supremacy.* New York: Pantheon Books, 2008.

Hobsbawm E. *The Age of Extremes: The Short Twentieth Century, 1914–1991.* London: Michael Joseph, 1994.

Hofrichter R (ed). *Health and Social Justice: Politics, Ideology, and Inequity in the Distribution of Disease*. San Francisco, CA: Jossey-Bass, 2003.

Huebner DM, Davis MC. Perceived antigay discrimination and physical health outcomes. *Health Psychology* 2007; 26:627–634.

Huebner DM, Rebchook GM, Kegeles SM. Experiences of harassment, discrimination, and physical violence among young gay and bisexual men. *Am J Public Health* 2004; 94:1200–1203.

Iriart C, Waitzkin H, Breilh J, Estrada A, Merhy EE. Medicina social latinoamericana: aportes y desafíos (Latin American social medicine: contributions and challenges). *Rev Panam Salud Publica* 2002; 12:128–136.

Isaac J. The human sciences in Cold War America. *The Historical Journal* 2007; 50:725–746.

Jaco EG. Introduction: Medicine and behavioral science. In: Jaco EG (ed). *Patients, Physicians and Illness: Sourcebook in Behavioral Science and Medicine*. Glencoe, IL: The Free Press, 1958; pp. 3–8.

Jaco EG. *The Social Epidemiology of Mental Disorders; A Psychiatric Survey of Texas*. New York: Russell Sage Foundation, 1960.

Jasanoff S. Ordering knowledge, ordering society. In: Jasanoff S (ed). *States of Knowledge: The Co-Production of Science and Social Order*. London: Routledge, 2004; pp. 13–45.

Kawachi I, Berkman L. Social cohesion, social capital, and health. In: Berkman LF, Kawachi I (eds). *Social Epidemiology*. New York: Oxford University Press, 2000; pp. 174–190.

Kawachi I, Kennedy BP, Wilkinson RG (eds). *The Society and Population Health Reader: Vol 1. Income Inequality and Health*. New York: New Press, 1999.

Kawachi I, Wamala S (eds). *Globalization and Health*. Oxford: Oxford University Press, 2007.

Kearns R, Moewaka-Barnes H, McCreanor T. Placing racism in public health: a perspective from Aotearoa/New Zealand. *Geojournal* 2009; 74:123–129.

Kelman S. Introduction to the theme: the political economy of health. *Int J Health Services* 1975; 5:535–538.

Kindig D, Stoddart G. What is population health? *Am J Public Health* 2003; 93:380–383.

Kindig DA. How do you define the health of populations? *Physician Exec* 1997; 23:6–11. (1997b)

Kindig DA. *Purchasing Population Health: Paying for Results*. Ann Arbor, MI: University of Michigan Press, 1997. (1997a)

Kindig DA. Understanding population health terminology. *Milbank Q* 2007; 85: 139–161.

King SH, Cobb S. Psychosocial factors in the epidemiology of rheumatoid arthritis. *J Chron Dis* 1958; 7:466–475.

Koob GF, Le Moal M. Drug addiction and allostasis. In: Shulkin J (ed). *Allostasis, Homeostasis and the Costs of Physiological Adaptation*. New York: Cambridge University Press, 2004; pp. 150–163.

Krieger N (ed). *Embodying Inequality: Epidemiologic Perspectives*. Amityville, NY: Baywood Pub, 2004.

Krieger N, Alegría M, Almeida-Filho N, Barbosa da Silva J Jr, Barreto ML, Beckfield J, Berkman L, Birn A-E, Duncan BB, Franco S, Garcia DA, Gruskin S, James SA, Laurell AC, Schmidt MI, Walters KL. Who, and what, causes health inequities? Reflections on emerging debates from an exploratory Latin American/North American workshop. *J Epidemiol Community Health* 2010; 64:747–749; doi:10.1136/jech.2009.106906.

Krieger N, Chen JT, Waterman PD, et al. The inverse hazard law: blood pressure, sexual harassment, racial discrimination, workplace abuse and occupational exposures in the *United for Health* study of US low-income black, white, and Latino workers (Greater Boston Area, Massachusetts, United States, 2003–2004). *Soc Sci Med* 2008; 67:1970–1981. (2008b)

Krieger N, Gruskin S. Frameworks matter: ecosocial and health & human rights perspectives on women and health—the case of tuberculosis. *J Am Women's Med Assoc* 2001; 56:137–142.

Krieger N, Northridge M, Gruskin S, Quinn M, Kriebel D, Davey Smith G, Bassett MT, Rehkopf DH, Miller C and the HIA "promise and pitfalls" conference group. Assessing health impact assessment: multidisciplinary & international perspectives. *J Epidemiol Community Health* 2003; 57:659–662.

Krieger N, Rehkopf DH, Chen JT, Waterman PD, Marcelli E, Kennedy M. The fall and rise of US inequities in premature mortality: 1960–2002. *PLoS Med* 2008; 5(2): e46. (2008a)

Krieger N, Rowley DL, Herman AA, Avery B, Phillips MT. Racism, sexism, and social class: implications for studies of health, disease, and well-being. *Am J Prev Med* 1993; 9 (Suppl):82–122.

Krieger N, Sidney S. Prevalence and health implications of anti-gay discrimination: a study of black and white women and men in the CARDIA cohort. Coronary Artery Risk Development in Young Adults. *Int J Health Services* 1997; 27:157–176.

Krieger N, Sidney S. Racial discrimination and blood pressure: The CARDIA study of young black and white adults. *Am J Public Health* 1996; 86:1370–1378.

Krieger N. A glossary for social epidemiology. *J Epidemiol Community Health* 2001; 55:693–700. (2001b)

Krieger N. Defining and investigating social disparities in cancer: critical issues. *Cancer Causes Control* 2005; 16:5–14.

Krieger N. Embodying inequality: a review of concepts, measures, and methods for studying health consequences of discrimination. *Int J Health Services* 1999; 29:295–352. (Revised and expanded: Krieger N. Discrimination and health. In: Berkman LF, Kawachi I [eds]. *Social Epidemiology.* Oxford: Oxford University Press, 2000; pp. 36–75.)

Krieger N. Epidemiology and social sciences: towards a critical reengagement in the 21st century. *Epidemiologic Reviews* 2000; 11:155–163.

Krieger N. Epidemiology and the web of causation: has anyone seen the spider? *Soc Sci Med* 1994; 39:887–903.

Krieger N. Ladders, pyramids, and champagne: the iconography of health inequities. *J Epidemiol Community Health* 2008; 62:1098–1104. (2008b)

Krieger N. Latin American Social Medicine: the quest for social justice & public health. *Am J Public Health* 2003; 93:1989–1991.

Krieger N. Proximal, distal, and the politics of causation: what's level got to do with it? *Am J Public Health* 2008; 98:221–230. (2008a)

Krieger N. Putting health inequities on the map: social epidemiology meets medical/health geography–an ecosocial perspective. *GeoJournal* 2009; 74:87–97.

Krieger N. Racial and gender discrimination: risk factors for high blood pressure? *Soc Sci Med* 1990; 30:1273–1281.

Krieger N. Special report - epidemiology in Latin America: the emerging perspective of Social medicine. *Epidemiology Monitor* 1988; 9:3–4.

Krieger N. Theories for social epidemiology in the 21st century: an ecosocial perspective. *Int J Epidemiol* 2001; 30:668–677. (2001a)

Krieger N. Ways of asking and ways of living: reflections on the 50th anniversary of Morris' ever-useful *Uses of Epidemiology. Int J Epidemiol* 2007; 36:1173–1180.

Krugman P. The market mystique. Op-ed. *New York Times*, March 26, 2009.

Kruse HD. The interplay of noxious agents, stress, and deprivation in the etiology of disease. In: Galdston I (ed). *Beyond the Germ Theory: The Roles of Deprivation and Stress in Health and Disease.* New York: Health Education Council, 1954; pp. 17–38.

Kubzansky LD, Kawachi I. Affective states and health. In: Berkman LF, Kawachi I (eds). *Social Epidemiology.* New York: Oxford University Press, 2000; pp. 213–241.

Kuh D, Ben-Shlomo Y, Lynch J, Hallqvist J, Power C. Life course epidemiology: glossary. *J Epidemiol Community Health* 2003; 57:778–783.

Kuh D, Davey Smith G. The life course and adult chronic disease: an historical perspective with particular reference to coronary heart disease. In: Kuh D, Ben-Shlomo Y (eds). *A Lifecourse Approach to Chronic Disease Epidemiology: Tracing the Origins of Ill-Health from Early to Adult Life.* Oxford: Oxford University Press, 1997; pp. 15–41.

Kunitz S. *The Health of Populations: General Theories and Particular Realities.* Oxford: Oxford University Press, 2007.

Labonte R, Polyani M, Muhajarine N, McIntosh T, Williams A. Beyond the divides: towards critical population health research. *Critical Public Health* 2005; 15:5–17.

Labonte R. Editorial: Towards a critical population health research. *Critical Public Health* 2005; 15: 1–3.

Labonte R. Population health and health promotion: what do they have to say to each other? *Canadian J Public Health* 1995; 86:165–168.

Latin American Social Medicine: Increasing access to publications. Available at: http://hsc.unm.edu/lasm (Accessed: April 9, 2009).

Laurell AC. Health reform in Mexico City, 2000–2006. *Social Medicine* 2008; 3:145–157.

Laurell AC. Social analysis of collective health in Latin America. *Soc Sci Med* 1989; 28:1183–1191.

Laurell AC. What does Latin American Social Medicine do when it governs? The case of the Mexico City Government. *Am J Public Health* 2003; 93:2028–2031.

LaVeist TA (ed). *Race, Ethnicity, and Health: A Public Health Reader.* San Francisco, CA: Jossey-Bass, 2002.

Lawrence C, Weisz G (eds). *Greater than the Parts: Holism in Biomedicine, 1920–1950.* New York: Oxford University Press, 1998.

Lefkowitz B. *Community Health Centers: A Movement and the People Who Made it Happen.* New Brunswick, NJ: Rutgers University Press, 2007.

Leon D, Walt G (eds). *Poverty, Inequality and Health: An International Perspective.* Oxford: Oxford University Press, 2001.

Levins R, Lewontin RC. *The Dialectical Biologist.* Cambridge, MA: Harvard University Press, 1985.

Levy BS, Sidel VW (eds). *Social Injustice and Public Health.* New York: Oxford University Press, 2006.

Lieberson S, Silverman AR. The precipitants and underlying conditions of race riots. *Am Sociol Rev* 1965; 30:887–898.

Lieberson S. *Making It Count: The Improvement of Social Research and Theory.* Berkeley, CA: University of California Press, 1985.

Link BG, Phelan J. Social conditions as fundamental causes of disease. *J Health Social Behav* 1995; 35:80–94.

Link BG, Phelan JC, Miech R, Westin EL. The resources that matter: fundamental social causes of health disparities and the challenge of intelligence. *J Health Social Behavior* 2008; 49:72–91.

Link BG, Phelan JC. Editorial: understanding sociodemographic differences in health—the role of fundamental social causes. *Am J Public Health* 1996; 86:471–473.

London L. Human rights, environmental justice, and the health of farm workers in South Africa. *Int J Occup Environ Health* 2003; 9:59–68.

Lurie P, Hintzen P, Lowe RA. Socioeconomic obstacles to HIV prevention and treatment in developing-countries—the roles of the International Monetary Fund and the World Bank. *AIDS* 1995; 9:539–546.

Lynch J, Smith GD. A life course approach to chronic disease epidemiology. *Annu Rev Public Health* 2005; 26:1–35.

Lynch JW, Davey Smith G, Kaplan GA, House JS. Income inequality and mortality: importance to health of individual incomes, psychological environment, or material conditions. *Br Med J* 2000; 320:1200–1204.

Maantay J. Asthma and air pollution in the Bronx: methodological and data considerations in using GIS for environmental justice and health research. *Health Place* 2007; 13:32–56.

MacArthur Network on Socioeconomic Status and Health. *Reaching for a healthier life: Facts on socioeconomic status and health in the United States.* San Francisco, CA: The John D. And Catherine T. MacArthur Foundation Network on Socioeconomic Status and Health, 2007. Available at: http://www.macses.ucsf.edu/Default.htm (Accessed: April 3, 2009).

Macleod J, Davey Smith G, Metcalfe C, Hart C. Is subjective social status a more important determinant of health than objective social status? Evidence from a prospective observational study of Scottish men. *Soc Sci Med* 2005; 61:1916–1929.

Macleod J, Davey Smith G, Metcalfe C, Hart C. Subjective and objectives status and health: A response to Adler's "When one's main effect is another's error." *Soc Sci Med* 2006; 63:851–857.

Malcoe LH, Lynch RA, Keger MC, Skaggs VJ. Lead sources, behaviors, and socioeconomic factors in relation to blood lead of Native American and white children: a community-based assessment of a former mining area. *Environ Health Perspect* 2002; 110(Suppl 2):221–231.

Mann J, Gostin L, Gruskin S, Brennan T, Lazzarini Z, Fineberg H. Health and Human Rights. *Health and Human Rights* 1994; 1:6–23.

Mann JM, Gruskin S, Grodin MA, Annas GJ (eds). *Health and Human Rights: A Reader.* New York: Routledge, 1999.

Marmot M, Wilkinson R (eds). *The Social Determinants of Health.* 1st ed. Oxford: Oxford University Press, 1999.

Marmot M. Psychosocial factors and cardiovascular disease: epidemiological approaches. *European Heart J* 1988; 9:690–697.

Marmot MG, Bell R. Action on health disparities: Commission on the Social Determinants of Health. *JAMA* 2009; 301:1169–1171.

Marmot MG. *The Status Syndrome: How Social Standing Affects our Health and Longevity.* 1st American ed. New York: Times Books/Henry Holt, 2004.

Mays VM, Cochran SD, Barnes NW. Race, race-based discrimination, and health outcomes among African Americans. *Ann Rev Psychol* 2007; 58:201–225.

Mays VM, Cochran SD. Mental health correlates of perceived discrimination among lesbian, gay, and bisexual adults in the United States. *Am J Public Health* 2001; 91:1869–1876.

McEwen B, Stellar E. Stress and the individual: mechanisms leading to disease. *Arch Intern Med* 1993; 153:2093–2101.

McEwen BS. Central effects of stress hormones in health and disease: understanding the protective and damaging effects of stress and stress mediators. *Eur J Pharmacol* 2008; 582:174–185.

McEwen BS. Physiology and neurobiology of stress and adaptation: central role of the brain. *Physiol Rev* 2007; 87:873–904.

McEwen BS. Protective and damaging effects of stress mediators: allostasis and allostatic load. *New Engl J Med* 1998; 338:171–179. (1998b)

McEwen BS. Protective and damaging effects of the mediators of stress and adaptation: allostasis and allostatic load. In: Shulkin J (ed). *Allostasis, Homeostasis and the Costs of Physiological Adaptation.* New York: Cambridge University Press, 2004; pp. 65–98.

McEwen BS. Stress, adaptation, and disease: allostasis and allostatic load. *Ann NY Acad Sci* 1998; 840:33–44. (1998a)

McFarland AS. Power: political. In: *International Encyclopedia of the Social & Behavioral Sciences* (online). Elsevier; 2004:11936–11939. Available at: http://www.sciencedirect.com.ezp1.harvard.edu/science (Accessed: March 28, 2009).

McLennan G. Power. In: Bennett T, Grossberg L, Morris M, eds. *New Keywords: A Revised Vocabulary of Culture and Society.* Malden, Mass: Blackwell Publishing, 2005; pp. 274–278.

Meyer IH. Minority stress and mental health in gay men. *J Health Social Behavior* 1995; 36:38–56.

Meyer IM, Northridge ME (eds). *The Health of Sexual Minorities: Public Health Perspectives on Lesbian, Gay, Bisexual, and Transgender Populations.* New York: Springer, 2007.

Moore S, Teixeira AC, Shiell A. The health of nations in a global context: Trade, global stratification, and infant mortality rates. *Soc Sci Med* 2006; 63:165–178.

Morello-Frosch R, Lopez R. The riskscape and the colorline: examining the role of segregation in environmental health disparities. *Environ Res* 2006; 102:181–196.

Morgan LM. Latin American social medicine and the politics of theory. In: Goodman AH, Leatherman TL (eds). *Building a New Biocultural Synthesis: Political-Economic Perspectives on Human Biology.* Ann Arbor, MI: University of Michigan Press, 1998; pp. 407–424.

Morris J. Uses of epidemiology. *Br Med J* 1955; 2:395–401.

Morris J. *Uses of Epidemiology.* Edinburgh: E. & S. Livingston, Ltd, 1957.

Morris JN, Wilkinson P, Dangour AD, Deeming C, Fletcher A. Defining a minimum income for health living (MIHL): older age, England. *Int J Epidemiol* 2007; 36:1300–1307.

Mullany LC, Richards AK, Lee CI, Suwanvanichkj V, Maung C, Mahn M, Beyrer C, Lee TJ. Population-based survey methods to quantify associations between human rights violations and health outcomes among internally displaced persons in eastern Burma. *J Epidemiol Community Health* 2007; 61:908–914.

National Conference on Preventive Medicine. *Theory, Practice and Application of Prevention in Environmental Health Services: Social Determinants of Human Health.* Sponsored by The John E. Fogarty International Center for Advanced Study in Health Sciences, National Institutes of Health and the American College of Preventive Medicine. New York: Prodist, 1976.

National Research Council and Institute of Medicine. *From Neurons to Neighborhoods: The Science of Early Childhood Development.* Committee on Integrating the Science of Early Childhood Development. Jack P. Shonkoff and Deborah A. Phillips, eds. Board on Children, Youth, and

Families, Commission on Behavioral and Social Sciences and Education. Washington, D.C.: National Academy Press, 2000.

Navarro V (ed). *Neoliberalism, Globalization, and Inequalities: Consequences for Health and Quality of Life*. Amityville, NY: Baywood Pub. Co., 2007.

Navarro V (ed). *The Political Economy of Social Inequalities: Consequences for Health and Quality of Life*. Amityville, NY: Baywood Pub. Co., 2002.

Navarro V, Borrell C, Benach J, Muntaner C, Quiroga A, Rodríguez-Sanz M, Vergés N, Gumá J, Pasarín MI. The importance of the political and the social in explaining mortality differentials among the countries of the OECD, 1950-1998. *Int J Health Serv* 2003; 33:419–494.

Navarro V, Muntaner C (eds). *Political and Economic Determinants of Population Health and Well-Being: Controversies and Development*. Amityville, NY: Baywood Pub, 2004.

Navarro V, Muntaner C, Borrell C, Benach J, Quiroga A, Rodríguez-Sanz M, Vergés N, Pasarín MI. Politics and health outcomes. *Lancet* 2006; 368:1033–1037.

Navarro V, Shi LY. The political context of social inequalities and health. *Soc Sci Med* 2001; 52: 481–491.

Navarro V. *Crisis, Health, and Medicine: A Social Critique*. New York: Tavistock, 1986. (1986b)

Navarro V. Editorial: a beginning. *Int J Health Services* 1971; 1:1–2.

Navarro V. U.S. Marxist scholarship in the analysis of health and medicine. In: Ollman B, Vernoff E (eds). *The Left Academy: Marxist Scholarship on American Campuses, Volume III*. New York: Praeger, 1986; 208–236. (1986a)

Navarro V. What we mean by social determinants of health. *Promot Educ* 2009; 16:5–16.

Norton JM, Wing S, Lipscomb HJ, Kaufman JS, Marshall SW, Cravey AJ. Race, wealth, and solid waste facilities in North Carolina. *Environ Health Perspect* 2007; 115:1344–1350.

Oakley A. Appreciation: Jerry (Jeremiah Noah) Morris, 1910-2009. *Int J Epidemiol* 2010; 39: 274–276.

Oliver HC. In the wake of structural adjustment programs - exploring the relationship between domestic policies and health outcomes in Argentina and Uruguay. *Can J Public Health-Rev Can Sante Publ* 2006; 97:217–221.

Oxford English Dictionary (on line). "Psychosocial." Available at: http://dictionary.oed.com. ezp-prod1.hul.harvard.edu/entrance.dtl (Accessed: May 19, 2009).

Packard RM. *White Plague, Black Labor: Tuberculosis and the Political Economy of Health and Disease in South Africa*. Berkeley, CA: University of California at Berkeley Press, 1989.

Paim JS, de Almeida Filho N. Collective health: a "new public health" or field open to new paradigms? *Rev Saude Publica* 1998; 32:299–316.

Paradies Y. A systematic review of empirical research on self-reported racism and health. *Int J Epidemiol* 2006; 35:888–901.

Phelan JC, Link BG, Diez-Roux A, Kawachi I, Levin B. "Fundamental causes" of social inequality in mortality: a test of the theory. *J Health Soc Behav* 2004; 45:265–285. Erratum in: J Health Soc Behav 2005; 46:v.

Phelan JC, Link BG. Controlling disease and creating disparities: a fundamental cause perspective. *J Gerontol B Psychol Sci Soc Sci* 2005; 60(Spec No 2):27–33.

Poland B, Coburn D, Robertson A, Eakin J. Wealth, equity and health care: a critique of a "population health" perspective on the determinants of health. *Soc Sci Med* 1998; 46:785–798.

Porta M (ed). *A Dictionary of Epidemiology*. 5th edition. New York: Oxford University Press, 2008.

Porter D. How did social medicine evolve, and where is it heading? *PLoS Med* 2006; 3(10):e399.

Porter D. The decline of social medicine in Britain in the 1960s. In: Porter D (ed). *Social Medicine and Medical Sociology in the Twentieth Century*. Amsterdam & Atlanta: Rodopi, 1997; pp. 97–119.

Power C, Hertzman C. Social and biological pathways linking early life and adult disease. *Br Med Bull* 1997; 53:210–221.

Psychosomatic Medicine. Available at: http://www.psychosomaticmedicine.org/misc/about.shtml (Accessed: May 18, 2009).

Pyramid of Capitalist System. Issued by Nedeljkovich, Brashick and Kuharich, for the International Workers of the World (IWW). Cleveland: The International Publishing Co., 1911. http:// laborarts.org/exhibits/iww/images/1/pyramid.jpg (Accessed: June 17, 2008).

Raphael D (ed). *Social Determinants of Health: Canadian Perspectives.* Toronto: Canadian Scholars' Press, 2004.

Raphael D, Bryant T. The limitations of population health as a model for a new public health. *Health Promotion Intl* 2002; 17:189–199.

Raphael D. Barriers to addressing the societal determinants of health: public health units and poverty in Ontario, Canada. *Health Promot Int* 2003; 18:397–405.

Reeder LG. Social epidemiology: an appraisal. (Revised version of a paper read at the annual meeting of the American Sociological Association, San Francisco, September, 1969). In: Jaco EG. *Patients, Physicians, and Illness.* 2nd ed. New York: The Free Press, 1972; pp. 97–101.

Regidor E. Social determinants of health: a veil that hides socioeconomic position and its relation with health. *J Epidemiol Community Health* 2006; 60:896–901.

Robert Wood Johnson Foundation. *Overcoming Obstacles to Health: Report from the Robert Wood Johnson Foundation to the Commission to Build a Healthier America.* Princeton, NJ: Robert Wood Johnson Foundation, 2008. http://www.commissiononhealth.org/Report.aspx?Publication=26244 (Accessed: June 17, 2008).

Romero RV, Ramirez NA, Mendez PAM, Velez MOR. Health policy in Bogota (2004–2008): an analysis of the experience with primary health care. *Social Medicine* 2008; 3:126–144.

Rose H, Rose S (eds). *The Political Economy of Science: Ideology of/in the Natural Sciences.* London: Macmillan, 1976; included, with introductory essay by Ruth Hubbard, as: Rose H, Rose S (eds). *Ideology of/in the Natural Sciences.* Cambridge, MA: Schenkman, 1980. (1976b)

Rose H, Rose S (eds). *The Radicalisation of Science: Ideology of/in the Natural Sciences.* London: Macmillan, 1976; included, with introductory essay by Ruth Hubbard, in: Rose H, Rose S (eds). *Ideology of/in the Natural Sciences.* Cambridge, MA: Schenkman, 1980. (1976b)

Rosen G. *From Medical Police to Social Medicine.* New York: Science History Publications, 1974.

Rosen G. What is social medicine? A genetic analysis of the concept. *Bull Hist Med* 1947; 21: 674–733.

Rosen JB, Schulkin J. Adaptive fear, allostasis, and the pathology of anxiety and depression. In: Shulkin J (ed). *Allostasis, Homeostasis and the Costs of Physiological Adaptation.* New York: Cambridge University Press, 2004; pp. 164–227.

Russo NF, Pirlott A. Gender-based violence: concepts, methods, and findings. *Ann NY Acad Sci* 2006; 1087:178–205.

Ruzek SB, Olesen VL, Clarke AE (eds). *Women's Health: Complexities and Differences.* Columbus, OH: Ohio State University Press, 1997.

Ryle JA. *Changing Disciplines: Lectures on the History, Method and Motives of Social Pathology.* London: Oxford University Press, 1948.

Ryle JA. Social medicine: its meaning and scope. *Milbank Memorial Fund* 1944; 22:58–71.

Sand R. *The Advance to Social Medicine.* London: Staples Press, 1952.

Sanders D. *The Struggle for Health: Medicine and the Politics of Underdevelopment.* London: MacMillan, 1985.

Sapolsky RM. Social status and health in humans and other animals. *Annu Rev Anthropol* 2004; 33:393–418.

Schnall P, Gaynor D, Guttmacher S, Hopper K, Kelman S, Stark E (eds). *HMO Packet 2: The Social Etiology of Disease – Part I.* New York: Health Pac, 1977. (1977a)

Schnall P, Stark E, Hopper K, Guttmacher S (eds). *HMO Packet 3: The Social Etiology of Disease – Part II – Implications and Applications of HME.* New York: Health Pac, 1977. (1977b)

Schnall P. An introduction to historical materialist epidemiology. In: *Health Movement Organization. Health Marxist Organization (HMO) Packet 2.* New York: Health/PAC, 1977; 1–9.

Schnall PL, Kern R. Hypertension in American society: an introduction to historical materialist epidemiology. In: Conrad P, Kern R (eds). *The Sociology of Health and Illness: Critical Perspectives.* New York: St. Martin's Press, 1981; pp. 97–122.

Schofield T. Health inequity and its social determinants: a sociological commentary. *Health Sociology Review* 2007; 16:105–114.

Schrecker E. *Many are the Crimes: McCarthyism in America.* Boston: Little Brown & Co, 1998.

Schulz AJ, Mullings L (eds). *Gender, Race, Class, and Health: Intersectional Approaches.* San Francisco, CA: Jossey-Bass, 2006.

Science for the People magazine (1970-1989): Tables of content. Available at: http://socrates.berkeley. edu/~schwrtz/SftP/MagTOCs.html (Accessed: March 28, 2009).

Selye H. A syndrome produced by diverse nocous agents. *Nature* 1936; 138:32.

Selye H. *Stress in Health and Disease*. Boston: Butterworths, 1976.

Selye H. The general adaptation syndrome and the diseases of adaptation. *J Allergy* 1946; 17:231–248, 289–323, 358–398.

Sen A. Capitalism beyond the crisis. *New York Review of Books*, 2009.

Sexton K, Olden K, Johnson BL. "Environmental justice": the central role of research in establishing a credible scientific foundation for informed decision making. *Toxicol Ind Health* 1993; 9:685–727.

Shaw M, Dorling D, Gordon D, Davey Smith G. *The Widening Gap: Health Inequalities and Policy in Britain*. Bristol, UK: The Policy Press, University of Bristol, 1999.

Shulkin J (ed). *Allostasis, Homeostasis and the Costs of Physiological Adaptation*. New York: Cambridge University Press, 2004. (Shulkin 2004a).

Shulkin J. Introduction. In: Shulkin J (ed). *Allostasis, Homeostasis and the Costs of Physiological Adaptation*. New York: Cambridge University Press, 2004; pp. 1–16. (Shulkin 2004b)

Singh-Manoux A, Adler NE, Marmot MG. Subjective social status: its determinants and its association with measures of ill-health in the Whitehall II study. *Soc Sci Med* 2003; 56:1321–1333.

Smith BE. Black lung: the social production of disease. *Int J Health Services* 1981; 11:343–359.

Smith EA, Mulder MB, Bowles S, Gurven M, Hertz T, Shenk MK. Production systems, inheritance, and inequality in premodern societies. *Current Anthropol* 2010; 51:85–94.

Solar O, Irwin A. Social determinants, political contexts and civil society action: a historical perspective on the Commission on Social Determinants of Health. *Health Promot J Austr* 2006; 17:180–185.

Stansfield SA. Social support and social cohesion. In: Marmot M, Wilkinson RG (eds). *Social Determinants of Health*. Oxford: Oxford University Press, 1999; 155–178.

Starfield B. Are social determinants of health the same as societal determinants of health? *Health Promotion Journal of Australia* 2007; 17:170–173.

Stark E, Flitcraft A. Killing the beast within: woman battering and female suicidality. *Int J Health Serv* 1995; 25:43–64.

Stark E. Introduction. In: *Health Movement Organization. Health Marxist Organization (HMO) Packet 2*. New York: Health/PAC, 1977; pp. i–ii.

Stebbins El. Epidemiology and social medicine. In: Galdston I (ed). *Social Medicine: Its Derivations and Objectives*. New York: Commonwealth Fund, 1949; pp. 101–104.

Sterling P, Eyer J. Allostasis: a new paradigm to explain arousal pathology. In: Fisher S, Reason J (eds). *Handbook of Life Stress, Cognition and Health*. New York: J. Wiley & Sons, 1988; pp. 629–649.

Sterling P, Eyer J. Biological basis of stress-related mortality. *Soc Sci Med (E)* 1981; 15:3–42.

Sterling P. Principles of allostasis. In: Shulkin J (ed). *Allostasis, Homeostasis and the Costs of Physiological Adaptation*. New York: Cambridge University Press, 2004; pp. 17–64.

Stiglitz J. Davos Man's depression. Project Syndicate. Available at: http://www.project-syndicate.org/ series/11/description (Accessed: April 4, 2009).

Stonington S, Holmes SM. Social medicine in the twenty-first century. *PLoS Med* 2006; 3(10):e445.

Sydenstricker E. *Health and Environment*. New York: McGraw-Hill, 1933.

Syme SL, Berkman LF. Social class, susceptibility and sickness. *Am J Epidemiol* 1976; 104:1–8.

Syme SL. Contributions of social epidemiology to the study of medical care systems: the need for cross-cultural research. *Med Care* 1971; 9:203–213.

Szreter S. The population health approach in historical perspective. *Am J Public Health* 2003; 93: 421–431.

Tajer D. Latin American Social Medicine: roots, developments during the 1990s, and current challenges. *Am J Public Health* 2003; 93:2023–2027.

Tesh S. *Hidden Arguments: Political Ideology and Disease Prevention Policy*. New Brunswick, NJ: Rutgers University Press, 1988.

Townsend P, Davidson N, Whitehead M. *Inequalities in Health: The Black Report and the Health Divide*. London: Penguin Books, 1990.

Townsend P. Why are the many poor? *Int J Health Services* 1986; 16:1–32.

Turshen M. *The Political Ecology of Disease in Tanzania.* New Brunswick, NJ: Rutgers University Press, 1984.

United Nations. *Recommendations by the Commission of Experts of the President of the General Assembly on reforms of the international monetary and financial system.* 63rd session, agenda item 48. Available at: http://www.un.org/ga/president/63/letters/recommendationExperts200309.pdf; (Accessed: April 4, 2009).

Universal Declaration of Human Rights, adopted and proclaimed by UN General Assembly Resolution 217A(III), December 10, 1948.

Viner R. Putting stress in life: Hans Selye and the making of Stress Theory. *Social Studies Science* 1999; 29:391–410.

Viniegra L. Towards a concept of collective health. *Salud Publica Mex* 1985; 27:410–418. (Spanish)

Wadsworth MEJ. Health inequalities in the life course perspective. *Soc Sci Med* 1997; 44:859–869.

Wainright H. There IS an alternative. Reimagining socialism: a Nation forum. *The Nation*, April 2, 2009.

Waitzkin H, Iriart C, Estrada A, Lamadrid S. Social medicine in Latin America: productivity and dangers facing the major national groups. *Lancet* 2001; 358:315–323. (2001b)

Waitzkin H, Iriart C, Estrada A, Lamadrid S. Social medicine then and now: lessons from Latin America. *Am J Public Health* 2001; 91:1592–1601. (2001a)

Waitzkin H. The social origins of illness: a neglected history. *Int J Health Services* 1981; 11:77–103.

Walters KL, Simoni JM, Evans-Campbell T. Substance use among American Indians and Alaska Natives: incorporating culture in an "indigenist" stress-coping paradigm. *Public Health Rep* 2002; 117 (Suppl 1):S104–S117.

Walters KL, Simoni JM. Reconceptualizing Native women's health: An "indigenist" stress coping model. *Am J Public Health* 2002; 92:520–524.

Ward A. The social epidemiologic concept of fundamental cause. *Theor Med Bioeth* 2007; 28: 465–485.

Warner J, McKeown E, Griffin M, Johnson K, Ramsay A, Cort C, King M. Rates and predictors of mental illness in gay men, lesbians and bisexual men and women: results from a survey based in England and Wales. *Br J Psychiatry* 2004; 185:479–485.

Watts C, Zimmerman C. Violence against women: global scope and magnitude. *Lancet* 2002; 359:1232–1237.

Werskey G. The Marxist critique of capitalist science: a history in three movements? *Science as Culture* 2007; 16:397–461.

Whitbeck LB, Adams GW, Hoyt DR, Chen X. Conceptualizing and measuring historical trauma among American Indian people. *Am J Community Psychol* 2004; 33:119–130.

Whitehead M, Scott-Samuel A, Dahlgren G. Setting targets to address inequalities in health. *Lancet* 1998; 351:1279–1282.

Wilkinson R, Marmot M (eds). *Social Determinants of Health: The Solid Facts.* 1st ed. Copenhagen: WHO Regional Office for Europe, 1998.

Wilkinson R, Pickett K. *The Spirit Level: Why More Equal Societies Almost Always Do Better.* London: Allen Lane, Penguin Books, 2009.

Wilkinson RG. *Mind the Gap: Hierarchies, Health and Human Evolution.* New Haven, CT: Yale University Press, 2001.

Wilkinson RG. *The Impact of Inequality: How to Make Sick Societies Healthier.* New York: The New Press, 2005.

Williams DR, Mohammed SA. Discrimination and racial disparities in health: evidence and needed research. *J Behav Med* 2009; 32:20–47.

Williams DR, Neighbors HW, Jackson JS. Racial/ethnic discrimination and health: findings from community studies. *Am J Public Health* 2003; 93:200–208.

Williams DR. Race, socioeconomic status, and health: the added effects of racism and discrimination. *Ann NY Acad Sci* 1999; 896:173–188.

Wing S, Horton RA, Muhammad N, Grant GR, Tajik M, Thu K. Integrating epidemiology, education, and organizing for educational justice: community health effects of industrial hog operations. *Am J Public Health* 2008; 98:1390–1397.

Wise P, Chavkin W, Romero D. Assessing the effects of welfare reform policies on reproductive and infant health. *Am J Public Health* 1999; 89:1514–1521.

Wise PH. Framework as metaphor: the promise and perils of MCH-lifecourse perspectives. *Maternal Child Health* 2003; 7:151–156.

Wolfe EL, Barger AC, Benison S. *Walter B. Cannon, Science and Society.* Cambridge, MA: Harvard University Press, 2000.

Woolf SH. Social policy as health policy. *JAMA* 2009; 301:1166–1169.

World Health Organization Commission on Social Determinants of Health (CSDH). *A Conceptual Framework for Action on the Social Determinants of Health.* Discussion paper for the Commission on the Social Determinants of Health, April 2007. http://www.who.int/social_determinants/resources/csdh_framework_action_05_07.pdf (Accessed: June 17, 2008).

World Health Organization, CSDH. *Closing the gap in a generation: health equity through action on the social determinants of health. Final Report of the Commission on Social Determinants of Health.* Geneva: World Health Organization, 2008.

XIV Conference of the Latin American and Caribbean Association of Schools of Public Health. Final Report and Recommendations. *Epidemiological Bulletin* 1988; 9:1–8.

Yankauer A. The relationship of fetal and infant mortality to residential segregation: an inquiry into social epidemiology. *Am Sociol Review* 1950; 15:644–648.

Young TK. *Population Health: Concepts and Methods.* New York: Oxford University Press, 1998.

Zinn H. *A People's History of the United States.* New York: HarperCollins, 2003.

Chapter 7

Abrums M. Faith and feminism: how African American women from a storefront church resist oppression in health care. *Advances in Nursing Science, Advances in Research Methods (Part II)* 2004; 27:187–201.

Adler NE, Ostrove JM. Socioeconomic status and health: what we know and what we don't. *Ann NY Acad Sci* 1999; 986:3–15.

Adler NE, Rehkopf DH. U.S. disparities in health: descriptions, causes, and mechanisms. *Annu Rev Public Health* 2008; 29:235–252.

Aoki Y. Polychlorinated biphenyls, polychlorinated dibenzo-p-dioxins, and polychlorinated dibenzofurans as endocrine disrupters—what we have learned from Yusho disease. *Environ Res* 2001; 86:2–11.

Archer A, Bhaskar R, Collier R, Lawson T, Norrie A. *Critical Realism: Essential Readings.* London: Routledge, 1998.

Atkinson A. *Principles of Political Ecology.* London: Belhaven Press, 1993.

Azambuja MIR, Duncan BB. Capturing determinants of vulnerability from modifications in disease occurrence. *Cad. Saúde Pública, Rio de Janeiro* 2002; 18:571–577.

Baer HA, Singer M. *Global Warming and the Political Ecology of Health: Emerging Crises and Systemic Solutions.* Walnut Creek, CA: Left Coast Press, 2009.

Baer HA. Bringing political ecology into critical medical anthropology: a challenge to biocultural approaches. *Med Anthropol* 1996; 17:129–141.

Ball P. *Flow: Nature's Patterns: A Tapestry in Three Parts.* Oxford: Oxford University Press, 2009.

Barbeau EM, McLellan D, Levenstein C, DeLaurier GF, Kelder G, Sorensen G. Reducing occupation-based disparities related to tobacco: roles for occupational health and organized labor. *Am J Industrial Med* 2004; 46:170–179.

Barbour MG. Ecological fragmentation in the fifties. In: Cronon W (ed). *Uncommon Ground: Rethinking the Human Place in Nature.* New York: W.W. Norton, 1996; pp. 233–255.

Bauer G, Davies JK, Pelikan J, Noack H, Broesskamp U, Hill C. Advancing a theoretical model for public health and health promotion indicator development. *Eur J Public Health* 2003; 13(Suppl 10):107–113.

Bellinger DC. Lead neurotoxicity and socioeconomic status: conceptual and analytical issues. *Neurotoxicology* 2008; 29:823–828.

Ben-Shlomo Y, Kuh D. A life course approach to chronic disease epidemiology: conceptual models, empirical challenges and interdisciplinary perspectives. *Int J Epidemiol* 2002; 31:285–293.

Berkman LF, Kawachi I (eds). *Social Epidemiology*. Oxford: Oxford University Press, 2000.

Bernardi SM, Ebi KL. Comments on the process and product of the health impacts assessment components of the National Assessment of the Potential Consequences of Climate Variability and Change for the United States. *Environ Health Perspect* 2001; 109(suppl 2):177–184.

Bhaskar R. *A Realist Theory of Science*. 2nd ed. Sussex: The Harvester Press, 1978.

Biersack A, Greenberg JB (eds). *Reimagining Political Ecology*. Durham, NC: Duke University press, 2006.

Biersack A. Reimagining political ecology: culture/power/history/nature. In: Biersack A, Greenberg JB. *Reimagining Political Ecology*. Durham, NC: Duke University Press, 2006; pp. 3–40.

Birn AE, Pillay Y, Holtz TH. *Textbook of International Health: Global Health in a Dynamic World*. Oxford: Oxford University Press, 2009.

Bock GR, Goode JA. *The Limits of Reductionism in Biology*. (Novartis Foundation Symposium 213). Chichester, UK: John Wiley & Sons, 1998.

Bourdieu P. *Distinction: A Social Critique of the Judgment of Taste*. (Translated by Richard Nice). Cambridge, MA: Harvard University Press, 1984.

Bramwell A. *Ecology in the 20th century: a history*. New Haven: Yale University Press, 1989.

Brandt A. *The Cigarette Century: The Rise, Fall, and Deadly Persistence of the Product that Defined America*. New York: Basic Books, 2007.

Bronfenbrenner U (ed). *Making Human Beings Human: Bioecological Perspectives on Human Development*. Thousand Oaks, CA: Sage Publications, 2005.

Bronfenbrenner U. The bioecological theory of human development. In: Smelser NJ, Baltes PB (eds). *International Encyclopedia of the Social and Behavioral Sciences*. New York: Elsevier, 2001; pp. 6963–6970.

Bronfenbrenner U. *The Ecology of Human Development: Experiments by Nature and Design*. Cambridge, MA: Harvard University Press, 1979.

Brothwell D (ed). *Biosocial Man: Studies Related to the Interaction of Biological and Cultural Factors in Human Populations*. London: Institute of Biology for the Eugenics Society, 1977.

Buerton PJ, Falk R, Rheinberger H-J (eds). *The Concept of the Gene in Development and Evolution: Historical and Epistemological Perspectives*. Cambridge: Cambridge University Press, 2000.

Buffardi AL, Thomas KK, Holmes KK, Manhart LE. Moving upstream: ecosocial and psychosocial correlates of sexually transmitted infections among young adults in the United States. *Am J Public Health* 2008; 98:1128–1136.

Burris S, Blankenship KM, Donoghoe M, Sherman S, Vernick JS, Case P, Lazzarini Z, Koester S. Addressing the "Risk Environment" for injection drug users: the mysterious case of the missing cop. *Milbank Quarterly* 2004; 82:125–156.

Calvo P, Gomila T (eds). *Handbook of Cognitive Science: An Embodied Approach*. Amsterdam: Elsevier, 2008.

Carter-Pokras O, Zamabrana RE, Poppell CF, Logie LA, Guerrero-Preston R. The environmental health of Latino children. *J Pediatr Health Care* 2007; 21:307–314.

Cassel J. Social science theory as a source of hypotheses in epidemiologic research. *Am J Public Health* 1964; 54:1482–1488.

Chew MK, Laubichler MD. Natural enemies–metaphors or misconceptions? *Science* 2003; 301: 52–53.

Chilton M. Developing a measure of dignity for stress-related health outcomes. *Health Hum Rights* 2006; 9:208–233.

Cockburn A, Ridgeway J (eds). *Political Ecology*. New York: New York Times, 1979.

Cook R. *The Tree of Life: Image for the Cosmos*. New York: Thames and Hudson, 1988.

Corburn J. Confronting the challenges in reconnecting urban planning and public health. *Am J Public Health* 2004; 94:541–546.

Cregan K. *The Sociology of the Body: Mapping the Abstraction of Embodiment*. London: Sage, 2006.

Cronon W (ed). *Uncommon Ground: Rethinking the Human Place in Nature*. New York: W.W. Norton, 1996.

Crossley N. Sociology and the body. In: Calhoun C, Rojek C, Turner B (eds). *The Sage Handbook of Sociology*. Thousand Oaks, CA: Sage Publications, 2005; pp. 442–456.

Csordas TJ. Introduction: the body as representation and being-in-the-world. In: Csordas TJ (ed). *Embodiment and Experience: The Existential Ground of Culture and Self*. Cambridge: Cambridge University Press, 1994; pp. 1–24.

Damasio A. *Looking for Spinoza: Joy, Sorrow, and the Feeling Brain*. Orlando, FL: Harcourt, 2003.

Darwin C. *The Origin of Species By Means of Natural Selection or the Preservation of Favoured Races in the Struggle for Life* (1859). Edison, NJ: Castle Books, 2004.

Doolittle WF, Bapteste. Pattern pluralism and the Tree of Life hypothesis. *PNAS* 2007; 104: 2043–2049.

Doyal L. *The Political Economy of Health*. London: Pluto Press, 1979.

Doyal L. *What Makes Women Sick? Gender and The Political Economy of Health*. New Brunswick, NJ: Rutgers University Press, 1995.

Earls F. The social ecology of child health and well-being. *Annual Review Public Health* 2001; 22:143–166.

Edwards N, Mill J, Kothari AR. Multiple intervention research programs in community health. *Canadian J Nursing Research* 2004; 36:40–54.

Eldredge N, Grene M. *Interactions: The Biological Context of Social Systems*. New York: Columbia University Press, 1992.

Eldredge N. *Darwin: Discovering the Tree of Life*. New York: W.W. Norton, 2005.

Eldredge N. *The Pattern of Evolution*. New York: W.H. Freeman & Co., 1999.

Ellis JC. On the search for a root cause: essentialist tendencies in environmental discourse. In: Cronon W (ed). *Uncommon Ground: Rethinking the Human Place in Nature*. New York: W.W. Norton, 1996; pp. 256–268.

Elreedy S, Krieger N, Ryan BP, Sparrow D, Weiss ST, Hu H. Relations between individual and neighborhood-based measures of socioeconomic position and bone lead concentrations among community-exposed men: the Normative Aging study. *Am J Epidemiol* 1999; 150:129–141.

Érdi P. *Complexity Explained*. Berlin: Springer, 2008.

Ernst W, Harris B (eds). *Race, Science and Medicine, 1700-1960*. London: Routledge, 1999.

Escobar A. After nature: steps to an antiessentialist political ecology. *Current Anthropology* 1999; 40:1–16.

Evans RG, Barer ML, Marmot TR (eds). *Why Are Some People Healthy and Others Not? The Determinants of Health of Populations*. New York: Aldine de Gruyter, 1994.

Evans RG, Stoddart GL. Consuming research, producing policy? *Am J Public Health* 2003; 93: 371–379.

Fassin D, Naudé AJ. Plumbism reinvented: childhood leading poisoning in France, 1985-1990. *Am J Public Health* 2004; 94:1854–1863.

Fee E, Krieger N. *Women's Health, Politics, and Power: Essays on Sex/Gender, medicine, and Public Policy*. Amityville, NY: Baywood Publishers, 1994.

Feldman T, Silver R. Gender differences and the outcome of interventions for acute coronary syndromes. *Cardiol Rev* 2000; 8:240–247.

Forsyth T. *Critical Political Ecology: The Politics of Environmental Science*. London: Routledge, 2003.

Fox NJ. *Beyond Health: Postmodernism and Embodiment*. London: Free Association Books, 1999.

Fox R (ed). *Biosocial Anthropology*. London: Malaby Press, 1975.

Franks P, Fiscella K. Reducing disparities downstream: prospects and challenges. *J Gen Intern Med* 2008; 23:672–677.

Frenk J, Bobadilla JL, Sepúlveda J, López-Cervantes M. Health transition in middle-income countries: new challenges for health care. *Health Policy Planning* 1989; 4:29–39.

Galea S, Vlahov D. Urban health: evidence, challenges, and directions. *Annu Rev Public Health* 2005; 26:341–365.

Gaylin DS, Kates J. Refocusing the lens: epidemiologic transition theory, mortality differentials, and the AIDS pandemic. *Soc Sci Med* 1997; 44:609–621.

Gehlert S, Sohmer D, Sacks T, Mininger C, McClintock M, Olopade O. Targeting health disparities: a model linking upstream determinants to downstream interventions. *Health Aff (Milwood)* 2008; 27:339–349.

Gilbert S. Ecological developmental biology: developmental biology meets the real world. *Developmental Biol* 2001; 233:1–12.

Gillespie S, Kadiyala S, Greener R. Is poverty or wealth driving HIV transmission? *AIDS* 2007; 21(Suppl 7):S5–S16.

Glass TA, McAtee MJ. Behavioral science at the crossroads in public health: extending horizons, envisioning the future. *Soc Sci Med* 2006; 62:1650–1671.

Gleick J. *Chaos: Making a New Science.* New York: Viking, 1987.

Godette DC, Headen S, Ford CL. Windows of opportunity: fundamental concepts for understanding alcohol-related disparities experienced by young Blacks in the United States. *Prev Sci* 2006; 7:377–387.

Goldberg M, Melchior M, Leclerc A, Lert F. Epidemiology and social determinants of health inequalities. *Rev Epidemiol Sante Publique* 2003; 51:381–401.

Goldberger AL, Amaral LA, Hausdorff JM, Ivanov PCh, Peng CK, Stanley HE. Fractal dynamics in physiology: alterations with disease and aging. *Proc Natl Acad Sci* USA 2002; 99 (suppl 1):2466–2472.

Goldberger AL, Rigney DR, West BJ. Chaos and fractals in human physiology. *Sci Am* 1990; February: 43–49.

Goldberger AL. Non-linear dynamics for clinicians: chaos theory, fractals, and complexity at the bedside. *Lancet* 1996; 347:1312–1314.

Goldstein LF (ed). *Contemporary Cases in Women's Rights.* Madison, WI: University of Wisconsin Press, 1994; pp. 3–32.

Gomila T, Calvo P. Directions for an embodied cognitive science: toward an integrated approach. In: Calvo P, Gomila A (eds). *Handbook of Cognitive Science: An Embodied Approach.* Amsterdam: Elsevier Science, 2008; pp. 1–25.

Graham H. Smoking prevalence among women in the European community 1950–1990. *Soc Sci Med* 1996; 43:243–254.

Graham H. *Unequal Lives: Health and Socio-Economic Inequalities.* Berkshire, England: Open University Press, 2007.

Graves JAM. The Tree of Life: view from a twig. *Science* 2003; 300:1621.

Gravlee CC. How race becomes biology: embodiment of social inequality. *Am J Phys Anthropol* 2009; doi: 10.1002/ajpa.20982

Greenberg JB, Park TK. Political ecology: editors preface. *J Political Ecology* 1994; 1:1–12.

Greenberg JB. The political ecology of fisheries in the Upper Gulf of California. In: Biersack A, Greenberg JB. *Reimagining Political Ecology.* Durham, NC: Duke University Press, 2006; pp. 121–147.

Grene M, Depew D. *The Philosophy of Biology: An Episodic History.* Cambridge, UK: Cambridge University Press, 2004.

Grene M. Historical realism and contextual objectivity: a developing perspective in the philosophy of science. In: Nersessian NJ (ed). *The Process of Science: Contemporary Philosophical Approaches to Understanding Scientific Practice.* Dordrecht: Martinus Nihhoff (Kluwer Academic Publishers), 1987; pp. 69–81.

Hader SL, Smith DK, Moore JS, Holmberg SD. HIV infection in women in the United States: status at the Millennium. *JAMA* 2001; 285:1186–1192.

Hall PA, Lamont M (eds). *Successful Societies: How Institutions and Culture Affect Health.* New York: Cambridge University Press, 2009.

Hamlin C. STS: where the Marxist critique of capitalist science goes to die? *Science as Culture* 2007; 16:467–474.

Hanchette CL. The political ecology of lead poisoning in eastern North Carolina. *Health Place* 2008; 14:209–216.

Hannan MT. Population ecology. In: Smelser NJ, Baltes PB (eds). *International Encyclopedia of the Social & Behavioral Sciences.* Oxford, UK: Pergamon, 2001; pp. 11780–11784. DOI: 10.1016/B0-08-043076-7/02013-1.

Haraway DJ. *The Haraway Reader.* New York: Routledge, 2004.

Hargreaves JR, Bonell CP, Boler T, Boccia D, Birdthistle I, Fletcher A, Pronyk PM, Glynn JR. Systematic review exploring time trends in the association between educational attainment and risk of HIV infection in sub-Saharan Africa. *AIDS* 2008; 22:403–414.

Harper J. Breathless in Houston: a political ecology approach to understanding environmental health concerns. *Med Anthropol* 2004; 23:295–326.

Harrison GA, Peel J (eds). *Biosocial Aspects of Race: Proceedings of the Fifth Annual Symposium of the Eugenics Society.* Oxford: Blackwell Scientific, for the Galton Foundation, 1969.

Harrison GA, Peel J (eds). *Biosocial Aspects of Sex; Proceedings of the Sixth Annual Symposium of the Eugenics Society, London, September 1969.* Oxford: Blackwell Scientific Publications, for the Galton Foundation, 1970.

Hertzman C, Siddiqi A. Population health and the dynamics of collective development. In: Hall PA, Lamont M (eds). *Successful Societies: How Institutions and Culture Affect Health.* New York: Cambridge University Press, 2009; pp. 23–52.

Hertzman C. The biological embedding of early experience and its effects on health in adulthood. *Ann NY Acad Sci* 1999; 896:85–95.

Heuveline P, Guillot M, Gwatkin DR. The uneven tides of the health transition. *Soc Sci Med* 2002; 55: 313–322.

Hobbs RJ. Managing ecological systems and processes. In: Peterson DL, Parker VT (eds). *Ecological Scale: Theories and Application.* New York: Columbia University Press, 1998; pp. 459–484.

Hobsbawm E. *The Age of Extremes: The Short Twentieth Century, 1914-1991.* London: Michael Joseph, 1994.

Hofrichter R (ed). *Health and Social Justice: Politics, Ideology, and Inequity in the Distribution of Disease.* San Francisco, CA: Jossey-Bass, 2003.

Honori M, Boylen T (eds). *Health Ecology: Health, Culture, and Human-Environment Interactions.* London: Routledge, 1999.

Hvalkof S. Progress of the victims: political ecology in the Peruvian Amazon. In: Biersack A, Greenberg JB. *Reimagining Political Ecology.* Durham, NC: Duke University Press, 2006; pp. 195–231.

Institute of Medicine. *Legalized Abortion and the Public Health: Report of a Study, by a Committee of the Institute of Medicine.* Washington, DC: National Academy of Sciences, 1975.

Ippolito G, Puro V, Heptonstall J, Jagger J, De Carli G, Petrosillo N. Occupational human immunodeficiency virus infection in health care workers: worldwide cases through September 1997. *Clin Infect Dis* 1999; 28:365–383.

Jackson JP Jr, Weidman NM. *Race, Racism, and Science: Social Impact and Interaction.* Santa Barbara, CA: ABC-CLIO, 2004.

Jacobs DE, Kelly T, Sobolewski J. Linking public health, housing, and indoor environmental policy: successes and challenges at local and federal agencies in the United States. *Environ Health Perspect* 2007; 115:976–982.

Jasanaoff S. Ordering knowledge, ordering society. In: Jasanoff S (ed). *States of Knowledge: The Co-Production of Science and Social Order.* London: Routledge, 2004; pp. 13–45. (2004c)

Jasanaoff S. The idiom of co-production. In: Jasanoff S (ed). *States of Knowledge: The Co-Production of Science and Social Order.* London: Routledge, 2004; pp. 1–12. (2004b)

Jasanoff S (ed). *States of Knowledge: The Co-Production of Science and Social Order.* London: Routledge, 2004. (2004a)

Jax K. History of ecology. In: *Encyclopedia of Life Sciences (ELS).* Chichester, UK: John Wiley & Sons, Ltd, 2008; http://www.els.net/(doi: 10.1038/npg.els.0003084)

Journal of Biosocial Science. Available at: http://journals.cambridge.org/action/displayJournal?jid=JBS (Accessed: June 22, 2009).

Kauppi N. *The Politics of Embodiment: Habits, Power, and Pierre Bourdieu's Theory.* Frankfurt: Peter Lang, 2000.

Kearns R, Moewaka-Barnes, McCreanor T. Placing racism in public health: a perspective from Aotearoa/New Zealand. *GeoJournal* 2009; 74:123–129.

Kegler MC, Miner K. Environmental health promotion interventions: considerations for preparation and practice. *Health Educ & Behavior* 2004; 31:510–525.

Keil R, Bell DVJ, Penz P, Fawcett L (eds). *Political Ecology: Global and Local*. London: Routledge, 1998.

Keller EF. *Making Sense of Life: Explaining Biological Development with Models, Metaphors, and Machines*. Cambridge, MA: Harvard University Press, 2002.

Kelso JAS. Self-organizing dynamical systems. In: Smesler NJ, Baltes PB (eds). *International Encyclopedia of the Social & Behavioral Sciences*. Oxford, UK: Pergamon, 2002; pp. 13,844–13,850. doi: 10.1016/B0-080043076-7/00568-4.

Kickbush I. Approaches to an ecological base for public health. *Health Promotion* 1989; 4:265–268.

Kitcher P. *Science, Truth, and Democracy*. New York: Oxford University Press, 2001.

Kravdal O. Is the relationship between childbearing and cancer incidence due to biology or lifestyle? Examples of the importance of using data on men. *Int J Epidemiol* 1995; 4:477–484.

Krieger N (ed). *Embodying Inequality: Epidemiologic Perspectives*. Amityville, NY: Baywood Publishing Co., 2004. (2004a)

Krieger N, Bassett M. The health of black folk: disease, class and ideology in science. *Monthly Review* 1986; 38:74–85.

Krieger N, Birn AE. A vision of social justice as the foundation of public health: commemorating 150 years of the spirit of 1848. *Am J Public Health* 1998; 88:1603–1606.

Krieger N, Chen JT, Waterman PD, Soobader M-J, Subramanian SV, Carson R. Choosing area-based socioeconomic measures to monitor social inequalities in low birthweight and childhood lead poisoning—*The Public Health Disparities Geocoding Project* (US). *J Epidemiol Community Health* 2003; 57:186–199.

Krieger N, Davey Smith G. Bodies count & body counts: social epidemiology & embodying inequality. *Epidemiol Review* 2004; 26:92–103.

Krieger N, Gruskin S. Frameworks matter: ecosocial and health & human rights perspectives on women and health—the case of tuberculosis. *J Am Women's Med Assoc* 2001; 56:137–142.

Krieger N, Margo G (eds). *AIDS: The Politics of Survival*. Amityville, NY: Baywood Publications, Inc., 1994.

Krieger N, Rehkopf DH, Chen JT, Waterman PD, Marcelli E, Kennedy M. The fall and rise of US inequities in premature mortality: 1960–2002. *PLoS Med* 2008; 5(2): e46. doi:10.1371/journal.pmed.0050046.

Krieger N, Rowley DL, Herman AA, Avery B, Phillips MT. Racism, sexism, and social class: implications for studies of health, disease, and well-being. *Am J Prev Med* 1993; 9 (Suppl):82–122.

Krieger N. A glossary for social epidemiology. *J Epidemiol Community Health* 2001; 55:693–700. (2001c)

Krieger N. Commentary: society, biology, and the logic of social epidemiology. *Int J Epidemiol* 2001; 30:44–46. (2001b)

Krieger N. Defining and investigating social disparities in cancer: critical issues. *Cancer Causes Control* 2005; 16:5–14. (2005c)

Krieger N. Does racism harm health? did child abuse exist before 1962?—on explicit questions, critical science, and current controversies: an ecosocial perspective. *Am J Public Health* 2003; 93:194–199. (2003a)

Krieger N. Ecological urbanism & health equity: an ecosocial perspective. In: Mostafavi M, Doherty G (eds). *Ecological Urbanism*. Baden, Switzerland: Lard Muller, 2010; pp. 518–519 (2010a)

Krieger N. Ecosocial theory. In: Anderson N (ed). *Encyclopedia of Health and Behavior*. Thousand Oaks, CA: Sage, 2004; pp. 292–294. (2004b)

Krieger N. Embodiment: a conceptual glossary for epidemiology. *J Epidemiol Community Health* 2005; 59:350–355. (2005a)

Krieger N. Embodying inequality: a review of concepts, measures, and methods for studying health consequences of discrimination. *Int J Health Services* 1999; 29:295–352; slightly revised and republished as: Krieger N. Discrimination and health. In: Berkman L, Kawachi I (eds). Social Epidemiology. Oxford: Oxford University Press, 2000; pp. 36–75. (1999b)

Krieger N. Epidemiology and social sciences: towards a critical reengagement in the 21st century. *Epidemiologic Reviews* 2000; 11:155–163. (2000a)

Krieger N. Epidemiology and the web of causation: has anyone seen the spider? *Soc Sci Med* 1994; 39:887–903.

Krieger N. Genders, sexes, and health: what are the connections—and why does it matter? *Int J Epidemiol* 2003; 32:652–657. (2003b)

Krieger N. Ladders, pyramids, and champagne: the iconography of health inequities. *J Epidemiol Community Health* 2008; 62:1098–1104. (2008b)

Krieger N. Proximal, distal, and the politics of causation: what's level got to do with it? *Am J Public Health* 2008; 98:221–230. (2008a)

Krieger N. Putting health inequities on the map: social epidemiology meets medical/health geography–an ecosocial perspective. *GeoJournal* 2009; 74:87–97. (2009a)

Krieger N. Refiguring "race": epidemiology, racialized biology, and biological expressions of race relations. *Int J Health Services* 2000; 30:211–216. (2000b)

Krieger N. Researching critical questions on social justice and public health: an ecosocial perspective. In: Levy BS, Sidel VW (eds). *Social Injustice and Public Health*. New York: Oxford University Press, 2006; pp. 460–479.

Krieger N. Shades of difference: theoretical underpinnings of the medical controversy on black-white differences, 1830–1870. *Int J Health Services* 1987; 17:258–279.

Krieger N. Sticky webs, hungry spiders, buzzing flies, and fractal metaphors: on the misleading juxtaposition of "risk factor" vs "social" epidemiology. *J Epidemiol Community Health* 1999; 53:678–680. (1999a)

Krieger N. Stormy weather: "race," gene expression, and the science of health disparities. *Am J Public Health* 2005; 95:2155–2160. (2005b)

Krieger N. The ostrich, the albatross, and public health: an ecosocial perspective—or why an explicit focus on health consequences of discrimination and deprivation is vital for good science and public health practice. *Public Health Reports* 2001; 116:419–423. (2001d)

Krieger N. The science and epidemiology of racism and health: racial/ethnic categories, biological expressions of racism, and the embodiment of inequality–an ecosocial perspective. Whitmarsh I, Jones DS (eds). *What's the Use of Race? Genetics and Difference in Forensics, Medicine, and Scientific Research*. Cambridge, MA: MIT Press 2010; 225–255. (2010b)

Krieger N. Theories for social epidemiology in the 21st century: an ecosocial perspective. *Int J Epidemiol* 2001; 30:668–677. (2001a)

Krieger N. Ways of asking and ways of living: reflections on the 50th anniversary of Morris' ever-useful *Uses of Epidemiology*. *Int J Epidemiol* 2007; 36:1173–1180.

Krieger N. Workers are people too: societal aspects of occupational health disparities–an ecosocial perspective (commentary). *Am J Industrial Medicine* 2010; 53:104–115; doi:10.1002/ajim.20759. (2010c)

Kunitz S. *The Health of Populations: General Theories and Particular Realities*. Oxford: Oxford University Press, 2006.

Kunitz SJ. The value of particularism in the study of the cultural, social and behavioral determinants of mortality. In: Ledergerg J, Shope RE, Oaks SC Jr (eds). *What We Know About Health Transition." The Cultural, Social, and Behavioral Determinants of Health*, Proceedings of an International Workshop, Canberra, Vol. 1. Canberrra, Australia: The Australian National University, 1992; pp. 92–109.

Kuzawa CV, Sweet E. Epigenetics and the embodiment of race: developmental origins of US racial disparities in cardiovascular health. *Am J Hum Biol* 2009; 21:2–15.

Lajoi SP. Extending the scaffolding metaphor. *Instructional Sci* 2005; 33:541–557.

Lakoff G, Johnson M. *Philosophy in the Flesh: The Embodied Mind and its Challenge to Western Thought*. New York: Basic Books, 1999.

Lanham JT, Kohl SG, Bedell JH. Changes in pregnancy outcome after liberalization of the New York State abortion law. *Am J Obstet Gynecol* 1974; 118:485–492.

Lansing JS, Schoenfelder J, Scarborough V. Rappaport's rose: structure, agency, and historical contingency in ecological anthropology. In: Biersack A, Greenberg JB. *Reimagining Political Ecology*. Durham, NC: Duke University Press, 2006; pp. 325–357.

Lawlor DA, Emberson JR, Ebrahim S, Whincup PH, Wannamethee SG, Walker M, Smith GD. Is the association between parity and coronary heart disease due to biological effects of pregnancy or adverse lifestyle risk factors associated with child-rearing? *Circulation* 2003; 11:1260–1264.

Lawrence RJ. Can human ecology provide an integrative framework? The contribution of structuration theory to contemporary debate. In: Steiner D, Nauser M (eds). *Human Ecology: Fragments of Anti-Fragmentary Views of the World*. London: Routledge, 1993; pp. 213–228.

Lawton G. Why Darwin was wrong about the tree of life. *New Scientist* 2009; available at: http://www.newscientist.com/article/mg20126921.600-why-darwin-was-wrong-about-the-tree-of-life.html (Accessed: June 23, 2009).

Lee KW, Paneth N, Gartner LM, Pearlman MA, Gruss L. Neonatal mortality: an analysis of the recent improvement in the United States. *Am J Public Health* 1980; 70:15–21.

Lefkowitz B. *Community Health Centers: A Movement and the People Who Made it Happen*. New Brunswick, NJ: Rutgers University Press, 2007.

Leslie WD, Lentle B. Race/ethnicity and fracture risk assessment: an issue that is more than skin deep. *J Clinical Densitometry* 2006; 9:406–412.

Levin SA. The problem of pattern and scale in ecology: the Robert H. MacArthur Award lecture. *Ecology* 1992; 73:1943–1967.

Levins R, Lopez C. Toward an ecosocial view of health. *Int J Health Serv* 1999; 29:261–293.

Levins R. Ten propositions on science and antiscience. *Social Text* 1996; 46/47:101–111.

Lewontin R. *The Triple Helix: Gene, Organism, and Environment*. Cambridge, MA: Harvard University Press, 2000.

Lidicker WZ Jr. Levels of organization in biology: on the nature and nomenclature of ecology's fourth level. *Biol Rev Camb Philos Soc* 2008; 83:71–78.

Lieberman-Aiden E, van Berkum NL, Williams L, Imakeaev M, Ragoczy T, Telling A, Amit I, Lajoie BR, Sabo PJ, Dorschner MO, Sandstrom R, Bernstein B, Bender MA, Groudine M, Gnirke A, Stamatoyannopoulous J, Mirny LA, Lander ES, Dekker J. Comprehensive mapping of long-range interactions reveals folding principles of the human genome. *Science* 2009; 326:289–293.

Liesegang TJ. Contact lens-related microbial keratitis: Part I: Epidemiology. *Cornea* 1997; 16:125–131.

Lipsitz LA, Goldberger AL. Loss of "complexity" and aging: potential applications of fractals and chaos theory to senescence. *JAMA* 1992; 267:1806–1809.

López J. *Society and Its Metaphors: Language, Social Theory, and Social Structure*. New York: Continuum, 2003.

Low N, Gleeson B. *Justice, Society, and Nature: An Exploration of Political Ecology*. London; New York: Routledge, 1998.

Lupien SJ, King S, Meaney MJ, McEwen BS. Can poverty get under your skin? basal cortisol levels and cognitive function in children from low and high socioeconomic status. *Dev Psychopathol* 2001; 13:653–676.

Maas RP, Patch SC, Morgan DM, Pandolfo TJ. Reducing lead exposure from drinking water: recent history and current status. *Public Health Rep* 2005; 120:316–321.

MacDonald MA. From miasma to fractals: the epidemiology revolution and public health nursing. *Public Health Nurs* 2004; 21:380–391.

Mackenbach JP. The epidemiologic transition theory. *J Epidemiol Community Health* 1994; 48: 329–331.

Madden LV, Hughes G, van den Bosch X. *The Study of Plant Disease Epidemics*. St. Paul, Minnesota: American Phytopathological Society, 2007.

Maddison DR, Schulz KS. (eds.) The Tree of Life Web Project, 2007. Available at: http://tolweb.org (Accessed: June 22, 2009).

Mandelbrot B. *The Fractal Geometry of Nature*. New York: Freeman, 1982.

March D, Susser E. Invited commentary: taking the search for causes of schizophrenia to a different level. *Am J Epidemiol 2006*; 163:979–981. (2006b)

March D, Susser E. The eco- in eco-epidemiology. *Int J Epidemiol 2006*; 35:1379–1383. (editorial) (2006a)

Markowitz G, Rosner D. *Deceit and Denial: The Deadly Politics of Industrial Pollution*. University of California Press, Berkeley, 2002.

Marmot M, Wilkinson R (eds). *The Social Determinants of Health*. Oxford: Oxford University Press, 1999.

Mascie-Taylor CGN (ed). *Biosocial Aspects of Social Class*. Oxford: Oxford University Press, 1990.

Maupin JE JR, Schlundt D, Warren R, Miller S, Goldzweig I, Warren H. Reducing unintentional injuries on the nation's highways: research and program policy to increase seat belt use. *J Health Care Poor Underserved* 2004; 15:4–17.

May R. Levels of organization in ecological systems. In: Bock GR, Goode JA. *The Limits of Reductionism in Biology*. (Novartis Foundation Symposium 213). Chichester, UK: John Wiley & Sons, 1998; pp. 193–202.

Mayer JD. The political ecology of disease as one new focus for medical geography. *Progress in Human Geography* 1996; 20:441–456.

Mazumdar PMH. Essays in the History of Eugenics (review). *Bulletin History Medicine* 2000; 74:180–183.

McAdam D, Tarrows S, Tilly C. *Dynamics of Contention*. Cambridge: Cambridge University Press, 2001.

McIntosh RP. *The Background of Ecology: Concept and Theory*. New York: Cambridge University Press, 1985.

McKinlay JB, Marceau LD. To boldly go...*Am J Public Health* 2000; 90:25–33.

McLaren L, Hawe P. Ecological perspectives in health research. *J Epidemiol Community Health* 2005; 59:6–14.

McMichael AJ. Environmental and social influences on emerging infectious diseases: past, present, and future. *Philos Trans R Soc Lond B Biol Sci* 2004; 359:1049–1058.

McMichael AJ. *Human Frontiers, Environments, and Disease: Past Patterns, Uncertain Futures*. Cambridge: Cambridge University Press, 2001.

McMichael AJ. Population, environment, disease, and survival: past patterns, uncertain futures. *Lancet* 2002; 359:1145–1148.

McMichael AJ. Prisoners of the proximate: loosening the constraints on epidemiology in an age of change. *Am J Epidemiol* 1999; 149:887–897.

McMichael AJ. The health of persons, populations, and planets: epidemiology comes full circle. *Epidemiol* 1995; 6:633–636.

Melvin CL, Rogers M, Gilbert BC, Lipscomb L, Lorenz R, Ronck S, Casey S. Pregnancy Intention: How PRAMS Data Can Inform Programs and Policy. *Matern Child Health J* 2000; 4:197–201.

Merchant C. *The Columbia Guide to American Environmental History*. New York: Columbia University Press, 2002.

Mitchell M. *Complexity: A Guided Tour*. New York: Oxford, 2009.

Morello-Frosch R, Lopez R. The riskscape and the color line: examining the role of segregation in environmental health disparities. *Environ Res* 2006; 102:181–196.

Morris J. *Uses of Epidemiology*. Edinburgh: E. & S. Livingston, Ltd, 1957.

Mutch WA, Lefevre GR. Health, 'small worlds,' fractals, and complex networks: an emerging field. *Med Sci Monitor* 2003; 9:9–23.

Navarro V, Shi LY. The political context of social inequalities and health. *Soc Sci Med* 2001; 52: 481–491.

Needham J. *Order and Life*. Cambridge, MA: The MIT Press, 1968 (New Haven, CT: Yale University Press, 1936).

Nettleton S, Watson J. *The Body in Everyday Life*. London: Routledge, 1998.

Neumann RP. *Making Political Ecology*. New York: Oxford University Press, 2005.

Nichter M, Quintero G, Nichter M, Mock J, Shakib S. Qualitative research: contributions to the study of drug use, drug abuse, and drug-use(r)-related interventions. *Substance Use & Misuse* 2004; 39:1907–1969.

Niedenthal PM. Embodying emotion. *Science* 2007; 316:1002–1005.

Northridge ME, Sclar E. A joint urban planning and public health framework: contributions to health impact assessment. *Am J Public Health* 2003; 93:118–121.

Northridge ME, Sclar ED, Biswas P. Sorting out the connections between the built environment and health: a conceptual framework for navigating pathways and planning healthy cities. *J Urban Health* 2003; 80:556–568.

Northridge ME, Stover GN, Rosenthal JE, Sherard D. Environmental equity and health: understanding complexity and moving forward. *Am J Public Health* 2003; 93:209–214.

O'Donovan-Anderson M (ed). *The Incorporated Self: Interdisciplinary Perspectives on Embodiment.* Lanham, MD: Rowman & Littlefield, 1996.

O'Neill RV, King AW. Homage to St. Michael; or, why are there so many books on scale? In: Peterson DL, Parker VT (eds). *Ecological Scale: Theories and Application.* New York: Columbia University Press, 1998; pp. 3–15.

Odum EP. *Fundamentals of Ecology.* 3rd ed. Philadelphia: Saunders, 1971.

Omran AR. A century of epidemiologic transition in the United States. *Prev Med* 1977; 6:30–51.

Omran AR. The epidemiologic transition theory: a preliminary update. *J Trop Pediatr* 1983; 29:305–316.

Omran AR. The epidemiologic transition: a theory of the epidemiology of population change. *Milbank Q* 1971; 49:509–538.

Oxford English Dictionary On-Line. Ecology. Draft revision June 2009. Available at: http://dictionary.oed.com.ezp-prod1.hul.harvard.edu/ (Accessed on: June 16, 2009).

Pakter J, Nelson F. Factors in the unprecedented decline in infant mortality in New York City. *Bull N Y Acad Med* 1975; 50:839–868.

Palazzo L, Guest A, Almgren G. Economic distress and cause-of-death patterns for black and non-black men in Chicago: reconsidering the relevance of classic epidemiologic transition theory. *Soc Biol* 2003; 50:102–126.

Pálsson G. Nature and society in the age of postmodernity. In: Biersack A, Greenberg JB. *Reimagining Political Ecology.* Durham, NC: Duke University Press, 2006; pp. 70–93.

Park RE. Human ecology. *Am J Sociol* 1936; 42:1–15. (1936a)

Park RE. Succession, an ecological concept. *Am Sociol Rev* 1936; 1:171–179. (1936b)

Parkes M, Eyles R, Benwell G, Panelli R, Townsend C, Weinstein P. Integration of ecology and health research at the catchment scale: the Taieri River Catchment, New Zealand. *J Rural Tropical Public Health* 2004; 3:1–17.

Parkes M, Panelli R, Weinstein P. Converging paradigms for environmental health theory and practice. *Environ Health Perspect* 2003; 111:669–675.

Paulson S, Gezon LL. *Political Ecology across Spaces, Scales, and Social Groups.* New Brunswick, NJ: Rutgers University Press, 2005.

Peterson DL, Parker VT (eds). *Ecological Scale: Theories and Application.* New York: Columbia University Press, 1998.

Philippe P. Chaos, population biology, and epidemiology: Some research implications. *Human Biol* 1993; 65:525–546.

Pickle LW, Gillum RF. Geographic variation in cardiovascular disease mortality in US blacks and whites. *J Natl Med Assoc* 1999; 91:545–556.

Piot P, Greener R, Russell S. Squaring the circle: AIDS, poverty, and human development. *PLoS Med* 2007; 4:1571–1575.

Porter D. *Health, Civilization and the State: A History of Public Health from Ancient to Modern Times.* London: Routledge, 1999.

Porto MF, Martinez-Alier J. Political ecology, ecological economics, and public health: interfaces for the sustainability of development and health promotion. *Cad Saude Publica* 2007; 23(Suppl 4):S504–S512.

Porto MF. Pesticides, collective health and non-sustainability: a critical vision of political ecology. *Cien Saude Colet* 2007; 12:17–20; discussion:23–24.

Porto MF. Workers' health and the environmental challenge: contributions from the ecosocial approach, the political ecology and the movement for environmental justice. *Ciencia & Saude Coletiva* 2005; 10:829–839.

Poundstone KE, Strathdee SA, Celentano DD. The social epidemiology of Human Immunodeficiency Virus/Acquired Immunodeficiency Syndrome. *Epidemiol Rev* 2004; 26:22–35.

Prigogine I. *Order Out of Chaos: Man's New Dialogue with Nature.* Boulder, CO: New Science Library, 1984.

Prothrow-Stith D, Gibbs B, Allen A. Reducing health disparities: from theory to practice. *Cancer Epidemiology Biomarkers Prevention* 2003; 12:256S–260S.

Quinn MM. Occupational health, public health, worker health. *Am J Public Health* 2003; 93:526.

Ranke MG, Saenger P. Turner's syndrome. *Lancet* 2001; 358:309–314.

Raphael D. Barriers to addressing the societal determinants of health: public health units and poverty in Ontario, Canada. *Health Promotion Int* 2003; 18:397–405.

Rastogi S, Nandlike K, Fenster W. Elevated blood levels in pregnant women: identification of a high-risk population and interventions. *J Perinat Med* 2007; 35:492–496.

Rayner G. Conventional and ecological public health. *Public Health* 2009; 123:587–591. doi:10.1016/j.puhe.2009.07.012

Richard RJ. *The Tragic Sense of Life: Ernst Haeckel and the Struggle over Evolutionary Thought.* Chicago: University of Chicago Press, 2008.

Richards G. *Putting Psychology in its Place: An Introduction from a Critical Historical Perspective.* London: Routledge, 1996.

Richardson JW. *The Cost of Being Poor: Poverty, Lead Poisoning, and Policy Implementation.* Praeger, Westport, CT, 2005.

Richmond C, Elliott SJ, Matthews R, Elliott B. The political ecology of health: perceptions of environment, economy, health and well-being among 'Namgis First Nation. *Health Place* 2005; 11:349–365.

Robbins P. *Political Ecology: A Critical Introduction.* Malden, MA: Blackwell Pub., 2004.

Robert JS, Smith A. Toxic ethics: environmental genomics and the health of populations. *Bioethics* 2004; 18:493–514.

Rose S. What is wrong with reductionist explanations of behavior? In: Bock GR, Goode JA. *The Limits of Reductionism in Biology.* (Novartis Foundation Symposium 213). Chichester, UK: John Wiley & Sons, 1998; pp. 176–192.

Rosner D, Markowitz G. The politics of lead toxicology and the devastating consequences for children. *Am J Indust Med* 2007; 50:740–756.

Roughgarden J. *Primer of Ecological Theory.* Upper Saddle River, NJ: Prentice Hall, 1998.

Sanders D. *The Struggle for Health: Medicine and the Politics of Underdevelopment.* London: MacMillan, 1985.

Scheiner SM. Toward a conceptual framework for biology. *Quarterly Review Biology* 2010; 85:293–318.

Shonkoff JP, Boyce WT, McEwen BS. Neuroscience, molecular biology, and the childhood roots of health disparities: building a new framework for health promotion and disease prevention. *JAMA* 2009; 301:2252–2259.

Smith JP. Healthy bodies and thick wallets: the dual relation between health and economic status. *J Econ Perspect* 1999; 13:144–166.

Solar O, Irwin A. Social determinants, political contexts and civil society action: a historical perspective on the Commission on Social Determinants of Health. *Health Promot J Austr* 2006; 17:180–185.

Sommerfeld J. Plagues and people revisited: basic and strategic research for infectious disease control at the interface of the life, health and social sciences. *EMBO Reports* 2003; 4:S32–S34.

Sorensen G, Barbeau E, Hunt MK, Emmons K. Reducing social disparities in tobacco use: A social contextual model for reducing tobacco use among blue-collar workers. *Am J Public Health* 2004; 94:230–239.

Spitler HD. Medical sociology and public health: problems and prospects for collaboration in the new millennium. *Sociological Spectrum* 2001; 21:247–263.

Starbuck WH. *The Production of Knowledge: The Challenge of Social Science Research.* Oxford: Oxford University Press, 2006.

Stark E, Flaherty D, Kelman S, Lazonick W, Price L, Rodberg L (eds). Special issue: The Political Economy of Health. *Rev Radical Political Economy* 1977; pp. 1–140.

Stauffer RC. Haeckel, Darwin, and Ecology. *Quarterly Review Biology* 1957; 32:138–144.

Steiner D, Nauser M (eds). *Human Ecology: Fragments of Anti-Fragmentary Views of the World.* London: Routledge, 1991.

Stewart AL, Napoles-Springer AM. Advancing health disparities research: can we afford to ignore measurement issues? *Medical Care* 2003; 41:1207–1220.

Stokols D. Ecology and health. In: Smelser NJ, Baltes PB (eds). *International Encyclopedia of the Social & Behavioral Sciences.* Oxford, UK: Pergamon, 2001; pp. 4030–4035.

Stokols D. Translating social ecological theory into guidelines for community health promotion. *Am J Health Promot* 1996; 10:282–298.

Stonich SC. Political ecology. In: Smelser NJ, Baltes PB (eds). *International Encyclopedia of the Social & Behavioral Sciences.* Oxford, UK: Pergamon, 2001; pp. 4053–4058.

Susser E. Eco-epidemiology: thinking outside the black box. *Epidemiology* 2004; 15:519–520. (editorial)

Susser M, Stein Z. *Eras in Epidemiology: The Evolution of Ideas.* New York: Oxford University Press, 2009.

Susser M, Susser E. Choosing a future for epidemiology: II. From black box to Chinese boxes and eco-epidemiology. *Am J Public Health* 1996; 86:674–677. Erratum in: *Am J Public Health* 1996 Aug; 86:1093.

Sydenstricker E. *Health and Environment.* New York: McGraw-Hill, 1933.

Taylor P. *Unruly Complexity: Ecology, Interpretation, Engagement.* Chicago: University of Chicago Press, 2005.

Taylor PJ. Philosophy of Ecology. In: *Encyclopedia of Life Sciences.* Chichester, UK: John Wiley & Sons, Ltd, 2008; http://www.els.net/(doi: 10.1002/9780470015902.a0003607.pub2)

Tesh SN. *Hidden Arguments: Political Ideology and Disease Prevention Policy.* New Brunswick, NJ: Rutgers University Press, 1988.

Teti M, Chilton M, Lloyd L, Rubenstein S. Identifying the links between violence against women and HIV/AIDS: ecosocial and human rights frameworks offer insight into U.S. prevention policies. *Health Hum Rights* 2006; 9:40–61.

Thacker SB, Buffington J. Applied epidemiology for the 21st century. *Int J Epidemiol* 2001; 30: 320–325.

Thompson JJ, Ritenbaugh C, Nichter M. Reconsidering the placebo response from a broad anthropological perspective. *Culture Med Psychiatry* 2009; 33:112–152.

Tudge C. *The Secret Life of Trees.* London: Allen Lane, Penguin Books, 2005.

Turner JH, Boyns D. The return of grand theory. In: Turner JH (ed). *Handbook of Sociological Theory.* New York: Plenum Press, 2002; pp. 353–378.

Turner JH. A new approach for theoretically integrating micro and macro analyses. In: Calhoun C, Rojek C, Turner B (eds). *The Sage Handbook of Sociology.* Thousand Oaks, CA: Sage Publications, 2005; pp. 405–422.

Turshen M. *The Political Ecology of Disease in Tanzania.* New Brunswick, NJ: Rutgers University Press, 1984.

Turshen M. The political ecology of disease. *Review Radical Political Econ* 1977; 9:45–60.

Van Tongeren M, Nieuwenhuijsen MJ, Gardiner K, Armstrong B, Vrijheid M, Dolk H, Botting B. A job-exposure matrix for potential endocrine-disrupting chemicals developed for a study into the association between maternal occupational exposure and hypospadias. *Ann Occup Hyg* 2002; 46:465–477.

Vaziri ND. Mechanisms of lead-induced hypertension and cardiovascular disease. *Am J Physiol Heart Circ Physiol* 2008; 295:H454–H465.

Velasco S, Ruiz MT, Alvarez-Dardet C. Attention models to somatic symptoms without organic cause: from physiopathologic disorders to malaise of women. *Rev Esp Salud Publica* 2006; 80:317–333.

Villa F, Ceroni M. Community ecology: an introduction. In: *Encyclopedia Of Life Sciences.* Chichester, UK: John Wiley & Sons, Ltd, 2005; http://www.els.net/(doi:10.1038/npg.els. 0003174)

Vygotsky LS. *Mind in Society.* Cambridge, MA: Harvard University Press, 1978.

Walsh A, Beaver KM (eds). *Biosocial Criminology: New Directions in Theory and Research.* London: Routledge/Taylor and Francis Group, 2009.

Walsh A. *Race and Crime: A Biosocial Analysis.* New York: Nova Science Publishers, 2004.

Walters KL, Simoni JM. Reconceptualizing native women's health: an "indigenist" stress-coping model. *Am J Public Health* 2002; 92:520–524.

Watts C, Zimmerman C. Violence against women: global scope and magnitude. *Lancet* 2002; 359:1232–1237.

Weiss G, Haber HF (eds). *Perspectives on Embodiment: The Intersections of Nature and Culture.* New York: Routledge, 1999.

Werskey G. The Marxist critique of capitalist science: a history in three movements? *Science as Culture* 2007; 16:397–461.

Whiteside KH. *Divided Natures: French Contributions to Political Ecology.* Cambridge, MA: The MIT Press, 2002.

Wigle DT, Arbuckle TE, Turner MC, Bérubé A, Yang Q, Liu S, Krewski D. Epidemiologic evidence of relationships between reproductive and child health outcomes and environmental chemical contaminants. *J Toxicol Environ Health B Crit Rev* 2008; 11:373–517.

Wise LA, Krieger N, Zierler S, Harlow BL. Lifetime socioeconomic position in relation to onset of perimenopause: a prospective cohort study. *J Epidemiol Community Health* 2002; 56:851–860.

Wise PH. The anatomy of a disparity in infant mortality. *Annu Rev Public Health* 2003; 24:341–362.

World Health Organization, CSDH. *Closing the gap in a generation: health equity through action on the social determinants of health. Final Report of the Commission on Social Determinants of Health.* Geneva: World Health Organization, 2008.

Worster D. *Nature's Economy: A History of Ecological Ideas.* 2nd ed. New York: Cambridge University Press, 1994.

Wright AA, Katz IT. Roe versus reality–abortion and women's health. *New Engl J Med* 2006; 355:1–9.

Yamada S, Palmer W. An Ecosocial Approach to the Epidemic of Cholera in the Marshall Islands. *Social Medicine* 2007; 2:79–88.

Yen IH, Syme SL. The social environment and health: a discussion of the epidemiologic literature. *Annu Rev Public Health* 1999; 20:287–308.

Ziman J. *Real Science: What it is, and What it Means.* Cambridge, UK: Cambridge University Press, 2000.

Zinn H. *A People's History of the United States.* New York: HarperCollins, 2003.

Chapter 8

Ahmed N, Sechi LA. Helicobacter pylori and gastroduodenal pathology: new threats of the old friend. *Annals Clin Microbiol Antimicrob* 2005; 4:1. doi:10.1186/1476-0711-4-1.

Akhter Y, Ahmed I, Devi SM, Ahmed N. The co-evolved Helicobacter pylori and gastric cancer: trinity of bacterial virulence, host susceptibility and lifestyle. *Infectious Agent Cancer* 2007; 2:2. doi:10.1186/1750-9378-2-2.

Almond DV, Chay KY, Greenstone M. Civil Rights, the War on Poverty, and Black-White convergence in infant mortality in the rural South and Mississippi. December 31, 2006. MIT Economics Working Paper No. 07-04. Available at: http://papers.ssrn.com/sol3/papers.cfm?abstract_id=961021 (Accessed: July 30, 2009).

Applied Research Center and Northwest Federation of Community Organizations. *Closing the Gap: Solutions to Race-Based Health Disparities.* Oakland, CA: Applied Research Center, 2005. Available at: http://www.arc.org/content/view/291/47/ (Accessed: July 25, 2009).

Archibold RC. Indians' water rights give hope for better health. *New York Times*, August 31, 2008.

Atherton JC. The pathogenesis of Helicobacter pylori-induced gastro-duodenal diseases. *Annu Rev Pathol* 2006; 1:63–96.

Auerbach AJ, Card D, Quigley JM (eds). *Public Policy and Income Distribution.* New York: Russell Sage Foundation, 2006.

Ayerst Laboratories. *The Clinical Guide to the Menopause.* New York: Ayerst Laboratories, 1960.

Bakken K, Alsaker E, Eggen AE, Lund E. Hormone replacement therapy and incidence of hormone-dependent cancers in the Norwegian Women and Cancer study. *Int J Cancer* 2004; 112:130–134.

Banks E, Canfell K. Invited commentary: hormone therapy risks and benefits–the Women's Health Initiative findings and the postmenopausal estrogen timing hypothesis. *Am J Epidemiol* 2009; 170:24–28.

Barone J. Scientist of the Year Notable: Hans Rosling. *Discover Magazine*, December 6, 2007. Available at: http://discovermagazine.com/2007/dec/hans-rosling (Accessed: August 9, 2009).

Barreto ML. Epidemiologists and causation in an intricate world. *Emerging Themes Epidemiol* 2005; 2:3. doi:10.1186/1742-7622-2-3.

Barreto ML. The globalization of epidemiology: critical thoughts from Latin America. *Int J Epidemiol* 2004; 33:1132–1137.

Barrett-Connor E, Grady D, Stefanick ML. The rise and fall of menopausal hormone therapy. *Annu Rev Public Health* 2005; 26:115–140.

Barrett-Connor E. Commentary: Observation versus intervention—what's different? *Int J Epidemiol* 2004; 33:457–459.

Barrett-Connor E. Hormones and heart disease in women: the timing hypothesis. *Am J Epidemiol* 2007; 166:506–510.

Barrett-Connor E. Risks and benefits of replacement estrogen. *Annu Rev Med* 1992; 43:239–251.

Bartlett JG, Iwasaki Y, Gottlieb B, Hall D, Mannell R. Framework for Aboriginal-guided decolonizing research involving M'etis and First Nations persons with diabetes. *Soc Sci Med* 2007; 65: 2371–2382.

Baschetti R. Diabetes epidemics in newly westernized populations: is it due to thrifty genes or to genetically unknown foods? *J R Soc Med* 1998; 91:622–625.

Beckfield J, Krieger N. Epi + demos + cracy: linking political systems and priorities to the magnitude of health inequities–evidence, gaps, and a research agenda. *Epidemiol Review* 2009; 31: 152–177.

Bennett PH, Burch TA, Miller M. Diabetes mellitus in American (Pima) Indians. *Lancet* 1971; 298:125–128.

Bennett PH. Type 2 diabetes among the Pima Indians of Arizona: an epidemic attributable to environmental change? *Nutr Rev* 1999; 57:S51–S54.

Benyshek DC, Watson JT. Exploring the thrifty genotype's food-shortage assumptions: a cross-cultural comparison of ethnographic accounts of food security among foraging and agricultural societies. *Am J Phys Anthropol* 2006; 131:120–126.

Beral V; Million Women Study Collaborators. Breast cancer and hormone-replacement therapy in the Million Women Study. *Lancet* 2003; 362: 419–427.

Blair SN, Morris JN. Healthy hearts–and the universal benefits of being physically active: physical activity and health. *Ann Epidemiol* 2009; 19:253–256.

Blaser MJ, Chen Y, Reibman J. Does Helicobacter pylori protect against asthma and allergy? *Gut* 2008; 57:561–567.

Boslaugh S (ed). *Encyclopedia of Epidemiology.* Thousand Oaks, CA: Sage Publications, 2008.

Boston Women's Health Book Collective. *Our Bodies, Ourselves.* Revised and expanded. New York: Simon & Schuster, 1976.

Bouchardy C, Morabia A, Verkooijen HM, Fioretta G, Wespi Y, Schäfer P. Remarkable change in age-specific breast cancer incidence in the Swiss canton of Geneva and its possible relation with the use of hormone replacement therapy. *BMC Cancer* 2006; 6:78. doi: 10.1186/1471-2407-6-78.

Bradlow HL, Sepkovic DW. Steroids as procarcinogenic agents. *Ann NY Acad Sci* 2004; 1028: 216–232.

Brinton LA, Schairer C. Estrogen replacement therapy and breast cancer risk. *Epidemiol Rev* 1993; 15:66–79.

Buist DS, Newton KM, Miglioretti DL, et al. Hormone therapy prescribing patterns in the United States. *Obstet Gynecol* 2004; 104:1042–1050.

Busfield F, Duffy DL, Kesting JB, et al. A genomewide search for type 2 diabetes-susceptibility genes in indigenous Australians. *Am J Hum Genet* 2002; 70:349–357.

Bush T. The epidemiology of cardiovascular disease in postmenopausal women. *Ann NY Acad Sci* 1990; 592:263–271.

Candib LM. Obesity and diabetes in vulnerable populations: reflections on proximal and distal causes. *Ann Fam Med* 2007; 5:547–556.

Canfell K, Banks E, Moa AM, Beral V. Decrease in breast cancer incidence following a rapid fall in use of hormone therapy in Australia. *Med J Aust* 2008; 188:641–644.

Carney DR, Banaji MR, Krieger N. Implicit measures reveal evidence of personal discrimination. *Self and Identity* 2010; 9:162–176; DOI:10.1080/13594320902847927

Carson B, Dunbar T, Chenhall RD, Bailie R. *Social Determinants of Indigenous Health.* Crows Nest, NSW: Allen & Unwin, 2007.

Castallo MA. Modern management of the menopause; this deficiency disease, caused by lack of ovarian hormone, should be treated throughout life by estrogen replacement therapy. *Pa Med* 1967; 70:80–81.

Castetter EF, Underhill RM (eds). *The Ethnobiology of the Papago Indians.* (Reprint of the 1935 ed. published by the University of New Mexico press, issued originally as University of New Mexico Bulletin, No. 275, Biological Series, v. 4, no 3, and as Ethnobiological studies of the American Southwest, 2). New York: AMS Press, 1978.

Chakravarthy MV, Booth FM. Eating, exercise, and "thrifty" genotypes: connecting the dots toward an evolutionary understanding of modern chronic diseases. *J Appl Physiol* 2004; 96:3–10.

Chen JT, Rehkopf DH, Waterman PD, et al. Mapping and measuring social disparities in premature mortality: the impact of census tract poverty within and across Boston neighborhoods, 1999–2001. *J Urban Health* 2006; 83:1063–1084.

Chen Y, Blaser MJ. Inverse associations of *Helicobacter pylori* with asthma and allergy. *Arch Intern Med* 2007; 167:821–827.

Chlebowski RT, Kuller LH, Prentice RL, et al. Breast cancer after use of estrogen plus progestin in postmenopausal women. *New Engl J Med* 2009; 360:573–587.

Choung RS, Talley NJ. Epidemiology and clinical presentation of stress-related peptic damage and chronic peptic ulcer. *Curr Molec Med* 2008; 8:253–257.

Clarke CA, Glaser SL, Uratsu CS, Selby JV, Kushi LH, Herrinton JL. Recent declines in hormone therapy utilization and breast cancer incidence: clinical and population-based evidence. *J Clin Oncol* 2006; 24:e49–50; doi: 10.1200/jco.2006.08.6504

Clarke CA, Glaser SL. Declines in breast cancer after the WHI: apparent impact of hormone therapy. *Cancer Causes Control* 2007; 18:847–852.

Cohen IB. *Revolution in Science.* Cambridge, MA: Harvard University Press, 1985.

Cohen MN. *Health and the Rise of Civilization.* New Haven, CT: Yale University Press, 1989.

Conley D, Springer K. Welfare state and infant mortality. *Am J Sociol* 2001; 107:768–807.

Coombs NJ, Taylor R, Wilcken N, Boyages J. HRT and breast cancer: impact on population risk and incidence. *Eur J Cancer* 2005; 41:1755–1781. (2005a)

Coombs NJ, Taylor R, Wilcken N, Fiorica J, Boyages J. Hormone replacement therapy and breast cancer risk in California. *Breast J* 2005; 11: 410–415. (2005b)

Cooper R, Steinhauer M, Schatzkin A, Miller W. Improved mortality among US blacks, 1968–1978: the role of antiracist struggle. *Int J Health Services* 1981; 11:389–414.

Cordera F, Jordan VC. Steroid receptors and their role in the biology and control of breast cancer growth. *Semin Oncol* 2006; 33:631–641.

Coronary Drug Project. Findings leading to discontinuation of the 2.5-mg day estrogen group. The Coronary Drug Project Research Group. *JAMA* 1973; 226:652–657.

Coronary Drug Project. The Coronary Drug Project. Initial findings leading to modification of its research protocol. *JAMA* 1970; 214:1303–1313.

Crosby AW. *Ecological Imperialism: The Biological Expansion of Europe, 900–1900.* Cambridge: Cambridge University Press, 1986.

Cunningham M. Health. In: United Nations, Department of Economic and Social Affairs. *The State of the World's Indigenous Peoples.* New York: United Nations, 2009; pp. 156–187.

Cutler D, Deaton A, Lleras-Muney A. The determinants of mortality. *J Economic Perspectives* 2006; 20:97–120.

Danesh J. Is *Helicobacter pylori* infection a cause of gastric neoplasia? In: Newton R, Beral V, Weiss RA (eds). *Infections and Human Cancer.* (Cancer Survey *vol. 33*) Plainview, NY: Cold Spring Harbor Laboratory Press, 1999; pp. 263–289.

Davey Smith G, Ebrahim S, Frankel S. How policy informs the evidence: "evidence based" thinking can lead to debased policy making. *BMJ* 2001; 322:184–185.

Davey Smith G, Ebrahim S. Data dredging, bias, or confounding–they can all get you into the BMJ and the Friday papers. *BMJ* 2002; 325:1437–1438.

Davey Smith G, Ebrahim S. Epidemiology–is it time to call it a day? *Int J Epidemiol* 2001; 30: 1–11.

Davis K, Schoen C. *Health and the War on Poverty: A Ten-Year Appraisal.* Washington, DC: The Brookings Institute, 1978.

de Waard F, Thijssen JH. Hormonal aspects in the causation of human breast cancer: epidemiological hypotheses reviewed, with special reference to nutritional status and first pregnancy. *J Steroid Biochem Mol Biol* 2005; 97:451–458.

DESA: Department of Economic and Social Affairs, Statistics Division. *The World's Women 2005: Progress in Statistics.* New York: United Nations, 2006.

Detels R. The search for protection against HIV infection. *Ann Epidemiol* 2009; 19:250–252.

Dickson SP, Wang K, Krantz I, Hakonarson H, Goldstein DB. Rare Variants Create Synthetic Genome-Wide Associations. *PLoS Biol* 2010; 8(1): e1000294. doi:10.1371/journal.pbio.1000294

Dietel M, Lewis MA, Shapiro S. Hormone replacement therapy: pathobiological aspects of hormone-sensitive cancers in women relevant to epidemiological studies on HRT: a mini-review. *Hum Reprod* 2005; 20:2052–2060.

Dockery DW. Health effects of particulate air pollution. *Ann Epidemiol* 2009; 19:257–263.

Donaldson L. Ten tips for better health. In: *Saving Lives: Our Health Nation.* Presented to Parliament by the Secretary of State for Health by Command of Her Majesty, July 1999. London, UK: Stationary Office, 1999. Available at: http://www.archive.official-documents.co.uk/document/cm43/4386/4386-tp.htm (Accessed: August 8, 2009).

Dorling D. Worldmapper: the human anatomy of a small planet. *PLoS Med* 2007; 4(1): e1. doi:10.1371/journal.pmed.0040001

Doyal L. *What Makes Women Sick: Gender and the Political Economy of Health.* New Brunswick, NJ: Rutgers University Press, 1995.

Dreifus C (ed). *Seizing Our Bodies: The Politics of Women's Health.* New York: Vintage Books, 1977.

Duncan GJ, Chase-Landsdale L (eds). *For Better and For Worse: Welfare Reform and the Well-Being of Children and Families.* New York: Russell Sage Foundation, 2004.

Dwyer T, Ponsonby A-L. Sudden infant death syndrome and prone sleeping position. *Ann Epidemiol* 2009; 19:245–249.

Dykhuizen D, Kalia A. The population structure of pathogenic bacteria. In: Stearns SC, Koella JC (eds). *Evolution in Health and Disease.* 2nd ed. Oxford: Oxford University Press, 2008; pp. 185–198.

Ebrahim S, Clarke M. STROBE: new standards for reporting observational epidemiology, a chance to improve. *Int J Epidemiol* 2007; 36:946–948.

Ebrahim S, Davey Smith G. Mendelian randomization: can genetic epidemiology help redress the failures of observational epidemiology? *Hum Genet* 2008; 123:15–33.

Egger M, Altman DG, Vandenbroucke JP. Commentary: Strengthening the reporting of observational epidemiology–the STROBE statement. *Int J Epidemiol* 2007; 36:948–950.

Epstein FH. Contribution of epidemiology to understanding coronary heart disease. In: Marmot MT, Elliott P (eds). *Coronary Heart Disease Epidemiology: From Aetiology to Public Health.* 2nd ed. Oxford: Oxford University Press, 2005; pp. 8–17.

Ettinger B, Grady D, Tosteson AN, Pressman A, Macer JL. Effect of the Women's' Health Initiative on women's decision to discontinue postmenopausal hormone therapy. *Obstet Gynecol* 2003; 102: 1225–1232.

Ezzati M, Friedman AB, Kulkami SC, Murray CJ. The reversal of fortunes: trends in county mortality and cross-county mortality disparities in the United States. *PLoS Med* 2008; 5(4):e66. Erratum in: PLoS Med 2008; 5(5). doi: 10.1371/journal.pmed.0050119

Fairclough A. *Better Day Coming: Blacks and Equality, 1890-2000.* New York: Viking, 2001.

Fee E, Krieger N (eds). *Women's Health, Politics, and Power: Essays on Sex/Gender, Medicine, and Public Health.* Amytiville, NY: Baywood Pub Co., 1994.

Ferriera ML, Lang GC. Introduction: deconstructing diabetes. In: Ferriera ML, Lang CG (eds). *Indigenous Peoples and Diabetes: Community Empowerment and Wellness.* Durham, NC: Carolina Academic Press, 2006; pp. 3–32.

Ferriera ML, Sanchez T, Nix B. Touch the heart of the people: cultural rebuilding and the Potawot Health Village in California. In: Ferriera ML, Lang CG (eds). *Indigenous Peoples and Diabetes: Community Empowerment and Wellness.* Durham, NC: Carolina Academic Press, 2006; pp. 459–492.

Fleisher NL, Diez Roux AV. Using directed acyclic graphs to guide analyses of neighborhood effects: an introduction. *J Epidemiol Community Health* 2008; 62:842–846.

Foxcroft L. *Hot Flushes, Cold Science: A History of the Modern Menopause.* London: Granta Books, 2009.

Gapminder. Available at: http://www.gapminder.org/ (Accessed: August 8, 2009).

Gaudillière J-P. Hormones at risk: cancer and the medical uses of industrially-produced sex steroids in Germany, 1930-1960. In: Schlich T, Tröhler (eds). *Medical Innovation: Risk Perception and Assessment in Historical Context.* London: Routledge, 2006; pp. 148–169.

Gilliland FD, Owen C, Gilliland SS, Carter JS. Temporal trends in diabetes mortality among American Indians and Hispanics in New Mexico: birth cohort and period effects. *Am J Epidemiol* 1997; 145:422–431.

Glass G, Lacey JV Jr, Carreon JD, Hoover RN. Breast cancer incidence, 1980-2006: combined roles of menopausal hormone therapy, screening, mammography, and estrogen receptor status. *JNCI* 2007; 99:1152–1161.

Glymour MM. Using causal diagrams to understand common problems in social epidemiology. In: Oakes J M, Kaufman J S, eds. *Methods in Social Epidemiology.* San Francisco, CA: Jossey-Bass, 2006; pp. 393–428.

Gohdes DM, Acton K. Diabetes mellitus and its complications. In: Rhoades EP (ed). *American Indian Health: Innovations in Health Care, Promotion, and Policy.* Baltimore, MD: Johns Hopkins University Press, 2000; pp. 221–243.

Gordon D. Alternative 10 tips for better health (1999). Available at: http://www.bris.ac.uk/poverty/health%20inequalities.html (Accessed: August 8, 2009).

Gordon L. *Woman's Body, Woman's Rights: A Social History of Birth Control in America.* New York: Grossman, 1976.

Gracey M, King M. Indigenous health part 1: determinants and disease patterns. *Lancet* 2009; 374: 65–75.

Grady D, Herrington D, Bittner V, Blumenthal R, et al. Cardiovascular disease outcomes during 6.8 years of hormone therapy. Heart and Estrogen/progestin Replacement Study follow-up (HERS II). *JAMA* 2002; 288:49–57.

Grady D, Rubin SM, Petitti DB, et al. Hormone therapy to prevent disease and prolong life in post-menopausal women. *Ann Int Med* 1992; 117:1016–1037.

Greenland S, Pearl J, Robins JM. Causal diagrams for epidemiologic research. *Epidemiology* 1999; 10:37–48.

Greenwood M. *Epidemics and Crowd Diseases: An Introduction to the Study of Epidemiology.* London: Williams & Norgate, Ltd, 1935.

Grob GN. The rise of peptic ulcer, 1900-1950. *Perspectives Biol Med* 2003; 46:550–566.

Grodstein F, Clarkson TB, Manson JE. Understanding divergent data on posthormonal hormone therapy. *New Engl J Med* 2003; 348:645–650.

Guay MP, Dragomir A, Pilon D, Moride Y, Perreault S. Changes in pattern of use, clinical characteristics and persistence rate of hormone replacement therapy among postmenopausal women after the WHI publication. *Pharmocepidemiol Drug Saf* 2007; 16:17–27.

Haas JS, Kaplan CP, Gerstenberger EP, Kerlikowske K. Changes in the use of postmenopausal hormone therapy after the publication of clinical trial results. *Ann Intern Med* 2004; 140: 184–188.

Hales CN, Barker DJ. The thrifty phenotype hypothesis. *Br Med Bull* 2001; 60:5–20.

Hales CN, Barker DJP. Type 2 (non-insulin-dependent) diabetes mellitus: the thrifty phenotype hypothesis. *Diabetologia* 1992; 35:595–601.

Hales CN, Desai M, Ozanne SE. The Thrifty Phenotype hypothesis: how does it look after 5 years? *Diabet Med* 1997; 14:189–195.

Hausauer AK, Keegan THM, Chang ET, Clarke CA. Recent breast cancer trends among Asian/Pacific Islander, Hispanic, and African-American women in the US: changes by tumor subtype. *Breast Cancer Res* 2007; 9:R90. doi:10.1186/bcr1839

Hedman B, Perucci F, Sundström P. *Engendering Statistics: A Tool for Change.* Stockholm, Sweden: Statistics Sweden, 1996.

Hegele RA, Zinman B, Hanley AJ, Harris SB, Barrett PH, Cao H. Genes, environment and Oji-Cree type 2 diabetes. *Clin Biochem* 2003; 36:163–170.

Henderson BE, Ross RK, Pike MC. Hormonal chemoprevention of cancer in women. *Science* 1993; 259:633–638.

Henwood D. *After the New Economy: The Binge… and the Hangover that Won't Go Away.* New York: The New Press, 2003.

Hérnan MA, Hernandez-Diaz S, Werler MM, Mitchell AA. Causal knowledge as a prerequisite for confounding evaluation: an application to birth defects epidemiology. *Am J Epidemiol* 2002; 155: 176–184.

Hersh AL, Stefanick ML, Stafford RS. National use of postmenopausal hormone therapy: Annual trends and response to recent evidence. *JAMA* 2004; 291: 47–53.

Hetzel BS, Zimmet P, Seeman E. Endocrine and metabolic disorders. In: Detels R, McEwen J, Beaglehole R, Tanaka H (eds). *Oxford Textbook of Public Health*. Oxford: Oxford University Press, 2004. Available at: http://www.r2library.com (Accessed: July 25, 2009).

Hillemeier MM, Geronimus AT, Bound SJ. Widening black/white mortality differentials among US children during the 1980s. *Ethn Dis* 2001; 11:469–483.

Hillier TA, Pedula KL, Schmidt MM, Mullen JA, Charles MA, Pettit DJ. Childhood obesity and metabolic imprinting: the ongoing effect of maternal hyperglycemia. *Diabetes Care* 2007; 30:2287–2292.

Hing E, Brett KM. Changes in U.S. prescribing patterns of menopausal hormone therapy, 2001–2003. *Obstet Gynecol* 2006; 108:33–40.

Houck JA. *Hot and Bothered: Women, Medicine, and Menopause in Modern America*. Cambridge, MA: Harvard University Press, 2006.

Hubbard R, Henefin MS, Fried B (eds). *Biological Woman–The Convenient Myth: A Collection of Feminist Essays and a Comprehensive Bibliography*. Cambridge, MA: Schenkman Pub Co., 1982.

Hulley S, Grady D, Bush T, et al. Randomized trial of estrogen plus progestin for secondary prevention of coronary heart disease in postmenopausal women. Heart and Estrogen/progestin Replacement Study (HERS) Research Group. *JAMA* 1998; 280:605–613.

Humphrey LL, Chan BK, Sox HC. Postmenopausal hormone replacement therapy and the primary prevention of cardiovascular disease. *Ann Intern Med* 2002; 137:273–284.

Independent Inquiry into Inequalities in Health. Chairman: Sir Donald Acheson. London: Stationery Office, 1998. Available at: http://www.archive.official-documents.co.uk/document/doh/ih/ih.htm (Accessed: August 8, 2009).

Inzucchi SE, Sherwin RS. Type 2 diabetes mellitus. In: Goldman L, Ausiello D (eds). *Cecil Medicine*, 23rd ed. Philadelphia, PA: Saunders, 2007. Available at: http://www.mdconsult.com (Accessed: July 25, 2009).

IPC Food Sovereignty. Available at: http://www.foodsovereignty.org/new/whoweare.php (Accessed: August 4, 2009).

Jackson MY. Diet, culture, and diabetes. In: Joe JR, Young RS (eds). *Diabetes as a Disease of Civilization: The Impact of Culture Change on Indigenous Peoples*. Berlin Mouton de Gruyter, 1993; pp. 381–406.

Jara L. Integrating a gender perspective into health statistics: an ongoing process in Central America. *Int J Public Health* 2007; 52:S35–S40.

Jarvis D, Luczynska C, Chinn S, Burney P. The association of hepatitis A and *Helicobacter pylori* with sensitization to common allergens, asthma and hay fever in a population of young British adults. *Allergy* 2004; 59:1063–1067.

Jemal A, Ward E, Thun MJ. Recent trends in breast cancer incidence rates by age and tumor characteristics among U.S. women. *Breast Cancer Res* 2007; 9:R28. doi:10.1186/bcr1672

Joe JR, Young RS (eds). *Diabetes as a Disease of Civilization: The Impact of Culture Change on Indigenous Peoples*. Berlin Mouton de Gruyter, 1993.

Justice JW. The history of diabetes in the Desert People. In: Joe JR, Young RS (eds). *Diabetes as a Disease of Civilization: The Impact of Culture Change on Indigenous Peoples*. Berlin Mouton de Gruyter, 1993; pp. 69–128.

Kandulski A, Selgrad M, Malfertheiner P. *Helicobacter pylori* infection: a clinical overview. *Dig Liver Dis* 2008; 40:619–626.

Katalinic A, Rawal R. Decline in breast cancer incidence after decrease in utilization of hormone replacement therapy. *Breast Cancer Res Treat* 2008; 107: 427–430.

Kelly JP, Kaufman DW, Rosenberg L, Kelley K, Cooper SG, Mitchell AA. Use of postmenopausal hormone therapy since the Women's Health Initiative findings. *Pharmacoepidemiol Drug Saf* 2005; 14:837–842.

Kim N, Gross C, Curtis J, Stettin G, Wogen S, Choe N, Krumholtz HM. The impact of clinical trials on the use of hormone replacement therapy: a population-based study. *J Gen Intern Med* 2005;20:1026–1031.

Kimball AW. Errors of the third kind in statistical consulting. *J Am Stat Assoc* 1957; 52:133–142.

King M, Smith A, Gracey M. Indigenous health part 2: the underlying causes of the health gap. *Lancet* 2009; 374:76–85.

Kington RS, Nickens HW. Racial and ethnic differences in health: recent trends, current patterns, future directions. In: Smelser NJ, Wilson WJ, Mitchell F (eds). *America Becoming: Racial Trends and Their Consequences, Vol II*. Commission on Behavioral and Social Sciences and Education, National Research Council. Washington, DC: National Academy Press. 2001; pp. 253–310.

Knowler WC, Pettitt DJ, Bennett PH, Williams RC. Diabetes mellitus in the Pima Indians: genetic and evolutionary considerations. *Am J Phys Anthropol* 1983; 62:107–114.

Knowler WC, Pettitt DJ, Saad MF, Bennett PH. Diabetes mellitus in the Pima Indians: incidence, risk factors and pathogenesis. *Diabetes Metab Rev* 1990; 6:1–27.

Knowler WC, Saad MF, Pettitt DJ, Nelson RG, Bennett PH. Determinants of diabetes in the Pima Indians. *Diabetes Care* 1993; 16:216–227.

Koutsky L. The epidemiology behind the HPV vaccine discovery. *Ann Epidemiol* 2009; 19: 239–244.

Kraker D. The new water czars. *High Country News*, March 15, 2004.

Kressin NR, Raymond NL, Manze M. Perceptions of race/ethnicity-based discrimination: a review of measures and evaluation of their usefulness for the health care setting. *J Health Care Poor Underserved* 2008; 19:697–730.

Krieger N (ed). *Embodying Inequality: Epidemiologic Perspectives*. Amityville, NY: Baywood Pub, 2004. (2004a)

Krieger N, Carney D, Waterman PD, Kosheleva A, Banaji M. Combining implicit and explicit measures of racial discrimination in health research. *Am J Public Health* 2010; 100:1485-1492 (epub advance access: November 17, 2009; doi:10.2105/AJPH.2009.159517).

Krieger N, Chen JT, Ebel G. Can we monitor socioeconomic inequalities in health? A survey of U.S. Health Departments' data collection and reporting practices. *Public Health Reports* 1997; 112:481–491.

Krieger N, Chen JT, Waterman PD, Rehkopf DH, Subramanian SV. Painting a truer picture of US socioeconomic and racial/ethnic health inequalities: the *Public Health Disparities Geocoding Project. Am J Public Health* 2005; 95:312–323. (2005b)

Krieger N, Chen JT, Waterman PD, Rehkopf DH, Subramanian SV. Race/ethnicity, gender, and monitoring socioeconomic gradients in health: a comparison of area-based socioeconomic measures—*The Public Health Disparities Geocoding Project. Am J Public Health* 2003; 93:1655–1671. (2003c)

Krieger N, Chen JT, Waterman PD, Soobader MJ, Subramanian SV, Carson R. Choosing area based socioeconomic measures to monitor social inequalities in low birth weight and childhood lead poisoning: *The Public Health Disparities Geocoding Project* (US). *J Epidemiol Community Health* 2003; 57:186–199. (2003a)

Krieger N, Chen JT, Waterman PD, Soobader MJ, Subramanian SV, Carson R. Geocoding and monitoring of US socioeconomic inequalities in mortality and cancer incidence: does the choice of area-based measure and geographic level matter?: *The Public Health Disparities Geocoding Project. Am J Epidemiol* 2002; 156:471–482. (2002a)

Krieger N, Chen JT, Waterman PD. Decline in US breast cancer rates after the Women's Health Initiative: socioeconomic and racial/ethnic differentials. *Am J Public Health* 2010; 100: S132-139 (epub advance access: Feb 10, 2010). doi:10.2105/AJPH.2009.181628 NIHMS 171687.

Krieger N, Löwy I, the "Women, Hormones, and Cancer" group (Aronowitz R, Bigby J, Dickersin K, Garner E, Gaudillière J-P, Hinestrosa C, Hubbard R, Johnson PA, Missmer SA, Norsigian J, Pearson C, Rosenberg CE, Rosenberg L, Rosenkrantz BG, Seaman B, Sonnenschein C, Soto AM, Thorton J, Weisz G). Hormone replacement therapy, cancer, controversies & women's health: historical, epidemiological, biological, clinical and advocacy perspectives. *J Epidemiol Community Health* 2005; 59:740–748.

Krieger N, Rehkopf DH, Chen JT, Waterman PD, Marcelli E, Kennedy M. The fall and rise of US inequities in premature mortality: 1960-2002. *PLoS Med* 2008; 5(2): e46. doi:10.1371/journal.pmed.0050046 (2008a)

Krieger N, Rowley DL, Herman AA, Avery B, Phillips MT. Racism, sexism, and social class: implications for studies of health, disease, and well-being. *Am J Prev Med* 1993; 9 (Suppl):82–122.

Krieger N, Sidney S. Racial discrimination and blood pressure: The CARDIA study of young black and white adults. *Am J Public Health* 1996; 86:1370–1378.

Krieger N, Waterman P, Chen JT, Soobader MJ, Subramanian SV, Carson R. Zip code caveat: bias due to spatiotemporal mismatches between zip codes and US census-defined geographic areas—*The Public Health Disparities Geocoding Project. Am J Public Health* 2002; 92:1100–1102. (2002b)

Krieger N, Waterman P, Lemieux K, Zierler S, Hogan JW. On the wrong side of the tracts? Evaluating the accuracy of geocoding in public health research. *Am J Public Health* 2001; 91:1114–1116.

Krieger N, Waterman PD, Chen JT, Rehkopf DH, Subramanian SV. *Geocoding and monitoring US socioeconomic inequalities in health: an introduction to using area-based socioeconomic measures—The Public Health Disparities Geocoding Project monograph* (2004). Boston, MA: Harvard School of Public Health. Available at: http://www.hsph.harvard.edu/thegeocodingproject/; available as of July 1, 2004 and Accessed: August 6, 2009.

Krieger N, Waterman PD, Chen JT, Soobader MJ, Subramanian S. Monitoring Socioeconomic Inequalities in Sexually Transmitted Infections, Tuberculosis, and Violence: Geocoding and Choice of Area-Based Socioeconomic Measures—*The Public Health Disparities Geocoding Project* (US). *Public Health Rep* 2003; 118:240–260. (2003b)

Krieger N, Waterman PD, Chen JT, Subramanian SV, Rehkopf DH. Monitoring socioeconomic determinants for healthcare disparities: Tools from the *Public Health Disparities Geocoding Project.* In: Williams RA (ed). *Eliminating Healthcare Disparities in America: Beyond the IOM Report.* Totowa, NJ: Humana Press, 2007; pp. 259–306.

Krieger N, Zierler S, Hogan JW, Waterman P, Chen J, Lemieux K, Gjelsvik A. Geocoding and measurement of neighborhood socioeconomic position. In: Kawachi I, Berkman LF (eds). *Neighborhoods and Health.* New York: Oxford University Press, 2003; pp. 147–178. (2003d)

Krieger N. A century of census tracts: health and the body politic (1906-2006). *J Urban Health* 2006; 83:355–361.

Krieger N. Commentary: society, biology, and the logic of social epidemiology. *Int J Epidemiol* 2001; 30:44–46. (2001a)

Krieger N. Counting accountably: implications of the new approaches to classifying race/ethnicity in the 2000 Census. *Am J Public Health* 2000; 90:1687–1689.

Krieger N. Data, "race," and politics: a commentary on the epidemiologic significance of California's Proposition 54. *J Epidemiol Community Health* 2004; 58: 632–633. (2004b)

Krieger N. Does racism harm health? did child abuse exist before 1962?—on explicit questions, critical science, and current controversies: an ecosocial perspective. *Am J Public Health* 2003; 93:194–199. (2003c)

Krieger N. Embodying inequality: a review of concepts, measures, and methods for studying health consequences of discrimination. *Int J Health Services* 1999; 29:295–352; slightly revised and republished as: Krieger N. Discrimination and health. In: Berkman L, Kawachi I (eds). *Social Epidemiology.* Oxford: Oxford University Press, 2000; pp. 36–75.

Krieger N. Epidemiology and the web of causation: has anyone seen the spider? *Soc Sci Med* 1994; 39:887–903.

Krieger N. Genders, sexes, and health: what are the connections—and why does it matter? *Int J Epidemiol* 2003; 32:652–657. (2003b)

Krieger N. Hormone therapy and the rise and perhaps fall of US breast cancer incidence rates: critical reflections. *Int J Epidemiol* 2008; 37:627–637. (2008a)

Krieger N. Postmenopausal hormone therapy. (letter) *N Engl J Med* 2003; 348:2363–2363.

Krieger N. Putting health inequities on the map: social epidemiology meets medical/health geography–an ecosocial perspective. *GeoJournal* 2009; 74:87–97.

Krieger N. Racial and gender discrimination: risk factors for high blood pressure? *Soc Sci Med* 1990; 30:1273–1281.

Krieger N. Stormy weather: "race," gene expression, and the science of health disparities. *Am J Public Health* 2005; 95:2155–2160. (2005a)

Krieger N. The making of public health data: paradigms, politics, and policy. *J Public Health Policy* 1992; 13:412–427.

Krieger N. The science and epidemiology of racism and health: racial/ethnic categories, biological expressions of racism, and the embodiment of inequality–an ecosocial perspective. In: Whitmarsh I, Jones DS (eds). *What's the Use of Race? Genetics and Difference in Forensics, Medicine, and Scientific Research.* Cambridge, MA: MIT Press, 2010; pp. 225–255 (2010 a).

Krieger N. Theories for social epidemiology in the 21st century: an ecosocial perspective. *Int J Epidemiol* 2001; 30:668–677. (2001b)

Krieger N. Ways of asking and ways of living: reflections on the 50th anniversary of Morris' ever-useful *Uses of Epidemiology. Int J Epidemiol* 2007; 36:1173–1180.

Kuller LH. Commentary: Hazards of studying women: the oestrogen/progesterone dilemma. *Int J Epidemiol* 2004;33:459–460.

Kumle M. Declining breast cancer incidence and decreased HRT use. *Lancet* 2008; 372: 608–610.

Kunitz S. *Disease and Social Diversity: the European Impact on the Health of Non-Europeans.* New York: Oxford University Press, 1994.

Kunitz S. *The Health of Populations: General Theories and Particular Realities.* Oxford: Oxford University Press, 2006.

Kunitz SJ, Pesis-Katz I. Mortality of White Americans, African Americans, and Canadians: the causes and consequences for health of welfare state institutions and policies. *Milbank Q* 2005; 83: 5–39.

Kuzawa CW, Gluckman PD, Hanson MA, Beedle AS. Evolution, developmental plasticity, and metabolic disease. In: Stearns SC, Koella JC (eds). *Evolution in Health and Disease.* 2nd ed. Oxford: Oxford University Press, 2008; pp. 253–264.

La Via Campesina, International Peasant Movement. Food Sovereignty. Available at: http://viacampesina.org/main_en/index.php?option=com_content&task=view&id=47&Itemid=27 (Accessed: August 4, 2009).

Lang CG. Talking about a new illness with the Dakota: reflections on diabetes, foods, and culture. In: Ferriera ML, Lang CG (eds). *Indigenous Peoples and Diabetes: Community Empowerment and Wellness.* Durham, NC: Carolina Academic Press, 2006; pp. 203–230.

Larson NK, Story MT, Nelson MC. Neighborhood environments: disparities in access to healthy foods in the U.S. *Am J Prev Med* 2009; 36:74–81.

Laurance J. Experts' 10 steps to health equality. *Independent,* November 12, 1998.

Lawlor DA, Davey SG, Kundu D, Bruckdorfer KR, Ebrahim S. Those confounded vitamins: what can we learn from the differences between observational versus randomised trial evidence? *Lancet* 2004; 363:1724–1727. (2004c)

Lawlor DA, Davey Smith G, Ebrahim S. Commentary: the hormone-replacement-coronary heart disease conundrum: is the death of observational epidemiology? *Int J Epidemiol* 2004; 33:464–467. (2004ae)

Lawlor DA, Davey Smith G, Ebrahim S. Socioeconomic position and hormone replacement therapy use: explaining the discrepancy in evidence from observational and randomized controlled trials. *Am J Public Health* 2004; 94:2149–2154. (2004b)

Lefkowitz B. *Community Health Centers: A Movement and the People Who Made it Happen.* New Brunswick, NJ: Rutgers University Press, 2007.

Leidy LE. Menopause in evolutionary perspective. In: Trevathan WR, Smoth EO, McKenna JJ (eds). *Evolutionary Medicine.* New York: Oxford, 1999; pp. 407–427.

Leonard WR. Lifestyle, diet, and disease: comparative perspectives on the determinants of chronic health risks. In: Stearns SC, Koella JC (eds). *Evolution in Health and Disease.* 2nd ed. Oxford: Oxford University Press, 2008; pp. 265–276.

Leong RW. Differences in peptic ulcer between the East and the West. *Gastroenterol Clin N Am* 2009; 38:363–379.

Leung WK. *Helicobacter pylori* and gastric neoplasia. In: Dittmar T, Zaenker KS, Schmidt A (eds). *Infection and Inflammation: Impacts on Oncogenesis*. Basel: Karger, 2006; pp. 66–80.

Levenstein S. Commentary: peptic ulcer and its discontents. *Int J Epidemiol* 2002; 31:29–33.

Levenstein S. The very model of a modern etiology: a biopsychosocial view of peptic ulcer. *Psychosom Med* 2000; 62:176–185.

Levine RS, Foster JE, Fullilove RE, Fullilove MT, Briggs NC, Hull PC, Husaini BA, Hennekens CH. Black-white inequalities in mortality and life expectancy, 1933–1999: implications for healthy people 2020. *Public Health Rep* 2001; 116:474–483.

Lin V, Gruszin S, Ellickson C, Glover J, Silburn K, Wilson G, Poljski C. Comparative evaluation of indicators for gender equity and health. *Int J Public Health* 2007; 52:S19–S26.

Lindee S. James Van Gundia Neel (1915-2000). *Am Anthropol* 2001; 103:502–505.

Lindsay RS, Bennett PH. Type 2 diabetes, the thrifty phenotype–an overview. *Br Med Bull* 2001; 60:21–32.

Little J, Higgins JP, Ioannidis JP, et al. STrengthening the REporting of Genetic Association Studies (STREGA)—An Extension of the STROBE Statement. *PLoS Med* 2009; 6(2): e1000022. doi:10.1371/journal.pmed.1000022 (2009a)

Little J, Higgins JPT, Ioannidis JPA, et al. STrengthening the REporting of Genetic Association studies (STREGA)—an extension of the STROBE statement. *Hum Genet* 2009; 125:131-151; doi:10.1007/s00439-008-0592-7 (2009b)

Little J, Higgins JPT, Ioannidis JPA, et al. STrengthening the REporting of Genetic Association studies (STREGA)—an extension of the STROBE statement. *Ann Intern Med* 2009; 150:206–215. (2009c)

Little J, Higgins JPT, Ioannidis JPA, et al. STrengthening the REporting of Genetic Association studies (STREGA)—an extension of the STROBE statement. *Eur J Epidemiol* 2009; 24:37–55. (2009d)

Little J, Higgins JPT, Ioannidis JPA, et al. STrengthening the REporting of Genetic Association studies (STREGA)—an extension of the STROBE statement. *J Clin Epidemiol* 2009; 62:597–608. (2009e)

Little J, Higgins JPT, Ioannidis JPA, et al. STrengthening the REporting of Genetic Association studies (STREGA)—an extension of the STROBE statement. *Eur J Clin Invest* 2009; 39:247–266. (2009f)

Little J, Higgins JPT, Ioannidis JPA, et al. STrengthening the REporting of Genetic Association studies (STREGA)—an extension of the STROBE statement. *Genetic Epidemiol* 2009; 33:581-598; doi:10.1002/gepi.20410 (2009g)

Lock MM. *Encounters with Aging: Mythologies of Menopause in Japan and North America*. Berkeley, CA: University of California Press, 1993.

MacMahon B, Pugh TF, Ipsen J. *Epidemiologic Methods*. Boston: Little, Brown, & Co. 1960.

Majumdar SR, Almasi EA, Stafford R. Promotion and prescribing of hormone therapy after report of harm by the Women's Health Initiative. *JAMA* 2004; 292:1983–1988.

Mann CC. *1491: New Revelations of the Americas Before Columbus*. New York: Alfred A. Knopf, 2005.

Manson JE, Bassuk SS. Hormone therapy and risk of coronary heart disease–why renew focus on the early years of menopause? *Am J Epidemiol* 2007; 166:511–517.

Marmot M, Elliott P (eds). *Coronary Heart Disease: From Aetiology to Public Health*. 2nd ed. Oxford: Oxford University Press, 2005.

Marshall B. Commentary: *Helicobacter* as the 'environmental factor' in Susser and Stein's cohort theory of peptic ulcer disease. *Int J Epidemiol* 2002; 31:21–22.

Marshall BJ, Warren JR. Unidentified curved bacilli in the stomach of patients with gastritis and peptic ulceration. *Lancet* 1984; 1(8390):1311–1315.

Martinez D, Salmón E, Nelson MK. Restoring Indigenous history and culture to nature. In: Nelson MK (ed). *Original Instructions: Indigenous Teachings for a Sustainable Future*. Rochester, VT: Bear & Company, 2009; pp. 88–115.

Mayes LC, Horwitz RI, Feinstein AR. A collection of 56 topics with contradictory results in case-control research. *Int J Epidemiol* 1989; 3:725–727.

McCrea FB. The politics of menopause: the "discovery" of a deficiency disease. *Social Problems* 1983; 31:111–123.

McDermott R. Ethics, epidemiology and the thrifty gene: biological determinism as a health hazard. *Soc Sci Med* 1998; 47:1189–1195.

McMichael P. A food regime genealogy. *J Peasant Studies* 2009; 36:139–169.

McPherson K, Hemminki E. Synthesising licensing data to assess drug safety. *BMJ* 2004; 328:518–520.

Mechanic D. Policy challenges in addressing racial disparities and improving population health. *Health Affairs* 2005; 24:335–338.

Medina D. Mammary developmental fate and breast cancer risk. *Endocr Relat Cancer* 2005; 12: 483–495.

Mjøset L. Theory: conceptions in the social sciences. In: Smesler NJ, Baltes PB (eds). *International Encyclopedia of the Social & Behavioral Sciences*. Elsevier, 2002; 15641–15647. doi:10.1016/B0-08-043076-7/00702-6 (accessed: July 9, 2008)

Morris JN. Uses of epidemiology. *BMJ* 1955; 2: 395–401.

Morris JN. *Uses of Epidemiology*. Edinburgh: E. & S. Livingston Ltd., 1957.

Mosteller F. A *k*-Sample Slippage Test for an Extreme Population. *Annals Math Stat* 1948; 19:58–65.

Murray CJ, Kulkarni SC, Michaud C, Tomijima N, Bulzacchelli MT, Iandiorio TJ, Ezzati M. Eight Americas: investigating mortality disparities across races, counties, and race-counties in the United States. *PLoS Med* 2006; 3(9): e260.

Nabokov P (ed). *Native American Testimony: A Chronicle of Indian-White Relations from Prophecy to the Present, 1492–1992*. New York: Penguin Books, 1991.

National Institute for Diabetes and Digestive and Kidney Diseases (NIDDK). The Pima Indians: Pathfinders for Health. Available at: http://diabetes.niddk.nih.gov/DM/pubs/pima/index.htm; accessed on: July 22, 2009.

National Institutes of Health. *Helicobacter Pylori* in Peptic Ulcer Disease. Consensus Development Conference Statement (1994). Available at: http://consensus.nih.gov/1994/1994HelicobacterPyloriUlcer094html.htm; accessed on: July 20, 2009

National Research Council. *Measuring Racial Discrimination*. Panel on methods for assessing discrimination. R. M. Blank, M. Dabady, & C. F. Citro (Eds), Committee on national statistics, division of behavioral and social sciences and education. Washington, DC: The National Academies Press, 2004.

Navarro V, Muntaner C (eds). *Political and Economic Determinants of Population Health and Well-Being: Controversies and Developments*. Amityville, NY: Baywood Pub Co., 2004.

Needleman H. Low level lead exposure: history and discovery. *Ann Epidemiol* 2009; 19:235–238.

Neel JV, Weder AB, Julius S. Type II diabetes, essential hypertension, and obesity as "syndromes of impaired genetic homeostasis": the "thrifty genotype" hypothesis enters the 21st century. *Perspect Biol Med* 1998; 42:44–74.

Neel JV. Diabetes mellitus: a "thrifty" genotype rendered detrimental by "progress"? *Am J Hum Genet* 1962; 14:353–362.

Neel JV. The "thrifty genotype" in 1998. *Nutr Rev* 1999; 57:S2–S9.

Neel JV. The thrifty genotype revisited. In: Kobberling J, Tattersall J (eds). *The Genetics of Diabetes Mellitus*. New York: Academic Press, 1982; pp. 283–293.

Nelson HD, Humphrey LL, Nygren P, Teutsch SM, Allan JD. Postmenopausal hormone replacement therapy: scientific review. *JAMA* 2002; 288:872–881.

Ness R. Introduction: the "triumphs of epidemiology." *Ann Epidemiol* 2009; 19:225.

NIH State-of-the-Science Panel. National Institutes of Health State-of-the-Science Conference Statement: Management of Menopause-Related Symptoms. *Ann Intern Med* 2005; 142:1005–1013.

Nobles M. History counts: a comparative analysis of racial/color categorization in US and Brazilian censuses. *Am J Public Health* 2000; 90:1738–1745.

Nutton V. *Ancient Medicine*. London: Routledge, 2004.

Ó Gráda C. *Famine: A Short History*. Princeton, NJ: Princeton University Press, 2009.

O'Connor A. *Poverty Knowledge: Social Science, Social Policy, and the Poor in Twentieth-Century U.S. History*. Princeton, NJ: Princeton University Press, 2001.

Oakley GP Jr. The scientific basis for eliminating folic-acid preventable spina bifida: a modern miracle from epidemiology. *Ann Epidemiol* 2009; 19:226–230.

Omura E. Mino-Miijim's 'Good Food for the Future': beyond culturally appropriate diabetes programs. In: Ferriera ML, Lang CG (eds). *Indigenous Peoples and Diabetes: Community Empowerment and Wellness.* Durham, NC: Carolina Academic Press, 2006; pp. 139–166.

Oudshoorn N. *Beyond the Natural Body: An Archaeology of Sex Hormones.* London: Routledge, 1994.

Pachter LM, Garcia C. Racism and child health: a review of the literature and future directions. *J Develop Behav Pediatrics* 2009; 30:255–263.

Pager D, Sheperd D. The sociology of discrimination: racial discrimination in employment, housing, credit and consumer markets. *Annu Rev Sociol* 2008; 34:181–209.

PAHO. Division of Health and Human Development, Program on Public Policy and Health. *Final Report Experts Workshop: Cultural diversity and disaggregation of statistical health information.* Quito, Ecuador, 4-June 5, 2002. Washington, DC: Pan American Health Organization, 2002.

Paixão M. Waiting for the Sun: An Account of the (Precarious) Social Situation of the African Descendant Population in Contemporary Brazil. *J Black Studies* 2004; 34:743–765.

Palmer Beasley R. Rocks along the road to the control of HBV and HCC. *Ann Epidemiol* 2009; 19:231–234.

Pappas G, Queen S, Hadden W, Fischer G. The increasing disparity between socioeconomic groups in the United States, 1960 and 1986. *N Engl J Med* 1993; 329:103–109. Erratum in: *N Engl J Med* 1993; 329:1139.

Paradies Y. A systematic review of empirical research on self-reported racism and health. *Int J Epidemiol* 2006; 35:888–901.

Paradies YC, Montoya MJ, Fullerton SM. Racialized genetics and the study of complex diseases: the thrifty genotype revisited. *Perspect Biol Med* 2007; 50:203–227.

Parkin DM. Is the recent fall in incidence of post-menopausal breast cancer in UK related to changes in use of hormone replacement therapy? *Eur J Cancer* 2009;45:1649–1653.

Pavkov ME, Knowler WC, Hanson RL, Nelson RG. Diabetic nephropathy in American Indians, with a special emphasis on the Pima Indians. *Curr Diabetes Rep* 2008; 8:486–493.

Payne S. *The Health of Men and Women.* Cambridge, UK: Polity Press, 2006.

Petitti D. Commentary: hormone replacement therapy and coronary heart disease: four lessons. *Int J Epidemiol* 2004; 33: 461–463.

Petitti DB, Freedman DA. Invited commentary: how far can epidemiologists get with statistical adjustment? *Am J Epidemiol* 2005; 162:415–418.

Petitti DB, Perlman JA, Sidney S. Postmenopausal estrogen use and heart disease. *N Engl J Med* 1986; 315:131–132.

Phelan JC, Link BG. Controlling disease and creating disparities: a fundamental cause perspective. *J Gerontol Series B* 2005; 60B(Special Issue II):27–33.

Pike MC, Spicer DV. Hormonal contraception and chemoprevention of female cancers. *Endocr Relat Cancer* 2000; 27:73–83.

Pocock SJ, Collier TJ, Dandreo KJ, de Stavola BL, Goldman MB, Kalish LA, Kasten LE, McCormack VA. Issues in the reporting of epidemiological studies: a survey of recent practice. *BMJ* 2004; 329:883–887.

Porta M (ed). *A Dictionary of Epidemiology.* 5th ed. Oxford: Oxford University Press, 2008.

Prentice AM, Hennig BJ, Fulford AJ. Evolutionary origins of the obesity epidemic: natural selection of thrifty genes or genetic drift following predation release? *Int J Obes (Lond)* 2008; 32: 1607–1610.

Prentice AM, Rayco-Solon P, Moore SE. Insights from the developing world: thrifty genotypes and thrifty phenotypes. *Proc Nutr Soc* 2005; 64:153–161. (2005b)

Prentice RL, Langer R, Stefanick ML, et al. Combined postmenopausal hormone therapy and cardiovascular disease: toward resolving the discrepancy between observational studies and the Women's Health Initiative clinical trial. *Am J Epidemiol* 2005; 162:404–414. (2005a)

Prentice RL, Manson JE, Langer RD, et al. Benefits and risks of postmenopausal hormone therapy when it is initiated soon after menopause. *Am J Epidemiol* 2009; 170:12–23.

Quadagno J, McDonald S. Racial segregation in Southern hospitals: how Medicare "broke the back of segregated health services." In: Green EC (ed). *The New Deal and Beyond: Social Welfare in the South since 1930*. Athens, GA: University of Georgia Press, 2003; pp. 120–137.

Ravdin PM, Cronin KA, Howlader N, et al. The decrease in breast-cancer incidence in 2003 in the United States. *New Engl J Med* 2007; 356:1670–1674. (2007b)

Ravdin PM, Cronin KA, Howlader N, Chlebowski RT, Berry DA. A sharp decrease in breast cancer incidence in the United States in 2003. Presented at: The 29th annual San Antonio Breast Cancer Symposium, December 14-17, 2006. http://www.sabcs.org. February 8, 2007. (2007a)

Ravussin E, Valencia ME, Esparza J, Bennett PH, Schulz LO. Effects of a traditional lifestyle on obesity in Pima Indians. *Diabetes Care* 1994; 17:1067–1074.

Raymer T. Diabetes as metaphor: symbol, symptom, or both? In: Ferriera ML, Lang CG (eds). *Indigenous Peoples and Diabetes: Community Empowerment and Wellness*. Durham, NC: Carolina Academic Press, 2006; pp. 313–334.

Rehkopf DH, Haughton L, Chen JT, Waterman PD, Subramanian SV, Krieger N. Monitoring socioeconomic disparities in death: comparing individual-level education and area-based socioeconomic measures. *Am J Public Health* 2006; 96:2135–2138 (erratum: *AJPH* 2007; 97:1543).

Rhoades FP. The menopause, a deficiency disease. *Mich Med* 1965; 64:410–412.

Richardson CT. Pathogenetic factors in peptic ulcer disease. *Am J Med* 1985; 79 (2 Suppl 3):107.

Richiardi L, Barone-Adesi F, Merletti F, Pearce N. Using directed acyclic graphs to consider adjustment for socioeconomic status in occupational cancer studies. *J Epidemiol Community Health* 2008; 62:e14; doi:10.1136/jech.2007.065581

Roberts H. Reduced use of hormones and the drop in breast cancer. *Br Med J* 2009; 338:b2116.

Robins JM. Data, design, and background knowledge in etiologic inference. *Epidemiology* 2001; 12:313–320.

Romera DE, da Cunha CB. Quality of socioeconomic and demographic data in relation to infant mortality in the Brazilian Mortality Information System (1996/2001). *Cad Saúde Pública* 2006; 22:673–681.

Ronzio CR. Urban premature mortality in the U.S. between 1980 and 1990: changing roles of income inequality and social spending. *J Public Health Policy* 2003; 24:386–400.

Rose G. Sick individuals and sick populations. *Int J Epidemiol* 1985; 14:32–38.

Rosenberg L. Hormone replacement therapy: the need for reconsideration. *Am J Public Health* 1993; 83:1670–1673.

Rosset P. Agrofuels, food sovereignty, and the contemporary food crisis. *Bull Sci Tech Soc* 2009; 29:189–193.

Rossouw JE. Implications of recent clinical trials of postmenopausal hormone therapy for management of cardiovascular disease. *Ann NY Acad Sci* 2006; 1089: 444–453.

Roubideaux YD, Moore K, Avery C, Muneta B, Knight M, Buchwald D. Diabetes education materials: recommendations of tribal leaders, Indian health professionals, and American Indian community members. *Diabetes Educ* 2000; 26:290–294.

Ruzek SB. *The Women's Health Movement: Feminist Alternatives to Medical Control*. New York: Praeger, 1978.

Satcher D, Fryer GE Jr, McCann J, Troutman A, Woolf SH, Rust G. What if we were equal? A comparison of the black-white mortality gap in 1960 and 2000. *Health Aff (Millwood)* 2005; 24:459–464.

Satel SL. *PC, MD: How Political Correctness is Corrupting Medicine*. New York: Basic Books, 2000.

Schalick LM, Hadden WC, Pamuk E, Navarro V, Pappas G. The widening gap in death rates among income groups in the United States from 1967 to 1986. *Int J Health Services* 2000; 30:13–26.

Schnittker J, McLeod JD. The social psychology of health disparities. *Annu Rev Sociol* 2005; 31: 75–103.

Schwartz S, Carpenter KM. The right answer for the wrong question: consequences of Type III error for public health research. *Am J Public Health* 1999; 89:1175–1180.

Seaman B, Seaman G. *Women and the Crisis in Sex Hormones*. New York: Rawson Association Publishers, Inc., 1977.

Seaman B. *The Greatest Experiment Ever Performed on Women: Exploding the Estrogen Myth.* New York: Hyperion, 2003.

Servio M, Wells JC, Cizza G. The contribution of psychosocial stress to the obesity epidemic: an evolutionary approach. *Horm Metab Res* 2009; 41:261–270.

Shariff-Marco S, Gee GC, Breen N, et al. A mixed-methods approach to developing a self-reported racial/ethnic discrimination measure for use in multiethnic health surveys. *Ethnicity Disease* 2009; 19:447–453.

Shaw M, Dorling D, Gordon D, Davey Smith G. *The Widening Gap: Health Inequalities and Policy in Britain.* Bristol, UK: Policy Press, 1999.

Sheridan TE. *Landscapes of Fraud: Mission Tumacácori, the Baca Float, and the Betrayal of the O'odham.* Tuscon, AZ: University of Arizona Press, 2006.

Siddiqi A, Hertzman C. Towards an epidemiological understanding of the effects of long-term institutional changes on population health: a case study of Canada versus the USA. *Soc Sci Med* 2007; 64:589–603.

Sigerist H. *A History of Medicine. Volume I; Primitive and Archaic Medicine.* New York: Oxford University Press, 1951 (1979).

Singer N. Medical papers by ghostwriters pushed therapy. *New York Times,* August 5, 2009.

Singh GK, Kogan MD. Persistent socioeconomic disparities in infant, neonatal, and postneonatal mortality rates in the United States, 1969-2001. *Pediatrics* 2007; 119(4):e928–939.

Singh GK, Siahpush M. Increasing inequalities in all-cause and cardiovascular mortality among US adults aged 25–64 years by area socioeconomic status, 1969–1998. *Int J Epidemiol* 2002; 31: 600–613.

Singh GK, Yu SM. Infant mortality in the United States: trends, differentials, and projections, 1950 through 2010. *Am J Public Health* 1995; 85:957–964.

Singh GK, Yu SM. Trends and differentials in adolescent and young adult mortality in the United States, 1950 through 1993. *Am J Public Health* 1996; 86:560–564. (1996a)

Singh GK, Yu SM. US childhood mortality, 1950 through 1993: trends and socioeconomic differentials. *Am J Public Health* 1996; 86:505–512. (1996b)

Singh GK. Area deprivation and widening inequalities in US mortality, 1969–1998. *Am J Public Health* 2003; 93:1137–1143.

Smigal C, Jemal A, Ward E, Cokkinides V, Smith R, Howe HL, Thun M. Trends in breast cancer incidence by race and ethnicity: update 2006. *CA Cancer J Clin* 2006; 56:168–183.

Smith CJ, Manahan EM, Pablo SG. Food habit and cultural change among the Pima Indians. In: Joe JR, Young RS (eds). *Diabetes as a Disease of Civilization: The Impact of Culture Change on Indigenous Peoples.* Berlin Mouton de Gruyter, 1993; pp. 407–434.

Smith DB. Racial and ethnic health disparities and the unfinished Civil Rights agenda. *Health Affairs* 2005; 24:317–324.

Smith J, Cianfolane K, Biron S, Hould S, Lebel S, Marceau S, Lescelleru O, Biertho L, Smiard S, Kral JG, Marceau P. Effects of maternal surgical weight loss in mothers on intergenerational transmission of obesity. *J Clin Endocrinol Metab* 2009; 94:4275–4283.

Smith LT. *Decolonizing Methodologies.* London: Zed Books; Dunedin, New Zealand: University of Otago Press, 1999.

Smith MK. Enhancing gender equity in health programmes: monitoring and evaluation. *Gender Development* 2001; 9:95–105.

Snaith A, El-Omar EM. *Helicobacter pylori*: host genetics and disease outcomes. *Expert Rev Gastroenterol Hepatol* 2008; 2:577–585.

Snipp CM. Selected demographic characteristics of Indians. In: Rhoades EP (ed). *American Indian Health: Innovations in Health Care, Promotion, and Policy.* Baltimore, MD: Johns Hopkins University Press, 2000; pp. 41–57.

Sober E. *Evidence and Evolution: The Logic Behind the Science.* Cambridge: Cambridge University Press, 2008.

Sonnenberg A, Cucino C, Bauerfeind P. Commentary: the unresolved mystery of birth-cohort phenomena in gastroenterology. *Int J Epidemiol* 2002; 31:23–26.

Speakman JR. Thrifty genes for obesity and the metabolic syndrome–time to call off the search? *Diab Vasc Dis Res* 2006; 3:7–11.

Speakman JR. Thrifty genes for obesity, an attractive but flawed idea, and an alternative perspective: the 'drifty gene' hypothesis. *Int J Obes* 2008; 32:1611–1617.

Stamler J. Established major coronary risk factors: historical overview. In: Marmot MT, Elliott P (eds). *Coronary Heart Disease Epidemiology: From Aetiology to Public Health*. 2nd ed. Oxford: Oxford University Press, 2005; pp. 18–31.

Stampfer M. Commentary: Hormones and heart disease: do trials and observational studies address different questions? *Int J Epidemiol* 2004; 33:454–455.

Stampfer MJ, Colditz GA. Estrogen replacement therapy and coronary heart disease: a quantitative assessment of the epidemiologic evidence. *Prev Med* 1991; 20:47–63.

Stefanick ML. Estrogens and progestins: background and history, trends in use, and guidelines and regimens approved by the US Food and Drug Administration. *Am J Med* 2005; 118 (Suppl 12B):64S–73S.

Stewart SL, Sabatino SA, Foster SL, Richardson LC. Decline in breast cancer incidence–United States, 1999-2003. *MMWR* 2007; 56:549–553.

STREGA: strengthening the reporting of genetic associations. Available at: http://www.medicine.uottawa.ca/public-health-genomics/web/eng/strega.html (Accessed: August 5, 2009).

STROBE statements: strengthening the reporting of observational studies in epidemiology. Available at: http://www.strobe-statement.org/index.php?id=2504 (Accessed: August 5, 2009).

Ströhle A, Wolters M. Comment on the article "Genotype, obesity and cardiovascular disease–has technical and social advancement outstripped evolution?" *J Intern Med* 2004; 256:86–88.

Subramanian SV, Chen JT, Rehkopf DH, Waterman PD, Krieger N. Racial disparities in context: A multilevel analysis of neighborhood variations in poverty and excess mortality among black populations in Massachusetts. *Am J Public Health* 2005; 95:260–265.

Subramanian SV, Chen JT, Rehkopf DR, Waterman PD, Krieger N. Comparing individual and area-based socioeconomic measures for the surveillance of health disparities: a multilevel analysis of Massachusetts (US) births, 1988-92. *Am J Epidemiol* 2006; 164:832–834. (2006a)

Subramanian SV, Chen JT, Rehkopf DR, Waterman PD, Krieger N. Subramanian et al respond to: "Think Conceptually, Act Cautiously." *Am J Epidemiol* 2006; 164:841–844. (2006b)

Sundin J, Willner W. *Social Change and Health in Sweden: 250 Years of Politics and Practice*. Östersund, Sweden: Swedish National Institute of Public Health, 2007. Available at: http://www.fhi.se/en/Publications/All-publications-in-english/Social-change-and-health-in-Sweden—250-years-of-politics-and-practice/ (Accessed: August 8, 2009).

Susser M, Stein Z. Civilization and peptic ulcer. *Lancet* 1962; 20 January: 115–119.

Susser M, Stein Z. Commentary: civilization and peptic ulcer 40 years on. *Int J Epidemiol* 2002; 31:18–21.

Susser M, Stein Z. *Eras in Epidemiology: The Evolution of Ideas*. New York: Oxford University Press, 2009.

Swedish National Institute of Public Health. Public health policy–11 objectives. Updated March 12, 2009. Available at: http://www.fhi.se/en/About-FHI/Public-health-policy/ (Accessed: August 8, 2009).

Swedish National Institute of Public Health. *Sweden's New Public Health Policy: National Public Health Objectives for Sweden*. Revised edition: 2003. Available at: http://www.fhi.se/en/Publications/All-publications-in-english/Swedens-New-Public-Health-Policy—The-National-Institute-of-Public-Health/ (Accessed: August 8, 2009).

Swedish National Institute of Public Health. *The 2005 Public Health Policy Report: Summary*. Östersund, Sweden: Swedish National Institute of Public Health, 2005. Available at: http://www.fhi.se/en/Publications/All-publications-in-english/The-2005-Public-Health-Policy-Report/ (Accessed: August 8, 2009).

Swinburn BA. The thrifty genotype hypothesis: how does it look after 30 years? *Diabet Med* 1996; 13:695–699.

Sydenstricker E. *Hagerstown Morbidity Studies: A Study of Illness in a Typical Population Group*. Reprints Nos. 1113, 1116, 1134,1163, 1167, 1172, 1225, 1227, 1229, 1294, 1303, and 1312 from Public Health Reports. U.S.Treasury Department, U.S. Public Health Service. Washington, DC: Government Printing Office, 1930.

Sydenstricker E. The incidence of illness in a general population group: general results of a morbidity study from December 1, 1921 through March 31, 1924, Hagerstown, Md. *Public Health Rep* 1952; 40:279–291.

Tanumihardjo SA, Anderson C, Kaufer-Horwitz M, et al. Poverty, obesity, and malnutrition: an international perspective recognizing the paradox. *J Am Diet Assoc* 2007; 107:1966–1972.

Taubes G. Do we really know what makes us healthy? *New York Times Sunday Magazine*, September 16, 2007.

Taubes G. Epidemiology faces its limits. *Science* 1995; 269:164–165,167–169.

Thagard P. *How Scientists Explain Disease*. Princeton, NJ: Princeton University Press, 1999.

The Oath. In: Lloyd GER. *Hippocratic Writings*. London: Penguin Books, 1983; p. 67.

TOCA. Tohono O'Odham Community Action. Available at: http://www.tocaonline.org/www.tocaonline.org/Home.html; (Accessed: July 12, 2009).

Travassos C, Williams DR. The concept and measurement of race and their relationship to public health: a review focused on Brazil and the United States. *Cad Saúde Pública* 2004; 20:660–678.

Tsubura A, Uehara N, Matsuoka Y, Yoshizawa K, Yuri T. Estrogen and progesterone treatment mimicking pregnancy for protection from breast cancer. *In Vivo* 2008; 22:191–201.

Turncock BJ, Atchison C. Government public health in the United States: the implications of federalism. *Health Affairs* 2002; 21:68–78.

U.S. Department of Health and Human Services. *Healthy People 2010: Understanding and Improving Health*. 2nd ed. *Washington, DC: U.S. Government Printing Office*, 2000.

United States, Federal Security Agency, Public Health Service. *Menopause*. (Health Information Series No. 15). Washington, DC: US Govt Printing Office, 1950.

Unnatural Causes: Is Inequality Making Us Sick?–Case Studies: "Finding Hope for the Future by Reclaiming the Past." Available at: http://www.unnaturalcauses.org/case_studies_01_prob.php (Accessed: July 12, 2009).

Vandenbroucke JP, von Elm E, Altman DG, et al. Strengthening the Reporting of Observational Studies in Epidemiology (STROBE): explanation and elaboration. *Epidemiology* 2007; 18:805–835. (2007a)

Vandenbroucke JP, von Elm E, Altman DG, et al. Strengthening the Reporting of Observational Studies in Epidemiology (STROBE): explanation and elaboration. *Ann Intern Med* 2007; 147: W163–W194. (2007b)

Vandenbroucke JP, von Elm E, Altman DG, et al. Strengthening the Reporting of Observational Studies in Epidemiology (STROBE): explanation and elaboration. *PLos Med* 2007; 4(10):e297. (2007c)

Vandenbroucke JP. Commentary: The HRT story: vindication of old epidemiological theory. *Int J Epidemiol* 2004; 33:456–467.

Vandenbroucke JP. Observational research, randomized trials, and two views of medical science. *PLoS Med* 2008; 5:339–343.

Verkooijen HM, Koot VCM, Fioretta G, et al. Hormone replacement therapy, mammography screening and changing age-specific incidence rates of breast cancer: an ecological study comparing two European populations. *Breast Cancer Res Treat* 2008; 107:389–395.

Viola HJ, Margolis C (eds). *Seeds of Change: A Quincentennial Commemoration*. Washington, DC: Smithsonian Institution Press, 1991.

Vogel F, Motulsky AG. Human and medical genetics. In: Detels R, McEwen J, Beaglehole R, Tanaka H (eds). *Oxford Textbook of Public Health*. Oxford: Oxford University Press, 2004. Available at: http://www.r2library.com (Accessed: July 25, 2009).

von Elm E, Altman DG, Egger M, et al. The Strengthening the Reporting of Observational Studies in Epidemiology (STROBE) statement: guidelines for reporting observational studies. *J Clin Epidemiol* 2008; 61:344–349.

von Elm E, Altman DG, Egger M, et al. The Strengthening the Reporting of Observational Studies in Epidemiology (STROBE) statement: guidelines for reporting observational studies. *Lancet* 2007; 370:1453–1457. (2007a)

von Elm E, Altman DG, Egger M, et al. The Strengthening the Reporting of Observational Studies in Epidemiology (STROBE) statement: guidelines for reporting observational studies. *Epidemiology* 2007; 18:800–804. (2007b)

von Elm E, Altman DG, Egger M, et al. The Strengthening the Reporting of Observational Studies in Epidemiology (STROBE) statement: guidelines for reporting observational studies. *Bull World Health Organ* 2007; 85:867–872. (2007c)

von Elm E, Altman DG, Egger M, et al. The Strengthening the Reporting of Observational Studies in Epidemiology (STROBE) statement: guidelines for reporting observational studies. *Prev Med* 2007; 45:247–251. (2007d)

von Elm E, Altman DG, Egger M, et al. Strengthening the Reporting of Observational Studies in Epidemiology (STROBE) statement: guidelines for reporting observational studies. *BMJ* 2007; 335:806–808. (2007e)

von Elm E, Altman DG, Egger M, et al. The Strengthening the Reporting of Observational Studies in Epidemiology (STROBE) statement: guidelines for reporting observational studies. *PLoS Med* 2007; 4(10):e296. (2007f)

von Elm E, Altman DG, Egger M, et al. The Strengthening the Reporting of Observational Studies in Epidemiology (STROBE) statement: guidelines for reporting observational studies. *Ann Intern Med* 2007; 147:573–577. (2007g)

von elm E, Egger M. The scandal of poor epidemiological research. *BMJ* 2004; 329:868–869.

Wall S, Persson G, Weinehall L. Public health in Sweden: facts, visions and lessons. In: Beaglehole R (ed). *Global Public Health: A New Era.* Oxford: Oxford University Press, 2003; pp. 69–86.

Warner D. Research and educational approaches to reducing health disparities among American Indians and Alaska Natives. *J Transcult Nurs* 2006; 17:266–271.

Watkins ES. *The Estrogen Elixir: A History of Hormone Replacement Therapy in America.* Baltimore, MD: Johns Hopkins University Press, 2007.

Weatherford J. *Indian Givers: How the Indians of the Americas Transformed the World.* New York: Crown Publishers, 1988.

Wei F, Miglioretti DL, Connelly MT, et al. Changes in women's use of hormones after the Women's Health Initiative estrogen and progestin trial by race, education, and income. *JNCI Monograph* 2005; 35:106–112.

Wellcome Trust Centre for the History of Medicine at UCL: "The World Health Organization and the social determinants of health: assessing theory, policy and practice." Available at: http://www.ucl.ac.uk/histmed/centre_projects/social_determinants (Accessed: August 8, 2009).

WHO Commission on Social Determinants of Health. *Closing the gap in a generation: health equity through action on the social determinants of health. Final report of the Commission on Social Determinants of Health.* Geneva: WHO, 2008. Available at: http://www.who.int/social_determinants/final_report/en/index.html (Accessed: August 8, 2009).

Willett WC, Manson JE, Grodstein F, Stampfer MJ, Colditz GA. Re: "Combined postmenopausal hormone therapy and cardiovascular disease: toward resolving the discrepancy between observational studies and the Women's Health Initiative clinical trial" (letter to the editor). *Am J Epidemiol* 2006; 163:1067–1068.

Williams DR, Mohammed SA. Discrimination and racial disparities in health: evidence and needed research. *J Behav Med* 2009; 32:20–47.

Williams DR, Neighbors HW, Jackson JS. Racial/ethnic discrimination and health: findings from community studies. *Am J Public Health* 2003; 93:200–208.

Williams DR. Racial variations in adult health status: patterns, paradoxes, and prospects. In: Smelser NJ, Wilson WJ, Mitchell F (eds). *America Becoming: Racial Trends and Their Consequences, Vol II.* Commission on Behavioral and Social Sciences and Education, National Research Council. Washington, DC: National Academy Press, 2001; pp. 371–410.

Williams G. Disorders of glucose homeostasis. In: Warrell D, Cox T, Firth J, Benz E (eds). *Oxford Textbook of Medicine, 4th ed.* Oxford: Oxford University Press, 2003. Available at: R2 OnLine Library. http://www.R2Library.com/marc_frame.aspx?ResourceID=107 (Accessed: July 25, 2009).

Williams R. *Keywords: A Vocabulary of Culture and Society.* Rev. ed. New York: Oxford University Press, 1983. (1983a)

Williams R. *Towards 2000.* London: Chatto & Windus, The Hogarth Press, 1983. (1983b)

Wilson C, Gilliland S, Cullen T, Moore K, Roubideaux Y Valdez L, Vanderwagen W, Acton K. Diabetes outcomes in the Indian health system during the era of the Special Diabetes Program for Indians and the Government Performance and Results Act. *Am J Public Health* 2005; 59:1518–1522.

Wilson RA. *Feminine Forever.* New York: M. Evans (distributed in association with Lippincott), 1966.

World Health Organization Executive Board Resolution: "Reducing health inequities through action on the social determinants of health" (EB124.46) Available at: http://apps.who.int/gb/ebwha/pdf_files/EB124/B124_R6-en.pdf (Accessed: August 8, 2009).

World Medical Association (WMA). Declaration of Helsinki: Ethical Principles for Medical Research Involving Human Subjects. Initially adopted by the 18th WMA General Assembly, Helsinki, Finland, June 1964, and most recently amended at the 59th WMA General Assembly, Seoul, October 2008. Available at: http://www.wma.net/e/policy/b3.htm (Accessed: July 12, 2009).

World Social Forum Charter of Principles (2001). Available at: http://www.forumsocialmundial.org.br/main.php?id_menu=4&cd_language=2 (Accessed: August 6, 2009).

Worldmapper: The World As You've Never Seen it Before. Available at: http://www.worldmapper.org/index.html (Accessed: August 8, 2009).

Writing Group for the Women's Health Initiative Investigators. Risk and benefits of estrogen plus progestin in healthy postmenopausal women: principal results from the Women's Health Initiative randomized controlled trial. *JAMA* 2002; 288:321–333.

Yager JD, Davidson NE. Estrogen carcinogenesis in breast cancer. *N Engl J Med* 2006; 354: 270–282.

Young TK, Reading J, Elias B, O'Neil JD. Type 2 diabetes mellitus in Canada's first nations: status of an epidemic in progress. *CMAJ* 2000; 163:561–566.

Young TK. *The Health of Native Americans: Toward a Biocultural Epidemiology.* New York: Oxford University Press, 1994.

Ziman J. *Real Science: What it is, and What it Means.* Cambridge, UK: Cambridge University Press, 2000.

Zimmet P, Thomas CR. Genotype, obesity and cardiovascular disease–has technical and social advancement outstripped evolution? *J Intern Med* 2003; 254:114–125.

Index

Note: Page references followed by "*f*" and "*t*" denote figures and tables, respectively.